# Herd Health and Production Management in Dairy Practice

# Herd Health and Production Management in Dairy Practice

A. Brand, J.P.T.M. Noordhuizen, Y.H. Schukken

Wageningen Pers

**CIP-data Koninklijke Bibliotheek, Den Haag**

**ISBN 90-74134-34-3 paperback**

**Subject headings: dairy practice, production management, herd health**

**First published, 1996**
**Second reprint, 1997**

**Cover design: Mrs. H.J. Brand - van den Berg**



**Printed in The Netherlands**

# CONTENTS

## FOREWORD

Times are changing and so is veterinary medicine. From an academic standpoint, the veterinarian is becoming more of a consultant to the food animal industry. (We must remember, however, that the individual animal is still the basis of herd medicine). Such factors as complex management functions, narrow economic margins, and modern accounting practices make it even more necessary for dairy and beef operations to have available experienced and qualified consultants in production medicine. In most cases the veterinarian can be the best qualified individual to meet these needs. The dairy industry, as an example, is highly consumer driven, especially in the area of food safety. The properly educated veterinarian can be invaluable to the dairy producer as he/she strives to produce the most wholesome, least expensive product for the consumer. This veterinatian must have a multi-disciplinary education that focuses on both farm profitability and safe wholesome products.

This book is authored by many individuals with longterm experience in herd health and production medicine. It can make a valuable contribution to any veterinarians' continuing education in areas mentioned above. It provides a methodical blue print to implement a consulting service and adequately aiding farm management. Handy protocols for the major areas of dairy farming are elaborated and further visualized in case studies.

I can recommend this book for veterinarians interested in improving their knowledge in dairy production as well as animal scientists interested in this information. It can also be valuable to students as they increase their knowledge of practical veterinary medicine.

*James A. Jarrett, D.V.M.*
*Executive Vice President*
*American Association of Bovine Practitioners*

# PREFACE OF THE EDITORS

## INTRODUCTION

Technological and genetic developments in dairy farming have been tremendous over the last decades. These developments have resulted in more cows handled per man and per unit area, and have increased productivity, making dairy farming more intensified and larger scaled. At the same time markets became more competitive which resulted in a smaller profit margin per animal unit. Today's markets are also strongly consumer driven which includes higher demands on animal welfare, and on process and product quality. Due to these developments, farmers are forced to produce more efficiently and at higher quality levels, primarily through better management. As a consequence, farm managers require support in their management strategies in order to survive in an economically and ecologically viable way.

## HERD HEALTH AND PRODUCTION MANAGEMENT

Management support to dairy farmers can best be offered within the frame work of Herd Health and Production Management (HH & PM) services that are aimed at optimizing animal health and production. The term HH & PM is chosen instead of preventive medicine or production medicine, because the word medicine directs veterinary service primarily to curing infectious or metabolic diseases and to a much lesser extent to support of farm management which is essential for every dairy farmer in the current economic environment. The term production in HH & PM is added because even when animals in a herd are considered to be healthy, it does not mean that production is optimal. The effort towards management support should not replace traditional curative veterinary approach. However, a clinical diagnosis and treatment should not be an end point but a starting point to search for underlying causal risk factors in management and in environmental conditions that are contributing to the health and/or production disturbances.

With regard to health care the major epidemic diseases of livestock have either been eliminated, or effectively controlled in the past. In contrast, endemic diseases and production inefficiences have not responded to traditional veterinary treatments due, in part, to the fact that these diseases or functional disorders frequently have multifactorial causes. They are now recognized as part of a complex host-agent-environment interaction, rather than simply host-agent entities. This means that for successful control and preventive measures to be developed, not only the interaction of the noxious agent and host, but also the interactions of the host and agent with management practices and/or environmental conditions must be taken into account and be manipulated if necessary. Development of effective and repeatable procedures and strategies that will regularly and predictably minimize the effects of endemic diseases on livestock productivity, presently is the most important disease control need of the food animal industry in the more intensive production areas.

## SCOPE OF THE BOOK

The main aim of the book is to teach students, veterinary practitioners, and farm advisors how to support the dairy farmer in his/her management in order to optimize health, productivity, and animal welfare of the herd. For that reason much attention is paid to management practices and farm conditions that influence health, production and welfare of dairy cattle in a positive or negative way. Instead of paying attention to specific diseases much more attention is paid to the methodology for optimizing health, animal welfare and production. Primary area of concern is the intensive dairy industry as encountered in the USA and Europe. However, major elements in the described methodology will also apply to other regions.

To accomplish this a structural approach is used. The core element in this methodology is the protocol. In this protocol, a sequence of steps is followed. At each step relevant herd performance issues are assessed in relation to farm management and farm conditions. With the standard protocol the practitioner and farm advisor are lead step by step through a farm visit, during which operational and problem-solving issues are addressed. Among these issues are: replacement rearing, nutrition, milk production, reproduction, health care, and farm economics.

A prerequisite for effective HH & PM services is that data are recorded, processed into performance indices, and analyzed. The HH & PM practitioner and farm advisor must be able to intelligently interpret the collected information, and to translate conclusions into practical advice for the benefit of the client. For that reason attention has been paid not only to data collection and data processing, but also to decision making, and follow up.

Growth and development of HH & PM services depend on adoption by producers, veterinary practitioners and farm advisors. The acceptance of this concept within the farming community will depend on the ability of practitioners and farm advisors to visualize the potentials of application and to solve problems and optimize health and productivity in a way that is acceptable to consumers and economically beneficial to the producer.

# HERD HEALTH AND PRODUCTION MANAGEMENT PROGRAMS

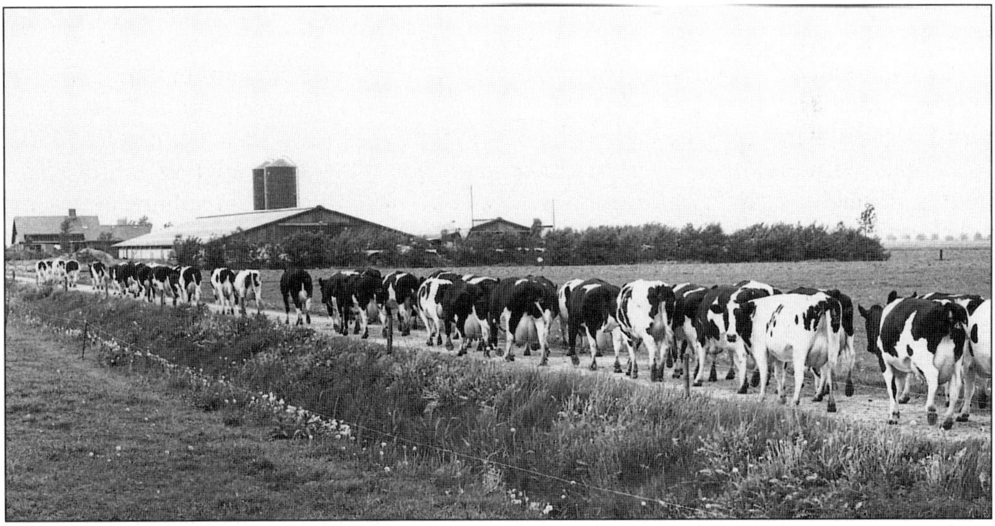

# 1.1 PRINCIPLES OF HERD HEALTH AND PRODUCTION MANAGEMENT PROGRAMS

Arie Brand[1] and Chuck L. Guard[2]

[1] Department of Herd Health and Reproduction, School of Veterinary Medicine, University of Utrecht, Yalelaan 7, 3584 CL Utrecht, The Netherlands

[2] Department of Clinical Sciences, New York State College of Veterinary Medicine, Cornell University, Ithaca, New York, USA 14853

## 1.1.1 INTRODUCTION

Herd health and production management (HH & PM) service is a complex of integrated veterinary and animal husbandry activities, centered around regularly planned farm visits, and based on a protocol approach to operational farm management functions. There are some important differences between HH & PM services and the traditional services of veterinary medicine, which were focused solely on the clinically diseased animal. These differences include a comprehensive concern for the herd and the entire farm enterprise, and the importance of general and herd-specific information needed for decision making in daily management. HH & PM services are ultimately meant to improve farm income and\or to reduce costs (Noordhuizen, 1984; Nelson and Redlus, 1989). Therefore, disease, health, and production should be regarded in an economic perspective.

Dairymen use many professionals to help manage their business. They include agricultural farm advisors such as nutritionists, geneticists, economists, service and sales representatives and last but not least veterinarians interested in HH & PM. Together they must be able to actively guide the management of a dairy enterprise instead of passively following it. Therefore, cooperation between the various advisors is crucial to successful guiding of related management functions and processes. Only then, HH & PM services can be translated into optimal animal health, food production, animal well being, and environmentally sustainable production methods.

In order to cooperate with other disciplines the practitioner has to broaden his/her purely veterinary technical and theoretical approaches, familiar in individual animal care. As a consequence, the practitioner must be willing and able to look beyond traditional boundaries of thought and practice in veterinary medicine in the development of HH & PM services. This new role for the veterinarian is an addition to, and not a substitute for, traditional practice activities.

This chapter discusses the objectives of HH & PM services, the skills required, the management structure of a dairy farm and the HH & PM protocol used in HH & PM services.

## 1.1.2 OBJECTIVES OF HERD HEALTH AND PRODUCTION MANAGEMENT PROGRAMS

The practitioner offering HH & PM services should know the primary objectives of these services. In general HH & PM services are directed at the maximum expression of the genetic potential of the individual animal and of the herd as a whole by optimizing farm management and farm conditions and subsequently farm income (Braun et al., 1983). In a more specific way the primary objectives of HH & PM services are aimed at optimization of:

* the health status of the herd, by prevention of health and (re)productive problems,
* the productivity of the herd by improving management practices,
* the production process in relation to animal welfare and ecological quality of the environment and the maintenance of a sustainable dairy industry,
* the quality and safety of dairy and meat products and,
* the profitability of the dairy enterprise.

If herd health and production management is to form part of a sustainable approach, for example expressed in an ecosystem's health, then the farm is to be considered as an eco-unit (Nielsen, 1993). In this situation herd health and production management are extended from the farm and the herd to the environment around the farm including soil types, water streams, forests etc. This situation, however, is not addressed in this book.

## 1.1.3 REQUIREMENTS OF PARTICIPANTS

For successful HH & PM services the following contributions from the farmer and the veterinary practitioner are expected:

**A. Contributions of the farmer or herd manager:**

* skills to operate a dairy farm using contemporary techniques in animal husbandry and management,
* knowledge and interests to be able to:
  - implement a management cycle (see Figure 1) on his farm,
  - communicate and cooperate with external experts for support in farm management,
* physical presence of:
  - accurate and up-to-date data recording of individual animal events and of herd events,
  - participation in artificial insemination and in regular milk recording and analyses services, offered by the Dairy Herd Improvement Association (DHIA) or similar organizations. Meaningful evaluations of farm performance cannot be made without milk production records. As a general rule, farmers not willing to participate in a standard milk recording system will not be appropriately motivated candidates for HH & PM services,

* permanent and legible animal identification. This is essential for correctly recording individual animal events.

**B. Contributions of the veterinary practitioner:**

* skills to implement and to operate HH & PM protocols,
* broad knowledge, and interest in:
  - the functional structure of dairy farm management and the convergence of operational farm management functions in relation to health, productivity, economy, animal welfare, and environment,
  - the pathophysiology, dynamics, diagnosis and prevention of diseases and production deficiences at herd level,
  - utilization and interpretation of diagnostic tests,
  - basic computer handling and data processing techniques,
  - communication and client education that enable him/her to stimulate and motivate the farmer in record keeping, improvement of management procedures, and adoption of recommendations.
* Physical presence of:

- computer facilities,
- a farm file of reports, analyses, conclusions, and recommendations, made during farm visits,
- a strong and current base of scientific information on dairy farm management, and in the sciences related to the HH & PM services,
- a practice structure for making appointments for regularly scheduled, non-interrupted farm visits. A group practice is almost essential for implementing HH & PM services.

Furthermore a practitioner should:

- have basic understanding of epidemiological principles including test characteristics, and observational surveys. He/she should be skilled in interpreting not only clinical or subclinical disease data but also production data and environment related observations in an epidemiological way,
- be a sentinel and advocate for the welfare of cattle;
- serve as both a source and critic for new information delivered to the farmer,
- serve as an intermediate between primary farm production and public health interests related to products delivered (milk, meat). He/she should know diseases and management practices which are important in relation to public health and quality of products (Nelson and Redlus, 1989).

The costs of the proposed HH & PM services should be discussed with the farmer beforehand and their breakdown clarified. There are several modes of fee structure currently in use. They vary from a straight hourly fee to a fee per cow per year divided into installments. There are insurance-like programs where the farmer pays a per cow fee that covers all veterinary expenses including routine and emergency procedures and supplies. Existing methods of charging for veterinary service might not include fees for HH & PM services, but they can usually be added very easily.

The benefits of overall HH & PM services should exceed the costs (Sol et al., 1984; Hogeveen et al., 1992) although specific proof of this relationship in many circumstances will be very difficult.

### 1.1.4 THE MANAGEMENT STRUCTURE OF A DAIRY FARM

Veterinary education begins with the study of anatomy of an animal in order to understand normal and abnormal functioning of an individual. By analogy, knowledge of the overall and operational management structure of a dairy farm, is needed to adequately provide HH & PM services by both the practitioner and farm advisor.

Farm objectives. The overall organization of a dairy farm, as in every industrial enterprise, is first of all based on defining farm objectives. Farm objectives are usually not defined quantitatively by many dairy farmers. Therefore, the first task of the HH & PM practitioner, starting HH & PM services, is to define financial and technical objectives. Examples of farm objectives are: an increase of income of 5 to 10% per year, an expansion of the farm, automation of farm activities, or just the construction of an extra farm building. The definition of farm objectives may be dependent on a number of factors, such as: the number of hectares of land available, the subdivisions or topography of the land, the existence or absence of a quota system for milk, the prospects of the farm in relation to the zoning scheme of local government, the capital and the size of the labour forces available, and the perception (knowledge and vision) and the wishes of the farmer. By taking these factors into account the farmer can try, either by himself or in cooperation with third parties, to formulate the optimal farm objectives. Differences in farm objectives, and consequently in farm organization, lead to different management styles. This may have an impact on the way HH & PM services are executed.

Management. Management of a dairy farm is structured around the farm objectives and should be based on three activities: planning of methods and tools needed to realize farm objectives, putting plans into operation, and assessment of overall performance. Planning, operation, and overall assessment are all interconnected and together with the definition of farm objectives, they form a management cycle (Figure 1).

**A. Planning.** Planning is the most basic management tool used to guide the conduct of operations for the accomplishment of the farms' objectives, and at a lower level at

*Figure 1. Management cycle*

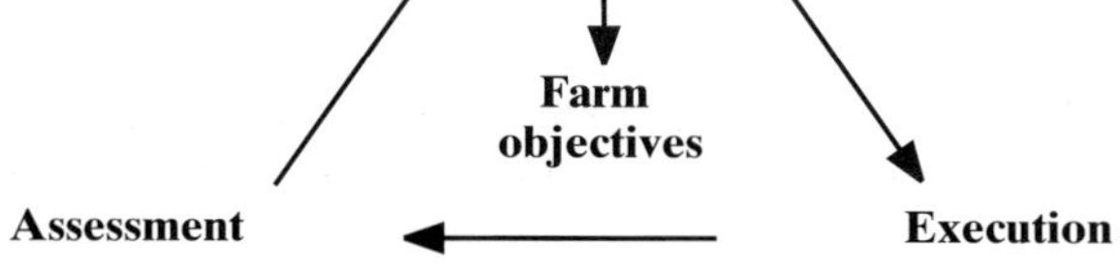

the accomplishment of preset targets in the various operational management functions. Together with farm objectives, planning activities define the organization of the farm in the future. Planning is done at strategic (long term), tactical (medium term), and operational or short term levels (Brand et al., 1995). Strategic planning defines the organization of the farm and tools and activities for years ahead. Tactical planning outlines plans for a year, or months, and operational planning for a few days or a week ahead in the various operational management functions. Planning of tools and activities differs between farms (Brand et al., 1995).

**Strategic planning**. Strategic planning is usually not a primary interest of the herd health practitioner but one has to realize that strategic planning is an integral and essential part of HH & PM services. Examples of strategic planning activities may include expansion of the farm via purchase of land, and/or milk quota if a quota system exists, automation of labor via purchase of a mixer magon. The HH & PM practitioner should be a discussion partner for the farmer e.g. to assess health and production consequences of chosen strategies.

**Tactical planning.** Within each operational management function, the farm objectives must be translated into specific objectives called preset targets, which must be achieved within a predetermined time period. Examples of tactical planning are: shortening of the calving to conception interval to < 90 days, an abortion rate < 4%, the proportion of the herd culled for subfertility < 6%, an age at first calving of 740 days, an increase in milk production of 5%, an improvement in the protein fat ratio and/or lowering the production cost of milk by 10%, lowering of the Bulk Milk Somatic Cell Count by 25%, purchase of a management computer system, hiring extra labor or starting to perform A.I. oneself, etc. After defining preset targets, the farmer should plan and implement activities to reach the preset targets.

**Operational planning.** Examples of short term operational planning are: implementing deworming programs, culling of diseased cows or young stock, harvesting grass for silage making based on prevailing weather conditions, etc.

**B. Operational management.** Operational management of the dairy enterprise can be divided into eight separate functions which include most of the farm activities (Brand et al., 1995). These individual functions are: 1) crop production, 2) nutrition, 3) health care, 4) reproduction, 5) milk production, 6) herd replacement, 7) fixed assets and labor, and 8) cash flow (Figure 2). In each operational management function several subfunctions can be distinguished. For example, within the function of health care many diseases are included, each needing its own management approach. The 3 overall, and 8 operational management functions can each be divided in a number of processes. This is shown in Figure 2 where the 11 management functions are divided into 56 processes.

There are at least 13 processes within the planning functions, 4 processes in overall assessment and 39 processes in the 8 operational management functions. Some processes

*Figure 2. Outline of the management structure of a dairy farm*

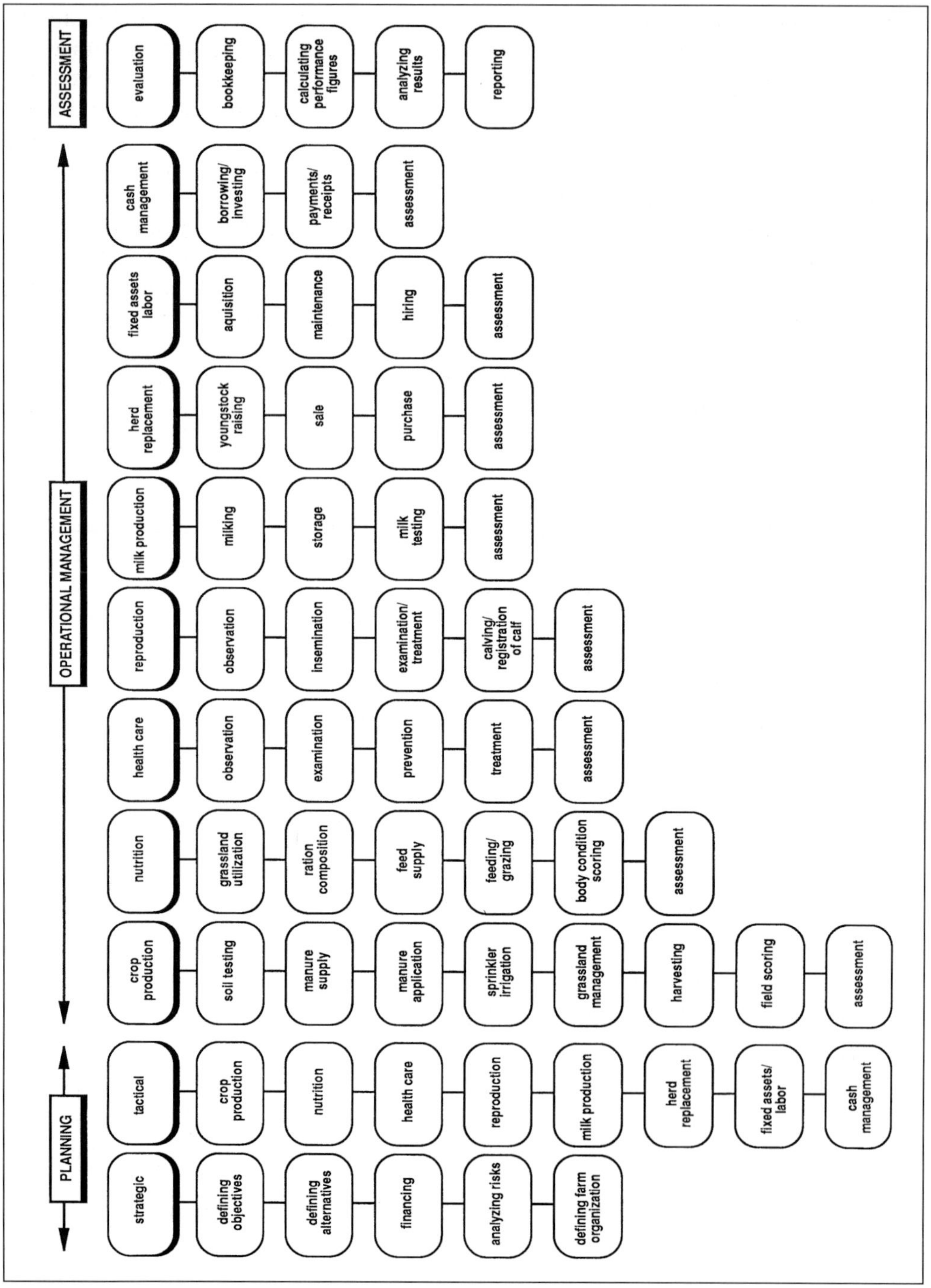

require daily activity and others seasonal. All the management functions and their processes are inexorably related and dependent on each other. For this reason practitioners providing HH & PM services, must not only pay attention to reproduction, as is still the case in many veterinary practices, but also to other operational management functions and their processes. If, for example, the practitioner suggests that more time be devoted to estrous detection then less time will be available for crop production or milking management. Allocation of the limited resources of the farmer must always consider a balance of all distinct and interrelated processes. In addition, the practitioner must have an understanding of how performance in one process is biologically or technically connected to other processes. For example, the decision to allocate the best forage to the milking cows may lead to reduced growth rates in the replacement stock fed the poorer forage. It is like putting a finger in communicating vessels. If more volume is added somewhere the water will rise elsewhere, producing either positive or negative effects.

**C. Overall assessment.** Overall assessment closes the management cycle. This assessment evaluates the technical and economic performance of the whole dairy enterprise by comparing actual performance indices with the farm objectives. For that purpose

*Figure 3. Herd Health and Production Management Protocol*

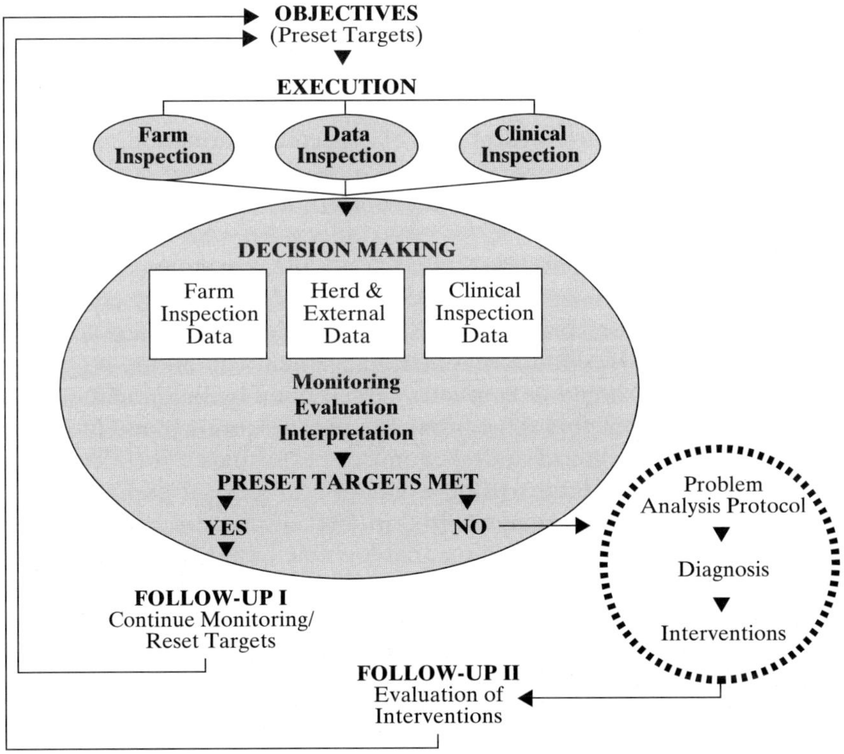

the performances within the individual operational management functions must be integrated. If the actual performance indices differ in a negative way from the farm objectives, measures must be taken within the operational management functions to diagnose and correct inefficiences in management. Another outcome could be to reset farm objectives. Generally, the financial planning and evaluation activities are not part of the HH & PM services, but practitioners should realize that they are of primary importance to the farmer. Optimally the implementation of any corrective actions should be evaluated in the overall economic assessment. However, the authors are not aware of an available economic monitoring program that can evaluate all the separate management functions identified in Figure 2 except the farmer's bank account. In doing this, farmers manage their enterprise intuitively.

### 1.1.5 SYSTEMATIC STRATEGIES IN HERD HEALTH AND PRODUCTION MANAGEMENT SERVICES: THE PROTOCOL

Clinical examination of a diseased individual cow follows a system that contains a sequence of steps in which attention is paid to every relevant aspect of the whole body or organ level function that can lead to a diagnosis. In HH & PM services, the examination of the whole enterprise or of the various operational management functions should also make use of a systematic approach. By analogy, HH & PM services make use of protocols to monitor and\or to solve problems with animal health or production. A HH & PM protocol consists of 4 main components:

1. defining objectives or preset targets,
2. execution or materials and methods,
3. decision making, based on interpretation of collected information, and
4. follow up (Figure 3).

In addition to this, a problem solving protocol must be available.

**1. Objectives or preset targets.** Preset targets are the translation of the farm objectives in the various operational management functions of the dairy enterprise according to the "goals roll down" principle. Preset targets differ from farm to farm due to the different farm objectives and farm and management conditions. As soon as they have been defined they should be mutually agreed upon by the practitioner and farmer. Defining preset targets forces the farmer and his practitioner and/or farm advisor to discuss and to plan technical and economical performance for a predetermined period. They also form the basis for the evaluation process of performance later in time. Herd performance can be summarized in a set of primary indices. Such a set is defined as the smallest number of indices that are able to indicate the current performance status within an operational management function. A set of primary fertility performance indices, together with their preset targets are presented in Table 1. The performance indices are calculated in a cumulative way over a 3, 6 or 12 month period. Comparison of the performance indices with preset targets enables the farmer to see if they fall short of expectations. In addition, trends in performance and/or seasonal performance problems can be visualized.

*Table 1. Primary preset targets and actual performance for fertility*

| Herd composition | Last 3 months | Last 6 months | Last 12 months | Preset target |
|---|---|---|---|---|
| # cows in herd | 87 | 88 | 91 | |
| # cows pregnant | 19 | 40 | 85 | |
| # heifers calved | 10 | 14 | 29 | |
| **Performance indices** | | | | |
| Expected C.I. (Days) | 458 | 477 | 448 | 400 |
| # Abortions | 5 | 7 | 7 | 4 |
| % culled for fertility | 27.6 | 31.9 | 24.1 | 10 |
| Age at 1st calving | 26.6 | 26.8 | 26.1 | 26 |

**2. Execution.** Execution or materials and methods includes the tools, activities, techniques, and management strategies used by both the practitioner and the farmer to help reach his/her preset targets. Standard activities of the practitioner include data, farm, and clinical inspections. A data inspection is only possible if the farmer records animal and farm data in a farm diary, on other forms, or directly in a computer. In the same way as the farmer is providing data about a diseased animal to be examined, herd data are required to examine the farm performance. Therefore, data are an absolute requirement for a quantitative assessment of herd performance, for judging whether planned preset targets are met as well as for proper decision-making. The HH & PM practitioner has to record his/her data resulting from the farm and clinical inspection during the farm visit. Collected data must be processed on a regular basis into herd and farm performance indices (Chapter 1, part 2)

Datasets from individual farms may serve as sentinel systems for disease or performance monitoring. These datasets can also serve as the basis for research in several fields. Whether the use is for improved individual herd performance or better understanding of broad principles, the concern for data quality remains vital.

The contents of a clinical and farm inspection depend on the operational management function(s) that are included in HH & PM services. Clinical inspection activities may include: genital examination, body condition scoring, claw trimming, blood sampling, identification of potential disease risk factors etc. Farm inspection activities may include: ration evaluation, checking milking machine function, general hygiene, evaluation of grassland management and of housing conditions etc.

**3. Decision making.** The third component of the HH & PM protocol is decision making, which is a key activity based on monitoring, evaluation, and interpretation of information (Stein, 1986). Monitoring is the regular compilation of data from several sources to detect early changes or trends in the performance of operational management functions over time. Evaluation consists of comparison of actual performance indices with preset targets and the determination of the significance of deviations and whether trends towards better or worse performance are present (Table 1). In this way, trends in performance become apparent. The outcomes of monitoring and evaluation can be either OK or not OK and should be explained to the farmer.

If performance indices in one or more operational management functions fall short, then these indices are further analyzed to determine whether deviations are real or by chance. Normal variation in the behavior of biological systems means that some deviations will require no action. Hence, primary performance indices should include estimates of variability. However, scientific background to determine whether deviations are true or chance based is currently only available for a limited number of indices e.g. bulk milk somatic cell count (Schukken et al., 1992). Experience and long term record keeping will enable recognition of seasonal patterns and non-significant deviations as long as no appropriate statistical methods are available in HH & PM software or applied. This means that most evaluations are conducted on the basis of experience, knowledge and heuristics.

**Problem solving.** If the evaluation suggests a real problem of performance, the HH & PM practitioner should follow a *problem solving protocol.* The problem solving protocol consists of: 1) detailed case history, 2) a relevant detailed data, clinical, and farm inspection, 3) evaluation of collected information, 4) differential diagnosis, and 5) additional (laboratory) investigations, which may be indicated if available data is inadequate for developing an acceptable herd level diagnosis. For example, there may be a need to examine milk samples bacteriologically or blood samples serologically. This is followed by 6) a herd performance related diagnosis. Finally, recommendations for changes in either management strategy or farm conditions are given or an intervention strategy is applied.

**4. Follow up.** The fourth component of the protocol is follow up. If the performance is adequate then follow up includes: a) continuing with the routine activities through the next farm visit and sometimes in b) re-setting the preset targets. If a problem exists and has been analyzed in the problem solving loop, follow up also includes assessment of the effects of recommended interventions at future farm visits.

The HH & PM protocol guides the practitioner step-by-step through the mental diagnostic processes of a farm visit in order to help meet the preset targets for farm performance using appropriate tools and methods. The system provides the structure used in HH & PM service to obtain optimal results.

The problem solving processes also can be used in farm problem investigations where no previous monitoring activity has occurred. The process may require significantly more time and effort than with herds for which a data base already exists. Following the problem solving protocol should lead to useful herd performance related diagnosis. The experience and knowledge of the practitioner can then be used to formulate interventions. Similar to herds participating in a HH & PM service, a method for evaluation of the response to management changes should be established.

### 1.1.6 THE IMPLEMENTATION OF HERD HEALTH AND PRODUCTION MANAGEMENT PROGRAMS: AN ILLUSTRATION

The involvement of the practitioner in HH & PM services within an operational management function can be seen by examining the information flow in management of reproduction (Figure 4). The 4 routine activities of observation, insemination, genital examination, and calving are generating data. At this level, the practitioner's role is to contribute data from the results of genital examinations. Tactical planning produces the overall preset targets of the reproductive program, i.e. desired number of cows and heifers calving in some future interval, the expected calving to conception interval, etc. Not shown are the necessary connections between tactical planning for reproductive activities and information from other operational management functions, e.g. planning for replacement heifer breeding will include consideration of housing, roughage availability, and perhaps anticipated culling of older cows. The practitioner also participates in the information flow by monitoring raw data, calculating performance indices, and by evaluating performance. If a suitable computer program is available, reproductive performance indices can be generated automatically. He/she may also initiate and direct an investigation into causal factors of poor performance, sometimes in other operational management functions, and ultimately help to formulate corrective actions.

The information processing within the function of reproduction often has to be completed with data from other operational management functions as is illustrated in the lower right corner of Figure 4. For example, if many cows are lame, reproductive performance will most likely be reduced (Barkema et al., 1994). If milk production is

*Figure 4. Diagram of information flow within the operational management function reproduction.*

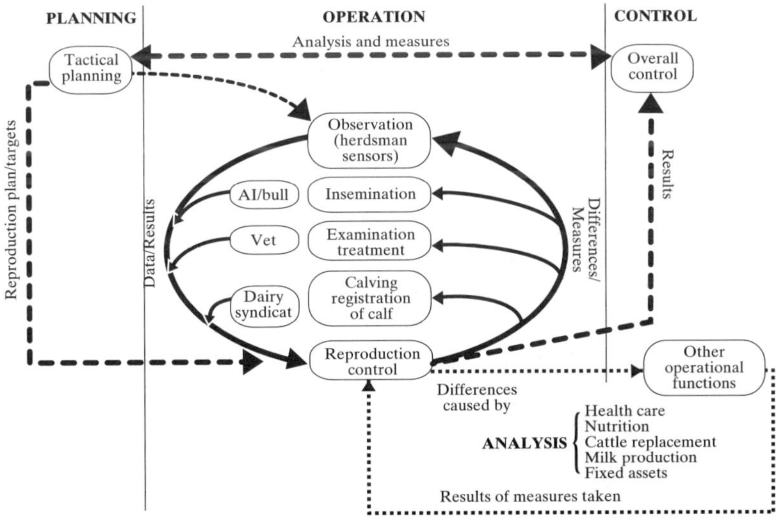

high, the interval from calving to first overt estrus may be prolonged (Britt, 1992). In principle, all the processes of the functional management structure of a dairy farm are interrelated either directly or indirectly. The practitioner must be aware of this when analyzing unacceptable performance and advising the farmer.

Reproduction is perhaps the most familiar operational management function to most dairy practitioners. HH & PM practitioners who are involved only in herd fertility services should do this in a broader perspective, rather than solely diagnosing and treating reproductive disorders. Reproductive performance can not be managed in isolation. Herd fertility services should be part of a total HH & PM service. Other operational management functions such as nutrition, health care, and housing facilities also play an important role in reproductive performance. The same degree of involvement of the practitioner in the guidance of other operational management functions may not seem so likely at first. However, when the interrelationships of different operational management functions are fully understood, the HH & PM practitioner will find it necessary to consider aspects of other operations.

## EPILOGUE

HH & PM services are evolving as an area of specialization in the veterinary profession. The implementation of these services on dairy farms relies on knowledge, skills, interests, and physical investments on the part of the practitioner and on a receptive and motivated attitude by the farmer. The relationship is a natural development of the practitioner's concern for the farmer's individual animals and the success of the farm. The veterinary profession began with treatment of overt illness and has progressed through attention to subclinical diseases, low productivity and the identification of risk factors for production and health disorders to concentrate on healthy animals. The entire dairy herd and the whole farm enterprise are now within the scope of the HH & PM practitioner. Health, production and management are key words in HH & PM services.

The farm enterprise can be compared to an industrial enterprise in having the same overall structure. However, an industrial company may have many individuals employed in planning, operational management, and assessment while a farm usually has a single individual performing these 3 activities. Due to the complexity of a modern dairy enterprise (Figure 2) the farmer is often looking for support from various resources to optimize his farm's performance. The HH & PM practitioner may be involved in many aspects of farm management with the overall concern of improving farm productivity through better management. Improvement of farm management should be achieved through integration of veterinary and animal husbandry knowledge and skills. Therefore the HH & PM professionals must combine understanding of farm management with knowledge and skills derived from veterinary science. The practitioner can be the primary advisor in the farm enterprise if he/she broadens his/her skills from disease diagnosis and treatment to support in health and production, process and product quality management and in farm economics.

*For references see part 3 of this Chapter.*

# 1.2 RECORD KEEPING

Chuck L. Guard[1] and Arie Brand[2]

[1] Department of Clinical Sciences, New York State College of Veterinary Medicine, Cornell University, Ithaca, New York, USA 14853

[2] Department of Herd Health and Reproduction, School of Veterinary Medicine, University of Utrecht, Yalelaan 7, 3584 CL Utrecht, The Netherlands

## 1.2.1 INTRODUCTION

In modern dairy farming, successful management relies on record keeping and on information which can be derived from it. The resulting information makes farm management issues more visible for the farmer and is of eminent importance to the veterinary practitioner and farm advisor. Without records, the practitioner is not able to provide the benefits of herd health and production management (HH & PM) services. With records, the practitioner and farm advisor can play a central role in the management decisions of the dairy by being an interpreter of on-farm information. This information is routinely utilized for everyday management and for easier problem solving when needed. Quantitative knowledge about the dairy provides the basis for understanding where the dairy has been, where it is today, and where it is going.

The practitioner must access a complex information system and be able to monitor, evaluate, analyze, and interpret the collected data in order to optimize health and production performance, and to forsee impending problems. The practitioner may use a computer to more easily interpret the information about the dairy just as he/she uses a stethoscope to diagnose a disease. The interpretation of the dataset available for a farm goes from the technological, e.g. average days open or bulk milk somatic cell count, to the biological basis for the observed performance. The practitioner is uniquely able to diagnose the underlying processes that cause the deviations from targets. Therefore, in HH & PM programs the practitioner must have skills in information handling, decision analysis, and epidemiological techniques. These skills allow the practitioner to monitor what is normal or diseased and to recognize what is optimal or suboptimal productivity at the herd level (Stein, 1986; Fetrow et al., 1987; Mueller, 1989; Lismore, 1989; Nelson, 1994).

In this part of Chapter 1 some guidelines for data recording, storage and processing are given, and specific items related to functional systems are discussed.

## 1.2.2 WHAT TO RECORD

The primary obligation of the farmer in contributing to the success of the HH & PM service is in accurate and complete, daily record keeping. Data may be only in the memory of the farmer or scattered in many different spots. For example, a problem with respiratory disease in calves may have been noticed by a farmer but no data on disease incidence or performance have been recorded. Without a correct assessment of the magnitude of the problem, quantitative improvement of heifer health, growth, and economics, after intervening actions, cannot be shown to the farmer. Therefore, the first step in a HH & PM service is to train the farmer or herdsman in accurate, and complete daily record keeping. The farmer should be encouraged by the practitioner to record data in a functional way. The data that should be recorded for the HH & PM service are generally those the farmer would logically keep anyway and include:

a. individual animal records of reproductive events, health disorders, condition scores, culling, and laboratory report data such as results of bacteriologic analyses of milk samples, etc.,
b. herd events such as vaccinations, ectoparasite control, anthelmintic treatment, routine claw trimming dates,
c. farm data such as grassland management data, relevant financial data, feedstuff purchases and inventories, and dates of fertilizer and manure application, forage analyses, dates and results of milking equipment evaluation.

The farmer should maintain additional information from external organizations which may include: milk production data and performance indices from DHIA (including summary reports) and from the milk company.

The practitioner makes important contributions to the herd database via clinical and farm inspections. Clinical data may include observations made during routine activities such as genital examinations and clinical examinations of diseased animals. Additionally, environmental and managerial factors observed during the farm inspection constitute valuable data. The data from farm inspections are not as easily structured nor quantified as individual cow data. Examples are observations on milking practices, air quality in confinement buildings, and the cleanliness of cows and stalls.

Data collection should at least lead to the calculation of primary indices (Chapter 1, part 1). With these indices farm performance can be evaluated. Further data collection to allow the calculation of secondary indices allow even more complex analysis which is at least required when deviations from what is acceptable are present in the primary indices. However, it is advisable to collect more complete data on every farm since further enhancements of performance always requires more detailed information on the underlying processes if problems occur.

### 1.2.3 RECORD KEEPING AND DATA STORAGE

Record keeping is important and will add to or detract from the ability of the farmer and HH & PM practitioner to make sound interpretations and decisions. Data recording can be done either manually or electronically. Manual recording is possible for almost all data routinely available on a farm but takes much time to perform. In the future, more farms will have automatic cow identification systems, making automated data recording in the milking parlor and in other places possible.

## a. Manual record keeping systems

In manual record keeping systems various forms are used varying from pocket-sized cards such as those provided by AI agencies to a more comprehensive farm diary or data logger.

*Figure 1. Example of a page from a farm diary*

| Date | Calving | Estrus | AI | Mastitis | Lameness | Diseased | Drying off | Other |
|---|---|---|---|---|---|---|---|---|
| 1/4 | (4) 41 ♀ fast 38 kg Afterbirth 3 hrs | | | | | | | |
| | | 280 | | | | 41 milk fever | | |
| 2/4 | | 280 Celsius | | | | | | |
| | | | | | 70 RR sole ulcer | | | |
| 4/4 | (4) 120 ♂ Caesarean section Afterbirth 3 days | | | | | | | |
| | | | | | | 162 Displaced | | |
| | | 45 metestrus bleeding | | | | Abomasum | | |
| | | | | | | | 50 } anti- | |
| 5/4 | | 171 Jabot | | | | | 121 } biot | |
| | | | 69 RF | | | | | |
| 6/4 | Claw Trimming herd | | | | | | | |
| | | | | | | | | |
| 8/4 | Milking system analysis | | | | | | | |
| | | | | | | | | |

A farm diary is used to record all individual cow actions and problems, especially those not recorded by third-party agencies, herd related data, and managerial events (Figure 1).

The data from the diary(ies) or pocket cards may be transferred to other media such as barn charts, individual cow cards, or computer files. Fertility barn charts (Figure 2) or 3-week calendars for recording reproductive events are in common use. A fertility barn chart can be extended to a fertility-health chart to record health data as well. Barn charts offer a line for each cow present, as well as an overview of performance of the whole herd or group, over a certain time period. Some farmers use for reproductive events a breeding wheel which provides an easily visible overview of the current reproductive status of the herd. These systems may pose limitations on analysis if the farmer fails to transfer the information to records that can be processed. The breeding wheel has the further disadvantage of losing information when a cow's peg is moved, e.g. when she is inseminated. Some farmers manually record all events directly on the individual cow or calf cards or in other appropriate systems without creating a daily diary or barn chart. On larger farms, different individuals may have daily responsibility for separate categories of herd management or different production groups, and keep separate records in various formats that are later combined. When records are kept in multiple formats and locations, it may take more time to collect the data for processing and analysis compared to records in one format.

*Figure 2. A fertility barn chart*

**Herd health program (VAMPP)**
**Fertility chart starting 1/1/1995**

| | | | Estrous | | Inseminations | | | | | | |
|---|---|---|---|---|---|---|---|---|---|---|---|
| **Calv.date** | **Cow** | **Par** | **1** | **2** | **1** | **2** | **3** | **4** | **Pregn.** | **Dry** | **Culled** |
| 2/1/95 | 12 | 8 | 16/2 | | 26/4 | | | | + | | 1/11/95 |
| 2/1/95 | 8513 | 2 | --- | | 8/6 - | 13/9 | 26/10 - | | kept open | | |
| 17/1/95 | 30 | 6 | --- | | 18/4 | 8/5 | | | twin | 18/11/95 | |
| 19/1/95 | 13 | 2 | 23/2 | | 18/3 | | | | + | 22/10/95 | |
| 19/1/95 | 45 | 2 | --- | | 24/4 | 8/6 | | | + | 4/1/96 | |
| 25/1/95 | 44 | 3 | --- | | 24/3 | | | | + | 27/11/95 | |
| 28/1/95 | 33 | 2 | --- | | 24/4 - | 29/6 | 2/9 | | + | 10/2/96 | |
| 2/2/95 | 22 | 2 | --- | | 3/4 | 27/4 | 8/6 | 29/6 | | | |
| | | | | | 12/8 | 2/9 | | | + | | |
| 17/2/95 | 76 | 3 | --- | | 13/5 | 3/6 | | | + | 9/1/96 | |
| 19/3/95 | 1 | 3 | --- | | 9/6 | | | | + | 4/1/96 | |
| 20/3/95 | 84 | 1 | --- | | 13/6 | 3/7 | 22/8 | 12/9 | | | |
| | | | | | 4/10 | | | | + | | |
| 5/4/95 | 11 | 3 | 9/5 | | 15/7 | 21/7 | 12/8 | 4/9 | + | | |
| 9/4/95 | 2 | 5 | --- | | 29/5 - | 12/7 | 5/8 | | + | 7/2/96 | |
| 27/4/95 | 39 | 4 | --- | | 28/6 | | | | + | 4/1/96 | |
| 28/4/95 | 42 | 5 | 30/5 | | 21/6 | | | | + | 4/1/96 | |
| 29/4/95 | 94 | 4 | --- | | --- | | | | | | 4/5/95 |
| 13/5/95 | 41 | 4 | --- | | 15/7 | 21/8 | 13/9 - | 7/11 | | | |
| | | | | | 12/12 - | 22/2 | | | | | |
| 25/5/95 | 62 | 2 | --- | | 31/7 | | | | + | 7/2/96 | |
| 11/6/95 | 54 | 1 | --- | | 22/8 | 12/9 - | 4/11 - | 1/1 | | | |
| | | | | | 25/1 | 15/2 | 27/2 | | | | |
| 15/6/95 | 21 | 3 | | | 21/8 - | 7/11 | 27/11 | 12/1 | + | | |
| 18/6/95 | 66 | 3 | 27/8 | | 13/9 | 25/10 | | | + | | |
| 25/6/95 | 81 | 3 | --- | | 13/9 | | | | + | | 9/3/96 |
| 25/6/95 | 89 | 1 | 13/8 | | 2/9 | | | | + | | |
| 27/6/95 | 32 | 1 | --- | | 30/9 | 27/11 | 8/1 | | + | | |

Often few individual animal health and young stock data are kept even on well managed farms. Therefore, a barn chart, called the calf rearing list, for routine events in the management of young stock should be used by all farmers (Chapter 2, part 1).

## b. Electronic record keeping systems

Automated milking parlors with continuous measurement of milk weight, milk electrical conductivity, milk temperature, and cow activity from pedometers are providing real-time data recording. All of these data are converted into instantaneous management-by-exception information using threshold values or more sophisticated algorithms. These systems may also measure concentrate consumption delivered via an automated concentrate feeder. This type of technology will become more widely adopted. Robotic milking parlors have all the features of the automated milking parlors and provide data about the frequency with which cows choose to be milked and milk produced per milking. This makes monitoring totally automatic. These systems can now be linked to expert systems for better interpretation of performance results (Devir et al., 1993).

Computerized systems for data storage may vary from on-farm computers to centralized databases such as provided by DHIA (Meuller, 1989; Nelson and Redlus, 1989). In the future, on-farm computers may be connected via modem to centralized databases at DHIA or equivalent organizations. Software for on-farm computer based dairy record processing is available with many features that are useful in HH & PM programs. Typical features include the ability to graphically portray data, to summarize data by demographic or productivity strata, and to generate lists of animals meeting either narror or broad criteria. Lists of cows requiring specific veterinary attention can be designed by the HH & PM practitioner in conjunction with the farmer. These lists can further be automated to prompt the farmer on the appropriate day for the action to occur. In large herds, the farm manager most often maintains the program by entering daily events. Milk recording technicians can enter milk data in their notebook computer and transfer this information to the farm computer directly or send a diskette later by mail. Artificial insemination technicians may enter breeding data directly into the farm computer rather than recording on the barn chart for later entry by the farmer. In some countries, they also may enter data in hand-held recorders (Data loggers) which connect to the central database via modem. In some veterinary practices, serving herds averaging less than 100 cows, the computer files are maintained in the clinic by the veterinary technician. Alternatively, notebook computers are carried to the farm by practitioners who enter all or some of the data at the time of the farm visit. Third-party systems, e.g. DHIA, usually record individual identification, dam and sire, milk production, calving and breeding dates. At present, these systems do not include the ability to record much of the managerial and health data which appear relevant to HH & PM services, although there are now 2 DHIA centers in the United States that store the complete herd data files including production, reproduction and health event data.

Future developments will probably include in-line or telemetric measuring of parameters on cow health, production, reproduction, and parameters currently inconceivable, which will allow instantaneous monitoring of the herd and individual cow. Sophisticated software is now in development to interpret the outputs of the in-line sensors. With wireless technology, data is now as mobile as we are, making exchange of information with any PC network or database possible, whenever and wherever we choose.

## 1.2.4 DATA PROCESSING

Record keeping and record storage is necessary but must be followed by computation of primary performance indices and, when required, by subsequent analyses. Data processing can be performed either manually or electronically. Electronic data processing is far more efficient than manual, but many performance figures can be manually computed. Hand calculations take time that is herd size dependent, and may be completely impractical for large herds. Moreover, with the increasing accessability of data in centralized systems, such as Dairy Herd Improvement databases, via personal computer and modem, the use of a computer with modem is becoming increasingly important in HH & PM services (Nelson, 1994). Furthermore, the time required for the practitioner to manually compute performance figures for all areas of interest for more than 2 or 3 herds in the practice, would likely be impossible.

Availability of the right data is a key factor in whether or not HH & PM services remain useful and cost effective in the long run. Some of these data will be routinely computed into performance indices by the DHI center, others by the farmer, and some may be left to the HH & PM practitioner and/or farm advisor.

### Manual data processing

Manual data processing is, in a large number of farms, the only way to generate adequate information in the form of performance indices that can be used for decision making(Kristula and Uhlinger, 1995). Not all primary performance indices, such as predicted calving interval, age at first calving, etc., are easily calculated by hand. Manual data processing lacks the computational ease and flexibility of computerized systems. In case computerized data processing is not done, a so called 12-monthly list can be used. This list is a useful form to monitor herd performance indices for small herds over time (Figure 3). It is optional to change the frequency with which this report is calculated depending on the interval between farm visits. The first column of this form lists performance indices (Noordhuizen et al., 1982/1983 a and b; Noordhuizen and Meurs, 1983/1984; Noordhuizen et al., 1984/1985). Some of them may be manually calculated during the farm visit. During each farm visit a new column of indices is added to the list. See the Appendix for an explanation of the items on the list.

Each index can be traced from month to month by scanning horizontally. After a few months, trends in behavior of a given index are easily followed by scanning across a row. This report makes it possible to monitor, at a glance, fluctuations in performance of relevant operational farm function indices, which differ from preset targets.

*Figure 3. The monthly list or monitor*

| | | | | | | | | | | | | | | | |
|---|---|---|---|---|---|---|---|---|---|---|---|---|---|---|---|
| **DATE OF VISIT** | | | | | | | | | | | | | | | |
| HERD STANDARD COW | | | | | | | | | | | | | | | |
| FAT % | | | | | | | | | | | | | | | |
| PROTEIN % | | | | | | | | | | | | | | | |
| COWS MILKING | | | | | | | | | | | | | | | |
| COWS DRY | | | | | | | | | | | | | | | |
| YOUNG STOCK | | | | | | | | | | | | | | | |
| **REPRODUCTION** | | | | | | | | | | | | | | | |
| COWS CALVED | | | | | | | | | | | | | | | |
| – RET PLACENTA | | | | | | | | | | | | | | | |
| – ABNORMAL VAG DISCHARGE | | | | | | | | | | | | | | | |
| – METRITIS | | | | | | | | | | | | | | | |
| – CYSTIC OVARY | | | | | | | | | | | | | | | |
| – TRUE ANESTRUS | | | | | | | | | | | | | | | |
| – ABORTIONS | | | | | | | | | | | | | | | |
| – 1ST SERVICE | | | | | | | | | | | | | | | |
| – 2ND & + SERVICE | | | | | | | | | | | | | | | |
| – % PREG/PREG EXAMINATIONS | | | | | | | | | | | | | | | |
| – SERVICES/PREGNANCY | | | | | | | | | | | | | | | |
| – RATIO / SERV/PREG | | | | | | | | | | | | | | | |
| – DIM AT 1ST SERVICE | | | | | | | | | | | | | | | |
| – DIM AT CONCEPTION | | | | | | | | | | | | | | | |
| – COWS > 85 DIM & NOT BRED | | | | | | | | | | | | | | | |
| – AGE AT 1ST BREEDING | | | | | | | | | | | | | | | |
| **MILK QUALITY & MASTITIS** | | | | | | | | | | | | | | | |
| – BULK TANK SCC X10000 | | | | | | | | | | | | | | | |
| – BULK TANK BACT COUNT | | | | | | | | | | | | | | | |
| – 1ST MASTITIS CASES | | | | | | | | | | | | | | | |
| – REPEAT CASES | | | | | | | | | | | | | | | |
| – COWS LS-SCC>5 (>500,000) | | | | | | | | | | | | | | | |
| **COW HEALTH & NUTRITION** | | | | | | | | | | | | | | | |
| – MILK FEVER/AT RISK | | | | | | | | | | | | | | | |
| – NO COWS < 60 DIM | | | | | | | | | | | | | | | |
| – KETOSIS | | | | | | | | | | | | | | | |
| – LDA | | | | | | | | | | | | | | | |
| – OFF FEED | | | | | | | | | | | | | | | |
| – DIARRHEA | | | | | | | | | | | | | | | |
| – LAMENESS | | | | | | | | | | | | | | | |
| **CULLING** | | | | | | | | | | | | | | | |
| – MASTITIS – UDDER | | | | | | | | | | | | | | | |
| – REPRO FAILURE | | | | | | | | | | | | | | | |
| – FEET – LEGS | | | | | | | | | | | | | | | |
| – DISEASE – INJURY | | | | | | | | | | | | | | | |
| – LOW PRODUCITON | | | | | | | | | | | | | | | |
| **CALF & HEIFER HEALTH** | | | | | | | | | | | | | | | |
| – CALVES KEPT | | | | | | | | | | | | | | | |
| – DIARRHEA TREATED | | | | | | | | | | | | | | | |
| – PNEUMONIA TREATED | | | | | | | | | | | | | | | |
| – DEAD 1ST MONTH | | | | | | | | | | | | | | | |
| – DEAD 1 MONTH TO CALVING | | | | | | | | | | | | | | | |

Seasonal influences on farm functions may produce repeatable changes in performance that can only be easily recognized with a record spanning more than one year. For instance, bulk milk somatic cell count is higher in August and September in the north temperate zone of North America and western Europe due to increased density of infectious agents from seasonal temperature and humidity factors. For other deviations from pre-set targets further analysis will be required to arrive at a herd level diagnosis (Chapter 1, part 1). Although most of the data for this report can be easily processed manually, a comprehensive and electronically computed spreadsheet version has been developed by Fetrow et al, (1988).

A convenient manual form for following the outcome of some frequently recurring events is the Q-sum graph (Kristula and Uhlinger, 1995). For example, the success of all (first) inseminations can be tracked by recording first the breedings and later the outcome, either return to estrus or diagnosed open at pregnancy examination (Figure 4). The same can be done for estrus observations. These graphs give an up-to-date, cumulative mean value for a dichotomous variable. This graphical technique is also performed by some dairy management software, eg. Daisy (Esslemont et al., 1981), and Dairy Comp 305. 1993. (User's Manual. Valley Agricultural Software, Tulare, California)

## 1.2.5 ELECTRONIC DATA PROCESSING

Use of computers with appropriate software to store, process, and analyze the very large volume of data that has been collected is of immense value to HH & PM services. Computer use is essential for reducing the burden of manual routine and time in these processes. The software may differ between countries, regions, and even from farm to farm. The HH & PM practitioner, however, must be able to intelligently interpret the results produced by the computer regardless of the software program used. As an example, all commercial software vendors in the Netherlands have agreed upon calculating and presenting identical calculated primary indices.

Computerization helps make HH & PM services feasible, cost effective, practical, and manageable. For the farmer, it helps reveal information that was previously difficult to obtain using farmers' common manual data processing practices. Computerized evaluation can be exciting for the farmer and the practitioner; it often adds to the pleasure they derive from their endeavors.

Computerized dairy records provide the opportunity to make lists of cows by demographic or production parameters for subsequent action. For example, a weekly list of milking cows pregnant 220 to 227 days may be produced for drying off procedures. Cows falling below 25 kg of milk may be moved to a different production group. Lists of cows meeting multiple criteria of reproduction status may be generated for veterinary examination. In addition, individual cows can be identified that fail to meet certain criteria (management by exception) such as milk production more than 10 kg below projected targets, a somatic cell count above 400,000 cells per ml, or days in milk more than 75 and not bred. Most HH & PM software includes capability for graphical presentation of individual or summary indices.

*Figure 4. Q-sum graph*

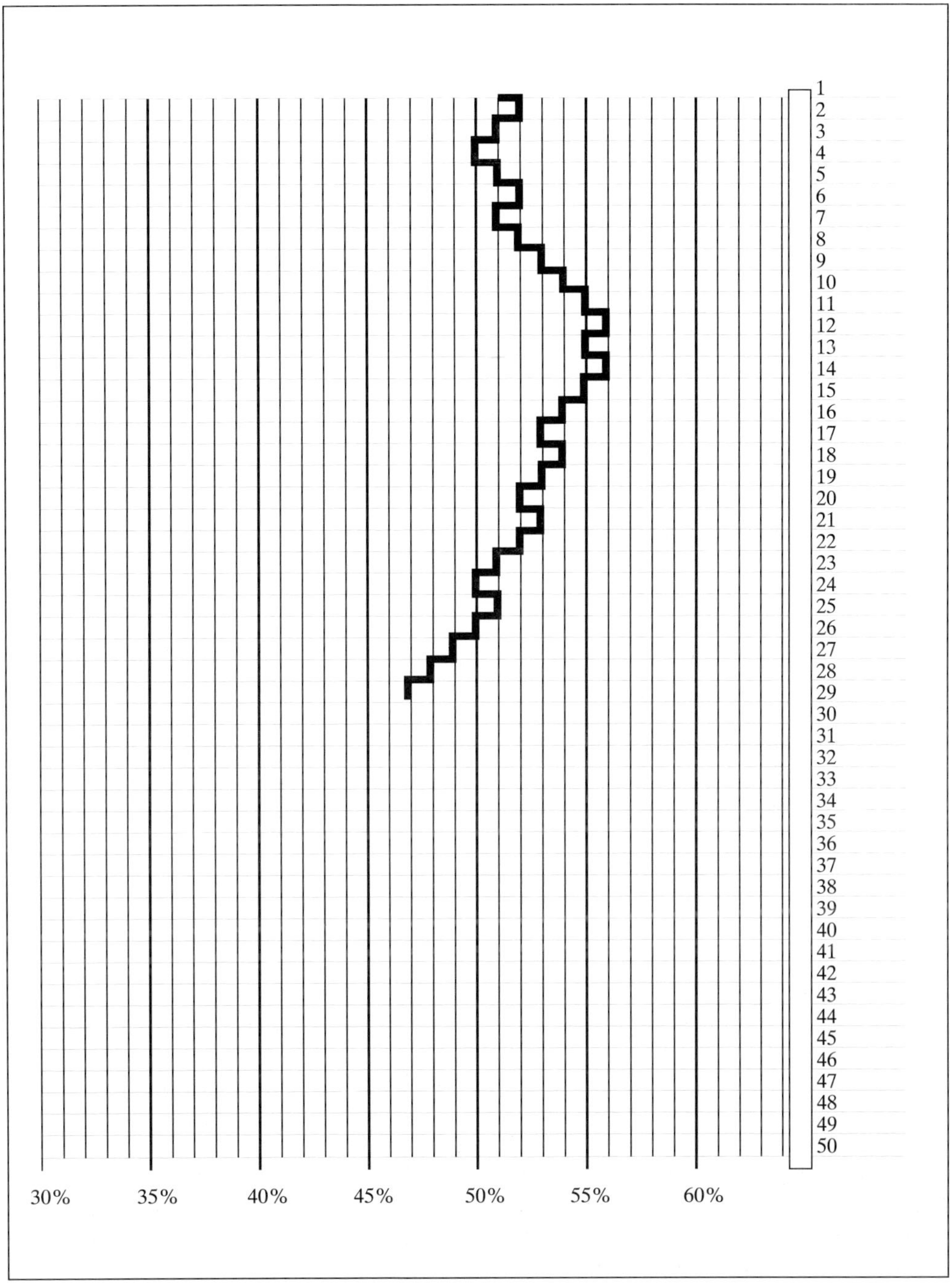

*Figure 5. Monthly summary report of DHIA with calculated performance figures (Source: Cornell Dairy Records, 1990)*

CDR 537L 4/12/94

| ST. | CO. | HERD NO. | REG. | CIRC. |
|---|---|---|---|---|
| | | | 25 | 32 |

| TYPE OF SAMPLING | STRING OPTION |
|---|---|
| DHIR-APT | |
| SPECIES: COW | |

# Herd Summary

**E — Genetics**

This herd is genetically better than percent of herds processed at Cornell Dairy Records and has an average Estimated Transmitting Ability (ETA) of $

**F — Herd Turnover**

| | Left Herd Animals | Left Herd % | New Animals | New % |
|---|---|---|---|---|
| This Period | 7 | 3 | 7 | 3 |
| This Year | 58 | 24 | 89 | 37 |

D 5 3 7

**G — Days Dry**

| | Number of Animals <40 | 40 to 70 | >70 | Avg. Days |
|---|---|---|---|---|
| This Period | | | | |
| 1st Lactation | | 6 | | 53 |
| 2nd+ Lactation | 1 | 6 | 2 | 59 |
| This Year | | | | |
| 1st Lactation | 2 * | 47 * | 2 * | 58* |
| 2nd+ Lactation | 10* | 82 * | 16* | 58* |

**H — Projected Herd Inventory**

| | May | Jun | Jul | Aug | Sep | Oct |
|---|---|---|---|---|---|---|
| Animals Milking* | 211 | 219 | 241 | 254 | 258 | 263 |
| Animals to Dry Off | | 15 | 12 | 17 | 19 | 19 |
| Cows to Freshen | 18 | 18 | 22 | 19 | 14 | 15 |
| Heifers to Freshen | 6 | 5 | 12 | 11 | 9 | 9 |

* As of the last day of the month

**I — Daily Feeding**

| | Milking Animals: Value of Milk | Value of Conc. | Total Feed Cost | Income over Feed | Feed Cost per cwt. of Milk | Lbs. Milk per lb. Conc. | Lbs. Forage Drymatter per cwt. BdyWt. | Dry Animals Feed Cost |
|---|---|---|---|---|---|---|---|---|
| This Sample Day | 10.82 | 2.06 | 2.95 | 7.87 | 3.56 | | | .94 |
| Last Sample Day | 10.63 | 2.06 | 2.95 | 7.68 | 3.58 | | | .94 |
| This Year | 10.30 | 2.05 | 2.94 | 7.36 | 3.71 | | | .95 |

**Feeding Notes**

**J — Reproduction**

| | Days to first Breeding | Days Open: Minimum Projected | Days Open: Likely Pregnant | Percent 1st Service Conception@ | Services per Concept. | Greater than 80 Days not Bred | Greater than 140 Days not Conf.@ | Calving Interval: Proj. | Calving Interval: Previous | Last Calving: Age | Last Calving: Weight |
|---|---|---|---|---|---|---|---|---|---|---|---|
| This Period | | | | | | | | | | | |
| 1st Lactation | 63 | XXX | XXX | XXX | XXX | 5 | 11 | 13.2 | XXX | 24 | 1250 |
| 2nd+ Lactation | 67 | XXX | XXX | XXX | XXX | 1 | 13 | 13.1 | 12.9 | 49 | 1250 |
| Overall | | | | | | | | | | | |
| 1st Lactation | 75 * | 129 | 132 | 40 * | 2.4 | 37 * | 11 * | 13.3* | XXX | 24 * | 1250* |
| 2nd+ Lactation | 76 * | 124 | 128 | 49 * | 2.2 | 78 * | 25 * | 13.3* | 13.2* | 53 * | 1250* |
| All | 76 * | 126 | 130 | 46 * | 2.3 | 115* | 36 * | 13.3* | 13.2* | 43 * | 1250* |

@ Requires that animals be reported confirmed pregnant

* To be included in Box G and Box J animals must have a calving date in the previous 18 months. The asterisk (*) indicates that animals culled in the last 365 days are also included.

The periodic reports of the milk recording service, e.g. DHIA, typically include calculated performance indices (Figure 5). These reports may also include values from earlier measurements to illustrate trends. However, the rolling 12-month calculations of many performance indices are relatively insensitive to potentially significant short term changes.

## EPILOGUE

The records kept by the farmer, practitioner and farm advisor are the basis of all information about herd and farm performance. Without good records, no meaningful evaluations and analyses can be undertaken, and therefore the processes of assessment and decision making can not be knowledgeably conducted. In the authors' experience, the weakest link in a HH & PM service is usually inaccurate or insufficient record keeping not only by the farmer but also by the practitioner. The practitioner should help the farmer design a record keeping system if he does not already have an appropriate one. Once the system is in place the practitioner might need to persistently encourage accuracy and thoroughness on the part of the farmer. The practitioner contributes clinical data and observations on management from the farm inspection to the database. The data can be preliminarily processed and summarized in the monthly list of performance indices. For many circumstances this will suffice. If unacceptable performance requires deeper analysis other information processing techniques may need to be employed.

*For references see part 3 of this Chapter.*

## APPENDIX

**Definition of terms in the monthly list of performance indices:**

*DATE OF VISIT* The date of the farm visit defines the end of the period included in the data in the column below.

**MILK PRODUCTION AND HERD DATA:**
*HERD STANDARD COW* Herd standard cow is a standarized milk production measure for the herd in the Netherlands, provided by the milk recording agency. Actual milk production corrected for age, season, and parity of calving. It may be calculated for each cow and the herd mean provided in the periodic report from the DHIA. [Canadian DHI use BCA or Breed Class Average that is an index corrected for breed, age and season of calving. It is calculated after 45 DIM.]
*FAT %* The fat % in milk is taken from the reports of either the milk testing agency or the milk purchaser.
*PROTEIN %* Protein % comes from the same source as fat %.
*COWS MILKING* The number of cows milking may be obtained from the DHIA

report or by direct counting. The number of cows milking serves as a denominator for proportions of cows with specific conditions in manual computations of incidence rates.
*COWS DRY* The number of cows dry may be determined in the same way as cows milking. The number of cows dry will give information on expected calvings.
*YOUNG STOCK* The number of young stock can be determined by census or by keeping a running total of additions and removals from the replacement herd. The young stock are the most valuable resource for the future of the herd and simultaneously a drain on all assets.

**REPRODUCTION:**
*COWS CALVED* The number of cows calved will come from the breeding wheel, barn chart or farm diary. The number of cows calved during the interval will serve as the reference point for periparturient disease incidence rates and reproduction management in the coming intervals.
*RET PLACENTA* The number of cows with placental retention beyond 24 hours after calving is obtained by either query of the farmer or by review of individual cow records or the farm diary.
*ABNORMAL VAG DISCH* The number of cows with abnormal vaginal discharge beyond 3 weeks after calving is recorded. The data come from both the farmer's observations and those of the practitioner during genital examinations.
*METRITIS* The number of cows with metritis is recorded from the observations of the practitioner during genital examinations. This category may be defined by the practitioner to include pyometra, delayed involution, endometritis or other abnormal uterine conditions.
*CYSTIC OVARIAN DISEASE* The number of cows with cystic ovarian disease is usually confined to those cows with abnormalities that are 35 days in milk or longer. Definition of cases may include milk progesterone testing to confirm the absence of functional luteal tissue.
*TRUE ANESTRUS* The number of cows with true anestrus is determined by review of rectal palpation data or milk progesterone measures. True anestrus is the absence of observed estrus, lack of secondary signs of estrus and small, inactive ovaries.
*ABORTIONS* Abortions are those cows and heifers which have been confirmed pregnant and subsequently return to estrus or are found open on reexamination. Many practitioners will restrict this class of reproductive problems to cows aborting between 100 and 260 days of gestation.
*1st SERVICE* The number of first inseminations of lactating cows is obtained from the records of the inseminator or the herd fertility-health barn chart or farm diary. This number serves as the denominator for calculation of conception rate.
*2nd & + SERVICE* The number of second or greater inseminations (repeat breedings) of lactating cows is taken from the same source as first inseminations. Total inseminations per pregnancy and number of repeat breeders may be determined with this number.
*PREG/PREG EXAM* The number of animals diagnosed pregnant divided by the number presented for pregnancy examination is one measure of heat detection efficiency

and conception rate. The data come from the genital examinations performed by the practitioner.
*SERVICES/PREGNANCY* The total number of inseminations for the cows diagnosed pregnant in the month is counted from the herd fertility-health barn chart or the insemination records. This number of inseminations divided by the number found pregnant is a measure of both fertility and costs to produce a pregnancy.
*RATIO SERV/PREG* The ratio of services per pregnancy is easier to compare by month than the whole number fraction in the above item.
*DIM AT 1st SERV* The average days in milk at first insemination is usually provided by the DHIA. It is probably too time consuming to calculate this from individual cow records in larger herds but may be feasible if less than 10 cows were inseminated in the month. Interval calculators are available from AI organizations or pharmaceutical companies.
*DIM AT CONCEPTION* The average number of days in milk at conception for the cows diagnosed pregnant during the month is either available from the DHIA or must be calculated as the preceding item.
*COWS > 85 DIM & NOT BRED* The number of cows more than 85 days in milk (or some other interval chosen by the practitioner) and not yet inseminated is obtained from individual cow records or the herd fertility-health barn chart. This group represents problem cows and will often be further examined.
*AGE AT 1st BREEDING* The age at first breeding of the replacement heifers will determine their earliest possible calving age. It may be time consuming to calculate, but the age at calving, which is usually provided by DHIA, is more historical than current. It is an indicator of the performance of the young stock rearing program.

**MILK QUALITY & MASTITIS:**
*BULK TANK SCC X 1000* The bulk milk somatic cell count is obtained from the agency purchasing the milk. Depending on the country one or several determinations are made each month and reported to the farmer with his payment.
*BULK TANK BACT COUNT* There are several types of testing for bacterial counts performed on milk and whatever is available from the milk company and appropriate for monitoring the functioning of the milking and storage system can be used.
*1st MASTITIS CASES* The number of first cases of clinical mastitis within the current lactation can be tabulated from individual cow records, the farm diary, or a separate mastitis treatment list.
*REPEAT CASES* Second or subsequent cases of clinical mastitis are noted from the same sources as first cases.
*COWS LS-SCC > 5 (> 400,000)* Individual cows with milk somatic cell counts above 400,000 cells per milliliter or with a linear score of > 5 can be enumerated from the reports of the milk testing service.

**COW HEALTH & NUTRITION:**

*MILK FEVER/AT RISK* The number of cows treated for milk fever can be counted from the farm diary or individual cow records. The cows at risk are those calving for the second or subsequent time.

*NO COWS < 60 DIM* The number of cows less than 60 days in milk represent the portion of the herd at greatest risk for metabolic disorders and nutritional upsets. This number can be obtained by adding the number of calvings in the current and previous months.

*KETOSIS* The number of cows treated for ketosis in the month can be found in the farm diary or from individual cow records.

DA The number of cows with left or right displacement of the abomasum can be tallied from the farm diary, fertility- health barn chart, or individual cow records.

*OFF FEED* The number of cows off feed without further specification will come from the same source as other health disorders. This category of disorder presumably reflects some cases of acute ruminal acidosis and is both a monitor of the general feeding program and of the management of the transition from dry cow to early lactation rations. It is also a management observation indicator.

*DIARRHEA* Diarrhea of unspecified etiology is also presumably indicative of feeding management errors.

*LAMENESS* Clinical lameness cases will be recorded by the practitioner or farmer after treatment.

**CULLING:**

*MASTITIS – UDDER* Cows culled for mastitis, slow or difficult milking, teat lesions, or poor udder conformation.

*REPRO FAILURE* Cows culled for failure to become pregnant or after aborting.

*FEET – LEGS* Cows culled for lameness, including painful musculo-skeletal conditions.

*DISEASE – INJURY* Cows culled for disease or injury, such as abomasal volvulus, wounds, or chronic pneumonia.

*LOW PRODUCTION* Cows culled for low milk production potential, including cows with low fat or protein concentrations.

**CALF & HEIFER HEALTH:**

*CALVES KEPT* The number of calves kept to raise as replacement heifers will be available by census. This number will be the denominator for incidence rates of health disorders in calves.

*DIARRHEA TREATED* The number of calves or heifers treated for diarrhea will come from the calf rearing chart.

*PENUMONIA TREATED* The number of calves or heifers treated for pneumonia will come from the heifer rearing chart.

*DEAD 1st MONTH* The number of calves dead from birth (born alive) until 1 month of age will come from the calf rearing chart.

*DEAD 1 MONTH TO CALVING* The number of calves and heifers dead from 1 month of age to first calving will come from the calf rearing chart.

# 1.3 THE FARM VISIT

Chuck L. Guard[1] and Arie Brand[2]

[1] Department of Clinical Sciences, New York State College of Veterinary Medicine, Cornell University, Ithaca, New York, USA 14853

[2] Department of Herd Health and Reproduction, School of Veterinary Medicine, University of Utrecht, Yalelaan 7, 3584 CL Utrecht, The Netherlands

## 1.3.1 INTRODUCTION

The time spent on the farm by the veterinary practitioner conducting a herd health and production management (HH & PM) service should be organized around the primary activities of rendering clinical and preventive service, data collection, decision making, and advising. In this chapter an outline of general items to consider for examination as part of the farm visit is presented. The items to examine are directed at optimization of health and production performance of the dairy herd. In addition some activities of the practitioner and the client in preparation for the first and then for subsequent visits are suggested. Each practitioner must find his/her own way in organizing these events so that time is spent efficiently and a thorough, mutually satisfactory job is done. The outline presented here is based on more than 10 years of herd health and production management experiences. Individual practice and farm circumstances may require adjustments or additional areas of concern.

## 1.3.2 PREPARATIONS FOR THE FARM VISIT

In an era of emerging HH & PM services, the initiation of a program often occurs during a discussion between the practitioner and client about the relevance of an individual animal problem or a herd problem. In such circumstances, the practitioner will have visited the farm for a variety of consultative or emergency services before a HH & PM program is discussed and initiated.

Some basic facts about the farm should be known prior to the first farm visit, for example: herd size, milk production level, barn type, milking system, feeding system, etc. In many cases most of these items are already known or can be determined by telephone interview. In addition the existing record keeping system(s) for animal health, reproduction, and general farm operations should be ascertained.

Usually the first facts and data acquired will relate to the specific problem identified by the farmer or practitioner. The initial problem or primary motivation to begin a program should be kept in focus when organizing the early efforts of the HH & PM service. For example, short term objectives may differ depending on whether the farm is embracing a HH & PM service to correct a single, serious problem or for general management support. In addition, from a long-term perspective the practitioner must have some understanding of the overall goals of the farmer (Chapter 1, part 1). Is maximizing profit or production the most important aim? HH & PM services are usually begun because of concern for a single area such as subfertility, calf health problems, or mastitis. At later stages of the relationship, other operational management functions can be included in the HH & PM services which may seem quite important to the practitioner but in the beginning not perceived as such by the farmer. A statement of understanding between the parties outlining the areas of concern and mutual expectations from the program should be agreed upon. The importance of thorough and efficient data recording systems to the success of HH & PM services should be stressed during early contacts with the farmer. Without accurate and up-to-date data an efficient HH & PM service is not possible. And finally, the anticipated costs of the HH & PM service should be discussed before any work is undertaken.

### 1.3.3 ACTIVITIES DURING THE FARM VISIT

Several activities have to be performed during the farm visits. They always include data inspection, clinical examinations and treatments, and a farm inspection. The objective of the first visit is to acquire an overview of general farm operations and an elementary inventory as the basis for future action. The first visit will usually require more time than later visits to observe management practices and farm conditions over the breadth of farm operations. Preparations for subsequent farm visits include updating of the data base, evaluating relevant performance indices, and further analysis of data when this is required. Also the advice of previous visits should be evaluated or checked during the current visit. Seasonal activities such as deworming, vaccination or planning of crop production should be included in the discussion when appropriate. The outcome of the farm visit should be discussed at the end of each visit. Finally an action list for the next farm visit is prepared.

### 1.3.4 DATA INSPECTION

Before the actual farm visit the existing data are inspected. This may include health and milk production data. Primary indices are useful to obtain an initial overview of performance. At the first farm visit special attention is required to obtain herd data, and to install an accurate data collection system. The farmer should be instructed to keep records (Chapter 1, part 2), and permission should be obtained to download data from central data bases such as milk recording, bulk milk quality and laboratory results, if access is possible.

## 1.3.5 CLINICAL INSPECTION

Primary attention during the first farm visit should be directed towards the major complaint which initiated the HH & PM service. Clinical examination and data collection relevant to the major complaint receive priority at the beginning of a HH & PM service. One of the reasons for immediately inspecting or treating the individual, when the ultimate concern of the HH & PM service is the status of the whole herd, is to assure the farmer that he will get service in addition to advice as part of the program. However, during future visits reproductive examinations and treatments will usually form the central part of the farm visit. The reason for their importance is the need they create to be on the farm at regular intervals and the value they provide in general management. For example, knowing the reproductive status of cows is essential for determining drying off and expected calving dates. Subsequent visits allow more thorough observations of farm conditions and further collection of current health and managerial data that can be helpful in solving or preventing the initial problem of concern to the farmer. For example, the clinical mastitis problem that was the farmer's major complaint may have been due primarily to dirty stall conditions but went by unnoticed or uncorrected by him. The practitioner may be able to monitor barn hygiene by inspection during reproductive examinations and improve the stall conditions by suggestions, reminders, or encouragement.

During the first visit, depending on the current information about the reproductive status of individual animals, the practitioner must decide whether to examine the reproductive tract of all cows or only those of unknown status (Chapter 5, part 2). The size of the herd and the restraint facilities will influence how this is handled.

The farmer may be asked to make a list in advance for subsequent visits that would include cows for genital examinations, clinically ill animals including lame cows, and other animals for routine procedures such as calves for dehorning. When the farmer provides this work list, the practitioner should always examine it for inclusion/exclusion rules and completeness. In some regions, the genital examination list might be an "action list" from the DHIA. These lists are usually based on flexible rules the practitioner may wish to modify.

The time spent in genital examinations can simultaneously be used to: do body condition scoring, examine and score fecal consistency, observe feet and legs for abnormalities, examine skin lesions, evaluate udder conformation and teat health, look for kicking animals, broken tails, nervous cows, or other evidence of stress or cruelty, and add to observations about cow and human activity patterns in the barn. After finishing genital examinations, the practitioner should demonstrate model hygienic standards when treating individuals for reproductive problems.

Clinical activities are continued by examination and treatment of sick, mastitic or lame cows. Blood, milk, feces, or urine may be collected for laboratory examination if the data obtained will be relevant to the problem initiating the HH & PM service, or if analyses are indicated by observations.

Young stock examination for the status of health, growth, and reproductive function is done following the same procedures as in adults (Chapter 2, part 2). Discussion of current replacement rearing policy can be incorporated into these activities.

## 1.3.6 FARM INSPECTION AND GENERAL DISCUSSION OF OPERATIONS

In addition to clinical examinations of individuals and groups of animals, a general farm inspection will be conducted that will be repeated in some form at each visit. Initially, the practitioner should become familiar with all aspects of the operation that might influence herd performance. However, those areas of farm operation that relate most closely to the initial focus of the HH & PM service should again receive greatest attention. Repeated assessment at subsequent visits of the same areas may be important; changes in activity patterns, herd composition, season, or other factors may significantly alter farm conditions and management practices. Furthermore, the specific concerns of this part of the farm inspection may change with the occurrence of new problems or with the advent of new information on the relationships of health, productivity, environment and management practices.

The farm inspection is critical; it is focused on management and farm conditions. It is based on the knowledge that diseases under the skin are influenced by conditions outside the skin. All senses are employed in evaluating environmental conditions and in developing an understanding of the underlying management philosophies that influence animal health and performance. The information derived from the farm inspection must be recognized as forming a crucial part of the data on the farm's management even though some parts will be difficult to quantify. Results of the farm inspection may be pivotal in the decision making process. Examination of some of the items listed below may be deferred to subsequent visits.

### A. General (barn) inspection

In herds housed all year, or during the winter for seasonally housed cattle, the following may be considered as an example of an inspection checklist. Many of these items may also be relevant for animals on pasture (under F. at page 35).

*Upon entering the barn:*

* current barn climatic conditions, e.g. temperature, humidity, drafts and air quality,
* presence and use of ventilation system components to handle seasonal extremes of weather, presence of barn insulation, evidence of condensation on insulation,
* artificial and natural illumination sources,
* presence of head locks or other group animal restraint facilities.

*From in front of the cows:*

* per cow availability of feed bunk space,
* presence of computerized feeding systems and animal density,
* grouping of lactating and/or dry cows,
* estimation of quality of feedstuffs provided,
* availability of fresh roughage or total mixed ration (TMR),
* legibility and prevalence of visible cow identification,
* general cow attitude, e.g. dull or alert?
* ocular or nasal discharge?
* presence of horned cows.

*From behind the cows:*
* general inspection of body condition and rumen fill,
* cleanliness of cows and their environment,
* skin and hair condition,
* vaginal discharges,
* consistency and color of feces,
* presence of lame cows,
* number of stalls in relation to number of cows,
* dimensions of stalls and alleys in relation to cow size,
* bedding use and stall hygiene.
* floor type, condition, and maintenance level,
* source and cleanliness of drinking water,
* type of manure handling system,
* use of grates over manure gutter.

*Further inspection of the facilities:*
* presence and condition of foot bath and contents,
* presence and cleanliness of maternity facilities,
* presence, conditions, and use of sick cow housing,
* condition of holding pen and crowd gate,
* concentrate fed in milking parlor, yes or no,
* young stock housing facilities (with a repeat of several of the specific concerns as listed above for milking cows),
* young stock size, heterogeneity within groups,
* general state of repair/maintenance of barn, stalls, etc.
* drug storage and labeling; what?, where?, how?

Although there are no hard criteria to quantify some of the aspects just listed, the practitioner should be able to give his/her opinion about these farm conditions in a qualitative manner.

### B. Daily schedule and activity patterns

The details of the daily routine for cow observation (estrus and health), milking, feeding, and barn cleaning should be determined (Chapter 4, part 2). An estimate should be made of the time that cows are away from feeding and resting areas while waiting to be milked, being milked, and in transit. The time constraints imposed on cows will influence dry matter intake. Relationships between when fresh feed is available, and which cattle have the first opportunity to consume it, may explain deviations from expectations in productivity. Some farmers are heavily involved in external organizational activities and are thus frequently away at meetings. Their absence must be considered in evaluating the daily work patterns on the farm.

### C. Milking system

The milking equipment and parlor, if present, should be examined for cleanliness and appropriateness of scale and design for the overall herd operation. Teat cup liners and rubber hoses should be examined for quality and condition. What supplies for pre- and post-milking hygiene are present (e.g. water, towels, sponges, buckets, teat dips, spray systems, and containers)? Temperature level of hot water for cleaning the milking system should be checked. The holding area should be evaluated for crowding, overheating, and potential for cow injury. At some early stage of the HH & PM service it will be useful to observe the milking process to monitor cow handling, milking procedures, and milking time per cow. The proportion of cows defecating in the parlor is an indirect measure of the stress of the milking environment and process. Only by direct observations can the quality of milking practices be determined (Chapter 6). Depending on the services supplied by third-party organizations, milking system performance should be measured by the practitioner. However performance evaluation will require specialized equipment and technical skills.

**D. Feeding program**

Examination of the feed itself will reveal whether appropriate harvesting and storing practices were employed. The quality of the forage should be estimated and these estimates compared with the laboratory analyses. Repeat analyses may be requested if the characteristics of the forage seem at odds with the reported tests. Inspection of feed storage facilities and areas will also provide information on potential feed quality deficiencies. This may include damage of plastic coverings by birds, rats or even cows. Muddy access lanes and lack of concrete floors and walls in bunker silos contribute foreign material to the feed offered to the cows. Permanent storage structures should be inspected for damage or wear that would decrease forage quality.

The details of the feeding program should be recorded. If concentrates are fed individually, how are amounts calculated and measured? Has the output of computer controlled concentrate stalls been calibrated? For TMR feeding is dry matter intake known? It is important to know who purchases the commodities, who formulates the rations, how often they are updated, what information from the farm is used, what forage analyses are performed and by whom. Does the nutritional consultant also sell ingredients? Does the responsible individual visit the farm and how often? Are recommendations provided for all age groups? What feeds and supplements are purchased and from whom? Copies of forage analysis reports and ration formulations should be obtained for the farm file. For further information on nutrition in relation to milk production see Chapter 4, part 2.

**E. Manure handling**

Manure handling is important in 3 ways. Removal of manure from the cow's immediate environment contributes to hygiene and general health by limiting exposure to potential pathogens. Secondly, the techniques of handling manure can significantly affect: (a) emission of nitrogen into the atmosphere as ammonia; (b) leaching of potassium, nitrate, and phosphate into either groundwater or surface water. These hazards of manure disposal may affect the health of humans, livestock and wildlife. Animal agriculture is increasingly scrutinized for non-point source pollution; farmers must be increasingly aware of possible environmental degradation due to manure management practices. Thirdly, the same nutrients that may represent environmental hazards are also potentially valuable for crops. Their conservation is an economic aspect of crop production and thus of interest to the practitioner. Therefore, the farmer's techniques and policies for manure removal, storage, and disposal should be discussed.

**F. Pasture management**

Pasture management is important because it affects roughage quality for both the housing and the grazing period. Harvesting of roughage is one of the key decisions in farming and influences milk production potential for the housing period. Grassland management may be evaluated using the following areas of attention:

* suitable record keeping of grassland utilization and manure or fertilizer application,
* length of grass in the current pasture,
* smell, color and leafiness of grass in current pasture,
* appropriateness of botanical composition of pasture,
* predominance of spots not eaten due to e.g. manure piles,
* appearance of the just finished and the next to be used plots,
* length of the time period in same plot, related to number of animals in plot,
* condition of cows and rumen fill,
* distance walked to pasture and condition of paths,
* presence of adequate shade if necessary,
* access to and quality of drinking water.

**G. Drylot corral management**

In drylots, environmental conditions of cows are an essential component of farm management. For drylot type dairies the examinations should include:

* corral conditions, e.g. mud, manure, mounds,
* adequate shade,
* additional cooling devices,
* grouping strategy,
* feed storage areas,
* cleanliness and surface of cattle lanes,
* operation of wash pens and holding areas,
* facilities for individual animal attention,

## 1.3.7 ON-GOING ACTIVITIES

A scheme for activities during the farm visit is usually established that follows a logical sequence and efficiently covers all the following aspects:

A. Routine genital examinations, clinical examination of sick or lame animals, and treatments. An action list of cows to be examined should be made in advance. Body condition scoring may be done on selected animals or at selected stages of the production cycle.

B. Dehorning of calves. Young stock growth monitoring. Attention focused on areas identified as problems from previous evaluation of health or growth monitoring.

C. Collection of samples for laboratory evaluation for disease diagnosis, monitoring, or surveillance. Samples should also be collected, if there is no agency routinely doing so, of forage or other feed samples for analysis of dry matter and nutrient content.

D. Farm inspection to monitor progress in planned changes and to check for managerial or environmental risk factors. Attention is focused on observing activities related to previously identified problems and in detecting potential problems.

E. Collection of farmer recorded data not available from third-party systems such as DHIA. This may be in the form of copies of farm diaries or files from the on-farm computer. The farm diary may be mailed to the practitioner to be entered in his computer prior to the next farm visit. This practice has the advantage of including the most recent data in those calculations made prior to the visit.

F. Review of performance indices. In addition to reviewing previously calculated indices, the farm visit usually includes interpretation of data gathered during the farm visit, eg. the monthly list (Chapter 1, part 2). All areas covered by the HH & PM service should be considered with discussion focusing on problem areas where performance failed to meet goals.

G. Planning for problems recognized during analyses or identified during farm inspection. Scheduling of next farm visit.

## 1.3.8 DECISION MAKING

Summary data on the status of some operational management functions may be available from DHIA or similar sources such as farmer-owned dairy records software. Other indicators will have to be calculated at the end of the farm visit, e.g. incidence of clinical cases of mastitis or prevalence of lame cows. This may be done manually in most circumstances or electronically in the case that a herd file has been pre-established in the computer system of the practitioner. The farmer will likely be most interested in those analyses that relate to the main problem he perceived when initiating the program. However, in some cases the events that motivated the farmer to act could have been normal random variation for that operational management function. It is useful for the HH & PM practitioner to appreciate that many measures of farm performance will have substantial inherent biological variation. Experience, plus the ability to calculate confidence intervals for targets of performance indices, will lead to reasonable assessment of short term performance. However, the performance in many areas will not be known until after the program has been in place for some time. Additionally, in some cases it will be more useful to observe the behavior of a performance index over a longer interval than between 2 successive visits to judge actual performance since the pattern of performance indices may vary considerably, especially in smaller herds or over short time intervals.

The performance indices calculated from this and subsequent visits should be listed in a columnar fashion for each month (Chapter 1, part 2). After a few farm visits actual performance can be easily traced over time by comparing indices within a row.

This makes it easy to observe fluctuations in performance at an early stage and to take actions if indicated. If computerized data processing is practised and sophisticated data management packages are used, the number of actual performance indices which can be calculated is increased significantly. However, it is always valuable to select the most relevant and important ones.

The observation of an unsatisfactory level of performance may be followed by any of several different analytical approaches to the existing data. The index in question may be divided into a frequency distribution to examine the dispersion of the data. Another approach is to divide the herd into demographic subgroups, e.g. first lactation, second lactation and older cows or early, middle and late lactation or summer versus winter calving cows to evaluate these effects on the index in question. A third possibility is to divide the herd into 2 subherds with performance for the index in question above or below some cut off point. The characteristics of these 2 subherds can then be contrasted for other risk factors potentially associated with poor performance.

## EPILOGUE

The traditional approach to dairy farming included consultative emergency farm visits by practitioners at irregular intervals during which diseased animals were examined and treated. In contrast, the regularly scheduled farm visit, when most time is devoted to healthy animals, is the foundation of HH & PM services. The routine farm visit forms the principal professional interaction between farmer and practitioner. The systematic approach described in Chapter 2, part 1 can help guide the practitioner in structuring the mental processes that accompany the clinical activities during the farm visit. The necessary overview of the whole farm operation involves considerable objective and subjective data evaluation. However, in many cases where major problems are not occurring, monitoring and routine clinical work will constitute the main activity.

Preparation for the farm visit includes the making of work lists, data acquisition or computer entry, and data analysis. The routine clinical work at the farm, performed at set intervals, provides regular, repeated opportunities for observation and data collection. The farm inspection part of the farm visit contributes to the awareness of specific environmental and managerial conditions, which can be assessed in more detail when problems appear to arise. Evaluation of the accumulated data will identify problem areas by comparing the actual performance with goals. It is the task of the practitioner to determine if the differences are caused by diseases or managerial inefficiencies and to suggest means of improving performance during discussion with the farmer. The visit is concluded with plans made for changes where they are indicated. The next routine visit will include reassessment of previously identified problems and action taken, and evaluation of current performance. A long term commitment to cooperation by both parties is necessary for success of the program.

## REFERENCES

*Barkema, H.W., J.D. Westrik, K.A.S. van Keulen, Y.H. Schukken, and A. Brand. 1994. The effects of lameness on reproductive performance and culling in Dutch dairy farms. Prev. Vet. Med. 20:249-259.*

*Blood, D.C., R.S. Morris, N.B. Williamson, C.M Cannon, and R.M. Cannon. 1978. A health program for commercial dairy herds. Parts 1-5. Australian Vet. J. 54:207-257.*

*Brand, A., H. Folkerts, W.J.A. Hanekamp, W.D. de Hoop, and G.M.A. Verheijen. 1995. Information model for dairy farms. Agricultural Telematics Centre. Wageningen, The Netherlands. pp.1-103.*

*Britt, J.H. 1992. Impacts of early postpartum metabolism on follicular developement and fertility. The Bovine Proceedings 24:39-42.*

*Braun, R.K., J.P.T.M. Noordhuizen, G.A. Donovan, and A. Brand. A goal oriented approach to herd health and production control. Proc. 15th Annual Convention of American Ass. of Bovine Practitioners. Nashville, Tennessee. pp.51-58.*

*Devir, S., J.A. Renkema, R.B.M. Huirne and A.H. Ipema. 1993. A new dairy control and management system in the automatic milking farm: basic concepts and components. J. Dairy Sci. 76:3607-3616.*

*Esselmont, R.J., A.J. Stephens, and P.R. Ellis. 1981. Daisy: Dairy information system, an aid to record keeping and health management. Proc. Am. Assoc. Bovine Pract. Toronto, 13:51-60.*

*Fetrow, J., B. Harrington, E. Henry, and K. Anderson. 1987. Dairy herd health monito ring. Part I. Description of monitoring systems and sources of data. Comp. Cont. Educ. Pract. Vet. 10:389-398.*

*Fetrow, J., B. Harrington, E. Henry, and K. Anderson. 1988. Dairy herd health monito ring. Part II. A computer spreadsheet for dairy herd monitoring. Comp. Cont. Educ. Pract. Vet. 10:75-81.*

*Hogeveen, H., A.A. Dijkhuizen, and J. Sol. 1992. Short- and long-term effects of a 2 year dairy herd health and management program. Prev. Vet. Med. 13:53-58.*

*Kristula, M. and C. Uhlinger, 1995. Dairy herd-health monitoring - Handwritten records to monitor disease events. The Comp. Cont. Educ. 17:1520-1525.*

*Lissemore, K.D. 1989. The use of computers in dairy herd health programs: A review. Can. Vet. J. 30:631-636.*

*Meuller, M. 1989. Computer aided dairy herd management. Agri-Practice. 10:3-10.*

*Nielsen, N.O. 1993. , Ecosystem health and veterinary medicine. Can. Vet. J. 33:23-26.*

*Nelson, A.J. and H.W. Redlus. 1989. The key role of records in a production medicine practice. Vet. Clinics of North America: Food Animal Practice. 5:517-552.*

*Nelson, A.J. 1994. Information needs of the dairy industry for health and nutrition management. J. Dairy Sci. 77:1984-1991.*

*Noordhuizen, J.P.T.M., A. Brand, P. Dobbelaar, and H. Wilbrink. 1982/1983a. Index list on milk production and udder health. Prev. Vet. Med. 1:201-213.*

*Noordhuizen, J.P.T.M. and A. Brand. 1982/1983b. Index list on reproduction and lameness. Prev. Vet. Med. 1:215-225.*

*Noordhuizen, J.P.T.M. and G.K. van Meurs. 1983/1984. Index list on calf rearing and cow culling. Prev. Vet. Med. 3:277-287.*

*Noordhuizen, J.P.T.M., H. Wilbrink, P. Dobbelaar, and A. Brand. 1984/1985. Index list on metabolic/nutritional diseases, body condition score and ration composition. Prev. Vet. Med. 3:289-300.*

*Noordhuizen, J.P.T.M. and J. Buurman. 1984. VAMPP: A veterinary automated management and production control programme for dairy farms. The Vet. Quart. 6:66-72.*

*Noordhuizen, J.P.T.M. 1984. Veterinary herd health and production control on dairy farms. Ph.D. Thesis, Veterinary School of Utrecht, The Netherlands.*

*Schukken, Y.H., K.E. Leslie, A.J. Weersink, and S.W. Martin. 1992. Ontario bulk milk somatic cell count reduction program. 2. dynamics of bulk milk somatic cell count. J. Dairy Sci. 75:3359-3366.*

*Sol, J., J.A. Renkema, J. Stelwagen, A.A. Dijkhuizen, and A. Brand. 1984. A three year herd health and management program on thirty dutch dairy herds. The Vet. Quart. 6:141-169.*

*Stein, T.E. 1986. Marketing health management to food animal enterprises. Part II. The structure of herd health mangement services. The Comp. on Cont. Educ. 8:330-336.*

# 1.4 APPLICATION OF EPIDEMIOLOGY IN HERD HEALTH AND PRODUCTION MANAGEMENT PROGRAMS

Ynte H. Schukken[1], Jos P.T.M. Noordhuizen[2], Hollis N. Erb[3]

[1] Department of Herd Health and Reproduction, School of Veterinary Medicine, University of Utrecht, Yalelaan 7, 3584 CL Utrecht, The Netherlands
[2] Department of Animal Husbandry, Animal Health & Reproduction division, Agricultural University of Wageningen, Prinses Marykeweg 40, 6709 PG Wageningen, The Netherlands
[3] Department of Clinical Sciences, New York State College of Veterinary Medicine, Cornell University, Ithaca, NY 14853-6401, USA

## 1.4.1 INTRODUCTION

Epidemiology is defined as the study of the distribution (occurrence and spread), the risk-indicators and the consequences of disorders in populations. Several types of epidemiology have been recognized, such as theoretical, observational, experimental. (Martin et al., 1987; Smith, 1995; Thrusfield, 1995). The applications of epidemiology in Herd Health and Production Management (HH & PM) services can be numerous. Already, various descriptive epidemiologic methods are used in current HH & PM programs.

Most computerized HH & PM systems are currently limited to descriptive analysis of the data. Means, medians, rates, ratios and graphical presentations play an important role in describing the current state of performance and disease on dairy farms. Performance indices are calculated for time periods, and are compared to those from previous periods and preset targets (see Chapter 1, part 2 and part 3). When indices deviate from the targets, the next steps in the protocol are to analyze the accumulated data and ultimately to identify risk indicators for disease occurrences. It is expected that advanced use of analytical epidemiology in the study of risk indicators and consequences of disorders, and the application of on-farm trials, will enhance the quality and benefits of HH & PM services.

This part deals with the application of some epidemiological principles and methods in HH & PM services. We will introduce some epidemiological terminology and explain a number of epidemiologic methods, while applications are illustrated with examples. In this text we will deal mostly with observational epidemiology.

## 1.4.2 MEASURING DISEASE

The distribution pattern of a disease can be described with epidemiological terminology. A disease can be described by its incidence, the distribution over seasons, the

*Figure 1. Annual incidence of clinical mastitis and the mean annual bulk milk somatic cell count in 23 dairy herds*

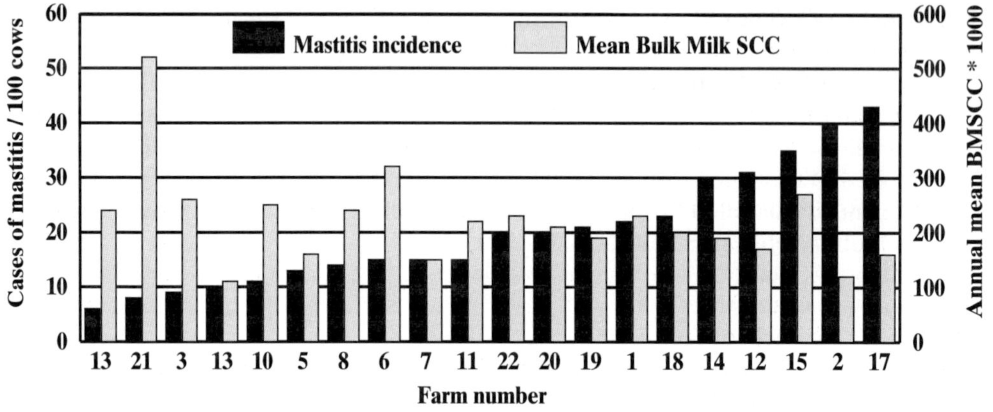


distribution per farm, the distribution over parities, the spatial distribution, etc. Descriptive epidemiology tells the farmer, practitioner and farm advisor what the current state of the particular disorder is on the farm. Descriptive epidemiology can be presented as numbers or can be collated in tables, and is very well suited for graphical presentations. In Figure 1 the incidence of clinical mastitis (Y-axis left) and the mean annual bulk milk somatic cell count (Y-axis right) of 23 herds is shown (after Schukken et al., 1989). It seems that there is a slightly negative correlation between clinical mastitis and bulk milk somatic cell count, and it may be hypothesized that clinical mastitis is predominantly caused by environmental pathogens. This illustrates a second purpose of descriptive epidemiology: by describing the data in certain patterns, hypotheses about disease occurrences may be generated.

Risk indicators are (animal, herd, management or farm) characteristics that are - at least mathematically - associated with disease. However, risk indicators need not always be biological causes of a disorder. There might be a common cause to both disease and the risk indicator, hampering a proper causal inference. Also, the risk indicator might be a proxy of the biological cause.

Herd Health and Production Management programs usually implement a variety of performance indices (see following Chapters). Commonly-used primary performance indices are the proportion of animals culled, expected calving interval, incidence of clinical mastitis or bulk milk somatic cell count. Apart from the question of whether a specific index is the best possible choice for practical use, indices differ in the way they are calculated, in the way the time component is included and in the way they can be interpreted.

It is highly recommended to measure disease in relation to the herd or population at-risk, because it is the probability of becoming diseased, not the disease event itself, that is of interest for preventive measures. "At-risk" means biologically capable of experiencing that particular disease. For example, the total dairy cattle population is not at-risk for abortion. A subtraction has to be made for male cattle and for non-pregnant animals. Often an animal is not counted in the population at-risk after having experienced the disease once. Including the at-risk population in the calculation means that formulas have a numerator and denominator. The time component in an index refers to a certain period of time or calendar period (e.g., monthly mastitis incidence or lactational mastitis incidence). This time component is relevant because disease patterns may change over time. On the other hand, disease itself has a time component; the disease duration itself is not necessarily one month. If incidence is calculated per lactation, then lactation is the internal time component. The population-at-risk and the internal time component can be combined through the determination of the number of lactations-at-risk, calving intervals-at-risk, animal-years-at-risk, etc. One animal-year-at-risk may result from 1 animal at-risk for 1 year, or 12 animals at-risk for 1 month each, or 365 animals each at-risk for 1 day.

The incidence of clinical mastitis in herds with a low bulk milk somatic cell count level was studied in Ohio, Pennsylvania and The Netherlands (Hogan et al., 1989; Erskine et al., 1988; Schukken et al., 1989). The incidence rates in the three studies were respectively 14.9, 13,9 and 5.2 cases per 10,000 cow-days-at-risk. Using the mastitis rate expressed as cases per cow-day-at-risk allows precise comparison of mastitis incidence.

### 1.4.3 MEASURES OF DISEASE OCCURRENCE

#### Prevalence P

The prevalence describes the number of existing disease cases in the population, either at a point of time (=point prevalence) or over a period (=period prevalence). It is the ratio between the number of diseased animals and the number of animals present at a certain moment (or in a certain period). Therefore, the prevalence is the probability that an animal has a given disease at a certain moment. Prevalence has values between 0 and 1, and is dependent on both disease duration and number of newly occurring cases per unit of time. A prevalence of 0.01% for mastitis cases of *S.aureus* means that 1 animal out of 10.000 was affected. Examples of prevalence studies may concern stillbirth surveys, national mastitis surveys, and seroprevalence studies of IBR/BHV-1.

#### Incidence I

The incidence describes the frequency of newly-occurring disease cases in the population during a certain period of time. In fact, it is the flow of animals from a disease-free status to a diseased status.

A cumulative incidence (CI) describes the ratio between the number of animals that were newly affected by the disease during a period and the number of healthy animals-at-risk in the population at the beginning of that period. The CI is the average risk of disease-free animals acquiring a given disease over a certain period. It is a proportion and presented in values between 0 and 1 (if the disease is only counted once per animal-at-risk). An example: if 20 calves out of 100 display symptoms of diarrhea X in one week, then the CI for that week is 20/100= 0.2. If in the second week another 15 calves are affected, then the CI for these 2 weeks is 0.35. The chance that any calf gets the disease during these 2 weeks is 35%. Note that the CI is highly influenced by the length of the observation period!

An incidence rate (IR) is the ratio between the number of new disease cases in a population during a certain period and the sum of the time-periods of all animals in the population-at-risk. It is the risk of acquiring disease per unit of time. The denominator includes a function of time (e.g. lactation months-at-risk).

In the example of diarrhea in 100 calves, there were 35 cases in 2 weeks: 20 in the first week and 15 in the second week. Assuming that the average calf got scours in the midpoint of the week, there were 90 weeks-at-risk in the first week and 73 in the second week. The number of weeks-at-risk is then 90 +73= 163. The IR is 35/163= 0.21 per week. Or, any healthy calf has a risk of 21% per week to get the disease.

The relationship between prevalence P and incidence rate IR can be expressed as P/(1-P) = IR * D, where D represents duration of the disease. At low disease frequencies, the value of (1-P) nears 1, which yields an approximate formula P= IR * D. Prevalence and incidence parameters calculated for the population as a whole are called "crude" prevalence or crude incidence rate. For subgroups or strata in the population we may calculate "specific" parameters, such as parity-specific incidence rate or region-specific prevalence.

### 1.4.4 EVALUATION OF DIAGNOSTIC TESTS

Diagnosis usually is made by subjectively interpreting signs and symptoms, by looking for causes and by additional diagnostic testing. The latter may lead to false interpretation and bias when these tests do not achieve a perfect result. However, perfect tests are often hard to develop in biological material, are expensive, and take time to perform. Alternative tests should be screened for validity (that is, for analytical sensitivity and specificity). The latter two characteristics determine the degree of misclassification and whether the test is really measuring what it is supposed to measure.

Sensitivity is the probability that a diseased animal is detected as being diseased (i.e., it is the number of diseased animals classified by the test as such, divided by the number of truly-diseased animals).

Specificity is the probability that a non-diseased animal is detected as being non-diseased (i.e., the number of non-diseased animals classified by the test as such, divided by the number of truly non-diseased animals).

Generally, these parameters are inversely associated: the higher the sensitivity, the lower the specificity, and vice versa. Due to this overlap, we have to declare threshold values above which a test result is called positive, and below which it is called negative (assuming higher values indicate disease; or vice versa for deficiencies). This threshold value determines the sensitivity and specificity, and can be manipulated. The objective of testing will define whether we need a high sensitivity or a high specificity. For zoonoses, we need a high sensitivity; we do not want many false negatives (diseased animals that test negative). In casc of eradication campaigns for non-zoonoses, we would not like to have many false positives (healthy animals that test positive), because otherwise many healthy animals would be slaughtered; we require a high specificity. Sensitive tests are used in screening programs, when diseased individuals should not be missed (e.g. disease treatment programs). Specific tests are used when a (clinical) diagnosis must be confirmed, or when a false-positive result causes considerable economic loss.

From a 2*2 table, the sensitivity and specificity can be calculated as follows:

| | | **True disease state** | | |
|---|---|---|---|---|
| | | Diseased | Healthy | |
| **Classified as diseased by the test** | Yes | a | b | |
| | No | c | d | |
| | | a+c | b+d | n |

Sensitivity = a / (a + c)
Specificity = d / (b + d)

As an example: The CBR (Complement Binding Reaction) for Johne's disease has a sensitivity of about 75% and specificity of about 70%. This means that 75% of the truly infected animals are detected as such (true positives), and that 30% of the non-infected animals will test positive (false positives).

When the disease prevalence in a population must be determined, we usually take a sample from the population. The number of test-positive animals divided by all sampled animals is the apparent prevalence ((a+b)/n). The number of the truly-diseased animals in the sample divided by all sampled animals is the true prevalence ((a+c)/n). The true prevalence does not necessarily equal the apparent prevalence, because the apparent prevalence depends on the sensitivity (SE) and specificity (SP) of the test. The relationship between the true (P) and apparent (AP) prevalence is shown by the formula:

$$P = (AP + SP - 1) / (SE + SP - 1).$$

In a herd of 70 cattle, 22 tested positive on the CBR for Johne's disease. Consequently, the AP was .31. Using the forenamed formula, the true prevalence (P)

*Figure 2. The predictive values of the M.johne CBR test versus the prevalence of the disease in the herd*

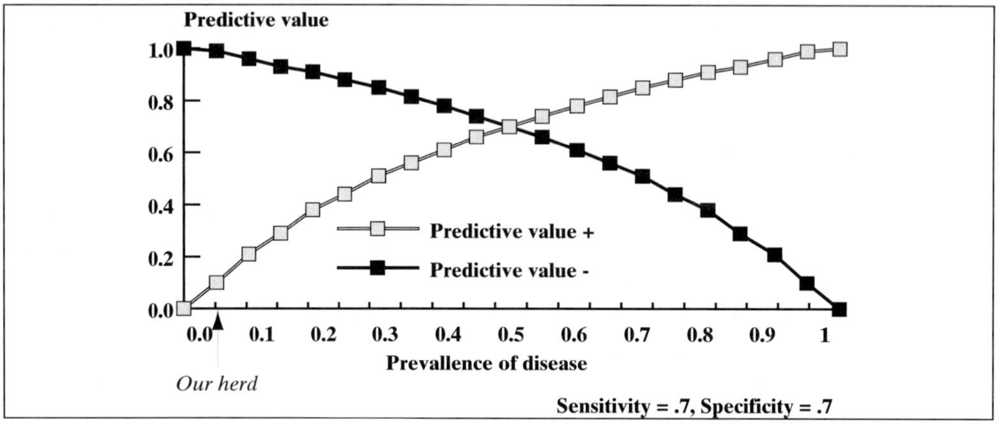


was calculated as (.31+.7-1)/(.75+.7-1)= .022, or 2.2% of the herd. At the herd level, we may conclude that the herd is infected, but the proportion of infected animals appears to be small.

**Predictive values**

The proportion of animals that are test positive and are truly positive (diseased) is called Predictive Value Positive; in terms of the 2*2 table above: PV+ = a/(a + b). Similarly, the Predictive Value Negative is: d/(c+d). The predictive value depends heavily on the prevalence of a disease in a region and is a population characteristic, whereas sensitivity and specificity are test characteristics independent of prevalence. For the herd mentioned above, the 2*2 table will look like:

| | | M.johne infected | | |
|---|---|---|---|---|
| | | Yes | No | Total |
| Classified positive by CBR | Yes | 1 | 21 | 22 |
| | No | 1 | 47 | 48 |
| | | 2 | 68 | 70 |

Hence, the PV+ = 1/22 = .045, and PV- = 47/48 = .98. This indicates that a negative test is fairly reliable, and that a positive test is not reliable at all. Currently, the CBR may be used to certify animals as disease negative, by requiring a negative test plus a written statement that clinical Johne's has not been seen in the herd recently. This seems a sensible use of this test.

In Figure 2, the predictive value of a test is depicted against the changing prevalence of the disease (X-axis). The test used in the graph is the *M. johne* CBR test, with a sensitivity and specificity of 70% each.

### 1.4.5 ANALYSIS OF HH & PM DATA

When a database is present on a dairy farm, analysis of data may take place according to epidemiological principles. For example, when the practitioner suspects a relationship between lameness and reproductive performance, he or she can do a cohort study where reproductive performance indices are analyzed separately for lame and non-lame animals (see Table 1). Principles behind the methods to analyze HH & PM data are introduced here. Further texts are available; among others, the textbooks by Martin et al. (1987), Thrusfield, (1995), Smith, (1995) and Noordhuizen et al. (1987) are recommended.

*Table 1. Reproductive performance of the complete herd (A), all cows with a history of lameness in the current lactation (A.1), and all cows without a history of lameness in the current lactation (A.2). Adapted from: Schukken et al., 1995*

| | A | A.1 | A.2 |
|---|---|---|---|
| (1) # Cows/Heifers calved | 69/23 | 22/7 | 47/16 |
| (2) # C/H inseminated | 52/20 | 17/7 | 35/13 |
| (3) Int. calving-conception (n) | 111(57) | 126(18) | 105(39) |
| (4) Expected calving interval | 391 | 406 | 385 |
| (5) # Inseminations | 143 | 47 | 96 |
| (6) # 1st inseminations | 72 | 24 | 48 |
| (7) Int. calving - 1st insem. | 79 | 81 | 78 |
| (8) Int. 1st insem.- conception | 33.2 | 47.2 | 26.7 |
| (9) Inseminations per conc. | 1.86 | 2.11 | 1.74 |
| (10) Days missed sub-oestrus | 15.1 | 23.9 | 11.1 |
| (11) Pregnancy % after 1st insem. | 44.4 | 29.2 | 52.1 |

### 1.4.6 STUDY TYPES

Usually, selections are made from the available animals to study certain characteristics. Several types of studies can be distinguished by that selection strategy. The selection strategy may be based on exposure to a factor status (cohort study),on outcome or disease status (case-control study) or on neither of the two (cross-sectional study).

In a cohort study, a proportion of the exposed animals and some proportion of the unexposed animals are selected. These proportions may be different, and this leads to one of the advantages of cohort studies: this is the best observational design to use if resources are limited and the exposure is rare. For example, all retained placenta cows are selected and evaluated for reproductive performance, but only a sample of the non-retained placenta animals are so used.

An example of a cohort study is found in the paper by Nielen et al., (1989) on the consequences of twinning in dairy cattle. A cohort of cows giving birth to twins, and a cohort of cows with singleton births were identified. Following both cohorts in time, it was observed that twin calvings increased the risks of retained placenta and of fertility-related treatment. The number of days open increased, as well as the inseminations per conception. After twin calving, cows produced less milk, and were culled more often than single-calving cows.

The second major selection strategy is that of the case-control study: selection is based on the disease status of the animals. Originally, the outcome was conceived of as disease, so that the animals with the outcome were named "cases" and those without the disease were the comparison group, or "controls" (hence the name "case-control").

The proportion of cases selected for study can be different from the proportion of controls selected. By an analogous argument to that used to explain the "rare-exposure" advantage of cohort studies, an advantage of case-control studies is that they are the most-efficient design for studying rare outcomes. Also, case-control studies are the best design to use when exploring the relationships between multiple exposures and the outcome. The disadvantages are roughly the converses of those of cohort studies: case-control studies are not efficient for rare exposures or multiple outcomes.

An example of a case-control study is a study from an HH & PM data base on risk factors for the occurrence of cystic ovarian disease (COD) (Laporte et al., 1994). Animals with and without COD were selected. Animals with COD had significantly higher milk production in the period preceding the diagnosis than did the control cows. Another example is about health disorders as risk factor for culling in dairy cattle (Beaudeau et al., 1994). In this study population in France specifically ketosis, teat injuries and other udder disorders were identified as increasing the risk of culling significantly.

The final selection strategy is the cross-sectional study. Subjects are selected without regard to either exposure status or disease status; rather, both statuses are determined simultaneously. The advantages are that this design tends to be the simplest, fastest, and cheapest of all to conduct, and that it tends to avoid the information biases of the cohort and case-control strategies. However, exposure and outcome statuses are determined at a single (same) point in time. This means that cause-effect relationships are hard to determine and that only prevalence data are obtained (hence, the sometimes-used name "prevalence studies").

An example would be to select cows on a given milk test, and to evaluate the body-condition score for each cow on the same day as the test. Then, the cows are cross-classified according to body-condition score on one axis, and on fat contents of their milk on the other axis. In the high-fat group the mean body condition score was 1.7, while it was 3.4 in the second group. Clearly there is a statistical association between fat content of milk and body-condition score, but it is not clear whether a high fat ratio leads to a low body-condition score, whether the opposite is true, or whether a third factor causes both high fat content and low body condition.

## 1.4.7 MEASURING EFFECT

To express the relation between a given risk factor (or treatment) and a disease, epidemiologists use measures of effect. These measures characterize the strength of the relation between the presence of a risk factor and the incidence of a disorder. Some measures of effect are absolute measures, i.e. the difference in incidence between animals with and without the risk factor—indicating the increase in risk due to the risk factor. Other measures are relative, i.e. the ratio of incidence in animals with and without the risk factor—indicating the relative increase in risk due to the risk factor. A third important measure of effect is the contribution of the risk factor to the total incidence of the disease in the population. These three major measures of effect will be discussed and illustrated. Further reading is recommended in Martin et al., (1987) and Rothman (1986). Throughout, an example is used of twinning as a risk factor for the cumulative incidence of retained placenta (Nielen et al., 1989).

### Absolute measures of effect

If the disease occurrence can be expressed as incidence rate or cumulative incidence (which is only true in cohort studies and clinical trials), then the difference between the incidence measures in the cohorts with and without the risk factor the (treatment) is the rate (risk) difference. This measure of effect is especially useful for estimating the magnitude of the health problem associated with the risk factor.

An example: the cumulative incidence of retained placenta among cows with a singleton birth was 5.2%, and the incidence among cows with twins was 15.3%. The risk difference is then 15.3 - 5.2 = 10.1%. Statistical significance of this risk difference can be estimated (Fleiss, 1981). The p-value of the risk difference in the example was .0034—indicating that it is very unlikely that the difference in incidence in the two cohorts can be attributed to chance alone. A 95% confidence interval (Fleiss, 1981) was calculated as: 6.4 < risk difference < 13.7 (hence, we may conclude with 95% certainty that the true risk difference lies in between 6.4 and 13.7 cases per 100 cows). The calculating formula's are shown in Table 2.

### Relative measures of effect

The relative measures of effect are based on the ratio of two disease incidences. The disease incidence in the cohort with the risk factor is divided by the disease incidence in a cohort without the risk factor (baseline incidence). If there is no effect due to the risk factor, the incidences in both groups are expected to be equal and the relative measure of effect is unity. A value larger than 1.0 means an increased risk due to the exposure, a value less than 1.0 means a protective effect due to exposure. In studies where a cumulative incidence is calculated, the relative measure of effect is called risk ratio or relative risk (RR). In studies where the disease occurrence is expressed as incidence rates, the relative measure of effect is called rate ratio or relative rate.

The cumulative incidences of retained placenta were 15.3 and 5.2 in the cohorts with twins and singletons, respectively. The relative risk is then 15.3/5.2 = 2.9. The interpretation is that cows experiencing a twin birth are 2.9 times more likely to retain their placenta than cows experiencing a singleton birth. This relative risk was significantly different from 1 at p=.001, and the 95% confidence interval for the relative risk was $1.8 < RR < 4.1$.

In case-control studies, cumulative incidences or incidence rates cannot be calculated. As a result, relative risks (rates) cannot be calculated. Instead, the odds ratio (OR) is used as the relative measure of effect. The odds ratio is the ratio of the odds of exposure (presence of the risk factor) among those with the disease and the odds of exposure among those without the disease (Table 2). The odds ratio is interpreted in a similar way as the relative risk, but is an estimate of the latter.

Suppose we sampled 100 cases of retained placenta and 100 cows without retained placenta. Among the 100 cases 9 had given birth to twins, while there were only three twin births in the controls. The odds of twinning was therefore 9:91 and 3:97 respectively. The odds ratio is then 9:91 / 3:97 = 3.2. The interpretation is the same as the interpretation of the relative risk: animals giving birth to a twin are 3 time more likely to retain their placenta than animals that gave birth to a single calf. The odds ratio was significantly different from 1 at p=.001 and the 95% confidence interval was: $1.6 < ORR < 5.8$. In this example, the odds ratio was calculated with a 2*2 table. However, in multifactorial diseases many interactions between factors may occur. For such diseases other, more complex, analytical techniques should be applied to account for multiple risk factors and interaction of risk factors (Rothman, 1986). An example of results obtained from such analyses is given in Chapter 7.

### Attributable proportion

The third measure of effect characterizes the proportion of cases that can be attributed to the risk factor. It is the proportion of cases that would not have occurred if the risk factor were not present in the population. More than the first two measures of effect, the attributable proportion (AP) relies heavily on causality in the implied relationship between risk factor and disease. The attributable proportion is calculated as the incidence in the total population minus the incidence in the cohort without the risk factor, divided by the incidence in the total population. With some algebra it can be shown that an alternative way of calculating the attributable proportion is:

$$AP = [(RR - 1) * P_{ce}] / RR,$$

where: RR = the relative risk (rate) or the odds ratio
$P_{ce}$ = the proportion of cases exposed to the risk factor.

Using the data from the case-control study above (and the OR in the place of the RR), the attributable proportion is:

AP = [(3.2-1) * .09] / 3.2 = .06.

Hence, 6 % of the retained placenta cases can be attributed to the presence of twinning.

*Table 2. Calculating formulas for measures of effect*

| | | Disease: Present | Disease: Absent | |
|---|---|---|---|---|
| **Risk factor** | Present(e) | A | B | A+B |
| | Absent(ne) | C | D | C+D |
| | | A+C | B+D | N |

Cohort study or clinical trial:

$I_e$ = A/(A+B) incidence in the cohort with the risk factor
$I_{ne}$ = C/(C+D) incidence in the cohort without the risk factor
$P_e$ = Occurrence of the risk factor in the population (in population wide studies this is (A+B)/N ).

then:
Risk difference = $I_e - I_{ne}$
Relative risk = $I_e / I_{ne}$
Attributable proportion = $[(RR-1) * P_{ce}] / RR$

Case-control studies

$P_{ce}$ = A/C odds of cases having the risk factor
$P_{cne}$ = B/D odds of controls not having the risk factor

then:
Odds Ratio = (A/C) / (B/D) = A * D / B * C
Attributable proportion = $(OR-1) * P_{ce} / OR$

Measures of effect are useful in examining the importance of a risk factor for the occurrence of the disease. If the interest is purely biological (clarifying the pathogenesis), then the relative measures of effect (RR, OR) are most useful. However, if any conclusions are made regarding the importance of the risk factor for the occurrence of disease, then both the relative measures of effect and the attributable proportion (AP) should be considered.

As an example, we carry the relation between multiple births and retained placenta to an extreme. Consider the situation that a cow giving birth to triplet calves has a 95% chance of retaining at least one placenta. Only 1 out of every 1000 calvings is triplets. The relative risk of triplet-birth for retained placenta is then 18 (.95/.052) and the risk difference will be .9 (.95 - .052)—but the proportion of retained placenta cases that may be attributed to this rare event will be small: 2%.

Only by examining both the relative measure of effect and the attributable proportion do we have sufficient information to decide on the importance of a given risk factor.

When data from herds are analyzed with the methods that were described, the practitioner should be careful with causal interpretations. For example, lame animals may have longer calving intervals than non-lame animals (Table 1). However, high-producing animals may be more lame, and high-producing animals are voluntarily kept open for a longer period of time by the farmer. Hence an association between lameness and fertility is present, but is caused by decisions of the farmer! It is not easy to distinguish causal and non-causal associations. In-depth knowledge of the underlying biological mechanisms and of the structure and management of a dairy farm are required to make causal judgments. Criteria for judging whether an association is causal are presented by Martin et al. (1987) but are beyond the scope of this book.

## 1.4.8 FIELD TRIALS ON FARMS

Field trials can be used by HH & PM practitioners to evaluate whether an intervention is efficacous in a dairy herd. Such an intervention may be an antibiotic or anthelmintic treatment or a feed additive—but also may be a management policy. Trials can often be performed rather easily in well-managed herds. For example, feed additives may rather easily be evaluated when animals can be grouped or when computerized feeders are available. Especially when no extra data need to be collected, trials require limited input from farmer and practitioner. Some general concepts of trials will be discussed here. Further details are available from textbooks (Friedman et al., 1985; Noordhuizen et al., 1994, Noordhuizen et al., 1997).

Some important issues in the design of field studies will be discussed here. This includes choice of the comparison group, randomization, blindness, losses to follow-up, sampling, and (briefly) some analytical procedures.

In trials there must be at least one comparison group, the "controls". As a rule, the controls should be studied concurrently with the animals getting the experimental treatment(s). This is because too many conditions (environmental stress, quality of forage, quality of management, medical technologies, etc.) can change across time to be sure that the conditions of the trial were similar for all treatments unless the treatments are studied concurrently. All treatments can be thought of as having both an "active ingredient" (the new drug, new protein level, new type of bedding, management, etc.) and a "delivery system" (the carrier solutions, the need for animal restraint, the need to change workers' habits, etc.). In every trial, it is necessary to decide whether it is only the active ingredient that is being tested, or whether the combination of active ingredient and delivery system. If the trial is of only the active ingredient, then the control animals should receive a placebo treatment. The placebo treatment mimics the delivery system, so that the active ingredient is the only thing that is different. If the trial instead is of both the active ingredient and the delivery system, then a placebo should not be used. Rather, the control animals should receive "usual management", even if usual management is to do nothing. When a currently- accepted therapy is available, a placebo or doing nothing would ethically be unacceptable. In such a situation, the new treatment will be compared to the current standard therapy.

"Randomization" refers to the use of a formal decision rule and a chance device (such as a lottery or a table of random numbers) to select animals. The selection could be to assign treatments, to determine the order in which animals will be examined, to select which of the available non-exposed animals will be used, etc. Randomization always is the preferred procedure, because it avoids the selection bias caused by the farmer or practitioner subjectively choosing each animal's assignment.

Blindness means that the treatment group assignment of each animal is not known (during the trial) by either the herdsperson caring for the animal or by the person making the outcome measurement. Blindness always is desirable but is not always necessary. Blinding the herdsperson assures that animals in one treatment group will not be treated differently (by an unconscious attempt to compensate for "only" getting the placebo vaccine, for instance); this avoids a source of confounding bias. Blinding the observer avoids a source of information bias, and is essential if there is subjectivity in the measurement, count, diagnosis, etc. However, if the measurement is precise and objective, blindness is less critical. This is important, because blindness sometimes cannot be achieved especially not in cost-benefit type trials where the comparison treatment is either to "do nothing" or to do a standard management that looks nothing like the experimental management. In such a situation, the solution is to use highly-objective data.

Losses always should be expected (and reported), but they can be minimized by improving informed consent (so there is a clear understanding of what the owners are getting into and so there is clear willingness to participate) and by simplifying the treatments and the follow-up procedures. The calculated sample sizes should be adjusted upwards to correct for the proportion of losses that can be anticipated.

An example of a clinical trial in a large beef herd is the comparison of penicillin, oxytetracycline (OTC) and trimethoprim-sulfadoxine (TMPS) in the treatment of acute undifferentiated bovine respiratory disease (Mechor et al., 1988). Animals with acute respiratory disease and a rectal temperature above 40.5°C were included in the trial. Animals were assigned to a treatment group according to a systematic procedure, i.e. every third animal presented received Penicillin. Animals were evaluated by rectal temperature decrease and clinical improvement, no blindness of the person evaluating the clinical improvement, or the herdsmen was reported. The treatment success was 50%, 50% and 59% for penicillin, OTC and TMPS respectively, mortality was 12%, 9% and 4% respectively. The authors concluded (based on the observed data), that in this population TMPS should be the treatment of choice.

Sampling of populations (e.g. dairy herds) is done often to get an estimate of a certain parameter (for example the serological status of the herd with respect to bacteriological or viral agents). Instead of measuring the whole population, a sample from that population is used for practical reasons.

Calculation of sample size is only useful and correct if random sampling is practiced. If samples are non-random, then inferences from the sample to the rest of the population are not valid, regardless of the size of the population. An example of non-random sampling is the collection of milk samples for bacteriological culturing of those quarters that are CMT positive. The results of the bacteriological culturing cannot be inferred as coming from the whole population, obviously; the results are only valid for the CMT positive animals. Another important assumption underlying sample size calculations is that the animals within a herd are independent of one another. This means that knowledge about the disease (infection, mineral etc.) status of one animal does not give any information on the disease status of another animal. If there is some dependence (i.e. heifers tend to be seronegative and cows tend to be seropositive), then the required sample size is always less than in the case of independence. In the extreme case that there is complete dependence between animals (i.e. if one animal is infected, then they are all infected) a single sample suffices.

Sample size calculations require guesses on certain population characteristics of the parameter that we wish to measure. It is not always possible to find a "best guess"; in those cases, calculations may be performed with several values of the required characteristics to get a rough idea of the estimated sample size. Textbooks with sample size tables are available (Friedman et al., 1985; Fleiss, 1981).

## EPILOGUE

In this section, an introduction to quantitative epidemiologic measures was presented. To be able to understand the underlying patterns of disease or suboptimal production in dairy herds, it is important that the HH & PM practitioner or farm advisor is able to use these tools. In combination with knowledge on pathophysiology of diseases, these tools are essential to better understand causes of disease or production problems. This introductory text is meant for those practitioners and farm advisors who have only recent experience in HH & PM. Those with longer-term experience in HH & PM services, are strongly advised to adopt and apply more-advanced quantitative epidemiological methods for high quality advisory activities.

## REFERENCES


*Beaudeau, F., K.Frankena, Ch.Fourichon, H. Seegers, B.Faye and J.P.T.M.Noordhuizen. 1994. Associations between health disorders during 2 consecutive lactations and culling in dairy cows. Livest.Prod.Sci.38: 207-216.*

*Erskine, R.J., R.J. Eberhart, L.J. Hutchinson, and S.B. Spencer. 1988. Incidence and types of clinical mastitis in dairy herds with high and low somatic cell counts. J.A.V.M.A. 192:761-764.*

*Fleiss, J.L. 1981. Statistical methods for rates and proportions. John Wiley and Sons, New York.*

*Friedman, L.M., C.D. Furberg, and D.L. DeMets. 1985. Fundamentals of Clinical Trials. PSGG Publishing Company, Inc., Littleton, MT.*

*Hogan, J.S., K.L. Smith, K.H. Hoblet, P.S. Schoenberger, D.A. Todhunter, W.D. Hueston, D.E. Pritchard, G.L. Bowman, L.E. Heider, B.L. Brockett, and H.R. Conrad. 1989. Field survey of clinical mastitis in low somatic cell count herds. J. Dairy Sci. 72:1547-1552*

*Laporte, H.M., H.H.Hogeveen, Y.H. Schukken, and J.P.T.M.Noordhuizen. 1994. Cystic ovarian disease in Dutch dairy cattle: incidence, risk factors and consequences. Livestock Production Science 38:191-197.*

*Martin, S.W., A.H.Meek, and P.Willeberg. 1987. Veterinary Epidemiology. Iowa State University Press, Ames. Iowa, USA.*

*Mechor, G.D., J.G.Kee, and D.Janzen. 1988. Comparison of Penicillin, Oxytetracycline and Trimethoprim-Sulfadoxine in the treatment of acute undifferentiated bovine respiratory disease. Can. Vet. J. 29:438-443.*

*Nielen, M., Y.H. Schukken, D.T. Scholl, H.J. Wilbrink and A. Brand. 1989. Twinning in Dairy Cattle, A study of risk factors and effects. Theriogenology 32:845-862.*

*Noordhuizen, J.P.T.M., K.Frankena, H.Ploeger, T.Nell (eds.) Field trial and error. Proc. of International seminar with workshops, Berg en Dal, Netherlands, 27-28 April 1993, EPIDECON/ Wageningen Agric. University Publ. 1994.*

*Noordhuizen, J.P.T.M., Frankena, K., Hoofd, C.M. van der, Graat, E.A.M. (eds.). Application of Quantitative Methods in Veterinary Epidemiology. Wageningen Pers, The Netherlands, 1997.*

*Rothman, K.J. Modern Epidemiology, Brown, Little and sons, Boston 1986.*

*Schukken, Y.H., F.J. Grommers, D. van de Geer, and A. Brand. 1989. Incidence of clinical mastitis on farms with low somatic cell counts in bulk milk. Veterinary Record 125:60-62.*

*Schukken, Y.H. and A. Brand. 1995. Health management in dairy herds. Vet. Research 25:160-164.*

*Smith, R.D., Veterinary Clinical Epidemiology. CRC press, 2-nd edition, Boca Raton, Florida. 1995.*

*Thrusfield, M., 1995. Veterinary Epidemiology. 2-nd edition. Blackwell Science Publ., Oxford, UK.*

## APPENDIX: STATISTICAL TESTS FOR MEASURES OF EFFECT

### *1. Risk difference*

$p_1$ and $p_2$ are the cumulative incidences of a disorder in two cohorts. The risk difference, RD = $p_1$ - p2. The standard error of the risk difference is equal to:

S.E.(RD) = $[(p_1 * (1\text{-}p_1)/n1) + (p_2 * (1\text{-}p_2)/n2)]^{.5}$.

The ratio RD/SE(RD) has an approximate normal distribution, and p-values may be found in statistical tables. Confidence intervals (95%) for RD can be calculated as: RD + 1.96 S.E.(RD).

### *2. Relative risk*

$p_1$ and $p_2$ are the cumulative incidences of a disorder in two cohorts. The relative risk, RR = $p_1$ / $p_2$. For reasons of normality the natural logarithm (ln) of the RR is used for calculations of statistical significance. The standard error of the ln(relative risk) is equal to:

$$\text{S.E. (lnRR)} = \left[\frac{(1-p_1)}{(n_1 * p_1)} + \frac{(1-p_2)}{(n_2 * p_2)}\right]^{.5}$$

Again, the ratio of the lnRR to the S.E.(lnRR) has an approximate normal distribution. The confidence interval (90%) of the lnRR may be calculated as: lnRR + 1.64 S.E.(lnRR).
Exponentiating the two boundaries yields the confidence interval in the scale of the RR.

### *3. Odds ratios*

$p_{ce}$ and $p_{cne}$ are the proportions of cases and non-cases that have the risk factor (exposed). The odds ratio is then:

OR = $(p_{ce} / (1 - p_{ce})) / (p_{cne}/(1 - p_{cne}))$. For normality reasons the natural logarithm of the odds ratio is used for calculations on statistical significance. The standard error of the lnOR is given by:

$$\text{S.E.(lnOr)} = \left[\frac{1}{p_{ce}} + \frac{1}{(1-p_{ce})} + \frac{1}{p_{cne}} + \frac{1}{(1-p_{cne})}\right]^{.5}$$

The ratio of the lnOR to its Standard Error has an approximate normal distribution, and the 95% confidence interval may be calculated by: lnOR + 1.96 * S.E.(lnOR). Exponentiating the boundaries yields the confidence interval in the original scale of the OR.

# 1.5 ECONOMIC ASPECTS OF HERD HEALTH AND PRODUCTION MANAGEMENT

Aalt.A. Dijkhuizen[1], Alien.W. Jalvingh[1], Ruud.B.M. Huirne[1] and David.T. Galligan[2]

[1] Department of Economics and Management, Farm Management Group, Animal Health and Management Economics Unit, Wageningen Agricultural University, Wageningen, The Netherlands

[2] Department of Clinical Studies, Section of Epidemiology and Health Economics, School of Veterinary Medicine, University of Pennsylvania, Kennett Square, USA

## 1.5.1 INTRODUCTION

Economics – as a science – deals primarily with decision making, in which money is only one of the elements of the system. Animal Health Economics can be described as the discipline that aims to provide a framework of concepts, procedures, and data to support the decision-making process in optimizing animal health management (Dijkhuizen, 1992).

Improving animal health and fertility can play a major role in achieving efficient and economically rewarding production. Current veterinary services are evolving to meet the needs of farmers through herd health and production management services. The application of these services is rarely an all-or-nothing affair. Usually several measures or programs are available, each of them offering a different degree of support and requiring a different level of investment. Determining the optimal input level, therefore, is to a large extent a matter of economic decision making. This is not only the case for the individual farmer, but also for a national government that must determine the optimal policy against specific infectious diseases.

In this part of Chapter 1 first the results of a field survey are presented and discussed, to show that herd health and production management control actually can improve the economic results of a farm. Then some basic techniques are presented that allow farmers and advisors to do simple economic calculations at the farm. Finally, two more advanced approaches, individual farm analysis to systematically search for strong and weak elements, and computer simulation to calculate the impact of management decisions and strategies on future farm performance, are introduced and discussed within the context of herd health and production management services.

## 1.5.2 ECONOMIC ANALYSIS OF A FIELD SURVEY

For a sound economic analysis of herd health and production management services, data from both the "with" and "without" situations should be available (Dijkhuizen,

1992). This may be realized in two ways: data from "before" (b) and "after" (a) application of the program, collected on farms participating in the program (P), as well as on comparable control farms (C). When available, these data make it possible to estimate the causal effects of the program more precisely, i.e., ($P_a$-$P_b$) - ($C_a$-$C_b$), especially when particular herds with obvious health and production management problems take part in the program. Collection of data in the "without" situation should be done concisely, however. Otherwise an interference with the program may occur, leading to an underestimation of the program effects.

In the Netherlands, a 2-year dairy herd health and management program was carried out along these lines from 1974/75 to 1976/77, including 30 program and 31 control farms (Sol et al., 1984). The year 1974/75 was used as a base year in which relevant data were collected from both groups before the program started. During the program years (1975/76 and 1976/77), the program farms were visited every six weeks by the veterinarian of the Animal Health Service, the local practitioner and the local extension officer. These visits primarily focused on reproduction, udder health, foot care, nutrition, cow culling, grassland exploitation and economic results. The control farms were visited twice a year, only to collect the necessary data.

Table 1 shows a comparison between the program and control group before and

*Table 1. Comparison of 30 program (P) and 31 control (C) farms before and during the field survey*

| | **Situation "before" (1974/75)** | | | **Changes during program (1976/77 - 1974/75)** | | |
|---|---|---|---|---|---|---|
| | **30P** | **31C** | **P-C** | **30P** | **31C** | **P-C** |
| Labor equivalents | 1.7 | 1.6 | 0.1 | -0.1 | 0.0 | -0.1 |
| Grassland area (ha) | 31.1 | 24.7 | 6.4* | 0.3 | 2.3 | -2.0 |
| Dairy cows (no) | 69.3 | 60.9 | 8.4* | 4.7 | 6.6 | -1.9 |
| Fertilizer (kg N/ha) | 300 | 351 | -51 | 42 | -24 | 66* |
| Milk per cow (kg) | 5121 | 5123 | -2 | 524 | 390 | 134 |
| Calving interval (d) | 378 | 376 | 2 | -5.3 | 3.3 | -8.6* |
| Cell count (x1000/ml) | 240 | 330 | -90 | -20 | 20 | -40 |
| Total culling rate (%) for reasons of: | 21.4 | 18.7 | 2.7 | 0.0 | 7.1 | -7.1* |
| - health/fertility probl. | 12.6 | 10.6 | 2.0 | 0.1 | 5.9 | -5.8* |
| Revenues (US$/cow) | 1740 | 1768 | -28 | 452 | 385 | 67 |
| Feed cost (US$/cow) | 569 | 576 | -7 | 198 | 227 | -29 |
| Margin (US$/cow) | 1171 | 1193 | -22 | 256 | 158 | 98 |

* $p < 0.05$

after two years of program application. In the preparatory year (1974/75), the groups showed no large differences. The farms of the program group were slightly larger (hectares of grassland and number of cows) and applied somewhat less nitrogen per hectare. Milk production per cow, and health and reproduction parameters (including culling data) did not differ between the groups, nor did the costs and returns per cow. The effects of the program were measured by comparing both groups for the changes in the various parameters per farm during the two successive years of program application. Neither group showed much difference in the development of farm structure (labor force, herd size, grassland area), although the program group increased nitrogen fertilization, compared to the control group. Statistically significant effects were found, regarding both calving interval and replacement rate of cows due to health problems and reproductive failure. Regarding udder health (i.e, somatic cell count) no significant effect was found. The average increase in the margin of revenues over feed cost per cow turned out to be US$256 in the program group, which is US$98 more than in the control group. Additional - veterinary - costs were estimated to average US$20 at the most, indicating that this herd health and production management program was a sound investment.

From both the farmers' and veterinarians' point of view it is also important to know whether or not such programs should be applied on a more than temporary basis. From these farms, therefore, data were gathered until ten years after the end of the program to see whether the initial effect on income had increased, decreased or remained the same. The necessary data were not available on all 61 farms. Therefore, two new groups were formed, consisting of 15 program farms and 20 control farms respectively (Hogeveen et al., 1992). Since the initial and new groups differed in number, the short-term program

*Table 2. Margin over feed cost per cow per year (US$) on the program (P) and control (C) farms*

| | **Initial groups** | | | **New groups** | | |
|---|---|---|---|---|---|---|
| | **30P** | **31C** | **P-C** | **15P** | **20C** | **P-C** |
| 1974/75 | 1170 | 1193 | -22 | 1156 | 1191 | -35 |
| 1976/77 - 1974/75 | 256 | 158 | 98* | 232 | 167 | 65 |
| 1976/77 | 1426 | 1351 | 75 | 1388 | 1358 | 30 |
| 1980/81 - 1976/77 | | | | 235 | 414 | -179* |
| 1980/81 | | | | 1623 | 1772 | -149* |
| 1985/86 - 1980/81 | | | | 599 | 575 | 24 |
| 1985/86 | | | | 2222 | 2347 | -125 |

* $p < 0.05$

effects were also re-evaluated. Results are summarized in Table 2.

During the years of program application (1975/76 to 1976/77) margin over feed cost per cow in the initial groups increased significantly more (US$98) on the program farms than on the control farms, as already stated before (Table 1). In the new groups the effect of the program on the income margin was smaller (US$65), and not statistically significant, but showed the same tendency as in the initial group. In the first few years after the program had finished (1976/77 to 1980/81), margin over feed cost per cow increased significantly more (US$179) on the control farms than on the program farms, as a result of both higher milk production and lower feed costs. In the period 1980/81 to 1985/86 the increase in income for both groups was almost the same, i.e, between US$575 and US$600 per cow. So, the initial increase in income soon had disappeared after the program had been finished. Such an outcome is not totally unexpected. Farmers' decisions have to be taken under continuously-changing price and production conditions, and in such dynamic circumstances, it seems to be profitable to apply herd health and production management programs on farms on a more than temporary basis.

## 1.5.3 BASIC TECHNIQUES FOR SIMPLE ECONOMIC CALCULATIONS AT THE FARM

There is a wide range of techniques available to help perform economic analysis of animal diseases and their control. These techniques and their possible applications are extensively described and illustrated in a textbook on Animal Health Economics (Dijkhuizen et al., 1996). Below, only the most common techniques are introduced and briefly described. That should at least give a better understanding of what they are and where they could be used for.

### Partial budgeting

If the proposed analysis concerns a simple economic comparison of disease control measures on a farm, and the outcome does not involve a specific time pattern nor a great degree of uncertainty, then partial budgeting is the method of choice.

Partial budgeting is simply a quantification of the economic consequences of a specific change in farm procedure and requires the simplest data collection of all the methods. It is particularly useful in analyzing relatively small changes within the production process, e.g. the effect of dry cow therapy to control mastitis. The general format for a partial budget is made up of four sections (Boehlje and Eidman, 1984):
1. additional returns realized from the change,
2. reduced costs as a result of the change,
3. returns foregone as a consequence of the change, and
4. extra costs incurred due to the implementation of the change.

The change should be adopted if the sum of (1) and (2) is greater than that of (3) and (4).

An example of a partial budget is presented in Table 3, quantifying the economics of a cesarean section in dairy cattle (Rougoor et al., 1994). The economic calculations are based on the differences in technical performances (i.e., milk production, feed intake, weight and survival rate of calves, and early replacement of cows) that were observed in field data between cows with and without cesarion section. The economic outcome is negative in this case, which means that cesarion section in dairy cattle turned out not to be profitable. Would the calf otherwise die, however, then its value should be included as additional returns of the surgery and then the net result may become positive.

*Table 3. The economics of caesarian section in dairy cattle*

| | | | | |
|---|---|---|---|---|
| 1. | **Additional returns** | US$25 | **Returns foregone** | US$ 30 |
| | – Heavier weights of calves | | – drop in milk production | |
| 2. | **Reduced costs** | US$10 | **Extra costs** | US$160 |
| | – Feed (less milk production) | | – surgery and culling | |
| | Total | US$35 | Total | US$190 |
| | Net result: US$35 - US$190 = US$-155 | | | |

**Cost-benefit analysis**

If the subject of research deals with more long-term measures and change in management strategies, then cost-benefit analysis is typically the analytical procedure of choice. Cost-benefit analysis is a procedure for determining the profitability of proposed courses of action over an extended period of time. Since the time at which costs or benefits occur may differ between the alternatives, it is important that these future costs and benefits are "discounted" to make them completely comparable, which results in the present value of costs and benefits. The reason for discounting is the time preference of money. A benefit of US$100 to be received immediately has more value than a benefit of US$100 received in one year, because of (potential) interest yields. The formula used to calculate the Present Value (PV) of a future cost or benefit (FV), where r is the annual "interest rate" (in %) and n is the number of years in the future, is:

$$PV = FV / (1 + r/100)^n$$

The "interest rate" used in cost-benefit analysis is called the discount rate, since it makes future values smaller than present values. The higher the discount rate the more a program with high initial costs and a low level of benefits over a long period of time will be penalized. Conventionally, the discount rate does not allow for inflation of prices, and future prices are calculated at current prices instead of inflated prices.

This avoids the difficulty of predicting future inflation rates, which would in any case have no effect on the real rate of return from the program under consideration. This discount rate then includes the so-called real rate of interest, being the difference between the market rate of interest and the inflation rate. An example of the cost-benefit approach is presented in Table 4, using a real interest rate of 5%. As can be seen from Table 4, the undiscounted benefits exceed the undiscounted cost in this example, whereas discounting induces the opposite.

*Table 4. Example of cost-benefit analysis*

| **Year** | **Discount factor** | **Undiscounted Costs** | **Undiscounted Benefits** | **Discounted Costs** | **Discounted Benefits** |
|---|---|---|---|---|---|
| 1 | 0.95[1] | 28 | 0 | 26.6[2] | 0.0 |
| 2 | 0.91 | 15 | 10 | 13.7 | 9.1 |
| 3 | 0.86 | 10 | 20 | 8.6 | 17.2 |
| 4 | 0.82 | 0 | 25 | 0.0 | 20.5 |
| **Total** | | **53** | **55** | **48.9** | **46.8** |

1 $0.95 = 1 / (1 + 5/100)^1$
2 $26.6 = 0.95 * 28$

### Decision-tree analysis

If there are multiple possible outcomes of the proposed courses of action, and chance is an important factor in determining which outcome occurs, then one of the various forms of decision analysis is the approach of choice. Decision-tree analysis is probably the most frequently used technique of decision analysis. A decision tree is defined as a graphical method of expressing, in chronological order, the alternative actions available to the decision maker and the choices determined by chance. An example is presented in Figure 1. Choices such as whether or not to vaccinate, are represented by squares called decision nodes. Chance events or states of nature, such as response to treatment, are represented by circles called chance nodes. The branches following each decision node must be exhaustive, that is, they must include all possible outcomes, and the outcomes must be mutually exhaustive. After each chance node, there is a probability ($P_j$) that an event occurs. The probabilities following a chance node must add up to 1.00, and can be taken from literature, experimental data, or expert opinion. The expected value of outcome for each action ($V_{ij}$) is entered at the far right of the tree branches, and expressed in dollars. The decision is then usually based on the expected monetary value (EMV). The EMV for each action (Ai) would be $EMV(A_i) = S_j(P_j V_{ij})$, with the highest EMV being preferred. In case of the example in Figure 1 the EMV of treatment A1 is the highest, i.e., 98 against 66 for treatment A2 and 57 for treatment $A_3$.

*Figure 1. A hypothetical decision tree representing action choices (treatment A1, A2, A3), states of nature (outbreaks in first, second, third or fourth quarter of the year), the associated probabilities and monetary values of outcome, e.g. US $.*

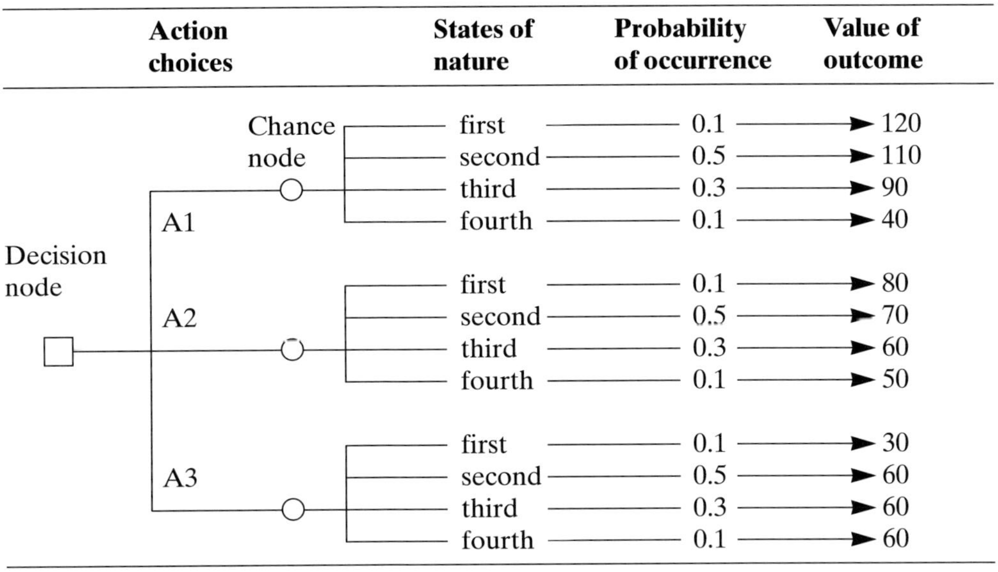


## 1.5.4 INDIVIDUAL FARM ANALYSIS

### Background

Farm records primarily reflect the historical performance on a farm. When analyzed carefully, however, they also provide signals for the future by highlighting current strengths to be exploited, and weaknesses to be eliminated or improved. False signals should be avoided and real problems not overlooked. As both strengths and weaknesses can be temporary, and easily be overlooked, appropriate analyses involve detailed examination of all issues contributing to a farm's success or failure. Potential underlying causes of changes should be examined as well. Hence, individual farm analysis requires a systematic approach.

Individual farm analysis can be defined as the comparison of the performance of an individual farm with a set of standards in order to identify strong and weak elements in farm management, and to determine the economic impact of these elements on current and future performance (Huirne et al., 1992). Individual farm analysis has different facets depending on the type of standards employed. First, standards for comparison can be derived from the farm itself. This type of analysis is commonly called **internal farm analysis**. If internal farm analysis is done on a multi-year basis, it is generally referred to as "trend analysis". The objective of trend analysis is to evaluate the development of the farm over time. Second, standards may be derived from another (similar) farm or a group of farms. This type of analysis, commonly called **external farm analysis** or "comparative analysis", is carried out primarily to determine the relative position of the farm. A third and last type of analysis includes a combination of these two, and is called "**comparative trend analysis**". The objective of comparative trend analysis is to evaluate differences between the development of the farm under consideration and the development of a group of (similar) farms.

Each of these three types of internal and external farm analyses can be divided into three interrelated stages: (1) tracing deviations, (2) weighting deviations, and (3) further analysis of deviations. The technique of individual farm analysis is a general one, and can basically be used for analyzing every type of agricultural enterprise.

### Tracing deviations

Tracing deviations involves three major aspects: (1) measuring farm performance, (2) establishing standards, and (3) comparing farm performance with standards. An important issue in the measurement of farm performance is data reliability. To be reliable, data must be accurate and consistent (see also Chapter 1, part 2). Practitioners play an important role in stimulating farmers to gather reliable data on animal health, reproduction, and milk production. The second aspect of tracing deviations concerns the establishment of performance standards; the preset targets. Because satisfactory values of performance vary by type of farm, a single set of standards can usually not be provided for all farms. Years and farms to be compared with should carefully be selected. During the third aspect of tracing deviations, farm performances and standards are compared. Because of the many uncertainties in agricultural production, deviations between performance and standards always exist. Questions concerning the relevance of deviations will be answered in the next sections.

### Economic importance of weighting deviations

The second stage of individual farm analysis firstly involves the economic weighting of traced performance deviations. Deviations between actual performance and standards will differ and the economic importance of one unit of deviation will vary between variables, depending on their impact on total economic farm performance. Furthermore the economic importance of deviations differs between farms and should ideally be calculated for each farm separately.

All deviations are initially assessed in their original dimensions. By calculating the economic importance of deviations, all deviations are converted to the same units (money values) and, therefore, comparisons can be made. The economic importance of deviations could be calculated using either common rules of thumb (e.g., one additional day of calving interval costs X dollars) or more advanced computer simulation tools (see next section).

### Statistical importance

As a measure of statistical importance, the traced deviation of a variable j ($TD_j$) could be related to its standard deviation ($SD_j$). The statistical importance ($SI_j$) of a deviation increases if the ratio between traced deviation and standard deviation increases, ie, $SI_j = TD_j / SD_j$. Standard deviations must be obtained for each of the three types of analysis. They are easily calculated from farm-specific databases, which are increasingly available on farms.

### Relevance of a deviation

In determining the relevance of a deviation, both the economic ($EI_j$) and statistical importance ($SI_j$) should be taken into account. The relevance of a deviation ($RD_j$) is calculated by multiplying the economic importance by the absolute value of the statistical importance of a deviation in performance variable j. In formula: $RD_j = EI_j * SI_j$. The absolute value in the formula is used only to avoid changes in sign in the economic importance of a deviation. Thus, economic importance and relevance of a deviation always have the same sign.

### Further analysis of deviations

In determining deviations that must be subject to further analysis, all deviations should be screened for relevance. As discussed before, deviations between performance and standards always exist. The question is at what level of deviation do they become relevant. For this purpose a so-called relevance diagram could be used (Figure 2).

The relevance diagram helps to determine important levels of traced deviations. Relevant deviations may be intolerable if they have a negative economic importance (weaknesses) or be desirable if they have a positive economic importance (strengths). The diagram is based on the principle of double relevance. If the calculated relevance of a deviation ($RD_j$) varies around zero (stage 0), it is presumed that the deviation is irrelevant, and no further analysis is needed. If the deviation falls into stage 1, it could be relevant and a previous time-period should be checked and the deviation is defined as relevant if it is the result of a slow change in performance. In case of stage 2, the deviation is considered to be relevant, and subject to further analysis. The diagram is symmetrical around zero, treating positive relevance of deviations in the same way as negative relevance. The choice of (user defined) boundaries, determines the level of analysis. If narrow boundaries are chosen, a greater number of differences will be relevant. If wide boundaries are chosen, the converse is true.

*Figure 2. The relevance diagram ($RD_j$ = Relevance of a Deviation in performance variable $_j$)*

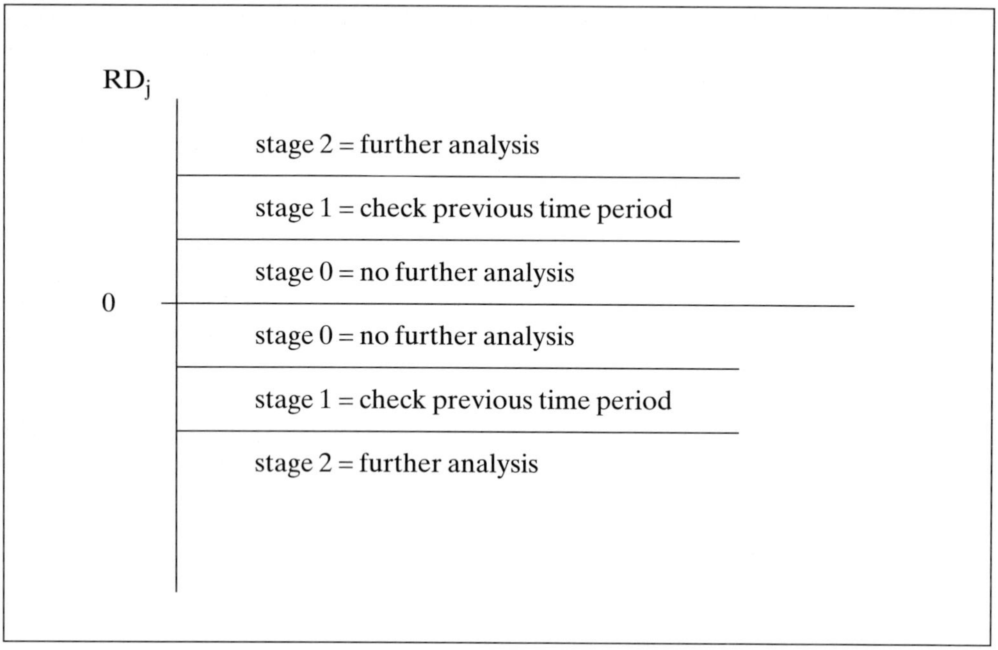


Performance deviations that are considered relevant should be subject to further analysis. In practice, analysis of deviations is not worthwhile unless the factors that caused them are identified. Therefore, further analysis of deviations requires the combination of deviations to find common causes. First, deviations should be divided into those that are to be controlled by an individual farm manager and those that are not. Because results of the analysis should be interpreted and used as a guide for management decisions, further analysis is performed only on those deviations that are under manager control. To find causes, deviations should be related to each other to see to what extent relevant deviations are associated. This is a difficult process, for which years of special training and experience are normally required.

In finding causes it may be valuable to find out that some deviations are relevant and others are not. So, information both on relevance and irrelevance of deviations can be very important. However, further analysis is started on the basis of relevant deviations. This is commonly called management by exception. The exceptions or relevant deviations between performance and standards are symptoms of strong and weak elements. These symptoms are then analyzed to pinpoint the cause of these elements. Management's attention is thus focused on a relatively small number of relevant deviations.

### Computerized analysis

Individual farm analysis can be performed manually. However, this is rather time consuming and, therefore, it would be more efficient to build the analysis into a computer model. Such a model works fast and can be used by different people, including those who lack the skills required to perform individual farm analysis manually.

For swine farms such a system, named CHESS (Computerized Herd Evaluation System for Sows) has been developed (Huirne et al., 1992). The system uses records of individual farms and of other (groups of) farms. As a supporting technique for the farm manager and his/her advisor, it can be used for early tracing of problems and for determining the maximum amount that could be spent in exploiting or improving farm performance. CHESS has the following features: it (1) has the ability to interface with both external simulation and optimization models for data exchange, and with management information systems for automated data input, (2) provides a basis for the three types of individual farm analysis, (3) is able to handle data from different time-intervals, and (4) is user friendly and suitable for use in the field. For dairy farms no such system exits yet, at least not along the lines described in this chapter.

## 1.5.5 COMPUTER SIMULATION

### Background

Management is becoming increasingly important in modern livestock farming and can be described as the decision-making process in which limited resources are allocated to a number of production alternatives (Kay and Edwards, 1994). The critical aspect of good management, therefore, is making the right decisions. The process of decision making is commonly described in five steps (Boehlje and Eidman, 1984): (1) define the problem or opportunity, (2) identify alternative courses of action, (3) gather information and analyze each of the alternative actions, (4) make the decision and take the action, and (5) evaluate the outcome.

Current management information systems are not yet well suited to support the various steps of the farmer's decision-making process. They are mainly restricted to recording and analysis of empirical data and do (also) not allow for calculation of the impact of alternative management strategies on future farm performance. In the Netherlands a project called TACT-Systems has been carried out to extend available systems in dairy cattle and swine with computer simulation, suitable to run on a PC (Jalvingh, 1993). For effective on-farm decision support it has been made possible that the input of the TACT computer simulation is farm-specific, representing the actual situation on the farm. Furthermore, the simulation model has the ability to evaluate a wide range of management strategies. The basic principle and some of the possible applications are presented and illustrated in the following sections.

*Figure 3. Schematic overview of the TACT-modeling approach*

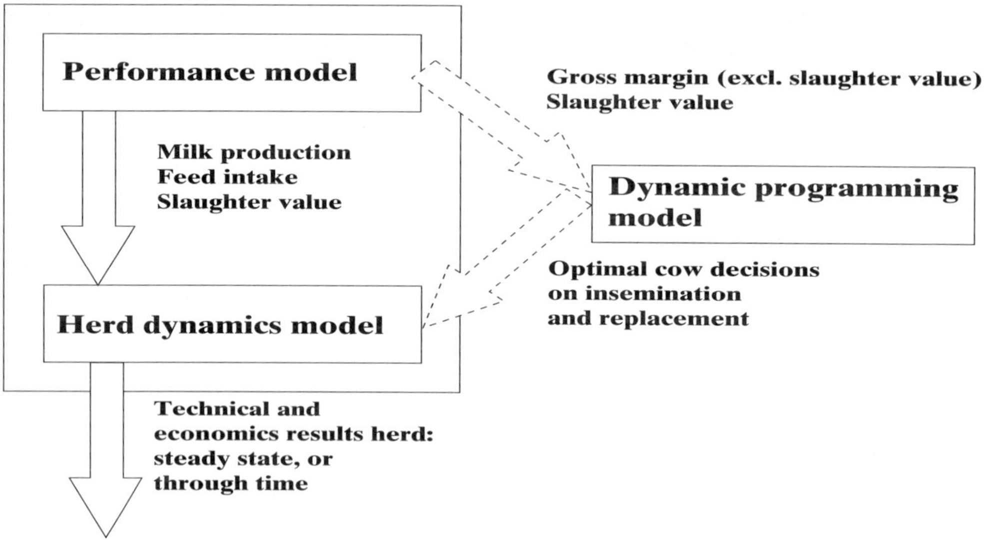


## Outline of the TACT-modeling approach

The TACT-modeling approach involves three separate models, as presented in Figure 3. Key issue in the model is the simulation of the flow of animals, and their performances, through time, taking into account farm-specific probabilities (e.g., estrous detection and pregnancy rate) and management strategies (e.g., insemination and replacement policy). Central in the approach are the concepts of states and state transitions. A state is defined as a condition in which an animal can be, such as "pregnant" or "culled". A transition means that an animal goes from one state to another, e.g., from open to pregnant. The distribution of animals over states at a certain moment can be derived from the distribution at the moment before and the transitions possible for each state. State variables used in the dairy simulation model are lactation number (1-10), stage of lactation (monthly base), milk production level during the present lactation (15 classes from 70 to 130% at Mature Equivalent), time of conception (2 to 8 months after calving) and month of calving. Uncertainty in future performance of the animals is represented in four groups of transition probabilities: production, reproduction, disposal, and replacement. An example of a transition probability in the reproduction area is the probability of conception, which determines whether an animal will go or not from "open" to "pregnant".

Technical and economic results of the herd are calculated by combining the number of animals per state with information from the performance model on milk production, feed intake, slaughter value and prices (Figure 3). Insemination and replacement of individual animals is determined by the outcome of a third model, ie, a dynamic programming model (Houben, 1995). The use of the results of the dynamic programming model in the herd dynamics model is optional, however, and to be replaced by more simple rules such as user-defined rules of thumb (e.g., cows older than 8 lactations are culled and replaced anyway). Technical and economic results can be generated for a herd in its steady state or for different consecutive years of the herd. The latter offers insight into the way the herd approaches a new steady state.

### Examples of model applications and outcome

The TACT-Dairy simulation model has various options for use in on-farm decision support of which two (ie, optimal calving interval and herd management comparisons) will be illustrated using typical Dutch input values for performance and prices (see Appendix).

### Optimal calving interval

The performance module can be used to calculate the optimum calving interval, and the losses of a sub-optimum calving interval for an individual farm. The outcome is summarized in Table 5.

*Table 5. Economic consequences of different calving intervals (US$)*

| | Calving interval (months) | | | | |
|---|---|---|---|---|---|
| | **11** | **12** | **13** | **15** | **17** |
| Optimal interval and losses per additional day | | | | | |
| First lactation | 0.20 | 0.00 | 0.90 | 1.40 | 1.70 |
| Older cows | 0.00 | 1.00 | 2.20 | 2.70 | 3.00 |
| Percentage in each interval of: | | | | | |
| All cows | 14.9 | 31.5 | 20.4 | 20.3 | 12.9 |
| Total losses | 0.0 | 6.2 | 15.2 | 34.9 | 43.7 |

If all relevant performances are considered, the optimal calving interval for first lactation cows is exactly one year. For older cows an optimal interval of less than one year is calculated, while the losses due to a longer calving interval is much more than for first lactation cows. The costs per day increases with the length of the calving interval, which is also shown in Table 5. In a typical herd, only a small percentage of the cows are in the highest calving intervals, In Table 5, for instance, 20.3% of the cows within the herd have a calving interval of 15 months and 12.9% of 17 months. These small percentages of the cows, however, cause a high proportion of the total losses in the herd, as is also indicated in Table 5. Consequently, one and the same average calving interval of a herd can lead to a difference in total losses, depending on the frequency distribution of which the average is composed. Hence, for a valid economic evaluation of the farm situation regarding fertility, an insight into this frequency distribution is necessary. In case additional kilograms retrieved from an improved calving interval would exceed the available quota, then the losses of an extended calving interval are considerably less.

**Herd management comparisons**

Application of the TACT-Dairy simulation model makes it also possible to gain insight into the effect of changes in biological variables and/or management strategies on the technical and economic results of the herd. The herd dynamics module is used to calculate for each alternative set of input values the steady state herd structure which will ultimately be reached with the respective input values, and its corresponding results. For a sample farm of 60 cows, the results of some calculations regarding improvements in herd management will be shown. The reproductive performance of the sample farm is below average in the basic situation. TACT-Dairy is used to obtain the technical and economic results of the farm in case reproductive management is improved. In Alternative I, the interval calving-first insemination is reduced from 90 days to 74 days. In Alterative II, the conception rate is increased from 40 to 60%. In Alternative III the

*Table 6. Major input data and results in the basic situation and in case of alternatives*

| | **Basic situation** | **Deviations from basic situation** | | |
|---|---|---|---|---|
| | | **I**[1] | **II** | **III** |
| **Input data** | | | | |
| – Interval calving-first ins. (days) | 90 | -14 | | -14 |
| – Conception rate (%) | 40 | | +20 | +20 |
| **Technical results** | | | | |
| – Average calving interval (days) | 399 | -11 | -16 | -28 |
| – % of animals with CI ≥ 14 months | 33.2 | -6.8 | -13.6 | -19.7 |
| – Annual culling rate | 34.2 | -1.2 | -5.7 | -6.5 |
| – Milk production (kg per cow) | 6840 | +76 | +162 | +247 |
| – Herd size (# of cows) | 61.4 | -0.7 | -1.4 | -2.1 |
| **Gross margin (US$)** | | | | |
| – per average cow | 2024 | 30 | 75 | 107 |
| – per 100 kg milk | 29.59 | +0.11 | +0.39 | +0.47 |
| – per farm | 124,295 | +480 | +1645 | +1995 |

1 Alternative I: first insemination earlier
Alternative II: conception rate increased
Alternative III: I + II

improvements of both Alternative I and II are realized. For each alternative, TACT-Dairy generates the corresponding herd structure and simulates the technical and economic results. The distribution of animals over calving intervals and lactation numbers will change due to the improvements in reproductive management, and with it the results. The major results of the basic situation and the alternatives are given in Table 6.

The average calving interval is reduced in all alternatives, as could be expected. In the basic situation one third of the cows had a calving interval of 14 months or more. In Alternative II this has been reduced to one fifth of the cows (33.2% minus 13.6%). Due to the increase in conception rate, culling rate is considerably reduced in Alternatives II and III, which has a large impact on replacement costs. Compared with the basic situation the increase in gross margin per average cow for the consecutive alternatives is US$30, 75 and 107 respectively. The economic results indicate the amount of money the farmer can spend at maximum on realizing the proposed improvement. It is also possible to mimic a milk quota system. The comparison of alternatives should then be based on gross margin per 100 kg milk. As milk production per average cow increases in each of the alternatives, herd size is decreased. Gross margin increases with US$ 0.11, 0.39 and 0.47 per 100 kg milk, respectively.

## EPILOGUE

Research in Animal Health and Management Economics focuses on the (further) development of simple as well as more advanced techniques that allow for the identification of strong and weak elements in the management on the one hand and to evaluate the impact of alternative decisions and strategies on the other, as illustrated in this part of Chapter 1. Such economic models can in the first place be helpful in a very early stage of farm advice, when almost no data of the farm under consideration are available. Calculations have then to rely on estimates of input values, to be obtained from literature and/or practical experiences, but these can systematically be varied to determine their impact on the results (sensitivity analysis). Such preliminary outcomes can be very helpful in setting priorities for further data gathering on the specific farm. Once available more reliable input values can be entered into the model to increase the realness of the outcome for the farm under consideration. This is an on-going process until no further significant improvement is made. A major challenge in future research is to integrate these models (where appropriate) into existing information systems, making them more accessible for actual use in herd health and production management services at the animal and herd level (Galligan et al., 1987). These systems in general and the economic models in particular should be flexible in their structure, and suitable to be tailored to individual farm and price conditions. That also opens the possibility for a sound international exchange and application. Once available, they can provide a solid and uniform basis for a mutual comparison of the economics of herd health and production management services, and may also be a starting point for further (and joint) research. Experiences gained so far in this respect with Dutch models are promising (Jalvingh et al., 1994).

## REFERENCES

*Boehlje, M.D. and V.R. Eidman, 1984. Farm management. Wiley, New York.*

*Dijkhuizen, A.A., 1992. Modelling animal health economics. Inaugural speech, Wageningen Agricultural University, Wageningen.*

*Dijkhuizen, A.A., R.S. Morris and R.B.M. Huirne, 1996. Animal Health Economics: Principles and Applications. The Postgraduate Foundation Publisher, Sydney (in press).*

*Galligan, D.T., W.E. Marsh and J.B. Madison, 1987. Decision making in veterinary practice: expected value and risk as dual utility scales. Preventive Veterinary Medicine, 5: 79-86.*

*Hogeveen, H., A.A. Dijkhuizen and J. Sol, 1992. Short and long term effects of a 2-year dairy herd health and management program. Preventive Veterinary Medicine, 13: 53-58.*

*Houben, E.H.P., 1995. Economic optimization of decisions with respect to dairy cow health management. Ph.D. thesis, Department of Farm Management, Wageningen Agricultural University, Wageningen.*

*Huirne, R.B.M., A.A. Dijkhuizen, J.A. Renkema and P. van Beek, 1992. Computerized analysis of individual sow-herd performance. American Journal of Agricultural Economics, 74: 388-399.*

*Jalvingh, A.W., 1993. Dynamic livestock modelling for on-farm decision support. Ph.D. thesis, Departments of Farm Management and Animal Breeding, Wageningen Agricultural University, Wageningen.*

*Jalvingh, A.W., I.R. Dohoo and A.A. Dijkhuizen, 1994. The use of computer simulation in teaching animal health and management economics. Proceedings 7th ISVEE-Congress, The Kenya Veterinarian, 18: 439-441, Nairobi.*

*Kay, R.D. and W.M. Edwards, 1994. Farm management. McGraw-Hill, New York.*

*Rougoor, C.W., A.A. Dijkhuizen, H.W. Barkema and Y.H. Schukken, 1994. The economics of cesarean section in dairy cattle. Preventive Veterinary Medicine, 19: 27-37.*

*Sol, J., J.A. Renkema, J. Stelwagen, A.A. Dijkhuizen and A. Brand, 1984. A three year herd health and management program on thirty Dutch dairy herds. The Veterinary Quarterly, 6: 141-169.*

## APPENDIX: MAJOR INPUT VALUE (DUTCH CONDITIONS)

| | |
|---|---|
| *Prices (US$):* | |
| milk fat (kg-1) | 4.72 |
| milk protein ($kg^{-1}$) | 7.78 |
| base price of milk (100 $kg^{-1}$) | -1.61 |
| female calves ($kg^{-1}$) | 3.67 |
| male calf | 5.86 |
| roughage ($kVEM^{-1}$) | 0.14 |
| concentrates ($kVEM^{-1}$) | 0.19 |
| carcass weight ($kg^{-1}$ for cow 7 months in first lactation) | 3.33 |
| price of replacement heifer | 1444 |
| insemination | 11 |
| *Mature Equivalent (8 years) herd level:* | |
| milk (kg) | 7750 |
| fat content (%) | 4.35 |
| protein content (%) | 3.39 |
| *Other:* | |
| age at first calving (months) | 24 |
| mature live weight (kg) | 650 |
| average estrus detection rate (%) | 70 |
| average conception rate after first insemination (%) | 60 |

# MONITORING REPLACEMENT REARING

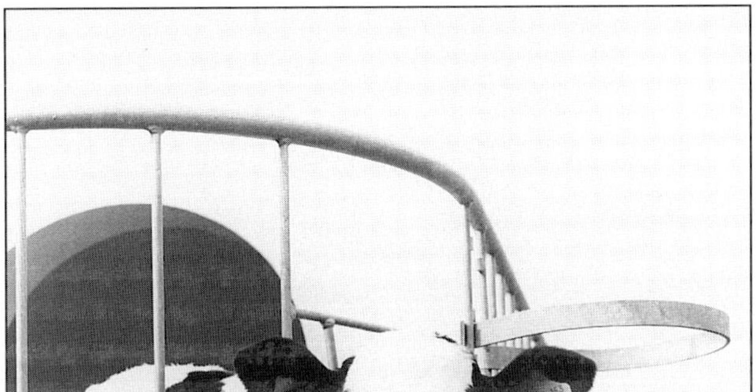

# 2.1 MONITORING REPLACEMENT REARING: OBJECTIVES AND MATERIALS AND METHODS

James D. Quigley III[1], Christopher S.T. Nyabadza[2], Geert Benedictus[3] and Arie Brand[4]

[1] Department of Animal Science, The University of Tennessee, P.O. Box 1071, Knoxville, TN 37901-1071, USA

[2] Department of Clinical Veterinary Science, University of Zimbabwe, Box M.P. 167, Harare, Zimbabwe

[3] Animal Health Service Noord Nederland, Morra 2, P.O. Box 361, 9200 AJ Drachten, The Netherlands

[4] Department of Herd Health and Reproduction, School of Veterinary Medicine, University of Utrecht, Yalelaan 7, 3485 CL Utrecht, The Netherlands

## 2.1.1 INTRODUCTION

An average of 25 to 35% of the dairy herd is culled each year and has to be replaced. Besides this, 10 to 12% of calves born die within the first two years of life (Remmen, 1976; National Animal Health Monitoring System, 1992). This makes replacement rearing an essential part of dairy farm management. Unfortunately, calf and heifer management is often overlooked in the dairy enterprise.

Calves are born with a predetermined genetic potential, which may be permanently affected by management decisions implemented throughout the rearing period and by environmental factors. A calf's genetic potential may be viewed as an upper limit that is expressed only if proper decisions are implemented at the appropriate time. Studies have shown that the level of management, estimated as herd milk production average, has a profound effect on calf morbidity and mortality (James et al., 1984; Curtis et al., 1985; Waltner-Toews et al., 1986a, 1986b; Perez, 1994; Jenny et al., 1981). Proper management of young stock, particularly during the neonatal period, can markedly reduce morbidity and mortality, whereas improper management will lead to economic losses from increased cost of veterinary intervention, death losses, growth retardation, and suboptimal reproductive performance. In addition, poor management of young stock can subsequently reduce the lifetime productivity of the individual cow and the herd as a whole.

Many management decisions implemented by the farmer in the various operational management functions may influence the success of replacement rearing. For example, decisions related to sire selection in the operational function of reproduction may influence calving ease and the ability of the calf to obtain adequate passive immunity. Therefore, it is important that replacement rearing decisions should be made within the context of management of the overall dairy operation.

Previously, veterinary practitioners have been consulted for specific complaints of young stock during the rearing period. Immediate advice, problem solving and treatments were requested and provided during these "as needed" consultations without due consideration to long term effects such as overall herd health and productivity. In the future, it will be increasingly important that both the practitioner, farm advisor and farmer become familiar and involved with a structured approach to replacement rearing so that problems are prevented and treatment and advice become relevant, meaningful, and functional within a long term replacement strategy (Donovan and Braun, 1987).

This chapter describes an integrated replacement rearing Herd Health and Production Management **(HH & PM)** protocol for use by practitioners, farm advisors and farmers in monitoring and evaluating health and development of young stock, from conception through birth of the calf, and to the first calving. Part 1 of this chapter deals with objectives and materials and methods of replacement rearing and with overall management strategies in the various developmental replacement rearing periods.

*Figure 1. Herd health and production management protocol for replacement rearing*

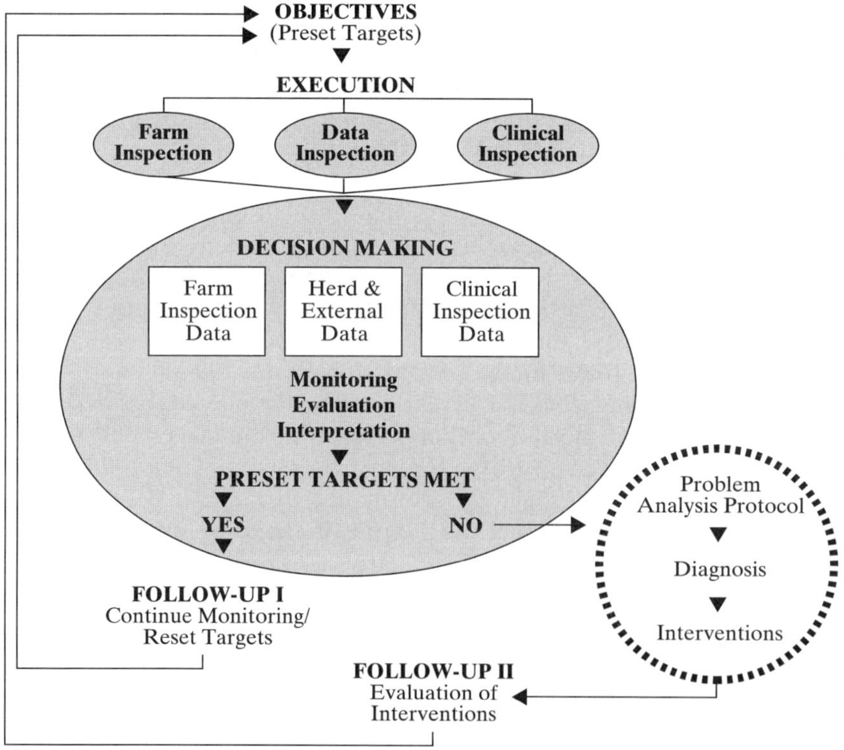

## 2.1.2 PROTOCOL

Young stock must be monitored throughout the rearing period, which covers 24 months on average, to guide optimal development and to identify and address deviations from optimal development at an early stage. A protocol as described in Chapter 1, part 1 is used as for other operational management functions (Figure 1).

## 2.1.3 GENERAL OBJECTIVES

The general objectives of replacement rearing should be:
1. to improve herd productivity through increased genetic value,
2. to rear healthy replacement heifers with a high total lifetime production,
3. to rear replacement heifers with low labour, fccd, and fixed overhead costs.

These objectives can be realised by the following management practices:

A) selecting the proper dams and sires to improve the genetic and phenotypic production potential of replacements,

B) optimizing health care through scrupulous record keeping, optimal housing, disease prevention, disease detection, and early and proper treatment of diseased young stock,

*Figure 2. Headings of a Calf Rearing Chart*

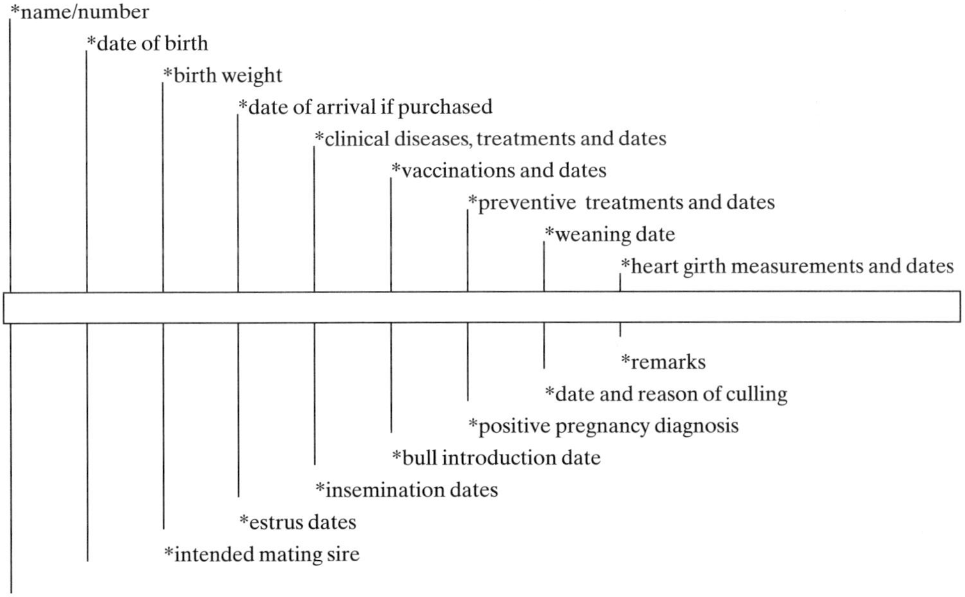

C) optimizing growth rates through adequate nutrition to ensure an optimal body size. expressed as a percentage of mature body size at first calving at 24 months or less.

For each farm the general objectives must be translated in preset targets which may differ from farm to farm.

## 2.1.4 PRESET TARGETS

Preset targets, expressed as performance indices, are the ultimate quantitative goals to achieve within a certain time period at a specific farm. They should be defined in conjunction with the farmer. To define preset targets, an inventory should be made

*Table 1. Primary and secondary performance indices for replacement rearing*

| PRIMARY INDICES | PERFORMANCE GOALS |
|---|---|
| – predicted minimum age at 1st calving | ≤ 24 months |
| – body weight postcalving | 570 kg |
| – wither height postcalving | 142 cm |
| – % mortality (total rearing period) | < 10 |
| – % abortions in heifers | < 4 |
| **SECONDARY INDICES** | |
| **% Mortality** | |
| – 0 - 24 hours | < 6 |
| – 1 - 30 days | < 2 |
| – 31 - 60 days | < 1 |
| – 3 - 24 months | < 1 |
| **% Morbidity (prevalence/pen)** | |
| % clinical diarrhea | < 20 |
| % clinical respiratory disease | < 6 |
| % clinical lameness | < 5 |
| % clinical mastitis | < 5 |
| **Body weight gain g/day** | |
| – prepubertal (≤ 10 months) | 800 |
| – postpubertal (> 10 months) | 825 |
| **Reproductive performance** | |
| – age at conception (months) | ≤ 15 |
| – % pregnant at first insemination | 70 |
| – # inseminations/pregnancy | 1.3 |
| – % dystocias in heifers | < 5 |

of all relevant data and information available on young stock present at the initiation of HH & PM services. This includes calculating herd size, number of replacements present, cow culling rates, young stock mortality and culling rates, age and body size at first calving and (if possible) cost of rearing replacements. This will enable the HH & PM practitioner to calculate actual performance indices. The calculated indices should then be compared with reference indices, followed by a redefinition of the calculated actual indices into preset targets for the forthcoming period. Performance indices and preset targets can be divided into primary and secondary indices (Table 1).

Primary performance indices in replacement rearing (Table 1) are related to health, growth and reproduction and must be calculated frequently. They form the smallest set of indices with which the replacement rearing performance can be evaluated quickly. Secondary indices provide more detailed information about subunits of primary indices and therefore are of diagnostic help.

## 2.1.5 MATERIAL AND METHODS

### Tools

1. Farm diary. A farm diary is necessary to record data on young stock and farm management events. These data must be transferred to a calf rearing chart or a barn fertility chart, and/or directly into a well designed computer program. All these data will generate a current overview and a dataset over time.
2. The calf rearing chart (CRC). On this chart the calves born are listed in a column in order of birth date. Data for each calf are recorded under a number of column headings (Figure 2).
3. A grassland management chart with both planned and realized pasture usage. Plots used by replacements should be evaluated carefully, due to the impact of internal parasites on young stock and on growth.
4. Computer software adequate for storing, processing and analysing data and generating action lists.
5. A list of current sire summaries from co-operatives or commercial semen distribution organisations. The list should include breeding values for production and conformation traits, calving ease, and predictions for fat and protein of offspring.
6. Milk production indices of the milk recording and testing organisation. These can be used for dam selection and for evaluation of milk production performance of first parity cows in the herd.
7. Nutrient requirement standards tables and forage analysis data.
8. Growth targets and a scale or a weight tape and a height stick for monitoring growth periodically.
9. Material for collecting nasal secretions, blood, urine and fecal samples for additional laboratory diagnostic examinations.
10. Relevant instrumentation for monitoring immunoglobulin content of colostrum and calf serum. Equipment includes a colostrometer and material to conduct blood

immunoglobulin measurements such as a refractometer, total serum protein, sodium sulfite precipitation test, or glutaraldehyde precipitation test.

11. Farm check list: a calendar with time-related veterinary and agricultural fields of attention to be examined or discussed with the farmer such as: vaccination schedules, internal and external parasite control programs, quarantine of purchased young stock and disinfection procedures (Noordhuizen, 1984).

**Methods**

During the farm visit the following activities must be performed:

1) Data inspection and calculation of relevant indices,
2) Farm inspection consisting of a diagnostic survey of the farm to discover potential risk situations,
3) Clinical examination and growth monitoring.

These activities must lead to prevention of health and growth disturbances.

## 2.1.6 DEVELOPMENTAL TIME SCALE

Replacement rearing consists of a number of successive phases in a developmental time scale (Figure 3). Each of the several age groups have their own management requirements and characteristic disease risks and growth rates. Disturbances in a certain age group may affect development later on. During a farm visit young stock will be found in nearly every age group. Attention must be paid to each of them. The developmental time scale of young stock rearing can be divided into several managerial time periods. The scale begins before conception, with selection of the appropriate genetic stock to produce offspring and ends at parturition with a live calf. The following periods are distinguished:

*Figure 3. Developmental time scale of replacement heifers*

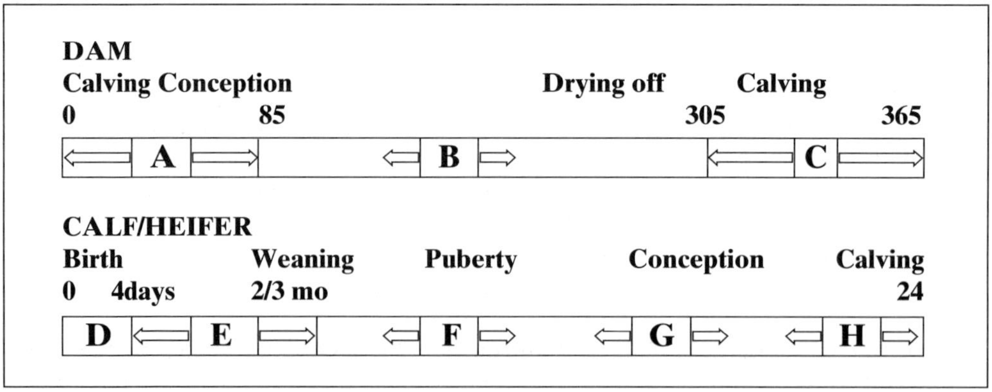

A/G. Breeding management cows/heifers,
B/H. Pregnant cow/heifer management,
C. Dry cow and calving management,
D. Calf management in the colostrum-feeding period (day 1 to 3),
E. Calf management in the milk-feeding period (day 4 to day 60 to 90 or shorter),
F. Growth period management (months 4 to 14).

Time periods A, B, and C are related to the dam and the others are related to the calf/heifer. In the next paragraphs, time periods A up to F will be addressed. For each management period, relevant background information will be presented.

## 2.1.7 BREEDING MANAGEMENT FOR COWS AND HEIFERS (A/G)

**Sire and dam selection**

Replacement rearing starts before conception with goal oriented selection of dam and sire based on production and conformation traits. Selection traits may include milk protein and fat content, mammary and locomotion system conformation, calving ease, etc. Milk production potential is the most important economic trait of the dairy cow. Therefore, more importance is usually given to the productive traits than to qualitative traits, as the latter are economically less important. HH & PM practitioners, farm advisors, and farmers should always evaluate production and conformation traits of heifers after calving. They also must know and correctly interpret sire summaries or sire selection programs. The choice of sires to use in a herd is determined by goals of the farmer and results of the evaluation of cows in the herd. Selected bulls must improve and correct deficiencies in the cows. Bulls chosen for use in the herd then must be matched to each cow. It is essential to use only progeny tested bulls, particularly for maiden heifers and dams selected to produce replacement heifers, as this will hasten the genetic improvement of the herd. In several countries, farmers can make use of cooperative or commercial organisations that manage advisory (non-)computerised breeding programs.

The genetic selection potential of cows for use in the replacement heifer rearing program is determined by:

1. Change in herd size - If herd size needs to be increased, more female calves must be retained even from dams with suboptimal genetic merit,
2. Total culling percentage and ratio between involuntary and voluntary culling. Involuntary culling reduces the selection potential,
3. Success of the rearing program - measured as the number of surviving healthy heifers that can be used as replacements,
4. Reproductive performance - subfertility reduces the number of calves born per year and limits the expression of the genetic potential of the herd.

With regard to heifer breeding management, health problems during the early rearing period, suboptimal nutrition and poor estrous detection will delay the time to breeding and conception (Hoffman, 1992). For optimal breeding management of cows and maiden heifers, a record keeping system which includes birth dates, estrous dates and weight measuring records of individual heifers is very important. Breeding attention lists based on accurate record keeping should be used. For an average body size of 570 kg post calving, a wither height of 142 cm, and a first calving age of 24 months or less, mating of heifers should start at about 350 kg body weight and a wither height of 125 cm, which should correspond with an age of 13 months or less. Frame size should be evaluated throughout the rearing period and nutrition should be focused on growth targets. Use of a sire advising list to improve the genetical potential of the herd should be encouraged. Bulls used for breeding heifers should be selected for calving ease. Use of non-tested bulls should be discouraged. Bulls used for natural breeding should be semen tested. Heifers in poor body condition should be fed properly before insemination.

**Participation in a herd fertility program**

After the selection of the parents, the dam's reproductive system should be checked before insemination to ensure that the ovaries and reproductive tract will be ready for the new pregnancy. Costly sperm can then be allocated to cows with a functional reproductive tract. These activities should all be included in a herd fertility program. If there are reproductive problems, they can be addressed immediately to maintain an adequate interval from calving to conception and a low involuntary culling rate due to fertility problems. estrous synchronization should be considered in case of shortage of labour in estrous detection. Cows and heifers inseminated should be examined for pregnancy from day 35 of pregnancy on. Body condition of cows should also be evaluated. Body condition scoring gives the practitioner and farmer an idea of the health and nutritional status of the dam. Severe body condition losses and anestrus indicates the cow has one or more nutritional deficiencies.

## 2.1.8 PREGNANT COW/HEIFER MANAGEMENT (B)

Ration formulation, feeding strategy and feed quality should be monitored and evaluated throughout pregnancy. The goal for heifers should be to obtain a post calving weight of 570 kg together with a wither height of 142 cm and an maximal body condition of 3.5. All pregnant heifers and cows should be identified properly. Udder health and feet and leg problems should be monitored regularly. Preventive measures (fly control) for summer mastitis should be taken.

**Loss of pregnancy**

Once a cow is pregnant, the main objective is to maintain the pregnancy to term. Health care of pregnant cows is an essential part of the rearing strategy within the framework of an integrated HH & PM service. Pregnancy can be terminated in one of four ways:

a) Early embryonic death. This is mostly unobserved and lengthens calving intervals,
b) Abortion up to 260 days of pregnancy. This is usually defined as any event resulting in the expulsion of a dead conceptus or a living conceptus unable to survive. Abortion may be caused by infectious agents, environmental, physical, genetic, nutritional, and hormonal factors,
c) Premature birth of a conceptus (alive or dead) from 260 days of pregnancy to term,
d) Parturition at term.

Early embryonic death, abortion, and premature birth will lengthen the generation interval, slow genetic improvement of the herd and lower the profitability of replacement rearing.

**Protection against non-infectious causes of abortion**

Protection against non-infectious abortion may be achieved by minimizing stress, especially in the last trimester of pregnancy. Stress may be, among others, caused by rigorous drying off practices and suboptimal cow comfort.

**Prevention of infectious causes of abortion: Vaccination strategy**

Abortion may be controlled by preventing exposure of the herd to specific infectious agents or with vaccination programs. Abortions may be caused directly by pathogens (e.g., *Brucella abortus*) or indirectly by pathogens that cause sudden and severe increases in body temperature (e.g., mastitis pathogens). Pathogens associated with both groups of causes of abortions should be regularly monitored as part of the HH & PM services. In addition, hygienic measures should be practised by the farmer, the veterinary practitioner/farm advisor and other visitors, including changing of clothing and boots after each farm visit.

A vaccination program must be based on the disease status of the herd, reproductive status of young stock and cows, potential interference by maternally derived antibodies, potential effects of vaccine-induced titres on suitability for export or introduction into bull studs, whether the herd is open or closed, prevailing farm and area conditions, national or regional vaccination strategies, the possible advantageous/disadvantageous postvaccination sequalae, and the cost benefit ratio of a vaccination program (Kahrs et al., 1986). Furthermore the vaccination schedule should be known, as well as the antigenic form of vaccine to be used (inactivated, modified live, live, or deletion vaccine), route of administration (intramuscularly, subcutaneously, or intranasally), and whether a booster vaccination is needed and when. A vaccination program to prevent infectious abortions could be directed against one or more of the following diseases: Infectious bovine rhinotracheitis (*Bovine Herpes Virus 1*), Bovine virus diarrhea/ mucosal disease, Para influenza, Leptospirosis (*Leptospira interrogans serovars*), Brucellosis (*Brucella abortus*), Campylobacteriosis (*C. fetus subsp. veneralis*), and Salmonellosis (*Salmonella dublin*). A vaccination program can be modified as diseases, farm conditions or available vaccines change. All vaccinations should be recorded on a calf rearing chart. Heifers should be vaccinated before initiation of the breeding period. Sick or stressed cattle should not be vaccinated. One of today's problems in farm management is the large dependence on vaccines and drugs, rather than on proper management practices and an optimal environment in which cows and calves are maintained. A first step in minimizing exposure of the herd to infectious agents should be accomplished by e.g. establishing a self-contained dairy not participating in exhibitions.

### 2.1.9 DRY COW AND CALVING MANAGEMENT (C)

Management of pregnant heifers and cows during the dry period is critical for optimal calf rearing performance, as it determines dam health and colostrum quality, which affect calf immune status and survival. Factors that must be monitored as part of the dry period and calving management in relation to replacement rearing are:

1. Breeding policy. Close-up heifers should be evaluated for proper size and pelvic development. This is affected by the previous rearing strategy. If deficient, these aspects should then also be checked in younger age groups and measures should be taken if needed. In addition, the use of bulls listed by AI organizations for easy calving for heifers already pregnant and currently for maiden heifers should be evaluated.
2. Grouping management. Heifers should be brought into contact with older dry cows 6 - 8 weeks before parturition to stimulate specific immune responses against micro-organisms present in the milking herd. Pregnant cows and heifers should be moved to a close-up group 2 to 3 weeks before expected calving date to gradually acclimate them to a ration provided in the upcoming lactation (Chapter 3).
3. Nutrition in the dry period. This should be considered an instrument to optimize health, reproductive, and milk production performance in the next lactation. During this period attention should be paid to feed and mineral intake.
   A) Insufficient energy intake in the close-up period will lead to a negative energy balance before calving, which may induce and/or enhance fatty liver disease after calving. A severe negative energy balance before calving may also disturb the calving process and may lead to metabolic diseases such as ketosis during lactation. Therefore, the energy content of the diet in the close-up period should be monitored and increased if necessary.
   B) Inadequate mineral balance in the diet, particularly in relation to Ca, may lead to milk fever and subsequently to disturbed calvings and a cascade of related diseases. Therefore, pregnant heifers and cows should be adequately fed, and anionic salts should be provided to prevent milk fever if necessary. To balance the ration, mineral content of the forage and concentrates must be known. See for more detailed information Chapter 3.

The nutrition program of the dams in late lactation and the dry period can, among others, be monitored by body condition scoring. Cows should calve with a body condition score of 3.25 to 3.75., and heifers with a score of 3 to 3.5. Cows and heifers with a score of 4 or more, generally are slow calvers that often need assistance (Maree, 1986). This can be associated with the birth of dead or weak calves.

Pregnant cows and heifers should be monitored for diseases - particularly mastitis.

A planned dry cow vaccination program to prevent diseases such as *Escherichia coli* K99 and Rota and Corona virus induced scours in the newborn calf should be considered in case improvement in management practices is not achievable on short term. Vaccinations result in increased titres of specific antibodies in colostrum (Saif and Smith, 1985). When this colostrum is fed, it provides increased passive immunity against the specific pathogen (Chapter 2, part 2).

### Use of a hygienic calving area and assistance

An hygienic environment at the time of birth is a prerequisite for optimal health performance of the new-born calf. For that reason legs and feet, hindquarters, perineum and udder of the dam should be cleaned before parturition. Maternity pens should follow the all-in-all-out system with disinfection in between to prevent transition of pathogens. Ideally, cows should calve in pasture which is clean and dry and which preferably has shade. A study in the U.S. (National Health Monitoring System, 1992) found that pasture resulted in low calf mortality. Obviously, the pasture must have good drainage to minimize mud and allow the cow to isolate herself for calving.

The incidence of dystocia should be $< 15\%$ in heifers and $< 8\%$ in multiparous cows. The percentage of dystocia is dependent on the gender of the calf, breed, bull choice, position at the time of birth, body condition of the dam and parity of the dam. Any calf born as a result of dystocia is much more prone to stillbirth, neonatal mortality and colostrum deprivation (Waltner-Toews et al., 1986 a, b). Where increased calf mortality and morbidity occur, calving supervision (including the competence of attendants and hygienic conditions) should be examined.

### Separation of calves from their dams

The calf should be separated immediately from her mother and transported to a clean and dry calf hutch to minimize transfer of infectious agents. This is important to prevent diarrhea caused by infections by bacteria (*E. coli, Salmonella*), viruses (Rota and Corona) and Protozoa (*Emeria* and *Cryptosporidiae*), and others. Neonatal calves infected with virulent enterotoxigenic *E. coli* during the first 24 hours after birth are very susceptible to develop diarrhea, and possibly, septicemia. Even very small infection doses can cause severe diarrhea, even at a later age as is the case with *Mycobacterium paratuberculosis.*

### Navel disinfection

The navel cord should be disinfected shortly after birth (Goodger and Theodore, 1986). This helps dry the cord and keeps organisms from entering the body. Studies have shown that calf morbidity (particularly enteritic and respiratory diseases) and mortality are reduced when the cord is dipped shortly after birth. A 5% iodine solution should be used and not dilute iodine solutions such as teat dip. Alcohol included in tincture of iodine can further reduce the risk of infection and speed drying of the cord.

A United States study (National Animal Health Monitoring System, 1992) revealed that approximately 47% of calves have their cords dipped. The stump should be rechecked for infection during the first 3 days after birth. If the umbilical cord should break just outside the abdominal wall, the naval should be stitched immediately. This is frequently seen when calves are born in a posterior position and in combination with a cesarean section.

**Calf identification and records**

After calving the date of birth and sex of calf born should be recorded. Complications of calving such as dystocia and conditions of significance should be recorded on the health record of the cow. Calves should be properly identified with a permanent identity immediately after birth. This makes subsequent record keeping possible on all events including health, growth and management. An identification system that is visible at a distance is a vital part of an efficient dairy management program. Early identification is important, especially in larger herds. It is advisable to use two ear tags and to follow a policy of replacing lost tags immediately.

## 2.1.10 CALF MANAGEMENT IN THE COLOSTRUM-FEEDING PERIOD(D)

Colostrum is defined as the secretion from the mammary gland of mammals during the first few days after parturition. Secretions from the cow's udder for one day after parturition are commonly referred to as colostrum. Secretions produced on the second and third day after parturition are called *transition milk*. Colostrum has an important nutritional role during the first 3 days of life when it differs from normal milk in many ways. It is markedly higher in solids [fat, protein, vitamins, and immunogobulins (**Ig**)], and lower in lactose. The amount of solids and protein (especially Ig) declines rapidly after the first day (Table 2), so that by day 4 the milk reaches normal composition.

Colostral feeding is crucial for calves because they are born without Ig, as the bovine epitheliochorial placenta is impermeable to proteins. Colostrum offers them their first immune response capability. The neonatal digestive system has the ability to absorb large molecules such as Ig without degrading them into their component amino acids and other components for a limited time after birth (approximately 24 hours). During this time, normal digestive enzymes in the abomasum and small intestine do not function or function with limited activity, allowing Ig to reach the small intestine for absorption. Further, colostrum contains enzyme inhibitors that allow Ig to escape intestinal degradation (Quigley et al., 1995a) and bacteriostatic proteins (lactoferrin, lysozyme) that directly inhibit the growth of bacteria in the intestine.

Research (Riedel-Caspari, 1993; Pitt et al., 1977) have indicated that leukocytes present in fresh colostrum may also contribute to the health of the calf. Leukocytes in colostrum can be absorbed directly into the circulation by the calf and reduce the effects of bacterial disease probably by enhancing cellular defense mechanisms. Leukocytes are killed by storage (freezing and refrigeration) and are only found in fresh colostrum and transition milk. Although additional research is needed, it appears that using fresh colostrum from the dam may be the optimal method to ensure absorption of maternal leukocytes.

*Table 2. Colostrum composition (From: Foley and Otterby, 1978)*

| | Milking Number | | | |
|---|---|---|---|---|
| Item | 1 | 2 | 3 | Milk |
| Specific gravity | 1.056 | 1.040 | 1.035 | 1.032 |
| Solids, % | 23.9 | 17.9 | 14.1 | 12.9 |
| Protein, % | 14.0 | 8.4 | 5.1 | 3.1 |
| Casein, % | 4.8 | 4.3 | 3.8 | 2.5 |
| IgG, mg/ml | 48.0 | 25.0 | 15.0 | .6 |
| Fat, % | 6.7 | 5.4 | 3.9 | 3.7 |
| Lactose, % | 2.7 | 3.9 | 4.4 | 5.0 |
| Vitamin A, mg/L | 2950 | 1900 | 1130 | 340 |
| Vitamin D, IU/g fat | .9 to 1.8 | | | .4 |
| Riboflavin, mg/ml | 4.8 | 2.7 | 1.9 | 1.5 |
| Choline, mg/ml | .70 | .34 | .23 | .13 |

Total Ig concentrations in neonatal calves represent a large repertoire of maternally derived antibodies to a huge variety of antigens. Calf serum Ig isotype concentrations peak at 24 to 36 hours after birth if colostrum is consumed by 24 hours. Subsequently, serum concentrations in calves gradually decline to minimal between 15 and 28 days of age. There is a gradual but steady increase for all serum isotypes from 4 to 7 weeks. Endogenous Ig synthesis is complicated by the presence of maternally derived antibody, which appears to delay such production. IgA is of little practical use in systemic defense although contributes of IgA at mucosal level may be significant (Burton et al., 1989).

Colostrum and transition milk contain IgG, IgA and non-specific antibacterial factors including lysozyme, lactoferrin and lactoperoxidase system that provide local protective immunity in the gastrointestinal tract. Recent research indicates that IgG in colostrum may provide local immunity in the gut (Fowler, 1995; Drew, 1994). In addition, IgG in the blood are released into the lumen of the intestine to provide immunity against enteric pathogens such as rotavirus (Besser et al., 1988 a, b).

It is difficult to overemphasize the importance of colostrum to the young calf. Calves receiving too little colostrum are at a much greater risk of morbidity and mortality than calves receiving sufficient colostrum. Insufficient consumption of colostrum reduces the concentration of IgG in serum, thereby increasing the risk of disease. A serum IgG concentration < 1,000 mg/dl by 48 hours of age has been defined as *failure of passive transfer* (**FPT**) and is associated with increased morbidity and mortality. In a U.S. study, mortality of calves with serum IgG less than 1,000 mg/dl was over twice that of calves with higher IgG levels (Figure 4). Important factors that contribute to FPT include:

1. Low Ig concentration in the dam's colostrum,
2. Poor colostral feeding technique:
   - too late after birth (6 - 8 h),
   - amount of colostrum per meal too small,
3. Calves not willingly to consume sufficient colostrum,
4. Dystocia.

Usually, disease prevalence is inversely related to neonatal serum Ig concentration. Risk of disease will be lessened by effective passive immunity at birth and perhaps efficient onset of endogenous Ig production between 2 and 4 weeks of age.

The two most important factors affecting serum IgG concentration are the amount of IgG consumed and age of the calf at the first colostrum feeding. The amount of IgG consumed is the colostral IgG concentration * the volume of colostrum consumed.

**Colostral quality**

The cow produces Ig in response to pathogens to which she has been exposed. Therefore, cows that have been exposed to a greater number of pathogens will produce colostrum with a broader spectrum of Ig than cows exposed to fewer pathogens. This is often why older cows will produce colostrum containing a broader spectrum of Ig than younger cows. Moreover, cattle raised on a farm will produce colostrum with antibodies *specific for the microorganisms on that farm* which is an added benefit.

*Figure 4. Calf survival by serum IgG concentration (National Animal Health Monitoring System, 1992)*

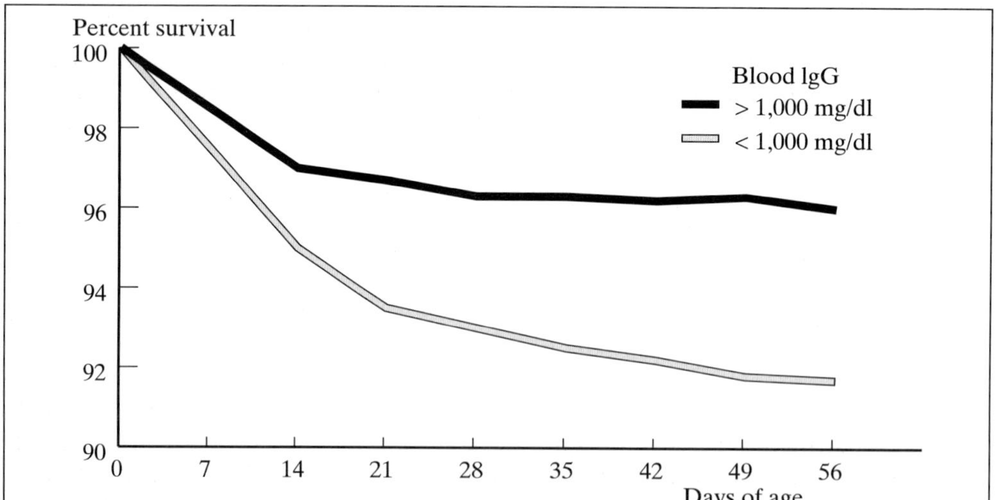

To improve colostral quality and subsequent health of calves dams should be immunized with *E.coli* and Rotavirus and Coronavirus vaccines during the dry period .

The large variation in Ig content of colostrum makes accurate colostrum management and feeding difficult. Colostral IgG can be measured in the laboratory with great accuracy; unfortunately, the assays involved are time-consuming and expensive. Measurement of colostral specific gravity using a device called a colostrometer is a method to estimate Ig content of colostrum on the farm. This device is based on the relationship between Ig in colostrum and specific gravity. The correlation between specific gravity and colostral IgG concentration has been reported to range from 0.6 to 0.9 (Fleenor and Stott, 1980; Quigley et al., 1994). Effective use of a colostrometer requires that the sample should be at room temperature when tested. Unfortunately, components of colostrum other than Ig may affect specific gravity (e.g. fat), so the relationship is variable (Pritchett et al., 1994). However, the colostrometer may give a reasonable qualitative estimate of colostrum quality - it is most effective when used to identify samples of poor quality.

The concentration of Ig in colostrum varies according to the cow's disease history, parity, volume of colostrum produced, season of the year, breed, length of dry period, degree of prepartum milking or milk leaking, and other factors (Roy, 1990). The average concentration of $IgG_1$ in colostrum from 919 Holstein cows was 48.2 mg/ml with a range of 20 to >100 mg/ml (Pritchett et al., 1991). A second study (Quigley et al., 1994) reported that colostrum from 96 Jersey cows averaged 66 mg/ml of IgG, with a range of 28 to 115 mg/ml. The difference between 20 and 100 mg/ml of IgG in colostrum can mean the difference between success and failure of passive transfer of immunity. If the quality of colostrum produced by the dam is insufficient (as measured by a colostrometer) one should check the drying off strategy, milk leakage, length of the dry period, udder health, premature calving and wether dystocia occurred. Dystocia reduces Ig absorption by calves due to a combination of decreased appetite and colostrum intake, hypothermia, and reduced plasma thyroid hormone levels (Vermorel et al., 1989).

Research has also indicated that the volume of colostrum produced will influence Ig in colostrum. Generally, colostrum produced in large volumes will have lower Ig concentration than colostrum produced in smaller volumes (Pritchett et al., 1991). This is only a general rule, however, and the relationship between Ig concentration and volume is not constant.

The dam produces enough colostrum in the first three milkings to feed a calf for the first four days. Therefore, colostrum collected under hygienic milking conditions should be stored frozen as a reserve (Foley and Otterby, 1978). Colostrum can be refrigerated for only about 1 week before quality (Ig concentration) declines. For long-term colostrum storage, freezing is the best alternative. Colostrum may be frozen for up to a year without significant decomposition of Ig (Roy, 1990). It should be noted that frost-free freezers are not optimal for long-term colostrum storage, as they go through freeze-thaw cycles that can allow the colostrum to thaw. This can markedly shorten colostrum storage life. Frozen colostrum should be placed in warm (not hot) water and allowed to thaw. Alternately, colostrum can be thawed in a microwave oven with little damage to the Ig. It is important to microwave the colostrum for short periods on low power and pour off the thawed liquid periodically to minimize heating. It is also important to avoid "hot spots" inside the frozen colostrum. Use of a turntable can help to minimize damage to Ig.

## Colostral feeding

The most important aspect of the colostral feeding period is the timely (before pathogens enter the digestive tract) provision of an adequate amount of high quality colostrum. The first feeding has by far the greatest influence on Ig absorption. At least 100 grams of pure Ig must be ingested at each of the first two feedings of colostrum to achieve a blood concentrations of at least 1,000 mg/dl of IgG to reduce the incidence of disease and death. The commonly recommended volume of 1.5 litres of colostrum for first feeding to Holstein calves does not provide sufficient Ig to protect most calves (Gay, 1994). To obtain an ingestion of 100 grams, 1 liter containing 100 mg/ml Ig must be fed. Voluntary intake of colostrum when fed by nipple bottle shortly after birth is 8 to 10% of body weight (Quigley, 1995 b). Offering more colostrum will usually be refused. In this situation, the volume of colostrum necessary to feed 100 grams of Ig should be offered in an additional feeding in the following 4 - 8 hours. This is important as colostral absorption decreases with time and determines the success of transfer passive immunity of the calf. It also means that the recommended rule of feeding 10% of body weight of colostrum during the first day of life should be replaced by feeding 100 grams of Ig as soon as possible after birth and again, 12 hours later. The temperature of the colostrum should be 39 ± 2°C to ensure good digestion and acceptance. Colostrum from the older cows should be fed to the calves in their first 24 hours of life and the heifer's colostrum to them after that time.

To feed an adequate amount of Ig the concentration in colostrum has to be measured with a colostrometer and the volume of colostrum must be adjusted to the concentration of colostrum Ig. Colostrum with adequate IgG concentration (≥ 50 mg/ml) has a specific gravity > 1.045 (Pritchett et al., 1994).

The timing of colostrum feeding is critically important because the intestine of the newborn is capable of absorbing large molecules intact for not more than 24 hours after birth. This absorptive ability is greatest at birth and declines thereafter due to maturation of the intestinal enterocytes (Bush and Staley, 1980). By 12 hours after birth nearly 50% of the the calf's ability to absorb Ig is lost. Another aspect is that the intestine does not discriminate among molecules. If absorptive sites in the intestine are not saturated by colostral proteins, other molecules, and possibly bacteria, may reach these sites and be absorbed (Logan, 1977). If bacteria reach absorptive sites before colostral proteins, the calf will be at great risk of septicemia, which is often fatal. Therefore, it is critical that colostrum be fed as soon as possible after birth, preferably, within the first 30 minutes. This is also a reason that calves should be separated from the dam and fed by nipple-bottle to minimize the risk of calves swallowing feces, bedding, or other contaminated material.

In many cases first or extra colostrum is provided by an esophageal tube. An esophageal feeder may be used when the calf will not consume colostrum voluntarily.

It should be noted that colostrum given by esophageal feeder enters the rumen and not the abomasum (via the esophageal groove). However, most of the colostrum will leave the rumen and flow to the abomasum within about 3 hours. Work of Lee et al. (1983) and Zaremba et al. (1985) indicated that feeding by esophageal feeder resulted in lower serum Ig concentrations compared to calves fed by nipple bottle. On the other hand, using an esophageal feeder is preferable to insufficient colostrum intake and development of FPT.

Colostral supplements have been introduced recently as a means to replace or increase the IgG concentration of colostrum. Most recent research suggests that these products do not contain sufficient Ig to significantly increase serum Ig when good quality colostrum is used (Abel Francisco et al., 1993). However, colostral supplements may be useful when colostrum is unavailable, of poor quality, or cannot be thawed in time to feed to a calf.

Care takers should feed every calf from its own clean bucket. Buckets must be cleaned and washed every day including the rubber teats. Research has shown that accumulation of solids in the nipples of buckets and bottles is a significant vector for infection and can increase morbidity and mortality (Lance et al., 1992). Boots or shoes should be cleaned and disinfected before entering the barn or pens. Hands should be washed beforehand. Calves should not be allowed to suckle hands of the care taker or other persons.

### Serum Ig tests

There is a number of tests used in laboratories which give detailed information of the immune status of a young calf. As hypo- and agammaglobulinaemia is often seen in calves a few days old, it is advisable to measure serum Ig levels of animals in a herd regularly. For veterinary practitioners there are several methods of estimating serum IgG concentration:

1. Commercial latex agglutination test (whole blood, results in five minutes, but expensive)
2. Sodium sulfite precipitation. The sodium sulfite precipitation test uses solutions of 14%, 16% and 18% sodium sulfite. Sodium sulfite causes precipitation of Ig. To each of three test tubes, 9 ml of one concentration of solution (14%, 16% and 18%) and then 0.1 ml serum are added, mixed well, and allowed to stand for 60 minutes. Samples that precipitate only with 18% sodium sulfite contain < 5 g Ig/liter, 2) Samples that precipitate with 16% and 18% sodium sulfite contain 5 to 10 g Ig/lit 3) Samples that precipitate with all three solutions contain > 15 g Ig/liter (Hopkins et al., 1984). It is not desirable to use plasma for tests that depend on precipitation of Ig, because of interference by fibrinogen.
3. Refractometer. A serum-refractometer will give information of the immune status of a young calf as there is a high correlation (r = 0,87) of whole serum protein and serum gammaglobulin levels. This test is reliable up to six days after birth. During this time total protein rises are due to the intake of colostrum. Interpretation of the total protein test results is as follows: < 4.9 g/dl high risk for disease, 5,0 - 5,4 medium risk for

disease, > 5,5 low risk for disease (Braun and Tennant, 1983). The refractometer cannot be used in hemolyzed blood. Another disadvantage is the low sensitivity of the test and the possibility of false negative results.

4. Glutaraldehyde test. Glutaraldehyde cross-links with certain blood proteins (particularly Ig and fibrinogen) to form a solid gel. Commercial kits are available that contain purified glutaraldehyde and can be run within 5 minutes. However, false positives results may occur if the calf is dehydrated or has elevated fibrinogen levels.

Other methods of measuring serum Ig concentration include radial immunodiffusion (**RID**) and enzyme-linked immunosorbent assay (**ELISA**). The RID assay is available in kit form. A small amount of serum is added to a small well in an agar-antibody matrix. The Ig in the serum reacts with the antibody in the agar, forming a precipitant ring. The diameter of the ring is proportional to the concentration of Ig in the sample. Advantages of the RID are high specificity and accuracy. However, the assay requires about 24 hours and is expensive. The ELISA is the most sensitive method of determining serum Ig concentration. It requires specific antibodies and microtiter plate readers, which makes it very expensive. This method also requires a significant amount of expertise.

## 2.1.11 CALF MANAGEMENT IN THE MILK-FEEDING PERIOD (E)

The milk feeding period starts between 2 and 4 days, depending on colostral management, and ends with the weaning decision which is based on the weight, age or feed intake of the calf. The milk feeding period should be characterized by rapid growth and good health, which are determined by the following:

1. Quality of milk or milk replacer,
2. Quantity and feeding practices.

### Quality of milk or milk replacer

After the colostral period, the calf is fed a liquid diet which may contain one or more of the following: excess colostrum, transition milk, unsaleable milk (contaminated with antibiotics, mastitic milk, or milk with unacceptably high somatic cell counts), normal milk, and/or milk replacer.

Colostrum and transition milk have the best nutritional value of all liquid feeds available to the calf if properly collected and stored. Colostrum can be frozen or fermented and conserved with e.g. bicarbonate. They are also the cheapest as they have no other use. Milk contaminated with antibiotics can be used but has several drawbacks which include effects on beneficial bacteria and high rejection rates which may slow growth. However, calves fed milk containing antibiotics cannot be sold for slaughter until all antibiotics have been eliminated.

Mastitic milk, if not contaminated with antibiotic, can safely be fed to calves (Kesler, 1981). Mastitic milk should not be fed to calves that suck each other due to the risk of transmission of mastitis pathogens. Moreover, milk from cows with mastitis caused by *E. coli* and *Pasteurella* should not be fed unless it has been pasteurized.

Milk replacers are commercially-produced milk substitutes which, when properly reconstituted with water, have a similar dry matter content as milk. Modern milk replacers contain high quality protein and energy and can provide rates of body weight gain similar to that of whole milk. However, the quality of milk replacer is difficult to determine without sophisticated laboratory testing, so care must be used to select only milk replacers known to be of excellent nutritional quality.

### Quantity and feeding practices

During the first days of life, the primary source of nutrients is colostrum followed by milk. During the transition period to a solid diet (the grey box in Figure 5), both liquid and solid feeds provide nutrients to the calf.

During the first 3 days calves should be fed high quality colostrum. The volume of colostrum fed per day should be 10% of body weight. Thereafter, calves are fed 1.5 litres of cow milk 3 times a day during 2 days as a transition to milk replacer. Milk replacer is fed at 8 to 10% of birth BW per day, usually divided into two feedings. This amount is held constant until weaning at 4, 6 or 8 weeks of age. Milk replacer should be fed at 40°C. The pH of milk replacer should be 6.2 to 6.6. To avoid problems of the alimentary tract, the milk must be warm and bottles or pails clean at each feeding. Choice of bottles or buckets does not affect intake of milk replacer or closure of the esophageal groove. High quality calf starter and fresh, clean water must be available from 3 days of age. Feeding a starter has the objective to meet energy and protein requirements for both maintenance and growth that can not be reached with milk alone, and to stimulate the development of the rumen flora. Starters can be split in grain and complete starters. A complete starter contains readily fermentable feed, and as much as 35 % good quality forage. If not a complete but a grain starter is fed, the best hay or grass should be fed in small amounts. When available for *ad libitum* consumption, calves will consume starter in excess of 700 grams/day by about 35 days of age.

When a starter is fed, provision of fresh clean drinking water is required from one week of age on. Feeding water also reduces scours scores thereby increasing body weight gain indirectly. Milk or milk replacer does not constitute "free water". When milk or milk replacer is fed to calves, it by-passes the rumen and reticulum by the

*Figure 5. Schematic diagram of calf growth and rumen development*

**Calf time line**

| | | | |
|---|---|---|---|
| **Diet** | **Liquid** | **Liquid + Solid** | **Solid** |
| **Organ** * | **Abomasum** | **Abo + Rumen** | **Rumen** |
| **Energy** ** | **Glucose** | **Glucose/VFA** | **VFA** |
| **Protein** ** | **Dietary** | **Dietary/Bacteria** | **Bacteria** |
| | | | ↑ **Weaning** |

* Primary organ  ** Primary nutrient

action of the esophageal groove. The esophageal groove is active in the calf until about 12 weeks of age. The groove closes in response to nervous stimulation, shunting milk past the reticulorumen and into the abomasum. Closure of the groove occurs whether calves are fed from buckets or bottles. Therefore, the feeding of milk replacer should not be construed as providing enough water.

Free water intake is essential for functioning of the rumen. Unfortunately, many producers do not provide free water to their calves until calves reach 4 or more weeks of age. In a U.S. study 39 % of producers provided water in the first week to their calves, but another 39 % waited until they reached an age of 5 weeks (NAHMS, 1992).

Offering water in winter can be a significant challenge in many parts of the world. However, calves still need water, even when it is cold. Sometimes, it may be necessary to bring warm water at an additional feeding to ensure that calves have enough liquid water available.

An alternative feeding method of young calves consists of *ad libitum* bulk feeding from a bucket with a teat. A disadvantage of this method of feeding is reduced consumption of concentrate, hay and water due to selective intake of milk. The sudden change from a ration with milk to a ration with water, hay and concentrate without adaptation may cause digestive problems and stress at the time of weaning.

**Development of the rumen**

Ruminal function is a key part of the development of the young calf. With the exception of veal calves, all calves are fed to promote ruminal development. This process begins shortly after birth and can be regulated by the producer. At 4 months of age calves must have a functional rumen and can be fed a growing ration. Early development of the rumen is important both to the calf (biologically) and to the producer (economically). An economic benefit is that after weaning, calves are less susceptible to disease and gain more body weight with lower labor and management costs. Therefore, it is in the producer's best interest to manage calves to promote early rumen development and to wean calves as early as is feasible.

## 2.1.12 GROWTH PERIOD MANAGEMENT (F)

**Growth**

Growth of young stock is related to both chronological and physiological age. Chronological age is defined in days, weeks, months, and years. Physiological age is defined as a percentage of mature body size. In replacement rearing optimal growth should be related to physiological age and not to chronological age (Skidmore, 1995; Van Amburgh et al., 1991). The recommended age at first calving has been 24 months for many years. Current research activities are now focussed at a calving age of < 24 months (Skidmore, 1995; Van Amburgh and Galton, 1994). Advantages are improved genetic progress, reduced length of the rearing period, reduced replacement herd size

**Processes that play a role in Rumen Development**

The following processes that play a role in rumen development will be discussed:

1. Functional and physical development of the rumen,
2. Establishment of a microflora in the rumen,
3. Outflow of material from the rumen (muscular action),
4. Absorptive ability of the tissue.

*Table 3. Change in the proportion of each compartment of the ruminant stomach (From: Church, 1976)*

| | Age in weeks | | | | | | |
|---|---|---|---|---|---|---|---|
| | **0** | **4** | **8** | **12** | **16** | **20** | **34** |
| Reticulo-rumen | 38 | 52 | 60 | 64 | 67 | 64 | 64 |
| Omasum | 13 | 12 | 13 | 14 | 18 | 22 | 25 |
| Abomasum | 49 | 36 | 27 | 22 | 15 | 14 | 11 |

A number of other changes occur in the rumen and other tissues during ruminal development, but we will consider the above factors as a requisite for the rumen to begin to function.

*Physical Development of the rumen.* At birth, the rumen and reticulum are under-developed, sterile and nonfunctional. Before solid feed is consumed, the abomasum is the primary compartment of the stomach and nutrients are digested by enzymes. Liquid feeds are shunted past the reticulorumen by the esophageal groove. By the time the calf is weaned, the rumen has become an important compartment of the stomach, and all feed consumed is exposed to bacterial fermentation prior to reaching the abomasum. A net result of this fermentation is a change in the type of energy and protein available to the calf. Figure 5 and Table 3 show a schematic diagram of the stomach development.

Not only does the activity of the stomach compartments change, the size of each compartment changes as well. Besides an increase in size, blood flow to the rumen also has increased. As seen in table 3, the percent of the stomach as reticulorumen increases from a low of about 38% to a high of 67% by 16 weeks of age. Note, however, that by 4 weeks of age, the reticulorumen has increased to 52% of the total stomach capacity. In contrast, the proportion of the stomach as abomasum declines from a high of 49% at birth to a low of 11% after 32 weeks of age. The absolute size of the abomasum does not decline - the reticulorumen simply grows at a much faster rate than the abomasum during ruminal development.

*Establishment of the rumen Microflora.* When the calf is born, the rumen is sterile. However, within 24 hours of age, a large concentration of mostly aerobic bacteria can be found for the fermentation of milk substrate that flows from the abomasum into the rumen. This continues as long as milk is fed. However, aerobic microbes decrease and anaerobes increase as soon as dry feed intake occurs. This is clearly shown in Figure 6. There is a dramatic decrease in the number of aerobic bacteria (solids lines) that occurs approximately 2 weeks after calves begin to consume grain at 1 week, when calves were offered grain from birth, and at 9 weeks when calves were fed only milk for 8 weeks and were then offered grain for the first time. The numbers of total bacteria (dashed lines) does not differ markedly between calves fed only milk to 8 weeks of age or those fed milk and grain. It can be concluded that the change in bacterial types is a function of changes in intake of substrate available for fermentation. The substrate ingested will also affect the types of ruminal bacteria that flourish in the rumen. For example, calves fed mostly hay develop a different flora from those fed mostly grain diets.

*Outflow of Material from the Rumen.* Proper ruminal development requires that material entering

*(continued)*

the rumen must be able to leave it. Measures of ruminal activity include rumen contractions, rumen pressure, and regurgitation (cud chewing). At birth, the rumen has little muscular activity, and few rumen contractions can be measured. Similarly, no regurgitation occurs in the first week or so of life. When calves are fed milk, hay, and grain from shortly after birth, rumen contractions can be measured as early as 3 weeks of age. However, when calves are fed only milk, rumen contractions may not be measurable for extended periods. Cud chewing has been observed as early as 7 days of age, and may not be related to ruminal development per se. However, calves will ruminate for increasing periods when dry feed (particularly hay) is fed.

*Figure 6. Numbers of bacteria in the rumen contents of calves fed milk and grain (From: Lengemann and Allen, 1959)*

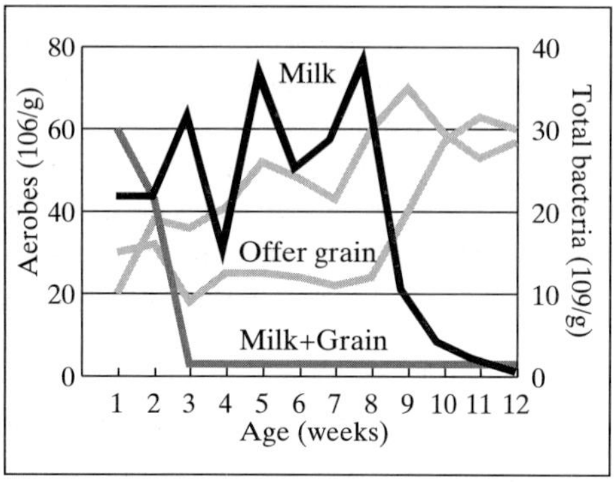


*Absorptive Ability of the Rumen Tissue.* Absorption of end-products of fermentation is an important criterion of ruminal development. End-products of fermentation, particularly the volatile fatty acids (**VFA**; acetate, propionate, and butyrate) are absorbed into the rumen epithelium, where propionate and butyrate are absorbed or metabolized in mature ruminants. Then, the VFA or end-products of metabolism (lactate and ß-hydroxybutyrate) are transported to the blood for use as energy substrates. However, there is little or no absorption or metabolism of VFA in neonatal calves. Therefore, the rumen must develop this ability prior to weaning. The absorptive function of the rumen is located in the epithelial layer. The epithelial layer is composed of a thin film of tissue holding many small finger-like projections called papillae. These papillae provide the absorptive surface for the rumen. At birth, the papillae are small and non-functional. They absorb very little and do not metabolize significant VFA.

The primary stimulus to development of the epithelium in relation to size and number of papillae and their ability to absorb and metabolize VFA are the VFA. Milk, grain, and hay added to the rumen are all fermented by the resident bacteria; therefore, they contribute VFA for epithelial development. Plastic sponges and inert particles - both added to the rumen to provide "scratch" - did not promote development of the epithelium. Thus, the primary factor determining ruminal development (defined as the development of the epithelium) is primarily driven by **chemical** (the availability of dry feed, particularly starter), and not **by physical** means. The absorption of VFA increased dramatically to 14 weeks of age when calves were fed milk, hay, and grain. However, when calves were fed only milk to 14 weeks, there was little absorption by epithelium.

When calves are given grain on week 15, the absorption of VFA began shortly after consumption of grain began. From these and other data, it appears that to promote early rumen development to allow early weaning, the key factor is early consumption of a diet to promote growth of the ruminal epithelium and ruminal motility. Because grains provide carbohydrates that are fermented to propionate and butyrate,

*(continued)*

they are a good choice to ensure early rumen development. On the other hand, the structural carbohydrate of forages tend to be fermented to a greater extent to acetate, which is less stimulatory to ruminal development. Although forage has less of an effect on ruminal epithelial development, forage is *very important* to promote the growth of the muscular layer of the rumen and to maintain the health of the epithelium.

*Figure 7. Intake of starter and hay by calves (From: Lengemann and Allen, 1959)*

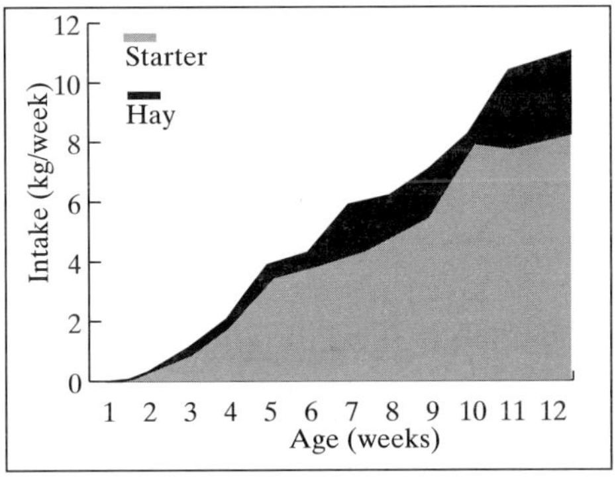


**Weaning**

*Biological Impact of Weaning.*

At weaning, the calf is forced to undergo several dramatic changes. Consider the following:

1. the primary source of nutrients changes from liquid to solids,
2. changes in housing and management often occur around weaning which can add to stress, such as moving calves from individual pens or hutches to group pens.

Stresses associated with this management change include social adaptation, introduction of different feeds (particularly forages), and exposure to pathogens. Generally, it is recommended that management changes such as housing should take place after weaning to minimize the overall stress to which the calf is exposed.

Many producers wean calves at 4 to 5 weeks of age and offer hay from 6 to 7 weeks of age. Effects of early weaning (4 to 6 weeks of age) on indices of stress in young dairy calves have been evaluated. Reddy et al., (1985) reported that early weaning (2 or 3 weeks of age) did not significantly affect lymphocyte blastogenesis, an indicator of immune response. Intake of dry matter and body weight gain of calves weaned at 3, 5, or 7 weeks of age did not differ significantly, although feed efficiency appeared to increase with increasing age of weaning.

If calves are not weaned until 8 to 10 weeks of age, it may be advised to feed a limited amount of hay (400 - 500 g/day) from about 6 weeks of age. In Figure 7, it is clear that most of the intake of hay occurred only after 6 to 7 weeks of age. However, the amount of hay should be limited to ensure that calves will consume sufficient starter. Most hay has too little energy for calves. The energy requirement for calves can usually be met when calves are fed high quality milk replacer, waste milk and/or excess colostrum and calf starter. Even good quality legume hay generally has too little energy to support growth of preweaned calves. Moreover most calves do not eat significant amounts of hay if grain is also offered (Figure 7). Therefore, producers feed calves the best quality hay available on the farm, only to have it turned into bedding. Moreover calves should be eating at least 1 kg of starter per 100 kg body weight before they are weaned.

Weaning age is also used to determine the number of calves to retain for replacement purposes. Table 4 provides the number of calves that should be retained at various culling rates. However periodic adjustment should be made to the number of young stock to more accurately reflect the farm's needs for replacements and for income from the sale of heifers.

(Table 5), decreased costs, increased herd turnover (making voluntary culling easier), greater lifetime productivity potential, increased rolling herd average and increased profitability. Disadvantages are a higher risk for dystocia and related health problems and a decreased first lactation yield (Hoffman, 1992; Hoffman and Funk, 1992). The most efficient and profitable time to achieve growth in young stock is from weaning to breeding. Lower levels of management and especially nutrition during this period will delay the time to breeding. As a result of delayed breeding, first lactation milk production is delayed which lowers income. Moreover, time and costs of maintaining the heifer increases as growth decreases in the second half of the rearing period (Van Amburgh and Galton, 1994).

There are three important concepts that must be understood when discussing growth rate during the rearing period:

1. it is important to distinghuish between true growth and fattening. True growth is defined as an increase in structural tissues such as muscle, bone, and vital organs, while fattening is defined as a disproportional increase of fat in fat depots (Skidmore, 1995),
2. growth rates should always be related to mature body size. Mature body size is a combination of weight and frame size of an adult cow. Average mature body size of a Holstein cow with a body condition score of 3.0 is 675 kg in body weight and 145 cm in height at the withers. It is assumed that the ultimate mature body size is normally reached in the 3rd lactation,
3. one should realize that growth rate varies with time. Growth starts slowly, reaches a maximum around puberty and slows down thereafter (Judge et al., 1989).

*Table 4. Number of heifers to maintain a herd size of 100 (Source: Menzi, 1995)*

| | Age at first calving (months) | | | | | | |
|---|---|---|---|---|---|---|---|
| | **20** | **22** | **24** | **26** | **28** | **30** | **32** |
| **Cull rate %** | | | **– Number of heifers –** | | | | |
| 20 | 37 | 40 | 44 | 48 | 51 | 55 | 59 |
| 22 | 40 | 44 | 48 | 52 | 56 | 61 | 65 |
| 24 | 44 | 48 | 53 | 57 | 62 | 66 | 70 |
| 26 | 48 | 52 | 57 | 62 | 67 | 72 | 76 |
| 28 | 51 | 56 | 62 | 67 | 72 | 77 | 82 |
| 30 | 55 | 61 | 66 | 72 | 77 | 83 | 88 |
| 32 | 59 | 65 | 70 | 76 | 82 | 88 | 94 |
| 34 | 62 | 69 | 75 | 81 | 87 | 94 | 100 |
| 36 | 66 | 73 | 79 | 86 | 92 | 99 | 106 |

Holstein heifers normally experience puberty (first estrus) at approximately 42% or 270 to 300 kg of mature body weight. This can occur between 7 and 11 months of age, depending on their prepubertal growth rate. Puberty is determined more by body weight than by age. Age at puberty declines with increased feed intake and body weight gain, so puberty can be manipulated by feeding (Stelwagen and Grieve, 1990). Independent of age at first calving, heifers should conceive at approximately 55% (370 kg), and have a postcalving weight of 85% (570 kg) of a mature body weight (675 kg). The goal for wither height and body condition at time of calving of heifers is 142 cm and 3 to 3.5 respectively. Target age at first calving may vary from farm to farm. A good average is 24 months (Hoffman and Funk, 1992), although some farms may target for less than 24 months age at first calving (Skidmore, 1995).

Age at first calving can only be manipulated by shortening or lengthening the interval between birth and conception. To achieve an age of first calving of 24 months the interval from birth to first breeding should not be longer than 13 months to get all heifers pregnant between 14 and 15 months of age. If the target age at first calving is 21 months, then breeding should start between 10 and 11 months of age and conception should occur by 12 months of age. An average daily gain of 900 grams from birth until conception is required to achieve a body weight of 370 kg at conception at 12 months of age. This average daily rate of gain is not desirable if body condition exceeds a score of 3.5. Different growth standards for replacement heifers have been published (Heinrichs and Hardgrove, 1987; Hoffman and Funk 1991; Skidmore, 1995 (Table 5).

Although it can be stated that at time of first calving larger heifers have higher first lactation milk production, after a certain body size incremental increases in milk production become much smaller in relation to incremental increases in postcalving body weight (Keown and Everett, 1986; Heinrich and Hargrove, 1987; Bucholtz, 1993). Optimal milk production (not maximum) occurs at that point when incremental increases of post calving body size results in smaller increases on milk production. This point of diminishing returns is about 85% of mature body weight or 570 kg for Holsteins at a body condition score of 3.0 (Skidmore, 1995). Since bone matures at an earlier age than other structural tissues, wither height at first calving should be about 95% of mature height or 142 cm for most Holsteins. It minimizes the necessary additional growth until the end of the third lactation. When first calf heifers calve at less than optimum body size they do not catch up in milk production with herd mates who calve at more optimum sizes (Fahr et al., 1985; Lin et al., 1985). To achieve a postcalving body weight of 570 kg in 24 or 21 months, an average daily gain of 729 or 821 grams respectively is required throughout the rearing period. However, the concept of optimal growth is related to how rates of gain during the prepubertal growth period affect mammary gland development (Hoffman and Funk, 1992; Skidmore, 1995). To ensure optimal mammary development, growth rate must be differentiated during the 24 month rearing period.

Mammary growth in heifers commences before puberty. At 2 to 3 months of age the mammary gland begins to develop at a rate that is faster (allometric) than body growth. After puberty, the rate of mammary development starts to slow down. By the second or third estrous cycle the mammary gland is once again developing at the same

*Table 5. Monthly body weights (BW, kg), average daily gains (ADG, g/day), and total weight (TW) for heifers calving at 570 kg, at 21, 24, and 27 months of age. TW includes BW and pregnancy weigth (PW) Pregnancy weight (PW) is only listed for calving at 21 months. Precalving weigth condition scores fall between 3.0 and 3.5; * postcalving, ** precalving (Adapted from Skidmore, 1995)*

| AGE | 21 Months AFC | | | | 24 Months AFC | | 27 Months AFC | |
|---|---|---|---|---|---|---|---|---|
| **MO** | **BW** | **ADG** | **PW** | **TW** | **TW** | **ADG** | **TW** | **ADG** |
| 0 | 41 | | 0 | 41 | 41 | | | 41 |
| 1 | 58 | 593 | 0 | 58 | 56 | 501 | 54 | 456 |
| 2 | 80 | 684 | 0 | 80 | 74 | 592 | 70 | 501 |
| 3 | 104 | 821 | 0 | 104 | 95 | 684 | 88 | 592 |
| 4 | 132 | 912 | 0 | 132 | 118 | 775 | 108 | 684 |
| 5 | 162 | 1003 | 0 | 162 | 144 | 866 | 130 | 729 |
| 6 | 194 | 1048 | 0 | 194 | 170 | 912 | 152 | 775 |
| 7 | 227 | 1095 | 0 | 227 | 99 | 957 | 177 | 820 |
| 8 | 260 | 1095 | 0 | 260 | 228 | 957 | 202 | 866 |
| 9 | 293 | 1095 | 0 | 293 | 257 | 957 | 228 | 866 |
| 10 | 329 | 1095 | 0 | 329 | 286 | 957 | 254 | 866 |
| 11 | 357 | 1095 | 0 | 357 | 315 | 957 | 280 | 866 |
| 12 | 387 | 1003 | 0 | 387 | 343 | 912 | 304 | 866 |
| 13 | 414 | 912 | 2 | 418 | 369 | 912 | 331 | 820 |
| 14 | 440 | 866 | 5 | 445 | 395 | 866 | 355 | 820 |
| 15 | 465 | 821 | 15 | 480 | 419 | 820 | 378 | 775 |
| 16 | 487 | 730 | 26 | 513 | 443 | 775 | 401 | 729 |
| 17 | 507 | 684 | 36 | 544 | 468 | 684 | 422 | 729 |
| 18 | 525 | 593 | 47 | 572 | 497 | 638 | 442 | 684 |
| 19 | 542 | 547 | 58 | 600 | 527 | 592 | 463 | 638 |
| 20 | 556 | 502 | 68 | 625 | 553 | 547 | 484 | 592 |
| 21 | 570* | 502 | 68 | 638** | 579 | 501 | 510 | 547 |
| 22 | | | | | 604 | 456 | 536 | 501 |
| 23 | | | | | 627 | 410 | 560 | 456 |
| 24 | | | | | 638 | 364 | 583 | 456 |
| 25 | | | | | | | 608 | 410 |
| 26 | | | | | | | 629 | 364 |
| 27 | | | | | | | 638** | 319 |
| AVG | | 821 | | | | 729 | | 638 |

proportionate rate as the rest of the body. This is referred to as isometric growth. Before puberty, mammary development is characterized by ductal development. After puberty and especially after conception, mammary development is characterized by elongation of ducts and alveolar development. Towards the end of gestation and early lactation, mammary parenchymal growth becomes allometric again (Tucker, 1987; Akers et al., 1981).

As already mentioned, the only way to shorten age at first calving, is by shortening the interval from birth to first breeding. This may be achieved by balancing nutrient intake from birth to first breeding. This period encompasses the prepubertal period during which mammary development may be adversely affected by high energy unbalanced diets. The critical period is from 3 through 10 months of age (Folgdager and Sejrsen, 1987). Sjersen et al. (1982) reported that heifers raised on high energy diets (1100 to 1200 g/day daily weight gain) with relatively low crude protein (14.6 to 16.5% of dry matter) during this critical period had less mammary parenchymal tissue than those raised on lower energy diets (daily gains of 600 to 740 g/day). Increased energy intakes after puberty have no effect on subsequent mammary gland development (Sejrsen et al., 1982; Peri et al., 1993). Others have reported similar observations (Harrison et al., 1983; Stelwagen and Grieve, 1990).

Sejrsen (1983) suggested that feeding high energy diets during the allometric period decreases growth hormone levels in blood causing a decrease in mammary secretory tissue development. Administration of exogenous growth hormone reversed these effects (Hoffman, 1992). Recently, Hovey et al., 1994, developed a new concept in which the fat pad plays an important role. The fat pad may be receiving hormonal signals which act upon the fat cell itself and the fat cell in turn responds by sending signals to the ductal tissue. Excessive energy intakes depress levels of these hormones thus reducing the development of parenchyma tissue during the prepubertal period.

Many have assumed that decreased parenchymal tissue before puberty causes reduced milk production (Gardner et al. (1977); Little and Kay, (1979); Harrison et al. (1983); Peri et al. (1993). In contrast Cappuco et al., (1995) raised heifers at different rates of gain and different diets. They demonstrated that high rates of gain on corn silage during the critical period decreased mammary development but had no effect on subsequent milk production.

Increasing dietary energy alone before puberty is not a useful approach to shorten the birth to conception interval and achieve maximal milk production (Tucker, 1987). In contrast, Kertz et al. (1987) concluded that body weight gains of 0.9 to 1.0 kg/day due to greater skeletal growth without fattening is feasible. Such body weight gain would not impair mammogenesis and subsequent lactation. A prerequisite is that an increased prepubertal energy intake is combined with a sufficient (17%) protein intake to provide nutrients for body weight gains of ≥ 0.8 kg/day without fattening (Kertz et al., 1987). However, one has to realize that there is still a great deal of controversy over the ideal postcalving target weight and frame size, and age at first calving.

## EPILOGUE

The protocol for monitoring replacement rearing should assist practitioners, farm advisors and farmers to identify weaknesses in management and offer strategies for improvement. Proper replacement management begins before birth with selection of genetics, ensuring cow health, and use of proper breeding techniques. At calving meticulous attention to cleanliness is essential to minimize the incidence of disease to both the dam and the calf. For the first 24 hours after birth, the calf can absorb large molecules without digestion, which allows acquisition of Ig from colostrum. The efficiency of Ig absorption declines rapidly, so early colostrum feeding is essential. Consumption of at least 100 g of IgG at each feeding is essential to minimize calf mobidity and mortality.

The next period is aimed at optimizing replacement growth up to a calving age of 24 months or less together with a body weight of about 570 kg and a wither height of 142 cm postcalving for Holstein cattle. To keep young stock on these targets, problems during the rearing period have to be identified and appropriate corrections have to be made in time and adequately. To prevent problems growth of young stock should constantly be monitored at regular intervals. A HH & PM program offers the frame work for an adequate monitoring system.

*For references see part 2 of this Chapter.*

# 2.2 MONITORING REPLACEMENT REARING: EXECUTION, DECISION MAKING AND FOLLOW-UP

James D. Quigley III[1], Arie Brand[2], Geert Benedictus[3] and Bram Kloosterman[4]

[1] III, Department of Animal Science, The University of Tennessee, P.O. Box 1071, Knoxville, TN 37901 1071, USA
[2] Department of Herd Health and Reproduction, School of Veterinary Medicine, University of Utrecht, Yalelaan 7, 3485 CL Utrecht, The Netherlands
[3] Animal Health Station Noord Nederland, Morra 2, P.O. Box 361, 9200 AJ Drachten, The Netherlands
[4] Department of Animal Husbandry, Animal Health & Reproduction division, Agricultural University of WageningeN, Marijkeweg 40, 6700 AH Wageningen, The Netherlands

## 2.2.1 INTRODUCTION

Replacement rearing is directed at developing the cow of the future. Many dairy farmers consider the rearing period as a nonproductive period in the replacement's life which requires little attention. However, the rearing period must be considered as an investment in the future of the dairy enterprise. In this period, adequate management practices must be exercised and environmental conditions created with the objective of achieving optimal productivity by exploiting the genetic make-up and biological processes of young stock. The total rearing period consists of several physiologic stages with different periods of susceptibility to disease that determine the expression of the genetic potential of the animal in adult life. The expression of the genetic potential should be monitored throughout the rearing period.

Part 1 of this Chapter dealt with preset targets and material and methods and with overall management strategies used in the various replacement rearing periods. In part 2 of this Chapter special attention will be paid to executional and decision making activities and to follow-up, within the framework of a replacement rearing protocol.

## 2.2.2 EXECUTION

The monitoring process of replacement rearing is made up of three activities:

1. Data inspection, inclusive data collection practices, and calculation of relevant indices,
2. Clinical examination of young stock that are diseased or whose performance indices are unsatisfactory, and implementation of protocols of preventive measures,

3. Farm inspection, consisting of a diagnostic stroll over the farm to discover risky situations.

The various aspects will be dicussed using the development time table presented in part 1.

### 2.2.3 DATA INSPECTION

Data inspection should include data in the farm diary, Calf Rearing Chart (CRC), grassland chart or computerized data records. Records must be inspected for timeliness and completeness. On many dairy farms data recording related to young stock rearing is inconsistent or incomplete because the rearing period is considered nonproductive. The best way to stimulate the farmer is to process recorded data into performance indices and provide information to the farmer in an understandable and practical way that can be used in daily management. Of all the performance indices on replacement rearing listed in Table 1 of Chapter 2, part 1, the primary indices should be calculated regularly or at least 3 to 4 times a year. The secondary indices should only be calculated if one or more primary indices deviate from the preset targets. For this reason data inspection should be done during each HH & PM farm visit and the HH & PM practitioner and/or farm advisor should stimulate the farmer to collect and process data for use in daily management.

### 2.2.4 CLINICAL INSPECTION

The high value of breeding material and the major expenses of labor, supplies, and feeds, demands daily concern for calf health and growth by the farmer. The clinical inspection of replacement heifers by the practitioner should begin by monitoring the CRC and farm diary for the incidence and current prevalence of diseases of the alimentary and respiratory tracts, infections of the umbilical cord, congenital abnormalities and other diseases up to the end of the rearing period.

Replacement heifers are often grouped and separated by age or stages of development. Examples of age groups are: 0 - 3 weeks; 3 weeks - 2 months; 3 - 9 months; 10 - 15 months; and > 15 months. Divisions in groups may differ from farm to farm. Each age group is subject to its own set of potential health problems influenced by managerial and environmental conditions.

During a clinical inspection the following should be checked within each age group:

#### Age group 0 - 2 weeks

Calves should be monitored both as a group and individually. Diseased calves should be examined clinically, and should be isolated from healthy calves and treated appropriately. This limits the horizontal spread of infection in the group and the rest of the herd. Early detection and treatment of diseases is important in calf rearing, as treatment is more successful in an early stage of the disease. Disease also has a great influence on performance in later life. Scours and respiratory diseases influence body weight gain negatively (Quigley et al., 1995).

Rates of calfhood morbidity and mortality are greatly influenced by: the management system, and quality of personnel implementing it, the calf's passive immunity level, burden of pathogens in the environment and the nutritional quality of the diet. In case of diarrhea problems, blood samples should be taken in the first week of life, to determine the immunoglobuline level and hence colostrum management.

* **alimentary tract diseases**

In case of alimentary tract diseases, feces consistency should always be scored (see method described by Larson et al., 1977). Important agents that cause alimentary tract diseases and their respective critical risk periods (Figure 1) are *E. coli*, Rota and Corona virus, *Salmonella sp.*, Coccidiosis sp., *Cryptosporidium* (see page 106 and 107).

* **prevention of alimentary tract diseases**

*E. coli.* The best defences against *E. coli* are sanitation of calving facilities, immediate separation of the calf from its dam and feeding a sufficient amount of high quality colostrum within the first hour after birth. Producers should work with their HH & PM practitioner to determine if any of the commercially available *E. coli* vaccines would be indicated in their herds.

**Enteric viruses**. Most pathogens that cause enteric diseases are noninvasive, such as Rota and Corona virus. However, to protect calves against these virus infections, continuing adequate amounts of specific IgG1 antibodies in the gut lumen must be present. IgG's in the gut are delivered in the gut in two ways: 1) via intake of colostrum and hence local deposition of IgG antibodies in the lumen of the gastrointestinal tract

*Figure 1. The most common ages at which scours are caused by various infectious organisms in dairy calves*

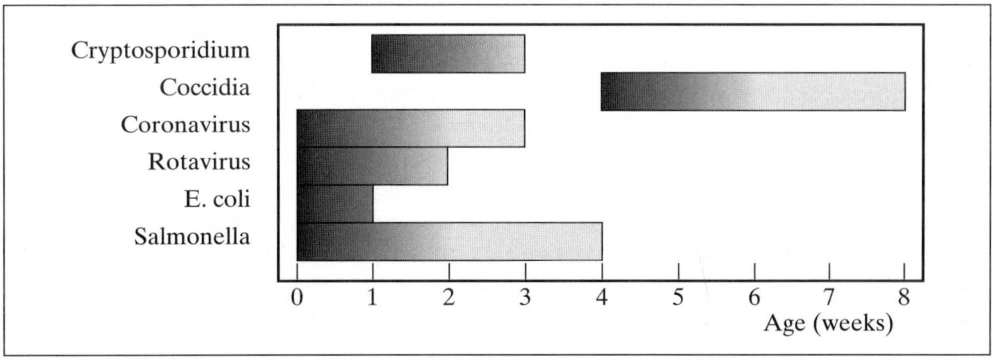

*Escherichia coli.* The two distinct disease conditions caused by *E. coli* are septicemia and enterotoxemia.

Septicemia occurs when the bacteria reach the small intestine before the calf consumes colostrum in sufficient quantity and of adequate quality. Disease occurs very quickly - usually calves show signs of diarrhea, depression, coma and die from septicemia within 24 to 36 hours after birth.

*Enterotoxemia,* or *E. coli* enteritis usually occurs within the first 7 days of life during which period bacteria attach to the receptors of mucosa cells of the intestinal wall of the calf and proliferate. By ageing, maturation of receptors on these mucosa cells occurs, which results in reduced susceptibility and faster excretion of pathogens (Gunther and Schulze, 1985). The bacteria produce toxins that causes the calf to move water into the intestine to flush toxins and bacteria out of the system and regain osmotic balance. Diarrhea produced by *E. coli* is profuse, watery and may contain blood.

*Rotavirus.* The virus which is transmitted through ingestion causes enteritis manifested by scours in calves, primarily from 3 to 19 days of age. Fecal samples may be positive up to about four weeks of age. Rotavirus attacks the villi of the epithelial cells of the small intestines; the large intestine is spared. Loss of villous epithelial cells and shortening of villi reduce the absorptive function of the small intestines, usually resulting in mild to moderate scours. Most calves will recover in uncomplicated cases. Often such complications are caused by *E. coli* infections. As with bovine Coronavirus, Rotavirus may be detected in both diarrhoeic and healthy calves. Rotavirus is widespread in the environment and resistant to many disinfectants except iodophores, so eliminating the virus from the farm is unlikely (Saif and Smith, 1985; Janke,1989; Bezek, 1994; Fagan et al., 1995).

*Coronavirus.* Bovine coronavirus (BCV) commonly causes scours in calves from three days to three weeks of age, although some calves may be affected up to three months of age. Calves may be infected with BCV by both the oral and respiratory routes. Subclinically persistent infected older calves and adult cows may harbor coronavirus and pass it to susceptible calves. Disease is more prevalent in cold winter months. The clinical signs associated with BCV enteritis are indistinguishable from those associated with rotavirus infection. Scours caused by the virus are profuse, yellowish and watery. The diarrhea is caused by a reduced absorptive and digestive capacity of the gut caused by damage of small intestinal villous epithelial cells and of epithelial cells of the colonic mucosa, including cells lining the crypts. Dehydration and acid-base imbalances can occur quickly in severe cases. The majority of calves recovers, but a few may die if diarrhoea is particularly severe (Clark, 1993).

*Salmonella.* Salmonella is one of the most common foodborne pathogens transmitted to humans (Losinger et al., 1995). Several species of the bacterium Salmonella can cause scours in young calves such as *S. typhimurium and S. dublin*. Salmonella causes scours in calves as early as 4 days of age (Figure 1), although it most commonly affects calves between one and four weeks. Salmonella strikes calves quickly, so youngest calves are at the greatest risk. Some calves may carry the organism but not show signs of disease. However, salmonella can also be found in older cattle and may cause disease or serve as a source of infection on the farm. Salmonella incidence varies by season, with greatest prevalence in late summer and fall, and lowest in late winter Hoorfar et al., 1993; Wray, 1993)

*Coccidia.* Scours caused by the most pathogenic coccidia *Eimeria bovis* and *Eimeria zuernii* usually occur after four weeks of age. Calves may be infected with coccidia as early as the first week of life, but the incubation period is about three weeks, so signs of infection (ie., diarrhea, often with blood) will not occur until then. Upon ingestion, coccidial oocysts multiply inside intestinal cells, causing damage to the intestinal wall. When the life cycle is complete, oocysts are excreted into the manure to repeat the process (Oetjen, 1993)

*Cryptosporidium.* Cryptosporidiosis is a zoonotic disease. The incubation period is two to seven days. This parasite causes scours in calves usually during the second and third weeks of life. Calves with cryptosporidiosis have pale, yellowish, nonhemorrhagic, watery faeces. The calves show signs of tenesmus, weight loss, anorexia, depression, weakness and dehydration. The oocytes are transmitted by the fecal-oral route and are immediately infective when shed. Scours caused by *Cryptosporidium* will clear up in 5 to 10 days if there is no secondary infection by enteric viruses. By the fourth week of life, the incidence of scours caused by *Cryptosporidium* declines as the calf develops immunity against the organism (Moore, 1989). Prevalence of *Cryptosporidium* (followed by prevalence of rotavirus) was the most significant factor influencing the incidence of scours, severity of scours and the number of days of scouring per week in a study in the U.S. (Quigley et al., 1994).

There are other micro-organisms that can cause scours in calves besides those listed here. A key component of proper diagnosis is the age of the calf. However, in some cases, more than one micro-organism is involved, so diagnosis is more difficult.

on day 1 of life, and 2) by a continuous secretion of circulating antibodies (IgG) from blood back to the intestine after day 1 (Saif and Smith, 1985; Besser et al., 1988a and 1988b; Clark, 1993; Bezek, 1994). Prolonged presence of protective levels of specific antibodies in the lumen of the small intestine over the first month of life can be established by: 1) production of colostrum with high concentrations of specific IgG's via vaccination of dams against relevant pathogens which should directly be fed after birth, and 2) prolonged feeding of colostrum with high titres of specific IgG's (Saif and Smith, 1985; Besser et al., 1988a and 1988b). In Rotavirus trials the highest specific IgG titres in colostrum against Rotavirus were obtained when pregnant dams were intramuscularly vaccinated at 9 weeks, and intramammary at two weeks before expected time of calving (Saif and Smith, 1985). The antibody response seems to depend on the adjuvant selected, virus titre, antigenic form (live or inactivated) and the route of administration (Saif et al., 1983). Both just mentioned approaches can prevent infection and diarrhea after Rotavirus challenge but high titres are necessary for complete protection (Saif and Smith, 1985; Besser et al., 1988 a and 1988 b). Diarrhea is most likely to occur if the passively acquired immunity declines before an adequate level of active immunity has developed. Therefore, it is advisable to have a bank of deep frozen high quality colostrum available, preferably from vaccinated older cows, for problem situations. Following natural exposure to Rotavirus and bovine coronavirus, BCV, infection, calves develop active immunity to the viruses.

Besides optimization of colostrum management to minimize scours caused by enteric viruses, further management practices should be directed at:

*) restriction of virus transmission in a herd. This can be achieved by providing optimal hygienic conditions at the time of birth, and implementation of proper hygiene practices during the colostrum and milk feeding period. Potential locations or management practices that serve as a source of infection should be identified and eliminated, and power washing of housing facilities, (feeding) equipment and boots should be practised before disinfection is performed. The rate of calf diarrhea is also influenced by overcrowding and calving pattern (Bezek, 1994; Fagan et al., 1995).

*) daily attention to good ventilation practices, including temperature, and humidity. Individual hutches may provide good isolation and dry, well-ventilated conditions for dairy calves (Janke, 1989; Bezek, 1994).

*) oral vaccination of neonatal calves to stimulate active immunity. This approach has not proved effective in field trials (Clark, 1993). The latter is probably because the virus in the vaccine is neutralized in the gut by passively acquired maternal antibodies (Bezek, 1994).

*Salmonella.* The primary sources of infection are contaminated feed, purchased infected calves and (latently) infected animals on the farm. An outbreak of salmonellosis in calf facilities can be devastating, with many calves being affected and dying. Calving in an individual area of a building, sanitation of utensils and facilities, provision of medicated milk replacer, feeding clean hay to nibble, and isolation of calves are the best prevention against salmonellosis (Losinger et al., 1995). Because salmonella generally affect young calves (± 4 weeks of age), the amount of colostrum calves consume can influence their resistance to the bacteria. There are also vaccines available that are effective against salmonella. Salmonella may be transmitted to humans, so calf raisers must be diligent in their personal hygiene when working with calves (see also Chapter 8).

*Coccidia.* Coccidia infect the calf through ingestion of oocysts originating from bedding or manure, making sanitation and isolation very critical. Housing calves in hutches is particularly effective against coccidia infections. Grouping of calves in small numbers together with an all-in-all-out system should be practised. Manure packs in loose housing groups should be removed continuously as these can provide ideal conditions for year round sporulation and survival of oocysts (Oetjen, 1993).

*Cryptosporidium.* Almost all herds are positive for *Cryptosporidium* and about 50% of all calves at any point in time from 1 to 3 weeks of age will be positive for the organism, so the goal is not to eliminate the pathogen, but to control or manage the disease. Due to the resistant nature of the *Cryptosporidium* oocysts, it is virtually impossible to eliminate the disease from a herd. Therefore, newborn calves should be separated from their dams immediately after birth and moved to completely different ground (Moore, 1989).

**Age group of 0.5 - 3 months**

As in the period of 0 to 2 weeks individual calves should be monitored for signs of diarrhea, including consistency and colour of feces and respiratory abnormalities. Prevalence of anaemic calves should be monitored. A clinically anaemic calf exhibits depressed appetite, reduced efficiency of body weight gain and greater susceptibility to disease. Blood haemoglobin concentration < 7.0 g/dl is considered clinically anaemic. Discharges from the nose, eyes and mouth or coughing should be monitored. The navel should be evaluated for swelling. The physical examination should also include inspection of the condition of the haircoat including moisture, dirtiness, shine and presence of skin lesions, and the rumen-fill.

Activities such as dehorning, removing extra teats and measuring chest circumferences should be performed on young calves. Diseased individuals may be treated or culled. Prophylactic and disease control measures should be instituted as needed. Calves must not be allowed to suck navels or ears as this predisposes calves to disease.

* **respiratory tract diseases**

The most critical period for respiratory disease in calves is between the second and tenth month of life. The most common infectious agents are:
- Bovine Respiratory Syncitial Virus (BRSV),
- Para Influenza-3 Virus (PI-3),
- Bovine Herpes Virus-1 (BHV-1),
- Bovine Virus Diarrhoea/Mucosal Disease virus (BVD/MD),
- Mycoplasma spp.,
- Pasteurella spp.,
- Haemophilus spp.,
- Salmonella spp.

On problem farms, a thorough clinical examination should be conducted and paired serum samples should be collected to examine for seroconversion to respiratory disease agents. These samples should also be taken from other calves to determine if they are subclinically affected. Nasal swabs and lung lavage samples for either virus isolation or immunofluorescent staining of epithelial cells for virus antigens should be used to reach a diagnosis of involved microbiological agents. For more details regarding some of the aforenamed diseases (see Chapter 2, part 4 and Chapter 8).

In addition to clinical and microbiological features regarding respiratory disease, attention should be paid also to managerial and environmental aspects. There are examples in literature dealing with these issues. For example the field study in 104 selected Ontario dairy herds (Canada) presented by Waltner-Toews et al. (1986). Among the risk indicators associated with an increased risk of pneumonia were: poor colostrum feeding method, night time feeding, poor navel disinfection, farm size. Several of these factors refer to the attention given to the calves. Another example refers to a field survey by Perez et al. (1994) in 42 Costa Rican dairy herds. Among risk indicators related to respiratory disease detected in their survey were: breeds other than Holstein, time of calving during the day, number of days colostrum was fed, housing conditions, milk replacer type, floor type. Although specific indicators may vary between geographical areas and production systems, it appears that several risk indicators are related to management and environment, which can be adjusted by changing farm management practices. Most respiratory infections in young stock are infectious in nature, but are multifactorial in causality. Therefore, these contributory aspects have to be addressed too. To a certain extent these are addressed under the heading of "farm inspection" during the routine farm visit.

**Age group of 3 - 15 months**

The physical examination is conducted as in the younger group. Chest circumference and wither height should be measured every two months by the farmer after instruction by the HH & PM practitioner. Body condition should be scored regularly on a scale of 1 to 5 (Wildman et al., 1982). The estimated weight, growth per day, and condition scores should be used to monitor replacement rearing performance. They are also indicators of the health status of individual calves and groups of calves and can be used to evaluate all aspects of management from the milk feeding period to calving and to culling. In this respect they can be compared with milk recording and milk quality data.

Rations should be formulated monthly. In addition, claw health should be evaluated regularly, especially with regard to dermatitis digitalis and interdigitalis (Chapter 7). Regular foot bathing with a 4% formalin solution should be practised. The reproductive tract must be checked for abnormalities before breeding is initiated.

Prevention of infectious diseases, including parasitic diseases, is an important field of attention. The vaccination strategy and the environmental conditions should therefore be evaluated periodically. The vaccination strategy may include vaccination against paratuberculosis, BRSV, PI-3, BHV-1, BVD/MD, leptospirosis, lungworm, clostridia and *Brucella abortus* if necessary. Blood, feces, and/or urine samples should be taken periodically or as indicated to monitor health and nutritional status of a representative group of young stock. Finally, young stock should be listed for breeding and a pre-breeding check should be performed.

* **parasitic diseases**

The parasitic diseases in calves to be dealt with here are the gastrointestinal nematodes, lungworms and liver fluke. The economic impact of fluke infections, which always occur at the subclinical level in bovines, is however less important in calves than in lactating animals, where they may cause production losses of 5 - 10%.

**Gastrointestinal nematodes**

These parasites comprise more than ten different species. In the cool and moist climates *Ostertagia ostertagi, Trichostrongylus axeí, Cooperia oncophora,* and *Nematodirus helvetianus,* are the most prevalent species, the first two mentioned parasitize the abomasum, and the last two the small intestine. In warm climates the very pathogenic and prolific abomasal parasite *Haemonchus contortus* and *Oesophagostomum radiatum* (in the large intestine) may also be found. This variety of species is less

## Epidemiology of trichostrongylosis

It can be safely assumed that all calves on pasture become infected with gastrointestinal worms. The calves infect themselves by the intake of infective larvae with the herbage. The origin of these larvae may be overwintered larvae in case cattle are housed during the winter and calves are reared saperated from their dam. This is the case for most dairy enterprises in the cooler climates of the USA and NW Europe. In warmer climates with year-round grazing the origin of the larvae often should be sought in fields that have previously been grazed by older stock. In beef enterprises the first larvae are picked up from eggs excreted by the dam, a situation comparable to sheep husbandry. After an initial infection calves begin to excrete eggs after 3 weeks. Depending on weather conditions infective larvae from these eggs can be expected in the faeces after one week. In the temperate climates the average conditions are such that the outcome of larvae accrues more or less, resulting in the so called mid-summer increase in larval herbage infestation followed sometimes by disease manifestation (Michel, 1969, 1976). There is a clear relationship between the level of initial (overwintered) infection and the level of herbage infestation in the mid-summer increase. The initial level can be kept low by starting on newly sown leys or on pasture that has not been grazed in the preceeding season by susceptible stock in the late summer and autumn, and has been mown for silage or hay before calves are introduced (Kloosterman, 1971). In temperate regions disease can be seen in first year grazing calves from late July onwards, but depending on the initial level of infection and the weather conditions, this is often postponed to the autumn, or clinical symptoms are not seen at all.

A special epidemiological feature is the occurrence of arrested development. This is especially true for the species Ostertagia ostertagi, which is arrested in the early fourth larval stage. Larvae picked up in the autumn are conditioned to enter this hypobiotic condition, they resume their development in the early spring, causing disease (Type two Ostertagiasis) if this occurs massively (Martin et al., 1957; Anderson et al., 1965). Other species manifest this arrested development also, (it is probably an adaptation of the parasite to survive difficult periods such as the winter in temperate climates and the dry period in tropical climates) but there is no disease entity connected with it, like in *O. ostertagi*.

Apart from the underlying biology of the parasites, the epidemiology is greatly influenced by environmental factors, which can be divided in those which can be influenced by the management of the farmer and other factors like climate and weather. The climate has a profound influence on the species distribution, and one of the first things to be determined is the species profile prevailing in the region. The weather is another condition that cannot be influenced by the farmer, but it is not structural or permanent, so it can only help to support advice given in a specific situation. From the weather conditions rainfall is undoubtedly the most important, because it enables the infective larvae to leave the fecal pat and migrate to the herbage. Temperature is also important for the development of eggs to larvae, but because this process takes place within the protected surroundings of the fecal pat, this is not as great a source of variation as rainfall. High temperatures are important because they decrease the longevity of infective larvae once they are on the herbage. The fecal pat serves as a reservoir for infective larvae under dry weather conditions, until sufficient rainfall causes them to migrate to the herbage in unusually high numbers. This is very pertinent in any situation where advice should be given for instance with respect to moving and/or treating animals.

problematic than it seems at first sight, because the life cycle is for all species very similar: direct, i.e. without an intermediate host, and with a prepatent period (the interval between uptake of infection and the start of fecal egg excretion) of around 21 days.
In addition the modern anthelmintics are nearly equally effective against all these species. However, the species differ greatly in pathogenicity as well as in prolificity, while their eggs in the feces cannot properly be distinguished from each other. This makes the interpretation of egg counts difficult as will be discussed later.

**Management factors**

These can be divided into grassland management and stock management and, where these two come together: grazing management.

- **grassland management.** Besides permanent grassland there are fields which are part of a rotation scheme with arable land, known as ley pastures. From the standpoint of parasitic diseases ley pastures offer great opportunities for prevention. Permanent pastures are more liable to create parasite problems, particularly in those areas of the world where all year round grazing is practised and no housing of young stock during the winter occurs and there is no need for mowing for silage or hay making. In areas where the latter is necessary, alternate mowing and grazing of pastures is a form of grassland management that greatly increases the productivity of permanent grassland and utilization of herbage. As will be seen later, it can also be used for the prevention of parasitism.
- **stock management**. The younger animals suffer most from gastrointestinal nematodes. Clinical disease is generally restricted to calves in the first grazing season. Even within this category, the older calves are much better able to withstand the parasites. If older and younger calves graze together in one group, the older ones may serve as as a source of contamination for the younger. This knowledge can be used to form groups of calves with a high uniformity of age, if herd size makes this possible. The supplemental feeding of calves varies considerably between farms (Ploeger, 1989). It depends on herbage availability, stocking rate, and is (unconsciously) used in many field situations as a tool to combat the effects of parasitism. A high feeding level does not offer a higher resistance to the parasites as such.
- **grazing management.** Stocking rate is undoubtedly the most important factor affecting an animal's exposure to parasites. It is defined as the number of young stock per hectare, more precisely: number of susceptible young stock per ha. The higher the stocking rate, the greater the risk of infection. A high general stocking rate on a farm does not necessarily mean a high stocking rate for the young stock most at-risk: this can be lowered by several measures.

The rotational grazing of calves is essentially a method of decreasing the stocking rate of susceptible young stock because by rotation the total area grazed by the calves is increased. If rotation is done on aftermath (i.e. the regrown herbage after mowing) the farmer has a very efficient prevention method.

The opposite of rotational grazing is set-stocking. This system, in which calves are turned out to pasture and remain there for the entire grazing period, is parasitologically undesirable, because animals are constantly in contact with their own contamination. A minor advantage, though rather theoretical, may be that the animals are better able to avoid the heavily infected grass around fecal pats. The system of set- stocking is also inferior with respect to the utilization of pasture, because the herbage production is largest during the first half of the season, when calves are young and their herbage intake low, whereas in the second half of the season the grass growth is low and the nutritional requirements of the calves have greatly increased. Set-stocking is unfortunately one of the prerequisites for the use of slow release bolusses, as will be discussed later.

Another method to achieve a lower stocking rate for susceptible animals is mixed grazing with either a different host species (sheep or horses) or with older, less susceptible cattle such as yearlings or milking cows. The term mixed grazing should not be taken literally: that calves are mixed with sheep or milking cows at the same time on the same pasture. It generally means that fields are grazed by a certain group and after re-growth of herbage are grazed by a different category of animals. In this way, the contamination and infestation of herbage is spread over as large an area as possible. In theory it is beneficial for calves as well as for other susceptible stock (lambs). Farmers sometimes object against grazing the milking cows after a field has been grazed by calves, due to insufficient herbage intake of cows later on.

### Diagnostic parameters

The diagnosis of gastrointestinal parasitism is preferentially done on *the* basis of parameters that can be measured in the live animal. In relatively unknown circumstances where the main problem is mortality, it is worthwhile to autopsy animals and record the species of nematodes involved, but in areas with a longstanding cattle tradition these fundamental features are probably known. In the live calf the diagnosis rests on clinical signs of infection, growth performance, fecal egg counts and blood parameters such as antibodies and pepsinogen.

### Control and prevention

**Therapy**. In the case of disease, when clinical signs of infection are unmistakebly present (see above), it is not difficult to decide what should be done. There is a great variety of broad spectrum anthelmintics available to treat affected young stock. It is wise to move the animals to a clean pasture after treatment, and to avoid regrazing of the same pasture with susceptible young stock during the months to come. It should be noted that appreciable economic damage has occurred, when the farmer is forced to treat the calves.

- **Clinical signs.** The clinical signs are loss of weight or diminished growth, diarrhea which may be intermittant, anorexia, anaemia, a dry and dull hair coat, listlessness. These signs are not specific and can be observed in a variety of other conditions as well.
- **Liveweight.** The liveweight can be obtained by weighing, but on most farms the equipment to do this is not available. A method much used is measuring the heart girth, and for many breeds tables are available to convert heart girth into kilograms of liveweight.
  Liveweight of calves has always to be seen in relation to the age of the animal. A good registration and identification system is a prerequisite for easily obtaining such data from the farmer. Without age data the weighing or measuring of young stock makes little sense and one has to rely solely on actual body condition scores, if present. It is remarkable that in many case reports on gastrointestinal parasitism in the literature, there is lack of data on liveweight or even body condition scores.
- **Fecal egg counts.** The demonstration of eggs in the feces is a more specific diagnostic parameter than those referred to above, although its specific nature is also questionable in the frequently occurring situations that simply every calf on pasture gets worms and excretes eggs with the feces. In that case one might hope that the number of eggs is a reflection of the number of parasites, or, at least a reflection of the severity of the parasitic problem. Much depends on the total parasite species profile prevailing in the region, because species differ widely not only in egg production, but also in immunological suppression of egg production.
  With two examples, Ostertagia and Cooperia, we will illustrate that this is sometimes, but not always the case.

A reasonably good impression of the severity of infection is obtained in haemonchosis in sheep. Not only is *Haemonchus* contortus a very prolific worm, but also a very pathogenic one. Despite the fact that other species are involved besides *H. contortus*, the number of eggs is a reflection of the severity of the infection. Gastrointestinal nematode infection of calves in the Netherlands consists predominantly of the species *Ostertagia ostertagi* and *Cooperia oncophora*. The first mentioned species is the most pathogenic of the two, whereas the latter is the most prolific. The eggs of the two species cannot be distinguished from each other. In addition *C. oncophora* elicits an effective immune response in the host, resulting in a decrease of egg production. This decrease occurs earlier and sooner in heavy infections than in small infections. Such an immune response does not occur for *O. ostertagi*, at least not during the first months after infection. It is clear that in such cases the fecal egg counts may be very misleading, there are even situations that the relationship between infection level and egg counts is significantly negative. For a good interpretation of egg counts it may be necessary to do larval differentiations in such fecal samples, which is a very laborious and specialistic procedure. Therefore, knowledge of the species profile, the egg production of the species involved, the immune response and the effects on egg production is needed to estimate when and under which conditions egg counts can be used for diagnostic purposes.

- **Serum antibodies.** Nematodes elicit a host immune reponse which is very complex and involves both cellular and humoral components. For protection of the host, the cellular components are probably more important than the humoral, and from these the local, mucosal antibodies are likely more important than the circulating. Nevertheless circulating antibodies are of great value for diagnostic purposes for the following reasons:

1. They are strongly related to the level of infection,
2. They are easily accessible,
3. Their assessment in the laboratory is possible in a quick and easy way, and if necessary it can be automated,
4. The course of antibody titres in time is not fluctuating as strongly as fecal egg counts.

In all four aspects serum antibodies are thus superior compared to egg counts. However, there are a few draw-backs to be mentioned. Serum antibodies appear three or four weeks after infection, depending on the infection level. The same disadvantage is found for egg counts, which do not appear before three weeks after infection. Antibodies are also not 100% specific because cross-reacting antibodies may be found with other helminth infections. The urge for specificity is however not as great as in infections where an all or none situation is existent, like many viral and bacterial infections. All calves on pasture get an infection, it is only the level of infection that really counts.

– **Other serum constituents**

*Pepsinogen.* In severe abomasal infections leakage of pepsinogen from the abomasal wall into the blood is found. The concentration of pepsinogen in the serum is therefore a good reflection of the damage to the abomasum caused by *O. ostertagi*. Because this is the most pathogenic species in cattle it is not a serious draw-back that other species are not involved in this parameter, although monospecific *C. oncophora* infections also are able to produce a slight increase in serum pepsinogen. The major disadvantage of the method is that it measures the presence of infection after much of the damage to the animal has already been done.

*Gastrine.* This is another enzyme from the abomasal wall that can be measured in the blood. Much of what has been said about pepsinogen applies for gastrine as well. With respect to the amount of damage that already has occurred, gastrin is inferior to pepsinogen.

Regular monitoring should include clinical inspection together with fecal egg counts and serology at crucial times. Fecal egg counts are best carried out 5 - 6 weeks after turn out. This gives a good impression of the inital infection resulting from overwintered larvae. Later in the season the fecal egg counts may yield misleading results, especially in the temperate regions where mixed infections of *O.ostertagi* and *C. oncophora* prevail. This inspection can be supplemented by serological methods estimating antibodies and pepsinogen in at least 5 animals of the group. This serology can be repeated every month, or every two months, depending on the weather conditions and the results of the liveweight measurements. The latter can be carried out by the farmer, provided that there is a good system of identification and registration so that the age of young stock (in days) is known.

Action should be taken if:

1. The fecal egg count exceeds a number of 300 e.p.g,
2. The Cooperia and Ostertagia titres exceed the value of 5 and 6 respectively,
3. The pepsinogen value exceeds the 1500 mU.,
4. The mean weight of the animals is 10 kilograms or more below the age adjusted mean of the norm weights,
5. Or a combination of the above mentioned threshold values.

**Preventive use of anthelmintics**

1. To prevent disease in first grazing season of calves a **slow release bolus** containing anthelmintic is given at turn-out. The objective is the prevention of pasture contamination with worm eggs during the first 3 months (McKellar, 1988). Prerequisites for this system are: 1. All young stock *are* treated at the start of the first grazing season, 2. They are not moved to other pastures (possibly heavily infected by other stock) and 3. no other untreated calves are introduced into the group. The method is efficient, safe and easy to apply. However, there are a few disadvantages to be mentioned. Firstly the method is rather costly. Secondly the method implies the use of the set-stocking grazing system, which is an inefficient system from the viewpoint of grassland care and -utilisation. In addition there are serious objections against the preventive use of anthelmintics with regard to: 1. the lack of stimulation of immunity in young stock, 2. the evoking of resistance of worms to anthelmintics, which is becoming a problem in the treatment of sheep and horses, and 3. the consumer's aversion towards the use of chemical means of food production.
2. Apart from slow release devices there are **strategic methods of anthelmintic application**, which aim at the same objective: prevention of pasture contamination with eggs by early season treatment. The most well known of these methods is the 3, 8 and 13 weeks treatment with ivermectin (McKellar, 1988). The timing of treatment is chosen with respect to the duration of the pre-patent period and a two-week long residual effect of these products. It is cheaper than a bolus treatment, but requires the collecting and handling of grazing animals. The other disadvantages of bolus treatments mentioned above, regarding immunity, resistance and consumers objections apply equally to this method.
3. **The dose and move system**. This very practical system was developed at Weybridge by Michel (1969). It is based upon the avoidance of the large numbers of larvae that are available at the so-called midsummer increase. Due to lower temperatures in the spring the eggs providing the new, disease producing generation of larvae, tend to accumulate until in the first weeks of July, when soil temperatures are high enough to allow the larvae to migrate onto the herbage in large numbers. This occurs under the condition of sufficient rainfall. At this time the calves are treated with an anthelmintic, and moved to another clean field were they may stay for the rest of the season.

**Management methods.** The prevention of economic damage due to gastrointestinal parasites is possible without the use of anthelmintics. In principle these methods are based on the avoiding the intake of too large numbers of larvae with the herbage. This should be done taking into account the age of the animals. Three examples are given: set stocking on clean field; rotation on aftermath; late turn out.

1. **Set stocking of calves on a clean field.** This grazing system prevents the sudden uptake by naive young stock of larvae that have been shed by older carrier animals, which is particularly important in lungworm infections. It can be applied if the farmer prefers to do so, but as stated earlier, set stocking is not highly efficient with

regard to grassland utilisation. This system is possible under the very strict condition that calves start on a clean field. As a clean field may be regarded a newly sown ley pasture, which has not carried stock during the last years, or a pasture that has been mown and has not carried young egg excreting stock during the preceeding summer and autumn. Under these conditions calves may build up an infection and immunity simultaneously, so that an equilibrium between immunity and parasite population is attained. The system requires regular monitoring.

2. **Rotation on aftermath.** This system was developed in the Netherlands in the sixties, and has been applied for several decades with great success. Aftermath is defined as the regrown grass after the paddock has been mown for silage or hay. The mowing of grass in the Netherlands starts end of May, depending on weather conditions. After mowing, fertilizer is applied to stimulate a quick regrowth of grass. After 3 - 4 weeks of normal weather the stage of grass growth is such that it offers optimal herbage for grazing. This is the time to start grazing calves. The mowing of pastures reduces any larval population *by* mechanical removal of larvae with the herbage, and leaves a short stubble where sun and wind reduces the larval population even further. The pasture can be safely grazed for 4 weeks, then the animals are rotated to another paddock, which also has been mown earlier, where they graze for 4 weeks, and this pattern continues until the end of the grazing season. It is a system that can be applied under very intensive grassland management prevailing in the Netherlands. The fields are relatively small, which is a disadvantage from the viewpoint of harvesting grass, but has great advantages with respect to the utilisation of grass by the milking cows. The small fields allow a frequent rotation of the cows. In this situation the systematic grazing of calves on aftermath offers no problems, although it requires some attention and careful planning of the farmer. It must be noted that the system is not effective against lungworms.
3. **Late turn out.** If the conditions on a farm are such that larval infestation of the fields has built up for years and the above mentioned systems are unlikely to work, it is always possible to keep the calves housed for a large part of the grazing season. Not only are the calves better able to withstand the worms at an older age, but there has also not been a build-up of larval populations during the season. The latter is of course only true if there are no age groups of calves present. It would be extremely dangerous for instance, to keep the younger age group indoors and allow the older calves to build up the grassland infestation, and then turn out the younger group in the autumn.

   There are some advantages of this system compared to entirely keeping the first year calves indoors, because in the former case the calves have the opportunity to acquire a certain degree of immunity, while in the latter case calves would be highly susceptible.

## Conclusions

Trying to get a good anamnesis of gastrointestinal parasites in calves is extremely difficult. To grasp all the above mentioned factors of species profile, grazing management, feeding, weather conditions, stocking rate, age and age distribution in one coherent picture which enables "predicting" the existence and severity of parasite problems in a given herd is virtually impossible. Investigations in the field where all the epidemiological and management factors were recorded together with the measuring of the growth performance of the calves, have been rather disappointing. Moreover the use of anthelmintics and high feed gifts mask any clear-cut effects of parasitism and preventive management practices on live weight gains. This does not mean that no effort should be made to understand the parasite situation on the farm. If combined with

1. What is the total number of calves to be reared yearly? Are they divided into age groups?
2. How many hectares are available for calf grazing?
3. Are the calves rotated on pasture? What frequency? To fields that have been mown before this grazing? To fields that have been grazed by other stock? Which type of stock? Do you expect contamination of these fields with trichostrongylid eggs by these earlier grazings?
4. When were the calves turned out (date) and what was their mean age? How is the uniformity in age?
5. How is the growth performance of the calves? Did you measure it? If yes, how?
6. What did the calves receive as supplementary feed (type of feed and quantity)?
7. Where there any anthelmintic treatments? If yes: when and on what grounds?

proper diagnostic data it should certainly be tried to get as much information from the farmer as possible. The questions of interest are brought together and listed below.

In the live animal diagnosis of gastrointestinal parasitism is difficult on the basis of clinical signs alone. It should be supported by laboratory assessment of fecal egg counts. Serology can be a valuable complement. Because in the highly developed dairy industry the economic impact of gastrointestinal parasitism is not primarily due to mortality or even overt disease, but predominantly to subclinical infections, the use of these prognostic tests is valuable to assist the practitioner in health surveillance at the herd level.

A great variety of control and prevention methods is available against gastrointestinal nematodes. They include the preventive use of anthelmintics and methods of pasture- and stock management which are based on the epidemiology of these infections.

### Lungworms

Lungworm disease or dictyocaulosis in the bovine is caused by *Dictyocaulus viviparus.* As for gastrointestinal nematodes its lifecycle is without an intermediate host. Infective larvae are ingested with the herbage, they pass the intestinal wall and migrate via the local lymph nodes to the lungs, where they grow to adults in three weeks. The females produce eggs, which are coughed up and swallowed with the sputum. During the passage through the digestive tract these eggs hatch to first stage larvae which can be found in the feces 3 - 4 weeks after infection.

**Epidemiology of dictyocaulosis**

Lungworms occur in almost every pastured calf in cool and moist climates. The signs consist of acute coughing and repiratory distress. This makes both farmers and veterinary practitioners much more alert to lungworm than to gastro-intestinal worms. Fecal examination for the presence of lungworm larvae is rather insensitive: the finding of one larva in one of a series of fecal samples taken from a herd of calves is sufficient to confirm the diagnosis of lungworm disease. It is quite possible that even this larva is missed due to inappropriate handling of the fecal samples during transport and stocking in the laboratory before they are processed. The infective larvae of lungworms are very immobile compared to those of gastrointestinal worms. This means that *D. viviparus* depends more on passive migration, for instance by: splashing of rain, the feet of grazing animals or foraging birds, and dissimination with the spores of the fungus *Pilobolus* which grows on fecal pats. Other bionomic characteristics of free living stages of lungworms are: 1. a rapid translation (i.e. the process by which eggs and larvae in the feces become infective larvae, available to the host) resulting in high herbage infestation within 1 - 3 weeks and 2. a high mortality rate which renders the pasture safe relatively soon after 9 - 10 weeks.

In comparison with gastrointestinal parasitism a solid protective immunity is build up quickly (Armour, 1989). In many cases of lungworm infections, the build-up of immunity holds pace with the build-up of herbage infestation, and disease does not occur. Therefore the role of carriers (older animals subclinically infected with lungworms that pass larvae with their feces) is of much greater importance in dictyocaulosis. Disease in young, relatively naive calves often results from the uptake of larvae originating from these carriers (Michel, 1969).

Like in gastrointestinal parasitism, there is some overwintering of infection on pasture, but to a much lesser degree. This overwintered pasture infection of lungworm larvae seldom results in disease, and is often enough to stimulate immunity. However, there are cases in which overwintered infections are so low that immunity is insufficient and disease is produced by the second or even the third generation of larvae (Michel, 1969; Eysker et al. 1993). Overwintering of lungworms may occur by arrested development of some worms in the lungs, which resume development in the spring and produce eggs when the host is on pasture again.

## Management factors

Much of what has been said about climate, weather and management factors for gastrointestinal nematodes also applies for lungworms. However, there are slight differences with respect to mixed grazing and rotation. Because lungworm disease often results from the uptake by naive young stock of infective larvae coming from carriers, mixed grazing of calves together with older cattle (yearlings or milking cows) is dangerous. Mixed grazing with other host species (sheep, horses) should be beneficial, because *D. viviparus* is a typical cattle species. For the same reason it is recommended not to add young calves to a grazing group of older calves. Age uniformity in a group is more important here than it is for gastrointestinal worm infections.

**Rotational grazing** can theoretically help to prevent lungworm disease, because the translation process to infective larvae on herbage is quick, and the longevity on herbage is short. This means that calves should be rotated to clean pasture every week, and that after 10 weeks of time the pasture can safely be regrazed by the same calves. This would require a lot of planning and, more importantly, does not prevent gastrointestinal worm infections. There is some evidence that the latter make the calves more susceptible to lungworms (Düwel,1971; Michel, 1976; Kloosterman et al., 1990).

## Diagnostic parameters

The diagnosis of lungworm is primarily based on the clinical signs during the grazing season, followed by the history of the herd and premisses with regard to lungworm infections, and the laboratory diagnosis of *Dictyocaulus viviparus* in feces or sputum.

## Control and prevention

- **Therapy.** In case of clinical disease, broad spectrum anthelmintics are available. It is possible that in some heavily infected young stock treatment may (temporarily) aggravate the clinical signs, even with fatal results. This condition, which is also seen in spontaneously recovering animals, is possibly caused by the aspiration of dead worm material.
- **Clinical signs**. They consist of deep, harsh coughing, particularly after exercise, high respiratory rate, salivation and anorexia. The calves may rapidly loose weight. These symptoms are relatively specific. Often the diagnosis can be based on clinical signs alone. If desirable it can be confirmed by examination of sputum, feces or serology.
- **Sputum examination**. A sputum collector can be introduced into the trachea to catch sputum which can be pressed between two glass slides for microscopical detection of embryonated eggs. The method is very quick and possibly more sensitive than fecal examination.
- **Fecal larval counts**. First stage larvae are extracted by Baermannisation from a weighed sample of fresh feces. This is the most widely used method, although larvae can also be flottated by centrifugation, which is not dependent on the activity of the larvae. As stated before, the sensitivity of the technique is relatively low. It can be increased by taking larger samples of feces, for instance 30 g., as used by Eysker et al. (1993). For research work, the advantage of fecal larval counts compared to examination of sputum is that the method is quantitative. It should be noted that during the prepatent period of heavy infections, clinical signs may be seen, while eggs in sputum or larvae in feces are not yet present.
- **Serology**. Depending on the level of infection, serum antibody titres begin to rise about three weeks after initial infection. For low level infections this may take longer, so that patent infections may be missed for 2 weeks or more (Eysker et al., 1993). Serology is of minor importance for the diagnosis of acute outbreaks, unless it is considered necessary to differentiate dictyocaulosis from viral respiratory diseases. For the detection of subclinical infections and for sero-epidemiological survey work, the antibody titres are useful. Because the unpredictability of lungworm disease, and its sudden, acute nature, serology can probably not play a role as a prognostic tool as it does in gastrointestinal parasitism.

- **Preventive use of anthelmintics.** Most slow release boluses, except those containing morantel, administered to young calves at the occasion of turn out, are also effective against *D. viviparus.* An obvious disadvantage is that they also prevent the development of immunity which is so essential in the whole epidemiological pattern of lungworm infections. The system is based on the prevention of the build up of large larval populations on the field where the calves are set-stocked. However accidental contamination by *D. viviparus* larvae from adjacent fields, by means of *Pilobolus* sporangiae cannot be excluded.
- **Prevention by grazing management.** Because of the unpredictable epidemiology, due to the very quick build-up of pasture infestation under suitable weather conditions and the sudden outbreak of symptoms, the grazing on aftermath and other grassland management systems do not work as they do against gastrointestinal nematodes.
- **Vaccination.** This has long been and remains the method of choice to prevent dictyocaulosis. The method is based on the administration of live *D. viviparus* larvae to calves from 2 months of age onwards. The larvae have been attenuated by irradiation to such a degree that they develop to adults in the lungs without the ability to reproduce. This results in a protective immune response and no further contamination of pastures occurs. A minor draw back is that the larvae have to be administered in two portions, four weeks apart, and the vaccinate should not be turned out to pasture within two weeks after administration of the second dose. This forces the farmer to keep the calves indoors for 6 weeks. Technically it is essential to keep the larvae alive (shelf life of the vaccine is limited) and to shake the bottle well before the larval suspension is administered. Sporadic outbreaks have been seen after vaccination, which could be explained either by technical errors or by unusually high levels of challenge infections. Under normal conditions a light challenge on pasture is desirable for boosting the immunity of the animals. Routine vaccination of all calves during several years might result in pastures that are virtually free of lungworm infestation. Perhaps outbreaks of dictyocaulosis incidentily seen in yearlings or even in milking cows could be attributed to insufficient challenge to maintain immunity. A method of natural immunisation has been advocated, which consists of introduction of calves to infected pasture, and by scrupulous monitoring calves for the very first clinical signs, whereupon the animals are treated with anthelmintic (Michel, 1969). The main advantage is that this method is cheap, but it is considered to be very risky.

## Conclusions

Although lungworm infections can be expected in the large majority of pastured calves, it does not always result in lungworm disease. The occurrence of disease is very unpredictable because of the precarious balance between the level of larval intake and the build-up of immunity. Moreover, if disease occurs it is often acute and very severe, and the clinical signs of infection are clear. Actions to be taken include chemotherapy when clinical signs are seen, and, for future prevention, vaccination. The questions to be asked in taking a history of lung worm problems include the following:

1. What is the number of calves to be reared yearly? Are they divided into age groups?
2. Are calves rotated on pasture? What frequency? To fields that have been grazed by older calves, yearlings or lactating cows?
3. Is there a history on the farm of coughing calves? Are there adjacent fields with a neighbour who has an actual or a a history of lungworms?
4. What are the levels of serum-antibody titres in older young stock?
5. Were the calves vaccinated against lung worm?
6. Where there any anthelmintic treatments? If yes: when and on what grounds?

## Liver fluke

Liver fluke disease or fascioliasis is caused by *Fasciola hepatica* or *Fasciola gigantica*. In W. Europe the latter does not occur. Because life cycle, pathogenesis, diagnosis and treatment are very similar for both parasites, the discussion is restricted to *F. hepatica*.

In bovines liver fluke infections are generally chronic in nature and many infections

**Epidemiology of liver fluke disease in general**

The life cycle is much more complicated than that of nematodes. The liver fluke uses a snail as intermediate host, and this has great consequences for the epidemiology and prevention. In contrast to nematodes (lungworms and gastrointestinal worms) farms can be free of liverfluke infections, simply because the intermediate host is not present. Furthermore, the snail is very sensitive to weather conditions, so that a dry year can decrease the snail population and hence the pasture infestation with flukes to a considerable degree. Any prevention method should account for these temporal and spatial restrictions in the occurence of infections.

Fluke eggs are passed in the feces and at optimal temperatures of 22 - 26°C. a motile, ciliated larva, the miracidium, is released in about 9 days. This takes longer at lower temperatures, and below 10°C. little development occurs. The miracidium larva has to find a snail within a few hours, to be able to penetrate into the snail. Via a sporocyst and rediae, cercariae are produced, which are shed into the environment. This process takes a minimum of 6 - 7 weeks, depending on the environmental temperatures, but can be extended to several months. This variation is favourable for the survival and infection chances of the parasites, but complicates the design of preventive management measures. One miracidium larva can produce over 600 cercariae. Within a few hours the motile cercariae must attach to herbage, and there it encapsulates to form metacercariae. Survival of metacercariae is possible for at least 6 months, depending on weather conditions. The whole process from egg shedding in the feces to infective metacercaria on the herbage takes a minimum of 12 weeks during the summer months. Metacercariae actively digest their own cyst wall, penetrate the intestinal wall and migrate via the peritoneal cavity to the liver, where the young flukes eat their way through the liverparenchym during 6 - 8 weeks, to arrive in the bile ducts. Here they become adult and start egg production, resulting in a prepatent period of 10 - 12 weeks. The minimum period for the completion of the entire life cycle is 17 - 18 weeks. The biology of liver fluke is characterized by a very high fecundity, and a high reproduction rate in the intermediate host, but also by a great vulnerability of miracidium larvae and cercariae.

The ecology of the intermediate host is very crucial in the epidemiology. In Europe *Lymnaea truncatula* is the common intermediate host, in other continents *L. tomentosa. L. humilis*, and other *Lymnaea* species may play a role as well. *L. truncatula* is the most widespread transmittor of liver fluke disease. It is an amphibious snail, living in places that are periodically wet and dry. They feed on algae, that grow on soils containing some clay material. They develop and reproduce at temperatures of 15 - 22°C., are able to withstand dry and cold circumstances. During the summer months they may produce a number of 100,000 offspring (Taylor,1964).

**Epidemiological factors**

Of decisive importance is the presence of **snail habitats**. These are spots that are alternately wet and dry, for instance the banks of ditches, low spots flooded by heavy rainfall, hoof marks and wheel tracks. The soil type and ground water level are structural factors on a farm, the rainfall and land use (grazing, heavy machinery, ditch cleaning) the more conjunctural factors which determine whether a potential snail habitat becomes an actual snail habitat. Very often a farm has fields where snails are present and other fields where they do not occur at all. This is a very important piece of information for the farmer, who can react by grazing management, reserving some fields for the harvest of hay or silage, and using other fields for grazing animals. The only way to get this information is to know and find the snails. This can be facilitated by looking at the vegetation, some plants like *Juncus* spp., *Glyceria fluitans* and *Ranunculus repens* having the same preference for soil type, pH, and moisture as the snails have (Taylor, 1964, Over, 1962), but it remains a specialist's job.

**Temperature** is important both for the development of free living stages of *F. hepatica* and for the development and reproduction of snails and of the fluke stages within the snails. The mean day and night temperature should be at least 10°C. which condition is usually met with from May to October. Most important is the summer infection of snails, which results in metacercariae on the herbage from August to October. In some countries, notably Britain, there may also occur a winter infection of snails, resulting in metacercariae in May - June, but even here the summer infection is of much greater importance. The seasonal pattern in warmer areas (Australia, Southern U.S. may be different, snail activity being greater during the cooler months. Here the metacercariae are most numerous on the herbage during the winter, but the epidemiological principles are the same.

**Moisture** is necessary for the development of miracidium larvae from the eggs, which have to be washed free from the feces before development takes place. The miracidium needs water films to migrate and find a snail, and the snail needs moisture for its development and reproduction. Apart from the general ground water level, the presence of moisture is largely determined by rainfall and evaporation. This is of such a crucial significance that fluke forecasting systems have been developed on the basis of meteorological data. The development of formulas in which rainfall, evapotranspiration and number if wet days during a certain period are correlated to a measure of incidence of fluke infections, have contributed considerably to the control of Fascioliasis in the United Kingdom and the Netherlands.

Much depends on the availability of data on incidence during a prolonged period of years. Such data are mortality rates in sheep (UK), or liver condemnation rates in cattle (the Netherlands). For bovine fascioliasis the presence of sheep on the farm may be a significant factor, as they contribute greatly to contamination of pastures with liver fluke.

remain at the subclinical level. This is in contrast to sheep, where acute and sub-acute infections occur and mortality is common. It should be recognized that subclinical infections of older animals cause most of the economic damage. Subclinical infections are the cause of lower growth rates, lower milk yields and condemnation of livers at slaughter (Oostendorp, 1990).

### Diagnostic parameters

In the live animal the diagnosis is based on clinical signs, growth retardation, reduced milk production, fecal egg counts and serological examinations.

### Control and prevention

- **Therapy.** Against chronic distomatosis as it occurs in cattle, several anthelmintics are available. Most of them work only against the adult flukes (rafoxanide, nitroxynil, acedist, chlorsulon and niclofolan) but triclabendazole is also effective against immature, parenchymal stages. Furthermore, most of these anthelmintics do not reach 100% efficacy, so that often a small proportion of the fluke population survives.

- **Clinical signs**. In bovines the subclinical form of the disease is most important, in contrast to sheep. In heavy infections of young animals there is loss of weight, anaemia and hypoalbuminaemia, resulting in submandibular oedema and pale mucous membranes. In the majority of cases the disease is subclinical, with effects on growth performance and milk production, which are difficult to differentiate from effects of suboptimal nutrition. Diarrhea is not seen.

- **Fecal egg counts**. The prepatent period is long and it is usually not before the end of the grazing season (November - December) that eggs can be found in the feces. Much of the damage has been done at that time, but it may be valuable to confirm the diagnosis.

- **Plasma levels of liver enzymes**. Enzymes are released by damaged liver cells. Glutamate dehydrogenase (GLDH) levels are increased when parenchmal liver cells are damaged, and levels become higher within a few weeks after infection. This could play a role in early detection of infections. Gamma glutamyl transpeptidase (GGT) is released when the epithelium of bile ducts is damaged, i.e. after maturation of the flukes is nearly completed. The advantage is that it remains high for a longer period.

- **Serum antibodies**. These can be detected about five weeks after infection, either with a passive haemagglutination test or an ELISA test. Because of its versatility and possible automation the latter is the method of choice. Contrary to nematode infections, where antibodies can be used to determine the relative level of infection in sero-epidemiological survey work, it is essential that the antibodies are highly specific because of the existence of infected and uninfected herds.

- **Preventive use of anthelmintics.** These are aimed at prevention of pasture contamination with eggs. Two treatments are generally recommended, the first at the beginning of the winter season when animals are stabled, which removes most of the adult population and a second treatment in early spring before animals are put on pasture, to remove the flukes that survived the first treatment.
- **Other prevention methods.** In regions where the disease is endemic and more specifically, on farms with a high proportion of fields containing snail habitats, the use of anthelmintics cannot be avoided, like in nematode infections.
- **Grassland management**. In low lying, flat fields, the application of tile draining has not only a positive influence on the grassland productivity, but this measure may also dramatically decrease the snail population. The system of ditches and furrows used in the Netherlands to remove excess water, promotes rather than eliminates snail populations. The modern highly mechanized methods of maintenance of this old drainage system may spread snail populations over much wider areas, as they were more spatially restricted to those ditch borders and furrows in former times. On farms where only a part of the fields harbour snails, it is often possible to design a scheme of grazing by which fluky fields are mown for hay or silage-making in spring or early summer so that they are not contaminated with eggs in that period. These fields will be safe for grazing in the autumn. It is also possible to fence off certain parts of a field, where snail habitats are restricted to very particular small zones, for instance near a ditch or brook. Often it is observed that by doing this, and thus preventing the grazing of cattle in those areas, the snail also disappears, because the hoof marks which are ideal habitats for snails are not there: it appears that the presence of the host is a prerequisite for the presence of the intermediate host. The cattle tracks along which cows travel each day to be milked, have a reputation of an ideal snail habitat; similarly, places where the movable milking machine is put, if milking is done in the field, can harbour snails.
  The use of molluscicides to kill the snails is detrimental to aquatic life, and should be abandoned on grounds of preserving the natural environment.
- **Vaccination.** Although cattle acquire some degree of immunity against liver fluke, experiments with irradiated larvae and other vaccination methods have not resulted in a sufficiently high degree of protection.

## Conclusions

The greatest problem with liver fluke infections in cattle is the unawareness of the farmer of any problem. To assist the practitioner in health surveillance the questions to be asked are brought together and listed next page.

If all or some of the answers to these questions are indicative for the presence of liver fluke on the farm, anthelmintic treatments should be given, both to remove existing infections and to prevent contamination of pastures in the next grazing season. Further preventive measures depend very much on the specific situation on the farm, notably the distribution of snail habitats.

1. Are potential snail habitats present on the farm (soil type and ground water)? If yes, are there actual snail habitats? How are these habitats distributed between and within fields? Are they restricted to specific sites which can be fenced off?
2. Have weather conditions been conducive for the development of fluke infections?
3. Is liveweight of young stock and milk yield of cows up to standards?
4. If sheep are present on the farm, does acute ovine fascioliasis occur? Have liver condemnations of slaughtered cattle or sheep of the farm ever occurred?
5. Is serology positive for liver enzymes and / or antibodies from August/September onwards?

### Age group of > 15 months

Pregnancy determination should be carried out after breeding as appropriate. Age of first breeding should be checked regularly to prevent a prolonged predicted minimum first calving age. Signs of lameness (Chapter 7) and mastitis (Chapter 6) must be evaluated during pregnancy. A few weeks before expected calving, heifers should be adapted to a close-up group and ration (Chapter 3).

After every inspection, the clinical findings must be processed into performance indices, either manually or electronically. If not computerized, indices should be listed on a 12-monthly list and be evaluated over time.

## 2.2.5 FARM INSPECTION

Diseases of young stock and growth disturbances often have a multifactorial background, even if caused by a specific agent. Rarely will a single factor cause clinical illness or growth retardation. Contemporary epidemiology recognizes that a sufficient cause for clinical disease consists of several contributing factors (Rothman, 1986). Contributing factors include the animal (genotype), farm management and farm conditions which may act to alter the health and growth status of young stock. For this reason, clinical inspection and diagnosis must be followed by a farm inspection during which all relevant animal, managerial and environmental risk factors for diseases and growth retardation should be considered. However, many risk factors are based on associations and do not necessarily indicate a biological cause and effect relationship. Against this background some general management aspects related to housing and nutrition will be discussed.

### Housing

Housing should be considered as an instrument to optimize the development of young stock and prevent spread of diseases. This is especially important during the first three months of life, which emcompasses the transition from passive immunity (maternally derived antibodies) to active immunity (antibodies produced by the calf itself). Aspects of housing to be monitored during a farm inspection include climatic conditions, type of housing, and spatial conditions.

## Climatic conditions

Calf health is influenced by air quality in young stock housing, which can be regulated by ventilation. Air quality is determined by the presence of pathogens, pollutants such as ammonia and other noxious gases, moisture level or relative humidity (RH) and temperature. Many pathogens are spread by the airborne route. Relative humidity is the most important factor influencing pathogen survival in aerosols. Relative humidity between 60 and 75% results in the shortest survival time for the greatest number of potential pathogens. However, its effects varies greatly between pathogens - some survive best in humid conditions, and others in dry air. Kelly et al. (1984) reported a higher incidence of scours but not of respiratory disease in 95% relative humidity housed calves compared to 75%. Relative humidity is dependent on temperature. As air is warmed, its capacity to pick up moisture produced by young stock from the barn environment is increased markedly (Bickert and Herdt, 1985). High RH may make lying conditions more uncomfortable due to decreased evaporation from the bed and absorption of moisture from the air by bedding material (Kelly et al., 1984). To remove moisture from the calf's environment, the inside temperature must be 5 to 10°C higher than the outside. However, the temperature inside the barn should not exceed 13 to 16°C.

Mitchell (1976) calculated the lower critical temperatures for a housed calf, adequately fed, protected from wind and rain and given a dry bed as follows:

- Calf on dry straw -13°C
- Calf on wet straw -10°C
- Calf on wood slats -10°C
- Calf on dry concrete 2°C

The effects of high temperatures are not significant below 26°C to 28°C.

Adjustments in ration formulation must be made during extremes in temperature. Dry matter intake is inversely related to temperature - during summer when temperatures are high, dry matter intake typically declines. Cattle will reduce feed intake, particularly of forages, to reduce heat of fermentation, thereby reducing body temperature. In cold weather, dry matter intake increases to allow increased energy intake and to maintain body temperature. An exception is extreme cold weather when intake will drop. Whenever the temperature reaches ± -15°C, allowances should be made for increased intake. Factors involved with cold stress include not only temperature and rain, but also wind, animal size and overall cleanliness. The amount of body mud affect the heifer's average daily gain. Heifers covered with mud, snow or manure on their legs, abdomen, sides or flanks or both, are much more likely to experience cold stress and reduced growth. Heifers raised under wet and muddy conditions gained 0.2 pound less a day (Price et al., 1994 a).

The goal of winter ventilation is to maintain suitable air quality by reducing the concentration of pathogens and removing excessive moisture produced by young stock and other pollutants (Bickert and Herdt, 1985). The flow of fresh air should be from younger, more susceptible young stock toward older heifers, reducing the exposure of younger animals to airborne organisms possibly carried subclinically by the older ones. Usual ventilation rates per calf up to 2 weeks of age are 0.4 $m^3$/min. in winter,

0.9 $m^3$/min. in mild weather and 1.4 $m^3$/min. in hot weather. For heifers these rates are 0.6 to 0.8 $m^3$/min. in cold weather, 1.7 to 2.2 $m^3$/min. in mild weather and 3.6 to 5 $m^3$/min. in hot weather (Bates et al., 1985). Cold barns must provide sufficient natural ventilation without exposing calves to direct drafts. Webster (1981) suggested that calves less than 12 weeks of age should not be exposed to air speeds greater than 0.5 m per sec.

**Housing of calves from birth to weaning**

The goal of calf housing is to create a dry, draft free micro-environment, that facilitates good disease control, manure handling and labor efficiency practices, especially in winter time.

**Outside barn housing**. Newborn calves should be separated from their dams immediately after birth and placed in a single isolated individual calf hutch outside the barn until a few days after weaning. Optimal transfer of passive immunity and housing in hutches appears to maximize health and growth. Calves left with the dam may be exposed to greater number of infectious micro-organisms associated with the dam and environment thereby increasing the risk of disease (Quigley et al., 1994). Hutches isolate calves from older cattle and prevent a buildup of gases and moisture. Hutches should be placed in a well drained area with a small fence, and if indicated, a covered yard may be attached. Outdoor pens provide space for exercise, facilitate observations, and encourage outside urination and defecation, thereby keeping hutches cleaner (MaCaulay et al., 1995). Hutches should be cleaned and disinfected thoroughly and moved to an uncontaminated area each time a new calf is moved in. This will reduce the risk of horizontal transmission of infection. Pens must be adequately distant from mature animals to prevent further horizontal exposure through direct contact or airborne transmission of pathogens. Individual housing of calves allows farmers to monitor calves for diseases individually and minimize a build up of pathogens in one area.

**Inside barn housing**. Newborn calves can also be kept in individual pens or crates in warm or cold barns. Warm barns are insulated and usually ventilated mechanically. The main disadvantages of warm buildings are costs, disease hazards, and the need to control temperature, ventilation and humidity. Cold barns are simply uninsulated buildings with natural ventilation. Any attempt to house young stock in an enclosed building with inadequate ventilation will result in excessively high humidity that complicate problems of air quality, disease transmission, and condensation; the net result will be generally unhealthy conditions (Bickert and Herdt, 1985).

The provision of a dry bed with good drainage to prevent chilling is important irrespective of type of housing - especially where air temperatures reach the lower critical temperature (Dodd, 1992). Dry bedding functions as thermal insulation when the calf lies down and reduces conductive heat loss; therefore, it must be provided continuously. A wet or damp lying surface increases conductive heat loss from the body due to reduced insulation of the hair coat and increased conductivity of the bedding material (Kelly et al., 1984).

Calves may be grouped in bedded packed pens from 4 weeks of age or a few days after weaning which usually takes place between 4 to 8 weeks of age. They should be grouped by size and not by age. Each group of calves needs its own micro-environment, i.e. protected from drafts and wet conditions, without physical contact and with minimum air-borne contact with older groups of cattle. The latter is important because young calves, up to 7 to 8 months of age are very susceptible to respiratory diseases. It is recommended to have small transition groups of 5 - 6 calves from weaning to 5 to 6 months of age with enough space and feeding places. Calves can later be grouped into larger groups of 10. The youngest calves should be placed nearest to traffic patterns to make checking easier. Providing transition housing reduces the setback in growth that often occurs after weaning. Young stock divided into groups can be cared for according to their specific needs and fed rations to meet their nutritional requirements. Calves to be grouped should be clinically free of disease.

After weaning young stock may be housed only during the winter or all year round. Housing conditions should meet environmental conditions as mentioned before. Thc floor should be solid and allow drainage of urine and should be covered with absorbent material such as straw or wood shavings which should be changed any time it gets wet. An all-in-all-out system with cleaning and disinfection between groups should be practised.

Byond the transition period, and depending on climatic conditions, various types of young stock housing facilities exist. They include: an open area with cement feeding area, bedded pack facility, counter-slope facility and freestall facility.

Allocation of space depends on the size of calves and size of the group (see Table 1).

*Table 1. Grouping, housing, and spatial requirements for older young stock (Menzi, 1995)*

| | AGE (months) | | | | |
|---|---|---|---|---|---|
| **Type of facility** | **3 - 4** | **5 - 8** | **9 - 12** | **13 - 15** | **16 - 25** |
| Square meter/animal | | | | | |
| Resting area ($m^2$/animal) | 1.8 | 2.3 | 2.6 | 2.9 | 3.7 |
| Paved outside lot($m^2$/ animal | 2.7 | 3.2 | 3.7 | 4.1 | 4.6-6.9 |
| Solid floor (total confinement, $m^2$/animal) | 1.8 | 2.3 | 2.7 | 3.7 | 5.5 |
| Slattedfloor (total confinement, $m^2$/animal) | 1.0 | 1.1 | 1.2 | 1.6 | 2.3 |
| Free stall dimensions (m) | 0.6 x 1,35 | 0.75 x 1.50 | 0.9 x 1.65 | 1.1 x 2.0 | 1.1 x 2.0 |
| Minimum manure alley width (m) | 1.5 | 2.7 | 2.7 | 2.7 | 2.7 |

## Nutrition

Nutrients required for adequate growth of young stock vary with increasing age. To optimize nutrition and subsequently body growth the following criteria should be met (VanAmburgh et al., 1991; VanAmburgh and Galton, 1994):

1. set goals for age and weight at first calving. Use these goals to develop targets for monitoring growth and the feeding program,
2. a target rate of gain that allows for optimal growth needs to be established for various age groups,
3. maintenance requirements must be determined and met before balancing for predicted weight gain,
4. feed intake and composition must be known to accurately balance the diet.

In Table 2, ration guidelines are presented for young stock in various weight groups. The values in Table 2 will allow for daily gains from 900 to 1000 g/day (Van Amburgh et al., 1991). Forage quality and forage analysis are very important keys for formulating rations Voluntary dry matter intake averages 3.0 to 2.3% of body weight for heifers from 100 to 500 kg. Many factors influence dry matter intake of heifers such as, feed quality and palatability, body weight, body weight gain, feed bunk management, availability of fresh and clean water, and environmental factors. Proper feed bunk management is necessary to allow adequate dry matter intake and growth. This in turn requires providing a fresh, complete mixed ration in a clean location where all heifers have equal access and a good opportunity to eat. A total mixed ration based on regular forage analysis is recommended. Use of ionophores improves utilization of dietary energy and protein, increasing growth rate, while allowing lower energy rations to be fed (Price et al., 1994 b). Ionophores also reduce the age at which heifers are ready to be bred (Steen et al., 1992). All heifers should be measured regularly (weighed or taped) to determine growth. When heifers are kept on pasture, regular monitoring of pasture management should be performed. This might include determination of nutrient content of pasture, extended grazing periods in autumn, excessive stocking rates, health

*Table 2. Ration guidelines for improved replacement growth (Source: Van Amburgh and Galton, 1994)*

| Weight (kg) | Dry matter intake (kg/day) | NE-gain (Mcal/kg) | Crude protein (%) | UIP % of CP |
|---|---|---|---|---|
| 91 - 181 | 3.2 - 4.1 | 1.15 - 1.23 | 17 | 35 - 45 |
| 181 - 272 | 4.5 - 6.4 | 1.06 - 1.15 | 16 - 17 | 35 - 40 |
| 272 - 363 | 6.8 - 8.2 | 0.93 - 0.99 | 15 - 16 | 25 - 35 |
| 363 - 456 | 8.6 - 10.9 | 0.84 - 0.93 | 14 - 15 | 15 - 20 |
| 454 - 612 | 11.4 - 15.9 | 0.66 - 0.77 | 12 - 14 | 10 - 15 |

care practices (deworming programs) and temperature stress, to allow producers to maintain excellent body weight gain during the rearing period.

Although the optimal growth rate to maximize both mammary development, first lactation milk production, and profitability is still unknown, milk production per cow will continue to increase. This suggests that the weight and frame size just postcalving need to be larger so that when in lactation, they have the ability to consume sufficient nutrients (Buchholtz, 1993).

To successfully achieve a calving age of 24 months or less (see part 1 of this Chapter), multiple planes of nutrition have to be balanced for energy and protein through out the rearing period (Hoffman and Funk,1992; Van Amburgh and Galton, 1994; Skidmore, 1995). This goal is only achievable when the growth of young stock is monitored, recorded and evaluated throughout the rearing period (Bucholtz, 1993). This means that monthly body taping, measuring withers heights, and body condition scoring of heifers is required (Buchholtz, 1993; VanAmburgh et al., 1991). Rations should be adjusted if heifers are not developing according to preset targets, for example a postcalving body weight of 570 kg, together with a wither height of 142 cm and a condition score of 3.5.

## 2.2.6 DECISION MAKING

Decision making is based on monitoring and evaluation of primary and secondary performance indices. During the evaluation process, primary performance indices are compared with pre-set targets for a specific herd. If the actual performance indices match the preset targets, no further action is undertaken and data collection by the farmer is continued. If the primary performance indices deviate from preset targets, secondary indices will be evaluated. This might reveal an impending or existing problem with regard to health, growth or reproductive performance relative to their age. Examples of problems are:

*) high morbidity and/or mortality rate,
*) growth retardation,
*) delayed first calving age,
*) suboptimal reproductive performance.

For decision making three sources of information are used: 1) herd data, 2) farm inspection data, and 3) clinical inspection data. Herd data is retrospective in nature. The two other data sources are actual but are not related to all animals in the herd. To demonstrate decision making an example farm is created.

### Example farm

Characteristics of the example farm are: Herd size: 205 lactating and dry cows, and 117 young stock (49 < 1 year, and 58 > 1 year). Labor force consists of the farmer and one hired person. Average milk yield per cow per year is 7300 kg. Calving interval 399 days. Cows are pastured in summer time. Forages fed in winter time consist mainly of grass silage and some corn silage and brewers grains. A mixer wagon is not available. In the milking herd, concentrates are provided via an automatic concentrate feeder, Young stock is kept on pasture in summer time and in an old, naturally ventilated barn in winter time. Normally young stock is not dewormed. The farmer decided to participate in a HH & PM service three months ago. At that time preset targets for replacement rearing were defined.

The first two farm visits revealed that nutrients fed to young stock, which were kept in a crowded pen, consisted of leftovers from the milking cows and/or grass silage of moderate quality plus an undefined amount of concentrates. Chest circumference measurements, body condition scoring and record keeping of young stock were initated at the first farm visit. Average body conditions of young stock were low and varied from 2 to 2.7.

The decision making proces starts with comparing actual primary performance indices, calculated from available recorded data and from clinical and farm inspections, with preset targets. The primary performance indices that could be calculated sofar (Table 3), indicate that the actual age at first calving, postcalving body weigth and wither heigth, which were measured during the last farm visit, are not meeting the preset targets. Mortality and abortion rate are in accordance with preset targets. The first conclusion that already can be drawn is that actual primary performance indices deviate from preset targets which necessitates an evaluation of secondary indices.

Relevant suboptimal secondary indices on the example farm are growth rates and reproductive performance indices, which are only based on some recently collected data. Alimentary tract and respiratory diseases are not a problem at this moment.

The main findings of this evaluation are that age at first calving is 3 months longer than the preset target of 24 months and that body weigth and frame size after calving is suboptimal.

To identify causal or contributing factors for suboptimal performance of these indices, retrospective information about these aspects in the various time periods of the developmental time scale (Figure 2, part 1 of this Chapter) should now be evaluated. In combination with secondary performance indices this might reveal certain risk periods. Secondly, detailed examinations/analyses of relevant primary and secundary indices should be conducted to arrive at a herd performance diagnosis. However, the problem is that data recording on replacement rearing started only recently on this farm. This means that a retrospective evaluation of information can only be performed with the recently collected data.

Trying to explain the delay in first calving and suboptimal body size, the following reasons could be thought of:

1. Poor estrous detection practices which could explain the delay in first insemination,
2. A delay in onset of puberty i.e. first estrus. A delay in onset of puberty may be caused by suboptimal growth rates or by diseases, and/or just by poor overall management,
3. other factors such as a seasonal calving pattern, which was not a goal on this farm.

Evaluating secondary reproductive performance indices in more detail reveals that

*Table 3. Primary and secondary performance indices (example herd)*

| PERFORMANCE INDICES | ACTUAL | TARGETS |
|---|---|---|
| Herd characteristics | | |
| – Herd size (cows and heifers) | 205 | — |
| – # Young stock | 107 | — |
| – # heifers calved last year | 50 | — |
| **PRIMARY INDICES** | | |
| – Predicted minimum age at 1st calving (mo) | 26 | ≤24 |
| – Body weight postcalving (kg) | 510 | 570 |
| – Wither height postcalving (cm) | 137 | 142 |
| – % mortality (total rearing period) | 7 | < 10 |
| – % abortions in heifers | 2 | < 4 |
| **SECONDARY INDICES** | | |
| **% Mortality** | | |
| – 0 - 24 hours | 3 | < 6 |
| – 1 - 30 days | 2 | < 2 |
| – 31 - 60 days | - | < 1 |
| – 3 - 24 months | 1 | < 1 |
| **% Morbidity rate (prevalence/pen)** | | |
| % clinical diarrhea | 14 | < 20 |
| % clinical respiratory disease | 20 | < 6 |
| % clinical lameness | 4 | < 5 |
| % clinical mastitis | 2 | < 5 |
| **Body weight gain g/day** | | |
| – prepubertal < 10 months | 523 | 800 |
| – postpubertal > 10 months | 418 | 825 |
| **Reproductive performance** | | |
| – Age at conception (months) | 16.9 | ≤15 |
| – % pregnant first insemination | 55 | 75 |
| – No. inseminations/pregnancy | 1.8 | 1.3 |
| – % Dystocias in heifers | 3 | < 5 |

reproductive performance is not optimal. The interval from first insemination of to conception is 37 days, 1.8 inseminations per pregnancy were needed and the pregnancy rate at first insemination is 55%. Due to these suboptimal indices, about 37 days are lost between first insemination and conception. However, this only partly explains the prolonged interval from birth to age of conception of three months.

Furthermore, although a suboptimal reproductive performance can be responsible for a delayed age at first calving, it does not explain the suboptimal body size at the time of calving. The next question then arises which other factors may be involved in the delay. Examining the secondary performance indices again, will focus our attention at growth rates of young stock. A disturbed growth rate caused by diseases or by suboptimal nutrition can be responsible for both a suboptimal performance in age at first calving and in body size. However chest circumference measurements are only available of a restricted number of young stock less than 1 year old. The results of the two chest circumference measurements (Table 4) indicate that the actual body weigths stay behind growth standards as presented in part 1 of this Chapter (Table 4) and also that growth rates of individual calves vary greatly. The average growth per calf per day between 3 and 10 months of age is only 523 grams. If this has been the case in the past this migth have caused a delayed onset of estrus and consequently a delayed first insemination. This necessitates to concentrate attention to nutrition of young stock throughout the rearing period and to frequent chest circumference measurements and body condition scoring during the next farm visits.

**Herd performance diagnosis**

The analysis of the available information of the example farm leads to a herd performance diagnosis, which concentrates on deficiencies in the field of nutrition, estrous detection, and possible health care, especially deworming. Existing knowledge and skills have to be applied to identify unwanted management factors or farm conditions that contribute to the problem in the specific areas. On a short term, advices should be given or treatments performed to solve actual problems. The recommendations should be based on the total analysis and economic impacts of suggested changes in management. At the end of the farm visit a report should be written with recommendations an or advices given.

## 2.2.7 FOLLOW-UP

The recommendations given or activities executed at previous visits should be evaluated at the subsequent visit by comparing the actual performance indices with the performance indices at the time of the previous visits. In case the recommendations/activities did not result in improvements of indices involved the reason why they failed should be examined. This could be due to improper recommendations/activities or to inadequate execution of them. If on a long term no problems occur and therefore no recommendations were given, the pre-set targets may be reset at a more appropriate level.

*Table 4. Results of two weight bandings (interval of 72 days) of calves and growth per day*

| Calf No. | Name | Age in months | Previous weigth (Kg) | Last weigth (Kg) | Gain/ day (gr) | Ref. weigth (Kg) | Difference (Kg) |
|---|---|---|---|---|---|---|---|
| 282 | Betje | 12.0 | 270 | 295 | 332 | 343 | -48 |
| 283 | Meggie | 11.7 | 270 | 301 | 430 | 335 | -34 |
| 284 | Rina 58 | 11.6 | 246 | 283 | 510 | 332 | -49 |
| 285 | Elza | 11.4 | 274 | 302 | 400 | 326 | -24 |
| 288 | Julia | 9.7 | 201 | 245 | 610 | 277 | -22 |
| 289 | Joke | 9.6 | 188 | 221 | 460 | 274 | -53 |
| 290 | Riek | 9.3 | 199 | 256 | 800 | 266 | -10 |
| 291 | Ida | 9.3 | 181 | 236 | 418 | 266 | 30 |
| 292 | Jannie | 8.3 | 170 | 209 | 548 | 237 | -28 |
| 293 | Bets | 8.3 | 171 | 199 | 400 | 237 | -38 |
| 294 | Marie | 7.8 | 165 | 200 | 500 | 222 | -22 |
| 295 | Jose | 7.8 | 149 | 186 | 514 | 222 | -35 |
| 296 | Cora | 7.7 | 153 | 219 | 917 | 219 | 0 |
| 297 | Rintje | 6.5 | 135 | 171 | 500 | 184 | -13 |
| 298 | Hetty | 5.9 | 126 | 160 | 472 | 167 | -7 |
| 299 | Thea | 5.7 | 129 | 139 | 139 | 162 | -23 |
| 300 | Beppie | 5.7 | 120 | 142 | 306 | 162 | -20 |
| 301 | Koos | 5.1 | 110 | 146 | 500 | 147 | -1 |
| 302 | Ditje | 5.1 | 103 | 126 | 319 | 147 | -21 |
| 303 | Corrie | 5.0 | 88 | 117 | 403 | 144 | -27 |
| 304 | Manon | 5.0 | 98 | 146 | 667 | 144 | +2 |
| 306 | Carla | 4.3 | 80 | 123 | 736 | 126 | -18 |
| 307 | Sophie | 4.2 | 74 | 123 | 681 | 123 | 0 |
| 308 | Rika | 4.1 | 78 | 117 | 542 | 121 | -4 |
| 310 | Sanne | 3.4 | 54 | 93 | 542 | 108 | -15 |
| 311 | Pieta | 3.3 | 68 | 106 | 528 | 105 | +1 |

## EPILOGUE

Replacement rearing starts at conception and ends at the time of first calving. The ultimate goal of replacement rearing is to reach first calving age at a predetermined time with less as posible health problems and with an optimal growth rate at minimal costs. To monitor this period a structured approach is needed. Such an approach is incorporated in the protocol described in Chapter 1, part 1 and demonstrated in this Chapter. The cornerstone of the protocol is formed by defining preset targets.

Once the targets are defined the available tools and methods must be implemented to reach the preset targets. Very essential tools in replacement rearing are record keeping, data monitoring, data processing into performance indices, and evaluation of these indices. They offer the farmer, the HH & PM practitioner, and the farm advisor the information on which continuously can be judged, whether the preset targets can be/are reached. With proper information also proper management decisions can be made in time to adjust the execution of replacement rearing activities if needed.

Besides to proper record keeping attention should be paid to proper health care and to an optimal growth rate of young stock. Optimal growth can only be established with well balanced and formulated rations. These essential aspects of replacement rearing are often neglected on many farms. It is the task of the HH & PM practitioner and farm advisor to monitor, to evaluate, and to manipulate these aspects continuously. For that reason chest circumference measurements and body condition scoring should be executed at regular intervals. They form, together with scrupulous record keeping and record analysis, the skeleton of an optimal replacement rearing. If executed in an adequate way replacement rearing will become a very profitable investment for the farmer.

## REFERENCES

*Abel Francisco, S.F. and J.D. Quigley, III. 1993. Serum immunoglobulin concentration in response to maternal colostrum and colostral supplementation in dairy calves. Am. J. Vet. Res. 54:1051-1054.*

*Akers, R,M., D.E. Bauman, G.T. Goodman, A.V. Capuco, and H.A. Tucker. 1981. Prolactin regulation of cytological differentiation of mammary epithelial cells in periparturient cows. Endocrinology. 109:31-40.*

*Anderson, N., J. Armour, F.W. Jennings, J.S.D. Ritchie and G.M.Urquhart. 1965. Inhibited development of Ostertagi ostertagi. Vet.Rec.77:146-147.*

*Anderson, M.J., M. Khoyloo, and J.L. Walters. 1982. Effect of feeding whole cottonseed on intake, body weight, and reticulorumen development of young Holstein calves. J. Dairy Sci. 65:764-772.*

*Armour, J. 1989. The influence of host immunity on the epidemiology of trichostrongy lus infections in cattle. Vet. Parasitol. 32:5-19.*

*Bates, D.W., W.G. Bickert, M.F. Brugger, G.R. Bodman, B.J. Holmes, D.L. Jones and T.J. Brevik. 1985. Dairy housing and equipment handbook. Midwest Plan service, Iowa State University, Ames, Iowa, USA.*

*Besser, T.E., T.C. McGuire, C.C. Gay, and L.C. Pritchett. 1988a. Transfer of functional immunoglobulin G (IgG) antibody into the gastrointestinal tract accounts for IgG clearance in calves. J. Virol. 62:2234- 2237.*

*Besser, T.E., C.C. Gay, T.C. McGuire, and J.F. Evermann. 1988b. Passive immunity to bovine rotavirus infection associated with transfer of serum antibody into the intestinal lumen. J. Virol. 62:2238- 2242.*

*Bezek, D. 1994. Rotavirus enteritis in food animals. Comp. Contin. Educ. 16:391-405.*

*Bickert, W.G. and T.H. Herdt. 1985. Environmental aspects of dairy calf housing. The Comp. Contin. Educ. 7:309-316.*

*Boon, J.H. 1980. Studies on the possible causes of cough in calves at pasture. Tijdschr. Diergeneeskd. 105:1077-1083.*

*Braun, R.K. and B.C. Tennant. 1983. The relationship of serum gamma globulin levels of assembled neonatal calves to mortality caused by enteritic diseases. Agri-Practice. 4:14-24.*

*Burton, J.L., B.W. Kennedy, E.B. Burnside, B.N. Wilkie, and J.H. Burton. 1989. Variation in serum concentrations of immunoglobulins G, A, and M in Canadian Holstein-Frisian calves. J. Dairy Sci. 72:135-149.*

*Bucholtz, H.F. 1993. Feeding for proper growth and age at first calving. Tri-state Dairy Nutrition Conference. Indiana University-Purdue University at Fort Wayne. May 18 and 19. pp.137-147.*

*Bush, L. J., and T. E. Staley. 1980. Absorption of colostral immunoglobulins in newborn calves. J. Dairy Sci. 63:672-680.*

*Capuco, A.V., J.J. Smith, D.R. Waldo, and C.E. Rexroad Jr. 1995. Influence of prepuber tal dietary regime on mammary growth of Holstein heifers. J. Dairy Sci. 78:2709-2725.*

*Church, D. C. 1976. Digestive Physiology and Nutrition of Ruminants. Vol. 1 - Digestive Physiology. 2nd ed. O & B Books, Inc., Corvallis, Oregon, USA.*

*Clarke, M.A. 1993. Bovine coronavirus. Br. Vet. J. 149:51-70.*

*Curtis, C.R., H.N. Erb, and M.E. White. 1985. Risk factors for calfhood morbidity and mortality on New York dairy farms. Proceedings of Cornell Nutrition Conference, pp 90-99.*

*Dodd, A. 1992. Calf housing: Principles and practice. Irish Vet. J. 45:91-104.*

*Donovan, G.A. and R.K. Braun. 1987. Evaluation of dairy heifer replacement-rearing programs. Compend. Cont. Educ. 9:F133-139.*

*Drew, M.D. 1994. Effects of immunoglobulin fortification of milk replacers on the per formance of calves challenged with Escherichia coli. J. Dairy Sci. 77 (Suppl. 1):298 (Abstr.).*

*Eysker, M., H.W. Saatkamp, and A. Kloosterman. 1993. Infection build up and develop ment of immunity in calves following primary Dictyocaulus viviparus infections of different levels at the beginning or in the middle of the grazing season. Vet. Parasitol. 49:243-254.*

*Fagan, J.G., P.J. Dwyer, and J.G. Quinlan. 1995. Factors that may affect the occurrence of enteropathogens in the feces of diarrhoeic calves in Ireland. Irish Vet. J. 48:17-21.*

*Fahr, R.D., K. Schmidt, and H.J. Schwark. 1985. Lebendmassenentwicklung und Lebendmasse - Leistungsbeziehungen bei Kuhe im Verlauf der Laktation. Arch. Tierzucht. 6:519-528.*

*Fleenor, W.A. and G.H. Stott. 1980. Hydrometer test for estimation of immunoglobulin concentration in bovine colostrum. J. Dairy Sci. 63:973-977.*

*Foldager, J. and K. Sejrsen. 1987. Mammary gland development and milk production in dairy cows in relation to feeding and hormone manipulation during rearing. Research in dairy cattle: Danish status and perspectives. Det kgl. danske Landhusholdningsselskab, Copenhagen, Denmark.*

*Foley, J.A. and D.E. Otterby. 1978. Availability, storage, treatment, composition, and fee ding value of surplus colostrum: A review. J. Dairy Sci. 61:1033-1060.*

*Fowler, M.A., R.L. Sweat, T.E. Johnson, and L.K. Seiser. 1995. Prevention of rotavirus scours in neonatal calves with colostrum feeding. J. Dairy Sci. 78 (Suppl. 1):235 (Abstr.).*

*Gardner, R.W., J.D. Schuh, L.G. Vargus. 1977. Accelerated growth and early breeding in Holstein heifers. J. Dairy Sci. 60:1941-1948.*

*Gay, C. 1994. Colostrum research says feed 4 quarts for healther calves. Hoards Dairyman, March 25, pp. 256.*

*Goodger W.J. and Theodore E.M. 1986. Calf management practices and health manage ment decisions on large dairies. J. Dairy Sci. 69:580-590.*

*Gunther, H. and F. Schulze. 1985. Zur Alterresistenz bei der Koliruhr des Kalbes. Monathefte Vet. Med. 40:419-422.*

*Harrison, R.D., I.P. Reynolds, and W. Little. 1983. A quantitative analysis of mammary glands of dairy heifers reared at different rates of live weight gain. J. Dairy Res. 50: 405-412.*

*Heinrichs, A.J. and G.L. Hargrove. 1987. Standards of weight and height for Holstein heifers. J. Dairy Sci. 70:653-660.*

*Hoffman, P.C. and D.A. Funk. 1991. Growth rates of Holstein replacement heifers in selected Wisconsin dairy herds. College of Agricultural and life Sciences Research Report. Univ. of Wisconsin-Madison. (cited by Hoffman, 1992).*

*Hoffman, P.C. 1992. Fundamentals of replacement heifer growth, Development, and production Potential. Dairy management Conference Proceedings. Prosperity in the 90's March 3-4 1992. Michigan. A.L. Skidmore editor pp. 119-131.*

*Hoffman, P.C. and D.A. Funk. 1992. Applied dynamics of dairy replacement growth and management. J. Dairy Sci. 75:2504-2516.*

*Hoorfar, J., N.C. Feld, A.L. Schirmer, V. Bitsch, and P. Lind. 1993. Serodiagnosis of Salmonella dublin infection in Danish dairy cattle herds using O-antigen based enzyme immunoabsorbent assay. Can. J. Vet. Res. 57:268-274.*

*Hopkins, F.M., D.F. Dean and W. Greene. 1984. Failure of passive tranfer in calves: Comparison of field diagnosis methods. Modern Vet. Practice. 1984. :625-628.*

*Hovey, R.C., T.B. McFadden, and D.D.S. Mackenzie. 1994. Response of mammary epit helial cells to ovarian steroids is modulated by the mammary fat pad during the estrous cycle. J. Anim. Sci. 72 (Suppl. 1), 68: (Abstr.)*

*James, R.E., M.L. McGilliard, and D.A. Hartman. 1984. Calf mortality in Virginia Dairy Herd Improvement herds. J. Dairy Sci. 67:908-911.*

*Janke, B.H. 1989. Protecting calves from diarrhea. Vet. Med. 84:803-811.*

*Jenny, B.F., G.E. Gramling, and T.M. Glaze. 1981. Management factors associated with calf mortality in South Carolina dairy herds. J. Dairy Sci. 64:2284-2289.*

*Judge, M.D., E.D. Aberle, J.L. Forest, H.B. Hedric, and R.A. Merkel. 1989. Principles of meat science. 2nd edition. Kendal/Hunt Publishing Company, Dubuque, IA.*

*Kahrs, R.F., D.T. Bechtol, and J.W. Morse. 1986. Council report. Bovine immunization guidelines. JAVMA, 189:281-284.*

*Kelly, T.G., V.A. Dodd, D.J. Ruan, R.J. Falon, and P.J. Tuite. 1984. An assessment of the influence of some house designs and environmental factors on calf performance. J. Agric. Engng. Res. 30:175-184.*

*Keown, J.F., and R.W. Everett. 1986. Effects of days carrier calf, days dry and weight of first calf heifers on yield. J.Dairy Sci. 69:1891-1896.*

*Kertz, A.F., L.F. Reutzel, and J.H. Mahony. 1984. Ad libitum water intake by neonatal calves and its relationship to calf starter intake, weight gain, feces score, and season. J. Dairy Sci. 67:2964-2972.*

*Kertz, A. F, Prewitt, L.R and J.M. Ballam. 1987. Increased weight gain and effects on growth parameters of Holstein heifer calves from 3 to 12 months of age. J. Dairy Sci. 70:1612-1622.*

*Kesler, E. M. 1981. Feeding mastitic milk to calves: Review. J. Dairy Sci. 64:719-723.*

*Kloosterman, A. 1971. Observations on the epidemiology of trichostrongylosis of calves. PhD thesis Wageningen Agricultural University.*

*Kloosterman, A., H.W. Ploeger, and K. Frankena. 1990. Increased establishment of lung worms after exposure to a combined infection of Ostertagi ostertagi and Cooperia oncophora. Vet. Parasitol. 36:117-122.*

*Lance, S.E., G.Y. Miller, D.D. Hancock, P.C. Bartlett, L.E. Heider, and M.L. Moeschberger. 1992. Effects of environment and management on mortality in preweaned dairy calves. J. Amer. Vet. Med. Assoc. 201:1197-1202.*

*Larson, L. L., F. G. Owen, J. L. Albright, R. D. Appleman, R. C. Lamb, and L. D. Muller. 1977. Guidelines toward more uniformity in measuring and reporting calf experimental data. J. Dairy Sci. 60:989-991.*

*Lee, R.B., T.E. Besser, C.C. Gay, and T.C. McGuire. 1983. The influence of method of fee ding on IgG concentrations acquired by calves. Proceedings, 4th International Symposium on Neonatal Diarrhea. VIDO, Saskatoon, Saskatchewan, Canada. pp. 373-377.*

*Lengemann, F. W. and N. N. Allen. 1959. Development of rumen function in the dairy calf. II. Effect of diet upon characteristics of the rumen flora and fauna of young calves. J. Dairy Sci. 42:1171-1181.*

*Lin, C.Y., A.J. Mallister, and A.J. Lee. 1985. Multitrait estimation of relationships of first-lactation yields to body weight changes in Holstein heifers. J.Dairy Sci. 68:2954-2963.*

*Little, W. and R.M. Kay. 1979. The efects of rapid rearing and early calving on the subse quent performance of dairy heifers. Anim. Prod. 29:131-142.*

*Little, W., C.B. Mallison, D.N. Gibbons, and G.J. Rowlands. 1981. Effects of plane of nut rition and season of birth on the age and body weight at puberty of British Frisian heifers. Anim. Prod. 33:273-279.*

*Losinger, W.C., S.J. Wells, L.P. Garber, H.S. Hurd, and L.A. Thomas. 1995. Management factors related to Salmonella shedding by dairy heifers. J. Dairy Sci. 78:2464-2472.*

*Logan, E.F., G.R. Pearson, and M.S. McNulty. 1977. Studies on the immunity of the calf to colibacillosis - VII: The experimental reproduction of enteric colibacillosis in colostrum-fed calves. Vet. Rec. 101:443-446.*

*MaCaulay, A.S., G.L. Hahn, D.H. Clark, and D.V. Sisson. 1995. Comparison of calf hou sing types and tympanic temperature rhytms in Holstein calves. J. Dairy Sci. 78:856-862.*

*Maree, C. 1986. The influence of high level feeding on the duration of parturition and the incidence of dystocia in dairy cows. J. South African Vet. Assoc. 38: 151-153.*

*Martin, W.B., B.A.C. Thomas, and G.M. Urquhart. 1957. Chronic diarrhoea in housed cattle due to atypical parasitic gastritis. Vet. Rec. 69:736-739.*

*McKellar, Q.A. 1988. Strategic use of anthelmintics for parasitic nematodes in cattle and sheep. Vet. Rec. 123:483-487.*

*Menzi, W. 1995. Heifer housing system for improved performance. AABP specialty seminars. Seminar 13. In: Optimizing dairy heifer replacement programs. San Antonio, Texas. September 12-13.*

*Michel, J.F. 1969. The epidemiology and control of some nematode infections in grazing animals. Adv. Parasitol. 7:211-282.*

*Michel, J.F. 1976. The epidemiology and control of some nematode infections in grazing animals. Adv. Parasitol. 14:355-397.*

*Mitchell, C.D. 1976. Calf housing handbook. Scotapress Publications.*

*Moore, D.A. 1989. Minimizing morbidity and mortality from cryptosporidiosis. Vet. Med. 84:811-815.*

*National Animal Health Monitoring System. 1992. Dairy herd management practices focusing on preweaned heifers, April 1991 - July 1992. U.S. Department of Agriculture, Animal and Plant Health Inspection Service, Veterinary Services, Ft. Collins, Colorado.*

*National Research Council. 1981. Effect of environment on nutrient requirement of domestic animals. Natl. Acad. Sci. Washington. D.C.*

*Noordhuizen, J.P.T.M. Veterinary herd health and production control on dairy farms. PhD Thesis, Utrecht, 1984.*

*Oostendorp, D. and H.E. Harmsen. 1968. Agricultural control measures against intestin al parasites in cattle. Neth. J. Agric. Sci. 16:177-185.*

*Oetjen, B.D. 1993. Management of coccidiosis in dairy calves and replacement heifers. Comp. Cont, Educ. 15:891-895.*

*Over, H.J. 1962. A method of determining the liver fluke environment by means of vege tation type. Bull. Office Internat. Epizoot. 58:297-304.*

*Perez, E. Epidemiological aspects of morbidity, mortality and growth of calves in Costa Rica. PhD Thesis, Utrecht, 1994.*

*Peri, I., A. Gertler, I. Bruckental, and H. Barash. 1993. The effect of manipulation in energy allowance during the rearing period of heifers on hormone concentrations and milk production in first lactation cows. J. Dairy Sci. 76:742-751.*

*Pitt, J., B. Barlow, and W.C. Heird. 1977. Protection against experimental necrotizing enterocolitis by maternal milk. I. Role of milk leukocytes. Pediatrics Res. 11:906-909.*

*Ploeger, H.W. 1989. Effect of nematode infections on productivity of young and adult cattle on commercial dairy farms. PhD thesis Wageningen Agricultural University.*

*Price, S., P. Hoffman, and J. Barmore. 1994a. Tailored rations help heifers grow. Hoard's Dairyman. October 10. pp.685.*

*Price, S., P. Hoffman and J. Barmore. 1994b. High and dry heifers... faster gains, lower cost. Hoard's Dairyman. September 25, pp.645.*

*Pritchett, L.C., C.L. Gay, T.E. Besser, and D.D. Hancock. 1991. Management and production factors influencing immunoglobulin G1 concentration in colostrum from Holstein cows. J. Dairy Sci. 74:2336-2341.*

*Pritchett, L.C., C.L. Gay, D.D. Hancock, and T.E. Besser. 1994. Evaluation of the hydro meter for testing immunoglobulin G1 concentrations in Holstein colostrum. J. Dairy Sci. 77:1761-1767.*

*Quigley, J. D., III, L. A. Caldwell, G. D. Sinks, and R. N. Heitmann. 1991. Changes in blood glucose, non-esterified fatty acids, and ketones in response to weaning and feed intake in young calves. J. Dairy Sci. 74:250-257.*

*Quigley, J.D., III, K.R. Martin, H.H. Dowlen, L.B. Wallis, and K. Lamar. 1994. Immunoglobulin concentration, specific gravity, and nitrogen fractions of colostrum from Jersey cattle. J. Dairy Sci. 77:264-269.*

*Quigley, J. D., III, K. R. Martin, D. A. Bemis. L.N.D. Potgieter, C. R. Reinemeyer, B.W. Rohrbach, H.H. Dowlen and K.C. Lamar. 1994. Effects of housing and colostrum feeding on the prevalence of selected infectious organisms in feces of Jersey calves. J. Dairy Sci. 77:3124-3131.*

*Quigley, J.D., III, K.R. Martin, D.A. Bemis, L.N.D. Potgieter, C.R. Reinemeyer, B.W. Rohrbach, H.H. Dowlen and K.C. Lamar. 1995b. Effects of housing and colostrum feeding on serum immunoglobulins, growth and fecal scores of Jersey calves. J. Dairy Sci. 78:893-901.*

*Quigley, J. D., III, K. R. Martin, and H. H. Dowlen. 1995a. Concentrations of trypsin inhibitor and immunoglobulins in colostrum of Jersey cattle. J. Dairy Sci. 78:1573-1575.*

*Quigley, J. D., III. 1995b. Effects of method of colostrum feeding and supplementation on serum IgG concentration in neonatal calves. J. Dairy Sci. 78 (Suppl. 1):234 (Abstr.).*

*Reddy, P. G., J. L. Morrill, and H. C. Minocha. 1985. Effect of early weaning on the cell mediated immune response of dairy calves. Nutr. Rep. Intl. 31:501-503.*

*Remmen, J.W.A. Een onderzoek naar mogelijkheden om perinatale sterfte bij het rund te beperken. Thesis, Utrecht, 1976.*

*Riedel-Caspari, G. 1993. The influence of colostral leukocytes on the course of an expe rimental Escherichia coli infection and serum antibodies in neonatal calves. Vet. Immunology and Immunopathology. 35:275-288.*

*Roy, J.H.B. 1990. The Calf. Vol. 1. Management of Health. 5th ed. Butterworth, London.*

*Rothman, K.J. 1986. Modern epidemiology. Little, Brown and company. Boston. USA.*

*Saif, L.J. and K.J. Smith. 1985. Enteric viral infections of calves and passive immunity. J. Dairy Sci. 68:206-228.*

*Saif, L.J., D.R. Redman, K.L. Smith, and K.W. Theil. 1983. Passive immunity to bovine rotavirus in newborn calves fed colostrum supplements from immunized or nonimmunized cows. Infect. & Immun. 41:1118-1131.*

*Saif, L.J. 1987. Development of nasal, fecal and serum isotype-specific antibodies in calves challenged with bovine coronavirus or rotavirus. Vet. Immunol. Immunopathol. 17:425-439.*

*Sjersen, K, J.T. Huber, H.A. Tucker, and R.M. Akers. 1982. Influence of nutrition on mammary development in pre- and postpubertal heifers. J. Dairy Sci. 65: 793-800.*

*Sjersen, K, J.T. Huber, and H.A. Tucker. 1983. Influence of amount fed on hormone con centrations and relationship to mammary growth in heifers. J. Dairy Sci. 66:845-855.*

*Skidmore, A.L. 1995. Growth management of dairy replacement heifers. Extension bul letin E-2580. September 1995.*

*Steen, T.M., J.D. Quigley, III, R.N. Heitmann, and J.D. Gresham. 1992. Effects of lasalo cid and undegradable protein on growth and body composition of Holstein heifers. J. Dairy Sci. 75:2517-2523.*

*Stelwagen, K. and D.G. Grieve. 1990. Effect of plane of nutrition on growth and mam mary gland development in Holstein heifers. J. Dairy Sci. 73:2333-2341.*

*Sutton, J. D., A. D. McGilliard, and N. L. Jacobson. 1963. Functional development of rumen mucosa. I. Absorptive ability. J. Dairy Sci. 46:426-436.*

*Taylor, E.L. 1964. Fascioliasis and the liver fluke. FAO Agricultural studies no. 64, FAO, Rome Italy.*

*Tucker H. A. 1987. Quantitative estimates of mammary growth during various physio logical states: A review. J. Dairy Sci. 70:1958-1966.*

*Vercruysse, J., H. Hilderson, and E. Claerebout. 1994. Effect of Chemoprophylaxis on immunity to gastrointestinal nematodes in cattle. Parasitology Today. 10:129-132.*

*VanAmburgh, M.E., D.M. Galton, D. Fox, and D. Bauman. 1991. Optimizing heifer growth. Proc. Cornell Nutrition Conference for feed Manufacturers. pp.85-93.*

*VanAmburgh, M.E. and D.M. Galton 1994. Growth and nutrition of heifers. Dairy management Conference Proceedings. Michigan State University Extention March 1-2 1992 Ed. A. Skidmore pp. 39-65*

*Vermorel, M., J. Vernet, C. Dardillat, D. Saido, and M. Davicco. 1989. Energy metabolism and thermoregulation in the newborn calf; effect of calving conditions. Can. J. Anim. Sci. 69:113-122.*

*Webster, A.J.F. 1981. Optimal housing criteria for ruminants. In: Environmental aspects of housing for animal production pp. 217-232. London: Butterworths.*

*Wildman E.E., G.M. Jones, P.E. Wagner, and R.L. Bowman. 1982. A dairy cow body condition scoring system and its relationship to selected production characteristics. J. Dairy Sci. 38:495-500.*

*Winter, K.A. 1985. Comparative performance and digestibility in dairy calves weaned at three, five, and seven weeks of age. Can. J. Anim. Sci. 65:445-450.*

*Wray, C. 1993. Bovine Salmonellosis: An Update. Irish Vet. J. 46:137-148.*

*Waltner-Toews, D., S.W. Martin, A.H. Meek, and I. McMillan. 1986a. Dairy calf manage ment, morbidity and mortality in Ontario Holstein herds. Prev. Vet. Med. 4:103-117.*

*Waltner-Toews, D., S.W. Martin, and A.H. Meek. 1986b. Dairy calf management, morbi dity and mortality in Ontario Holstein herds. IV. Association of management with mortality. Prev. Vet. Med. 4:159-171.*

*Zaremba, W., E. Grunert, W. Heuwieser and H. Schniffer-Mehrens. 1985. Untersuchungen über die Immunglobulinabsorption bei Kälbern nach Verabreichung von Kolostrum per Schlundsonde im Vergleich zur freiwilligen Aufnahme. Deutsch. tierarztl. Wschr. 1985 92:18-20.*

# 2.3 MONITORING REPLACEMENT REARING: CASE STUDY ON PERINATAL CALF DEATH

Daniel T. Scholl[1], Geert Benedictus[2] and Arie Brand[3]

[1] School of Veterinary Medicine, Louisiana State University, Baton Rouge, Louisiana 70803, USA
[2] Regional Animal Health Centre, Morra 2, 9200 AJ Drachten, The Netherlands
[3] Department of Herd Health and Reproduction, School of Veterinary Medicine, University of Utrecht, Yalelaan 7, 3485 CL Utrecht, The Netherlands

## 2.3.1 INTRODUCTION

The on-going success of a dairy enterprise rests in part on its replacement rearing program which begins with successful birth of live calves. In contrast, perinatal calf death results in genetics related opportunity cost, and culling restrictions by virtue of a reduced pool of replacements. Perinatal death, which is defined as calf death from the 270th day of gestation to 24 hours after birth, varies from 9 to 12% in heifers and from 2 to 4% in older cows in the Netherlands (Meyering, 1984). A survey in Norway estimated a 2.8% incidence of stillbirths and mortality within 24 hours of life (Simensen, 1982) and an 8.37% incidence was estimated in Ireland (Mee, 1988). One survey in the United States estimated a 1.2% incidence of death at birth among heifers (James, et al., 1984), which is an underestimate with respect to total perinatal death. Another study of 1459 pregnancies over 24 years on one farm showed that 4.2% of the fetuses that reached the 270th day of gestation experienced perinatal calf death (Leonard and Gardner, 1975).

Problem solving is a part of Herd Health and Production Management (HH & PM) services. Investigating a herd problem or complaint requires a top-down approach. The starting point is a search for potentially causal factors that can be retained or ruled out as potential contributors to the problem. The investigation works towards the ultimate cause or causes in successive steps. The following case study provides an example of how one might proceed investigating a perinatal calf death complaint using a methodical protocol for investigation.

## 2.3.2 DEFINITION OF CLIENT'S COMPLAINT

A 100 cow Holstein dairy herd is experiencing a high incidence of calves born dead near term or dying within 24 hours of birth. The farmer considers this an important problem and asks for a solution to the problem.

## 2.3.3 HISTORY

The history of the problem was obtained by asking the farmer a predetermined sequence of questions. The following answers were obtained:

* **Regarding the complaint:**
- Duration: The problem started about 1 year ago, was first noticed among calves of heifers and later of cows, and has steadily worsened.
- Incidence: The farmer estimated that more than 10% of the heifers and cows delivered dead calves over the last year. No seasonal distribution was evident. In previous years, dead calves were delivered only occasionally. Congenital abnormalities among the dead calves were not noticed.
- Dystocia: At least 15% of all calvings were assisted.

* **Characteristics of the farm:**
- Milk production: The rolling herd average is about 7,000 kg. According to the farmer milk production of both cows and heifers has gradually declined over the last year.
- Labor: The labor force consists of the farmer and his wife (35% time) and one person working on Saturdays only.
- Management support: The farmer participates in a national milk production recording and analysis scheme but not in HH & PM services. Pregnancy checks are occasionally performed by the producer's practitioner. Feed analyses are performed irregularly.
- Housing: During summer, the lactating herd is pastured and confined in a freestall setup during winter. The replacements and dry cows are maintained in a separate barn in winter and usually pastured in summer.
- Maternity area: One maternity pen is available and is used when possible. Cows are restrained when in the pen. If the pen is already in use, calving animals stay with the early lactation group.

* **Management changes:**
- Labor: A full time employee left one year ago and has not been replaced. A mixer wagon was purchased at that time.

* **Records:**
- Type of records: Reproductive data are recorded on a herd fertility barn chart (see Chapter 1, part 2). Disease records are not kept. Milk production/testing data are available from DHIA.
- Data quality: The producer considers record keeping adequate, up-to-date and accurate.

* **Health status:**
- Abortions: Abortions before the 270th day of gestation have occurred in 3 cows

over the last year (i.e., ± 3%). The aborted calves have not been necropsied and sera have not been collected from the dams.

- Disease incidence: About 2 cows per month experience ketosis in the winter and about 2 cows per month experience milk fever throughout the year. No other disease complaints except for some mastitis cases were given.
- Immunization: Replacements are immunized only against Brucella abortus. There is no adult cow vaccination program in place.

* **Insemination strategy:**

- Breeding methods: Mature cows are artificially inseminated up to three times and mated naturally thereafter. Heifers are bull bred. A new Holstein bull is purchased every two years. Maiden heifers are exposed to the bull beginning at 11 months of age.
- Sire selection: AI sires are selected on the basis of milk production potential, with calving ease considered secondarily. The calving ease potential of the bull used for natural mating is unknown.

* **Calving management:**

- Relocation: Cows and heifers are moved to the maternity pen (if it is free) when the onset of labor is observed. If the pen is in use, the cow is left with the early lactation string.
- Calving site: Calving is year round with about 30% of the calvings occurring in the maternity pen, and the remainder occurring in the barn or on pasture, depending on the season.
- Monitoring: Cows in the maternity pen are observed as frequently as possible. The same applies to the near term cows that are not in the maternity pen. However there is no specific monitoring plan in place.
- Assistance: The producer provides assistance if calving is not completed 4 to 5 hours after the observed onset of labor. The producer defines dystocia as the need for calving assistance.

* **Neonatal management:**

- Routine: Calves are left with their dams for 12 to 24 hours so that they can get colostrum. Calf navels are usually sprayed with a 4% iodine solution fairly soon after birth.
- Asphyxia: Vitality checks, such as measurement of time from birth to sternal recumbency (Schuyt, 1992) are not performed. Calves that appear to fail to begin respiration are washed with cold water and/or rubbed with straw over the chest. Medical treatment is not given. No necropsies were performed on dead calves.

* **Replacement management:**

- Purchases: When farm-raised replacements are expected to be inadequate, 10 - 12 month old females are purchased from other farms in the area.

* **Nutritional management:**

- Ration formulation: Rations are formulated by the farmer. Published nutrient requirement guidelines are not strictly adhered to.
- Nutrition during summer and winter: Cows are pastured on native grass pasture during the summer. When cows are pastured, extra concentrate is provided in the milking parlor according to recorded milk production levels and the farmer's impressions of production relative to production potential. In winter, two different total mixed rations (TMR) are fed to two lactation groups. Roughage consists of corn silage and alfalfa hay. Minerals are provided free choice to both lactating and dry cows. Body condition scoring (BCS) is not done.
- Heifer nutrition: Replacements are pastured in the summer and supplemented with lactating cow concentrates when it appears that their body condition or their growth rate is below standards. In winter, replacements are confined and are fed the same ration as the early lactation cows. Heartgirth measurements to monitor growth are not performed.
- Dry cow nutrition: Dry cows are fed the leftovers of the lactating groups, plus straw as a high fiber ingredient, up to 2 weeks before expected calving. They are then, together with the heifers, moved into the lactation group where alfalfa hay and corn silage comprise the roughage portion of the ration.

## 2.3.4 INSPECTIONS

After finishing taking the disease history an inspection of retrospective and current data recording and a farm and clinical inspection is performed in search of risk factors that may contribute to the problem.

**Data inspection:**

- Reproductive events: The following reproductive events were recorded on a herd fertility barn chart: calving dates, together with records of dystocias, abortions, sex of calves born, perinatal calf deaths, estrus and insemination dates of cows but not of maiden heifers, and results of pregnancy diagnoses if performed. Reproductive data are not closely monitored by the farmer and indices of reproductive performance are not calculated.

**Farm inspection:**

- General impression: General neatness of the farm was not impressive. Equipment was scattered about. Pieces of equipment in various states of repair were noted. Condition of facilities was moderate. Alleys and freestalls were not well cleaned. Cows were dirty.
- Replacement housing: Young stock (30 $<$ 1 year and 35 $\geq$ 1 year) is housed or pastured in 4 separate groups. The four groups consist of animals up to 5 months of age, 6 to 10 months, 11 to 20 months, and greater than 20 months. The 11 - 20 month old group is exposed to a Holstein bull.

- Cow grouping: Cows are kept in an early lactation group (up to 90 days in milk), a mid-to-late lactation group (greater than 90 days in milk), and a dry cow group. The number of cows currently in each group, were 30, 89 and 13 respectively. At the time of the farm inspection late gestation heifers and cows were mixed with the early lactation group. Submission to this group was based on udder development in heifers and on expected calving date in cows.
- Ration: Inspection of a recent nutrient analysis of the ration revealed an energy shortage (1.55 Mcal/kg DM net energy of lactation (NEL) for the higher producing cows in the early lactation group as well as excessive energy (1.54 Mcal/kg DM NEL) and inadequate protein (11% CP) in the mid-to-late lactation cow diet.
- Forage quality: Forage analysis data were not available. Smell, color and texture of alfalfa hay and corn silage was acceptable and no seepage was evident in the silage.

**Clinical inspection:**
- Calves: The only calf less than 1 week old that was present was unremarkable in terms of health and size. The older calves present appeared healthy. No current signs of diarrhea, respiratory disease or other clinical signs could be observed.
- Replacement heifer growth: During the inspection, replacement heifer weights were estimated by heartgirth measurements. Sixty-eight percent (44/65) of heifers were above target weights for their ages. Height at the withers, determined on heifers in late pregnancy, were variable, indicating non-uniform growth (see Figure 1).

*Figure 1. Weights estimated by heartgirth measurement and heights of heifers examined, with targets (Adapted from J.H. Clapp, Hoard's Dairyman, 15:1250-1251, 1981)*

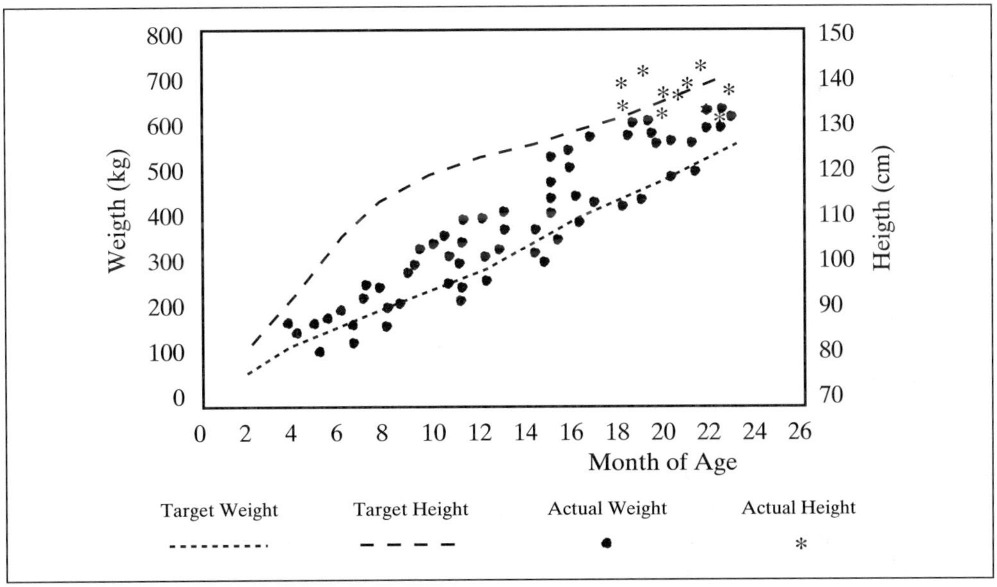

- Body condition: Mean BCS of late gestation heifers and cows was 3.85, ranging from 3 to 4.5 in heifers and from 2.5 to 4.5 in cows. In the early lactation group, the average BCS was 3.0, ranging from 2 to 4.0. The average BCS in the mid-to-late lactation group was 3.70 (range: 2.75 - 4.25).
- Genital examinations: Pregnancy examination of all dry cows and heifers in late pregnancy revealed two non-pregnant animals. Three heifers that calved within the last month had perivaginitis and a slight mucopurulent vaginal discharge. Seven cows that freshened in the same month appeared normal.

### 2.3.5 EVALUATION OF INFORMATION OBTAINED FROM HISTORY TAKING AND INSPECTIONS

In order to include or rule out potential risk or causal factors at an early stage, an evaluation of the generated information is performed. The evaluation comprises information derived from 1) history taking and data inspection, 2) farm inspection, and 3) clinical inspection.

**Evaluation of information from history taking and data inspection**

Breeding history of replacement heifers is unknown for all heifers due to the use of a bull. Expected calving dates are based on observed udder development. Inaccuracy of predicted heifer calving dates may contribute to suboptimal calving management.

The recorded data of cows on the barn fertility list will allow evaluation of some demographic patterns of perinatal calf loss with regard to parity of dams, farmer-diagnosed dystocia, and age at first calving. However, additional supportive data, such as historical cow BCS and necropsy findings of perinatal deaths are not available.

- Parity related perinatal deaths:
  * Thirty heifers and 70 cows calved in the last year.
  * Perinatal death was 14% (14/100) overall and much higher than the average level of 2% in Holsteins (Grunert, 1994). Eight of the 14 dead calves were males (57%). Five of the dams (36% of perinatal death cases) had retained placentas.
  * Perinatal death was 23% (7/30) among the first calf heifers and 10% (7/70) among the cows. This is high in both groups, but the relative percent is 2 times higher among heifers, suggesting a separate problem specific to the heifers (Auren, 1972). It is worthwhile to organize these data into a 2-by-2 table and estimate a crude relative risk and confidence interval (see also Chapter 1, part 4) of perinatal death in order to contrast the risks of cows and heifers.

    Doing this will avoid concluding that one subgroup of cows had a higher incidence than another when there is a substantial possibility that the differential incidences could have been produced by chance.

**Perinatal Death**

| | | Yes | No | Total |
|---|---|---|---|---|
| **Parity** | 1 | 7 | 23 | 30 |
| | >1 | 7 | 63 | 70 |
| | Total | 14 | 86 | 100 |

The relative risk of perinatal death among heifers, relative to cows is obtained by the following calculation (Rothman, 1986):

Relative Risk (RR) = 23.3% / 10.0% = 2.33.
A 90% confidence interval shows whether the RR differs from 1.0 (Rothman, 1986):

$$\exp\left( \ln RR \pm 1.64 * \sqrt{\frac{23}{7 * 30} + \frac{63}{7 * 70}} \right) = (1.05, 5.19)$$

The RR is greater than 1.0 and the 90% confidence interval excludes 1.0. This means that, with 90% confidence, the risk of perinatal deaths in heifers is between 1.05 and 5.19 times greater among heifers than cows. We can be reasonably certain that the estimated relative risk greater than 1.0 is not merely due to random biological variation and that heifers really were at greater risk than cows. However, this is a crude RR, meaning that other factors which may influence the risk of perinatal and that are associated with being a cow or heifer may be contributing to the RR estimate as well. For example, it may be that differences between heifer and cow management are partly or wholly responsible for higher perinatal calf death incidence among the heifer pregnancies.

- **Dystocia:**
  - Farmer diagnosed dystocia occurred in 19 calvings (19%). This is higher than the approximate average of 5% which was thought to be acceptable by the farmer.
  - Dystocia occurred among 23% (7/30) of the heifer calvings, and among 17% (12/70) of the cow calvings. The differences between the two is probably not significant.

| | | Dystocia | | |
|---|---|---|---|---|
| | | Yes | No | Total |
| **Parity** | 1 | 7 | 23 | 30 |
| | >1 | 12 | 58 | 70 |
| | Total: | 19 | 81 | 100 |

The RR is 23.3% / 17.1% = 1.36, and the 90% confidence interval (calculated as previously) is .68 to 2.72. It appears unlikely that an increased rate of dystocia among the heifers explains the increased occurrence of perinatal deaths among the heifer pregnancies. However, dystocia may have been a risk factor for perinatal death of calves among both cows and heifers.

- **Perinatal death by dystocia:**
  * Perinatal death loss occurred among 10 of the 19 dystocias (53%) and among 4 of the 81 non-dystocia calvings (5%).

| | | Perinatal Death | | |
|---|---|---|---|---|
| | | Yes | No | Total |
| **Dystocia** | Yes | 10 | 9 | 19 |
| | No | 4 | 77 | 81 |
| | Total: | 14 | 86 | 100 |

The crude RR was 52.6% / 4.9% = 10.66 (90% confidence interval: 4.44, 25.58). Animals experiencing dystocia were at increased risk of also experiencing perinatal loss of their calves.

The analysis of the subgroups has pointed to two possible determinants of perinatal death loss. One is management of heifers and the other is dystocia. The remainder of the investigation should focus on what is different about the heifers relative to the cows and on potential causes of dystocia.

- **Age at calving:**
  - Age at calving of the replacement heifers over the last year ranged from 20 to 28 months according to the DHIA records.
  - Sixteen point seven percent (5/30) of heifers calved at 20 - 22 months of age.
  - Perinatal death occurred among 60% (3/5) of the heifers that calved at 20 - 22 months of age, and among 16% (4/25) of the heifers that calved at greater than 22 months of age.

**Perinatal Death**

| Heifer Age at Calving | | Yes | No | Total |
|---|---|---|---|---|
| | 20 -22 months | 3 | 2 | 5 |
| | > 22 months | 4 | 21 | 25 |
| | | 7 | 23 | 30 |

The RR of perinatal death with respect to heifer age at calving was 60.0% / 16.0% = 3.75 and the 90% confidence interval was (1.43, 9.80). The heifers calving at younger ages were at increased risk of perinatal death loss among their calves. Heifer frame size may play a role with some of the perinatal death loss; although, some other factor associated with the heifers that calved at younger ages may be partly or wholly responsible for the significant RR as well.

**Evaluation of farm inspection findings**

- The suboptimal maintenance of facilities and equipment together with the disorganized appearance of the farm suggests that labor resources are inadequate. The departure and non-replacement of an employee about 1 year previous to the complaint suggests that the farm labor resources are inadequate to maintain proper dry cow and heifer management, monitoring of imminent calving and to provide adequate observation and assistance during calving. The availability of only one maternity pen worsens the calving monitoring problem.
- Replacement rearing. Purchasing young replacements creates an open farm situation, providing opportunity for introduction of infectious disease agents into the herd.
- Sires. Calving ease is a secondary selection factor for artificial insemination sires. It is not known what the calving ease scores were of the sires used in AI over the preceding 24 months. The calving ease scores of the natural service sires are also not known.
- There were two lactation groups. Over-conditioning and under-conditioning of cows is more difficult to prevent with only two nutrition groups.

### Evaluation of clinical examination findings

- Calf birth weights were not available to be evaluated.
- Birth trauma in perinatal death cases could not be evaluated because the calves had not been necropsied.
- Body condition of cows currently at the end of the dry period is excessive. Target BCS for this period are from 3.25 to 3.75. Excessive body condition may have been due to inappropriate ration formulation. Assuming that this was true for a substantial proportion of the cows that calved over the last 12 months, this may have resulted in reduced postpartum dry matter intake, ultimately leading to the relatively high clinical ketosis incidence as reported by the farmer. In addition, milk fever incidence as reported by the farmer is high, and possibly due to excessive late gestation calcium intake or low anion-cation ratio (see Chapter 3).
- The replacement heifer weight estimates generally exceed age-specific targets while height at the withers vary (Figure 1). These findings are indicative of excessive and/ or unbalanced replacement heifer nutrition.

The epidemiological evaluation, employing crude 2-by-2 Table analysis and holistic farm data and clinical inspections, has demonstrated that: 1) heifers were at greater risk for perinatal death than cows, 2) heifers calving at 22 months of age or younger were at greater risk than heifers calving at greater than 22 months of age, 3) dystocia among both cows and heifers increased the risk of perinatal death, 4) body condition of some dry cows and springing heifers is excessive, and 5) prepartum and intrapartum females are not regularly observed.

## 2.3.6 DIFFERENTIAL LIST OF CAUSES

Potential causes of perinatal death in general can be listed as follows:

- excessive body condition of dams at time of calving,
- insufficient frame size of some heifers at calving,
- use of sires with unknown calving ease scores,
- inadequate prepartum and intrapartum observation,
- dystocia followed by risky extractions,
- infectious diseases of dams,
- mineral deficiency,
- intoxications,

Using the data gathered up to this point in the investigation, the differential cause list can be narrowed to those causes that are likely to be affecting this farm.

- **Excessive body condition of dams at calving**. The body condition of dry cows and springing heifers and of recently calved cows is excessive and is a potential cause. We must assume that the body condition of the cows and heifers that calved over the preceding 12 months was also excessive. The high incidence of ketosis suggests that body condition was indeed excessive among those animals. Excessive body condition can lead to prolonged delivery time (Greene, 1978; Maree, 1986) and subsequently to perinatal death.

- **Insufficient frame size at calving of some heifers.** The heifers presently in the replacement inventory were not uniform in frame size, with some below target heights for their ages. Although the frame sizes of heifers that calved over the last 12 months are unknown, we may assume that some of them also had inadequate frame size at calving. Because heifers were at greater risk of perinatal death of their calves than cows, and heifers calving at < 22 months of age (who were presumably the smallest framed heifers) were at the greatest risk of perinatal death of their calves, frame size at calving may be an important risk factor for perinatal calf loss on this farm. This can be worsened by use of bulls with unknown calving ease.

- **Use of sires with unknown calving ease.** Cows and heifers that were bull bred, were bred to sires with unknown calving ease potential and the calving ease scores of the artificial insemination sires that had been used were unknown by the farmer at the time of the investigation. Thus, it is not possible to determine the role of sire calving ease in the perinatal death losses, but it certainly cannot be ruled out and should not be ignored. Calving ease is related to calf birth weight which is partly a product of sire effects (Philipson, 1976; Meijering, 1984; Notter et al., 1978).

- **Inadequate prepartum and intrapartum observation.** The onset and progress of calvings were probably inadequately monitored during the problem period. Limited labor resources combined with inadequate maternal facilities are largely to blame. Unknown heifer calving dates may have played a contributory role as well.

- **Dystocia followed by forced extractions.** Dystocia may be caused by several things, including heavy birth weights, narrow pelvic diameter, insufficient dilatation of the cervix, and abnormal fetal position. Dystocia is often followed by forced extraction which can lead to calf and dam trauma. Excessive traction is the most important cause of rib and vertebral fractures in calves dying perinatally (Schuijt, 1992). Forced extractions are often accompanied by perivaginitis, though unskilled obstetrical assistance, without fetal trauma, can cause perivaginitis as well.
  During the clinical inspection periparturient trauma in calves was not observed, although only one calf less than one week of age was present, and necropsies on previous perinatal death cases had not been performed. Perivaginitis was found in three of three recently calved heifers, but in none of seven recently calved cows, suggesting that some periparturient trauma had occurred.
  Although evidence of association of parturient trauma with perinatal death could not be observed directly, the fact that perinatal death was much more likely to occur among calvings with dystocia than among calvings without dystocia suggests that dystocia related parturient trauma may have indeed played a role.

- **Infectious diseases of dams.** Neither history nor clinical examinations of dams revealed evidence of infectious processes that can be implicated in the perinatal deaths. However, no objective infectious disease related information is available on cows that had calved during the last 12 months and no calf necropsy data is available.

- **Mineral deficiencies.** There are no farm data available at this time to support or rule out a mineral deficiency hypothesis.

- **Intoxications.** The limited number of affected animals and the restriction of symptoms to perinatal death do not suggest a point source exposure to a toxic substance.

The cause of the perinatal calf death problem is probably multifactorial. Based on observed evidence the items at the top of our list of potential causes include cow and heifer condition at calving, insufficient frame size of some parturient heifers, failure to select sires with desirable calving ease potential, inadequate prepartum and intrapartum observation and assistance, and forced or unskilled fetal extractions. These causes all act through the pathway of increasing calving time and/or difficulty, increasing the risk of parturient trauma and intrapartum calf anoxia. There is no indication of intoxications and mineral deficiencies are not highly suspect given the variety of likely causes that have already been identified. Infectious causes also seem unlikely, but further investigation can be performed to rule out bovine viral diarrhea virus, *Leptospira, Listeria* and *bovine herpes virus type 1*.

## 2.3.7 ADDITIONAL INVESTIGATIONS

Simple evaluations of the herd status with respect to exposure to BVDV, *Leptospira*, and BHV1 consist of taking a bulk tank milk sample to be tested for antibodies against these organisms. Perinatal death cases can also be necropsied and the placentae examined for evidence of placentitis and maternal and fetal tissues submitted for microbiological investigation. A negative result on the milk antibody assays would confirm that these infectious agents are unlikely to form a part of the perinatal calf mortality problem in cows because this is a non-vaccinated herd. A positive result should stimulate further investigation of the herd to detect carriers (see Chapter 8).

## 2.3.8 FINAL LIST OF CAUSES

Because thorough retrospective analysis of data was not possible, our final causal list may be incomplete. Factors that most likely contribute to the problem are: excessive body condition caused by suboptimal nutritional management in both heifers and cows, poor heifer management resulting in inadequate size at first calving, with use of sires with potentially poor calving ease leading to dystocia, failure to recognize dystocia early and failure to use proper technique in assisting dystocia cases.

At this point the restricted differential list of causes, pending milk anti-BVDV, -*Leptospira*, and -BHV1 antibody titers, is as follows:

- excessive body condition of dams at calving,
- insufficient frame size at calving of some heifers,
- use of sires with unknown calving ease,
- inadequate prepartum and intrapartum observation.

Infectious disease of dams might complicate the problem but evidence for this is lacking at this stage. This list, which contains several possible causes of perinatal deaths on this farm, reflects the probable multifactorial nature of this problem.

### 2.3.9 RECOMMENDATIONS

The following recommendations should be implemented immediately:

* Implement a HH & PM program that includes the following:
  - a thorough record keeping system that includes recording of heifer growth, bull use, reproduction, and disease event information (see Chapter 1, part 2),
  - necropsy examinations of perinatal death cases,
  - monitoring and management of reproductive performance,
  - monitoring and management of body condition (see Chapter 1, part 3 and Chapter 3),
  - monitoring and management of replacement heifer growth and breeding based on size and weight,
  - more thorough observation of late gestation cows and heifers coupled with more timely calving assistance or earlier calls for veterinary assistance with dystocias, and
  - definition of preset targets for the foregoing activities.

* Employ a nutritional management program that is specific to stage of lactation, is in accordance with nationally accepted nutrient composition guidelines and that insures proper nutrient delivery to the cows. In particular, avoid over-nutrition and aim at body condition scores of 3.2 to 3.7 at dry-off and at calving. Furthermore, feed late gestation cows and heifers as a separate group, rather than as early lactation cows. Establish three production groups: early lactation, mid lactation and late lactation.

* Hire additional labor and assign specific tasks.

* Increase the emphasis given to calving ease in sire selection.

* Estimate gestational length in cows and heifers regularly.

* Use a marking harness on the natural service bull; observe the heifers daily to record insemination dates.
* Improve general hygiene practices and implement a total closed herd policy together with an infectious disease control program that minimally includes an immunization protocol, quarantine of newly purchased animals (if a total closed herd is impossible to achieve) and isolation of clinical disease cases.

Further recommendations that should be considered include the following:

* Evaluate the feasibility of constructing an expanded maternity facility that will accommodate the majority of animals that could be near term at any one time. Cows should have free movement in the maternity pen at the time of calving.

* Submit two more bulk tank milk samples at three week intervals for quantification of BHV1, BVDV and Leptospira antibodies. Have dead calves necropsied.

It is important to realize that initially only some recommendations will be or can be implemented. Therefore, the recommendations should be prioritized and only those with the highest priority implemented immediately. Furthermore, it will take at least several months before the problem is solved. It is hoped also that the producer will be willing to engage the practitioner in follow-up and review of progress toward reducing perinatal calf death. If this is the case, a strategic plan can be laid out for the implementation of additional recommendations.

### 2.3.10 FOLLOW-UP

Assuming that the recommendations are adopted, the progress toward the goals and effectiveness of the recommendations should be assessed at future farm visits.

### EPILOGUE

Among other things, this case study demonstrates the fact that dairy health and productivity problems do not occur in isolation from one another. Problems often have multiple causes and interrelate with numerous aspects of a dairy's management. In this case study the following management factors were involved: over-conditioned cows in combination with inappropriate feeding strategy, breeding management, supervision of calving, and replacement rearing. Convincing evidence for infectious causes were not found, but were kept in mind as the problem was investigated. The recommendations included further exploration and monitoring relative to potential biological causes. It is important to note that management is at least partly to blame for many health and productivity complaints. Thus, the producer, as manager, may play an important causal role. The practitioner has the task of directing attention away from the animals to the role of management. This must be done cautiously and tactfully.

With respect to the 2-by-2 tables that were used for analyzing data gathered on the problem farm, note that a 2-by-2 table yields a single crude RR estimate (see chapter 1, part 4); that is, the relationship between only two variables is analyzed. Many factors and their interactions are involved in multifactorial problems, though. This requires that the practitioner analyzes multiple factors, looking beyond the RR estimate associated with one single factor when analyzing the data. In addition, epidemiologic confounding due to one or more variables, in addition to the two variables represented in the table, may have a biasing effect on the estimated RR. The result may be that the estimated RR is either larger than it really is or is smaller than it really is. Therefore, the investigator must by careful to use 2-by-2 table analyses as guides in an investigation while always making interpretations on the basis of the entire body of data and observations rather than on the basis of a small number of estimated crude RRs. Similar caution is recommended when the numbers of animals represented in a 2-by-2 table is rather low, as was the case in this case study. finally, it is strongly advised to design a cost-benefit analysis (see Chapter 1, part 5) on recommended measures, to further convince the farmer.

## REFERENCES

*Auran, T. 1972. Factors affecting the frequency of stillbirths in Norwegian cattle. Act. Agric. Scand. 22:178-182.*

*Berger, P.J. 1994. Genetic prediction for calving ease in the United States: Data, models, and use by the dairy industry. J. Dairy Sci. 77:1146-1153.*

*Greene H.J. 1978. Causes of dairy calf mortality. Irish J. Agric. Res. 17:295-301.*

*Grunert, E. 1994. Zur Aetiologie und Prophylaxe der perinatalen Mortalitat beim Kalb. Der Praktische Tierarzt. 73:67-69.*

*James, R.E., M.L. McGilliear, and D.A. Hartman. 1984. Calf mortality in Virginia dairy herd improvement herds. J. Dairy Sci. 67:908-911.*

*Leonard, H.A.0 and D.L. Gardner. 1975. Dairy calf and heifer mortality. J. Dairy Sci. Abstracts. 58:1240-1241.*

*Maree, C. 1986. The influence of high level feeding on the duration of parturition and the incidence of dystocia in dairy cows. J. So. Afr. Vet. Assoc. 57:151-153.*

*Mee, J.F. 1988. Bovine perinatal mortality and parturient problems in Irish dairy herds. J. Irish. Grassland Anim. Prod. Assoc. 22:106-110.*

*Meijering, A. 1984. Dystocia and stillbirth in cattle - a review of causes, relations and implications. Livestock Prod. Sci. 11:143-177.*

*Notter, D.R., L.V. Cundiff, G.M. Smith, D.B. Laster, and K.E. Gregory. 1978. Characterization of biological types of cattle. VI Transmitted and maternal effects on birth and survival traits in progeny of young cows. J. Anim. Sci. 46:892-907.*

*Philipsson, J. 1976. Studies on calving difficulty, stillbirth and associated factors in Swedish cattle breeds. II Effects of non-genetic factors. Acta Agric. Scand. 26:165-174.*

*Philipsson, J., J.L. Foulley, J. Lederer, T. Liboriussen and A. Osinga, A. 1976. Sire evaluation standards and breeding strategies for limiting dystocia and stillbirth. Report of an EEC/EAAP working group. Livest. Prod. Sci. 6: 111-127.*

*Rothman, K.J. 1986. Modern Epidemiology. Little, Brown and Co. Boston. pg.173.*

*Schuijt, G. 1992. Aspects of obstetrical perinatology in cattle. PhD Thesis, Veterinary school of Utrecht, The Netherlands.*

*Simensen, E. 1982. An epidemiological study of calf health and performance in Norwegian dairy herds. II. Factors affecting mortality. Acta. Agric. Scand. 32:421-427.*

# 2.4 MONITORING REPLACEMENT REARING: CASE STUDY RESPIRATORY DISEASES

Wim H. M. Van der Poel[1], Koos Verhoeff[2] and Arie Brand[1]

[1] Department of Herd Health and Reproduction, School of Veterinary Medicine, University of Utrecht, Yalelaan 7, 3485 CL Utrecht, The Netherlands
[2] Animal Health Service, P.O. Box 361, 9200 AJ Drachten, The Netherlands

## 2.4.1 INTRODUCTION

Respiratory disease is one of the most frequently seen and most costly multifactorial disease problems in young stock of dairy cattle (Kaneene et al., 1990). It is associated with an increased risk of culling (Dohoo et al., 1984), which involves the loss of production potential. Besides flaws in farm management and farm conditions, respiratory disease in cattle can be caused by a number of pathogens (Sharp et al., 1993; Stott et al., 1980). Veterinary practitioners can be confronted with respiratory disease problems in dairy herds both within and outside the framework of a HH & PM service. In this part of Chapter 2, a case study of respiratory disease in calves in a herd not participating in a Herd Health and Production Management (HH & PM) service, is discussed. The study follows a protocol consisting of the following items: definition of client's complaint, disease history, data-, farm-, and clinical- inspections, laboratory investigations, evaluation and synthesis of information derived from disease history, farm inspection, clinical investigations, and laboratory data, differential diagnosis list, additional laboratory investigations upon indication, final cause list, followed by recommendations, preventive measures, and follow up.

## 2.4.2 DEFINITION OF CLIENT'S COMPLAINT

In a herd of 100 cows and 60 young stock, 25 replacement calves less than 8 months old are experiencing a high incidence of respiratory disease. The problem becomes apparent every year during winter time but is now very severe. The farmer asks for veterinary help and strategies to prevent the problems in future.

## 2.4.3 DISEASE HISTORY

After questioning the farmer the following overview of the problem was obtained:

**Concerning the calves:** The problem started mid autumn. Calves of about 3 months of age were first affected, and within a few days most calves of 1 to 5 months old showed respiratory disease signs. Affected calves manifested coughing, increased respiratory rates, nasal discharges and a decrease of appetite. After 2 to 3 days of disease, appetite became normal again, but some calves continued coughing and/or manifested a relatively high respiratory rate. The disease spread from one group of calves, to the neighbouring group within a few days. Diseased calves had not been treated yet. Last year diseased calves were treated with antibiotics for one week. Three calves have died so far, two of them clearly manifested an abdominal type of breathing.

**Concerning housing and management**: Dry cows are housed in a loose housing system under one roof with the lactating cows. Near term dams are transferred to a maternity pen. An all-in-all-out system is used for the maternity pens. After birth, calves are immediately separated from their dams and housed in individual crates within a closed barn. Young stock has not been vaccinated, or treated with anthelmintics. According to the farmer no stressful situations occurred in the last month before the respiratory signs became apparent. The calves have not been out on pasture and have not been regrouped recently. Some calves were dehorned and weaned 2 to 3 weeks ago. Unfortunately the farmer did not keep any records on calf rearing.

## 2.4.4 INSPECTIONS

### Data inspection

Due to the fact that no records are kept on calves and heifers, no data inspection is possible. The only data that can be inspected are those generated from the farm and clinical inspections.

### Farm inspection

Ear tags are used for identification of calves. Young stock are housed in a closed barn separated from the adult lactating and dry group. The youngest calves are housed individually in crates up to three weeks of age. From that age on calves and young stock are housed in 3 age groups: 3 weeks - 6 months, 6 - 9 months, and 9 months and older. There is no physical separation between the age groups. The 3 weeks - 6 months old calves are grouped in pens consisting of 8 - 10 calves. Beddings are not dry and the entire floor is made out of concrete. Ventilation is suboptimal, based on the smell of ammonia, and condensed water dripping from the ceilings. The quality of hay and grass silage in the feed bunk was low.

### Clinical inspection

Calves are dirty and wet. Eight calves, out of a group of 10 calves, had a nasal discharge and started coughing when they exerted themselves. A clinical examination was performed on all 8 calves. Body temperatures ranged from 38.8 to 39.9°C and respiratory rates ranged from 50 to 110 per minute. Two calves clearly manifested an abdominal type of breathing. Increased respiratory sounds and rales were heard during auscultation, particularly over the cranioventral areas of the lungs of all 4 calves examined. Two calves had slightly red mucosae. Lacrimation was not observed. Feces were normal from all calves in the investigated group.

## 2.4.5 LABORATORY INVESTIGATIONS

### Samples

In addition to clinical inspection, laboratory investigations were performed. Blood samples for serologic and virologic examinations and nasal swabs were collected from 8 calves in the acute to subacute phase of the disease during the first visit. This offers the best chance to isolate causative pathogens, and to see if seropositive calves are present. To observe seroconversions, blood sampling should be repeated 3 to 4 weeks later, during the convalescent phase. Samples of feces were collected from 5 calves.

### Virological and serological examinations

In the acute phase of the disease, viruses may be isolated from blood samples. Bovine virus diarrhea virus (BVDV) also can be isolated from blood in persistently infected animals. Some respiratory viruses, like Bovine Herpesvirus Type 1 can be isolated from nasal swabs. This is more difficult for BRSV and PI-3. The culture time needed for a virus to develop a cytopathic effect (cpe) depends on the virus and the culture cells used. Culture usually takes 2 days for BHV1, 5 days for BVDV, and more than 2 weeks for other viruses like BRSV. Cell cultures can be examined for virus by

*Table 1. Results of body temperature measurement and virologic examinations*

| No. | Temp. | BHV1 virus isolation[1] | BVD virus isolation[2] |
|---|---|---|---|
| 22 | 38.8 | neg | neg |
| 23 | 38.9 | neg | neg |
| 24 | 38.8 | neg | neg |
| 25 | 39.1 | neg | neg |
| 26 | 39.8 | neg | neg |
| 27 | 39.9 | neg | neg |
| 28 | 38.9 | neg | neg |
| 29 | 39.0 | neg | neg |

1 Culture from nasal swabs
2 Culture from heparinized blood

*Table 2. Results of serologic examinations of blood samples*

| Nr. | Age | BVD B1 - (ELISA) | BRSV | BHV1 (ELISA) | PI3 (ELISA) |
|---|---|---|---|---|---|
| 22 | 4 mths | 20 | 1280 | 20 | 16 |
| 23 | 4 mths | 20 | 5120 | 20 | 32 |
| 24 | 4 1/2 mths | 10 | 5120 | 20 | 16 |
| 25 | 4 1/2 mths | 40 | > 5120 | 10 | 16 |
| 26 | 4 1/2 mths | < 5 | 2560 | 10 | <8 |
| 27 | 4 1/2 mths | < 5 | 2560 | 10 | <8 |
| 28 | 5 mths | < 5 | 640 | 10 | <8 |
| 29 | 5 mths | < 5 | 320 | < 10 | <8 |

immunoperoxidase monolayer assay (Wensvoort et al., 1986).

A large number of tests are available for diagnostic serology of respiratory infections in cattle. Enzyme linked immunosorbent assays (ELISA) are most popular for detection of specific antibodies in large numbers of blood samples obtained from cattle, because most of these tests are rapid, sensitive and easy to perform (Westenbrink et al., 1985; Westenbrink et al., 1986; Kramps et al., 1994).

Results of the virologic and serologic investigations and of body temperature measurements are presented in Tables 1 and 2.

### Nasal swabs

Nasal swabs of diseased calves can be used to culture bacteria, mycoplasmas and viruses. To prevent drying, nasal swabs should be kept in phosphate buffered saline when the pathogen is to be cultured, or in Eagle's minimum essential medium when antigen detection or antibody detection is to be performed. Fluids should be kept around 4°C until further processing. If specimens cannot be processed in a laboratory the day they are obtained, nasal swabs for serologic and bacteriological examinations should be frozen and stored at -20°C, and nasal swabs for virologic or mycoplasma examinations at -70°C.

### Bacteriological examinations

Pathogenic bacteria and mycoplasmas of the respiratory tract can also be cultured from lung lavage fluids, or nasopharyngeal/tracheal wash fluids (Ter Laak et al., 1993). Sterile collection of lung lavage fluid for bacteriologic examinations can be performed by trans-tracheal puncture (Espinasse et al., 1991).

*Table 3. Results of pathological and parasitologic examinations*

| | |
|---|---|
| **Calf A** | |
| Macroscopic findings: | Necrotic pleuropneumonia |
| Histological findings: | Some edema in the lungs<br>Hyperaemia of the lungs<br>*Pasteurella haemolytica* |
| **Calf B** | |
| Macroscopic findings: | Bronchopneumonia<br>Petechia in the trachea |
| Histological findings: | Some peribronchial cuffing |
| Bacteriologic examinations: | *Pasteurella multocida* |
| Parasitological examinations: | Parasites were not detected in any of the fecal samples. |

**Necropsy**

In the farm under study, two moribund calves were killed and were necropsied the same day. Necropsy findings are presented in Table 3. Macroscopic and microscopic lesions can be important indications for the final diagnosis of the respiratory disease. Respiratory pathogens can often be detected in, or cultured from tissues of dead calves if necropsied in a fresh state. Immunofluorescence assays are often used for antigen detection during histologic examinations; staining can be performed after tissues have been fixed to slides. PCR assays on tissue samples can be performed for an increasing number of tissues types (see additional investigations).

The next step is to evaluate and to synthesize information derived from disease history, farm inspection, clinical inspections, and laboratory investigations to get an indication of possible diseases that might be involved.

## 2.4.6 EVALUATION AND SYNTHESIS OF INFORMATION

Suboptimal ventilation and poor hygienic conditions as observed during the described farm inspection, can make calves more susceptible to respiratory disease. When all young stock are housed in one single large barn, respiratory pathogens, especially viruses, may easily be transmitted from one age group of calves to another.

Observed clinical respiratory symptoms are often not very specific. Most respiratory infections can cause coughing, fever, increased respiratory rates and nasal discharge. Some respiratory pathogens can cause diarrhea in addition to respiratory signs. In the examined calves alimentary tract problems were not observed.

Due to poor record keeping and the fact that most observed clinical signs are not very specific, laboratory results become extra important. Serologic results of single samples of the examined calves show antibody titers against BHV1 and PI-3 (Table 1), but these antibodies may very well be maternally derived. Four calves did not have an antibody titer against BVDV, whereas 4 of the 8 sampled calves were seropositive which also might be due to maternally derived antibodies. Antibody titers against BRSV of calves 23, 24, 25, 26 and 27, were so high that these titers are most likely the result of an infection. The isolated *Pasteurellae* may be secondary pathogens. Although interpretation of the disease history and clinical inspection findings, together with serological findings in single blood samples indicate BRSV as the most probable disease diagnosis, other potential diseases should not be overlooked. Therefore, the next step is to list and evaluate all potential diseases that might be involved in the respiratory disease problem.

### 2.4.7 DIFFERENTIAL DIAGNOSES

Frequently isolated pathogens in respiratory disease in young cattle are: BRSV, PI-3, BHV1 (IBRV), BVDV, *Pasteurellae*, *Salmonellae*, *Mycoplasmas*, and *Dictyocaulus viviparus*. All these respiratory pathogens have their own characteristics: BRSV infections may cause acute respiratory distress (Bryson et al., 1978) and are mainly found in calves 1 to 6 months of age. In BHV1 infections, respiratory signs are mainly of the upper respiratory tract (Wiseman et al.,1978). BVDV is normally not a primary pathogen in respiratory disease and can be associated with diarrhea. Because of immunosuppressive effects of the virus, BVDV infections may facilitate secondary infections (Duffell et al., 1985). As such, Pasteurella often causes respiratory disease in various ages of calves (Shoo, 1989). Salmonellosis is most often found in calves 2 to 4 weeks old. It can be a continuing problem on veal calf farms (Wray, 1993) and may be associated with diarrhea. *Hemophilus somnus* can be a primary respiratory pathogen in calves, but its prevalence is far below the prevalence of *Pasteurella* and *Salmonella* in cattle (Saunders et al., 1980). Lungworm infections will only be found in young stock that has been out in pasture. Mycoplasmas are also often secondary pathogens; they may cause chronic respiratory symptoms (Howard et al., 1987). Symptoms of PI-3 infections in cattle are usually aspecific (Stevenson et al., 1970). Other viruses, like Adeno-, Toro-, and Reo-virusses, that have been described as respiratory pathogens, are considered less pathogenic in the respiratory tract (Mattson, 1973; Woode et al., 1985).

Of the diseases listed, *Salmonellae*, and *Dictyocaulus viviparus* should be excluded as potential disease causes due to the fact that no diarrhea was observed and calves had not been pastured. Serologic results of single blood samples and virus isolation exclude BHV1 (IBRV), BVDV and PI-3. Pasteurellae and Mycoplasmas were detected in necropsied animals, whereas *Hemophilus somnus* was not detected. This means that BRSV, and Mycoplasmas are the most probable disease diagnoses that might have caused the respiratory problem.

For a definite disease diagnosis, detection of seroconversion or a fourfold rise in antibody titer, of a suspected causative pathogen, is needed. To do this acute phase samples and convalescent samples must be investigated. If a seroconversion is found it means that there must have been a significant contact with the antigen: virus replication or bacterial growth, etc., in the calf. Therefore, additional investigations which are complementary to those performed on a routine basis should be executed.

## 2.4.8 ADDITIONAL INVESTIGATIONS UPON INDICATION

### Lung lavage fluids

Due to the fact that many respiratory pathogens are found in higher concentrations in lung lavage fluid, these pathogens can easier be isolated from, or detected in lung lavage fluids than in nasal fluids or from blood (Kimman et al., 1987 a, b). Mucosal antibody titers against a number of respiratory pathogens can also be determined in lung lavage fluids. However, this is not routinely done in many laboratories. Lung lavage fluids are most easily obtained according to the method described by Fogarty et al. (1983).

### Antigen (virus, bacteria) detection

Immunofluorescence assays opolymerase chain reaction (PCR) assays can also be used to detect the antigen in nasal swabs or nasal fluids. These techniques are rapid assays and are available for many pathogens. Polymerase chain reaction assays (PCR) are usually more sensitive. Since 1990, PCR assays have become more and more popular in diagnostic laboratories. Nowadays, PCR assays can be performed on various kinds of samples (Hooft van Iddekinge et al., 1992; Van Engelenburg et al., 1994; Van der Poel et al., 1994).

*Table 4. Results of additional investigations*

| No. | BRSV IgM-ELISA (serum) | BRSV-PCR* | Fluorescent* Antybody Test (FAT) BRSV |
|---|---|---|---|
| 22 | pos | neg | neg |
| 23 | pos | neg | neg |
| 24 | pos | neg | neg |
| 25 | pos | neg | neg |
| 26 | neg | neg | neg |
| 27 | neg | pos | neg |
| 28 | neg | pos | pos |
| 29 | pos | neg | neg |

*Table 5. Results of BRSV and PI-3 serology*

| No. | BRSV | | PI-3 | |
|---|---|---|---|---|
| | S1 | S2 | S1 | S2 |
| 22 | 1280 | 2560 | 16 | 16 |
| 23 | 5120 | 2560 | 32 | 16 |
| 24 | 5120 | 2560 | 16 | 16 |
| 25 | >5120 | 5120 | 16 | 16 |
| 26 | 2560 | 5120 | 16 | 8 |
| 27 | 2560 | 5120 | <8 | <8 |
| 28 | 640 | 2560 | <8 | <8 |
| 29 | 320 | 1280 | <8 | <8 |

S1 = sample 1   S2 = sample 2

*Table 5. continued*

| No. | BVDV | | BHV1 | |
|---|---|---|---|---|
| | S1 | S2 | S1 | S2 |
| 22 | 20 | 20 | 20 | 10 |
| 23 | 20 | 40 | 20 | 20 |
| 24 | 10 | 20 | 20 | 10 |
| 25 | 40 | 20 | 10 | <10 |
| 26 | <5 | <5 | 10 | 10 |
| 27 | <5 | <5 | 10 | <10 |
| 28 | <5 | <5 | 10 | <10 |
| 29 | <5 | <5 | <10 | <10 |

S1 = sample 1   S2 = sample 2

**Further serologic examinations**

For a more definite diagnosis using serologic examinations, convalescent blood samples should be collected. For that reason blood samples should be collected 3 weeks after the first sampling. Mucosal antibody titers can be determined in nasal fluids and lung lavage fluids (Kimman et al., 1987b). In lactating cows, antibodies can also be detected in milk.

In young calves, detected antibodies are often maternally derived. In calves up to 6 months age, these maternally derived antibodies can prohibit or mask serocoversions and significant antibody-rises after infection. For diagnosis of infections in the presence of maternally derived antibodies, development of specific IgM can be determined. Serum samples for this purpose should be obtained around 10 days after the first clinical symptoms.

### 2.4.9 FINAL CAUSE LIST

In the herd studied, BRSV infections have been confirmed by polymerase chain reaction assay (PCR), fluorescent antibody test (FAT) and serology. BRSV antibody responses were detected in the BRSV IgM Elisa and fourfold antibody-rises were detected in the standard BRSV-Elisa. Fourfold antibody rises were detected in just a few animals because the first samples were obtained after the acute phase of the disease, and antibody levels probably already had elevated. The detected BRSV infections are the best explanation for the described respiratory problems. Secondary bacterial infections (*Pasteurella* and/or *Salmonella*, and mycoplasmal infections) may also play a role.

### 2.4.10 RECOMMENDATIONS

Calves showing respiratory distress should be treated with antibiotics if indicated. Meanwhile the dairy owner should be advised to keep a calf rearing chart and a farm diary, and further comply to a HH & PM service for young stock. Record keeping is an essential prerequisite to monitor the growth and health of replacement calves adequately. A 12-monthly list should be installed and filled in by the practitioner during every HH & PM farm visit. Important replacement rearing performance indices can then be monitored over time (Table 6).

*Table 6. Part of a 12-monthly list to monitor health aspects in replacement rearing*

| Month | Jan | Febr | March | April | May |
|---|---|---|---|---|---|
| Calves < 6 months | 15 | 13 | 14 | | |
| # diarrhea treated | 4/2 | 5/2 | 3/1 | | |
| # pneumonia treated | 2 | 0 | 0 | | |
| # died 1st month | 1 | 0 | 0 | | |
| # died 1 to 24 months | 1 | 0 | 0 | | |
| remarks | | | | | |

Calves and older young stock should be housed in age groups physically separated, and in a clean comfortable environment. An all-in-all-out system should be used if calves are moved to another pen. To provide adequate fresh air for all calves, ventilation must be improved.

## 2.4.11 PREVENTIVE MEASURES

After the final diagnosis has been made, adequate preventive measurements must be taken. Vaccines are available against many respiratory pathogens. Unfortunately not all of these vaccines are effective. The efficacy of some vaccines is unknown. Calves that are pastured should be vaccinated against lungworm if indicated. Vaccination against BRSV can best be performed before the beginning of autumn. High quality colostrum must be provided to newborn calves in sufficient quantities (see Chapter 2, part 1) within an hour after birth. Barns must be cleaned and disinfected regularly. Stress factors originating from housing, climatic and hygienic conditions, must be reduced as much as possible.

## 2.4.12 FOLLOW UP

During future farm visits, the practitioner should evaluate effects of preventive measures taken and/or recommendations given during previous visits. Results of treatments should be evaluated as well. When indicated, adjustments should be made.

## EPILOGUE

For a good performance of young stock later on during their productive lifetime, respiratory diseases must be prevented, or their incidence should be reduced to a minimum, during the rearing period. In case respiratory diseases occur, a structured evaluation of all potential causes is needed and a definite identification of causative pathogens should be performed. The diagnoses and treatments should be recorded on a Calf Rearing List. To prevent respiratory disease problems with a multifactorial background, farm management as well as housing conditions should be examined and optimized (Dodd et al., 1992). Vaccinations against specific pathogens should be executed, especially when it is proved that these pathogens are involved in the disease occurrence. Finally, growth of young stock should be monitored regularly (see Chapter 2, part 1).

## REFERENCES

*Bryson, D.G., J.B. Mcferran, H.J. Ball and, S.D. Neill. 1978. Observations on outbreaks of respiratory disease in housed calves; Epidemiological, clinical and microbiological findings. Vet. Rec. 103:485-489.*

*Dodd, V.A. 1992. Calf housing principles. Irish Vet. J. 45:91-104.*

*Dohoo, I.R. and S.W. Martin. 1984. Disease, production and culling in Holstein-Friesian cows. V. Survivorship. Prev. Vet. Med. 6:771-784.*

*Duffell S.J. and J.W. Harkness. 1985. Bovine virus diarrhea - Mucosal disease in cattle. Vet. Rec. 117:240-245.*

*Espinasse, J., J.P. Alzien, C. Patageorgion, J.C. Begum, and F. van Gool. 1991. Use of transtracheal aspiration to identify pathogens in pneumonic calves. Vet. Rec. 129:339.*

*Fogarty, U., P.J. Quinn, and J. Hannan. 1983. Bronchopulmonary lavage in the calf: a new technique. Irish Vet. J. 37:35-38.*

*Hooft van Iddekinge, B.J.L., J.L.B. Wamel, H.G.P. van Gennip, and R.J.M. Moormann. 1992. Application of the polymerase chain reaction to the detection of bovine viral diarrhea virus infections in cattle. Vet. Microbiol. 30:21-34.*

*Howard C.J., E.J. Stott, L.H. Thomas, R.N. Thomas, R.N. Gourlay, and G. Taylor. 1987. Protection against respiratory disease in calves induced by vaccines containing respiratory syncytial virus, parainfluenza type 3 virus, mycoplasma bovis and mycoplasma dispar. Vet. Rec. 121: 372-376.*

*Kaneene, J.B. and H.S. Hurd. 1990. The national animal health monitoring system in Michigan. III. Cost estimates of selected dairy cattle diseases. Prev. Vet. Med. 8:127-140.*

*Kimman, T.G., F. Westenbrink, P.J. Straver, D. van Zaane, and B.E.C. Schreuder. 1987. Isotype specific Elisas for the detection of antibodies to bovine respiratory syncytial virus. Res. Vet. Sci. 43:180-187.*

*Kimman, T.G., F. Westenbrink, B.E.C. Schreuder, and P.J. Straver. 1987. Local and systemic antibody response to bovine respiratory syncytial virus infection and reinfection in calves with and without maternal antibodies. J. Clin. Microb. 25:1097-1106.*

*Kramps, J.A., J. Magdalena, J. Quak, K. Weerdmeester, M.J. Kaashoek , M.A. Maris Veldhuis, F.A.M. Rijsewijk, G. Keil, and J.T. van Oirschot. 1994. A simple, specific, and highly sensitive blocking-enzyme immunosorbent assay for detection of antibodies to bovine herpesvirus 1. J. Clin. Microb. 32:2175-2181.*

*Mattson, D.E. 1973. Adenovirus infection in cattle. J. Am. Vet. Med. Ass. 163:894-896.*

*Sharp, M.W., R.L. Williams, and R. Munro. 1993. Acute respiratory distress syndrome in yearling cattle. Vet. Rec. 132:467-468.*

*Shoo, K. 1989. Experimental bovine pneumonic pasteurellosis: A review. Vet. Rec. 124:141-144.*

*Stevenson, R.G. and D.E. Hore. 1970. Comparative pathology of lambs and calves infected Parainfluenza type 3. J. Comp. Path. 8:613-618.*

*Stott, E.J., L.H. Thomas, A.P. Collins, S. Crough, J. Jebbet, G.S. Smith, P.D. Luther, and R.A. Caswell. 1980. Survey of virus infections of the respiratory tract of cattle and their association with disease. J. Hyg. 85:237-247.*

*Saunders, J.R., W.A. Thiessen, and E.D. Janzen. 1980. Haemophilus Somnus infections I. A ten year (1969-1978) retrospective study of losses in cattle herds in western Canada. Can. Vet. J. 21:119-123.*

*Ter laak, E.A., J.H. Noordergraaf, and R.P.J.W. Dieltjes. Prevalence of mycoplasmas in the respiratory tracts of pneumonic calves. J. Vet. Med. B39:553-562.*

*Van der Poel, W.H.M., J.P.M. Langedijk, J.A. Kramps, and J.T. van Oirschot. 1994. A sensitive reverse transcription polymerase chain reaction assay for detection of bovine respiratory syncytial virus in cattle. Proceedings of the third international congress of the European Society of Veterinary Virologists; Interlaken 1994, W5 p 2.*

*Van Engelenburg, F.A.C., R.K. Maes, J.T. van Oirschot, and F.A.M. Rijsewijk. 1993. Development of a rapid and sensitive polymerase chain reaction assay for detection of bovine herpesvirus type 1 in bovine semen. J. Clin. Microbiol. 31:3129-3135.*

*Wensvoort, G., C. Terpstra, J. Boonstra, M. Bloemraad, and D. van Zaane. 1986. Production of monoclonal antibodies against swine fever virus and their use in laboratory diagnosis. Vet. Microbiol. 12:101-108.*

*Westenbrink, F., J.M.A. Brinkhof, P.J. Straver, J. Quak, and P.W. de Leeuw. 1985. Comparison of a newly developed enzyme-linked immunosorbent assay with complement fixation and neutralisation tests for serology of bovine respiratory virus infections. Res. Vet. Sci. 38:334-340.*

*Westenbrink, F., W.G.J. Middel, P.J. Straver, and P.W. de Leeuw. 1986. A blocking enzyme-linked immunosorbent assay (ELISA) for bovine virus diarrhoea virus serolo gy. J. Vet. Med. B 33:354-361.*

*Wiseman, A., P.M. Msolla, I.E. Selman, E.M. Allan, H.J.C. Cornwell, H.M. Pirie, and W.S. Imsay. 1978. An severe outbraeak of infectious bovine rhinotracheitis: clinical, epidemilogical, microbiological and pathological aspects. Vet. Rec. 103:391-397.*

*Wray, C. 1993. Bovine Salmonellosis: an update. Irish Vet. J. 46:137-140.*

*Woode, G.N., L.J. Saif, M. Quesasa, N.J. Winand, J.F. Pohlenz, and N. Kelso Gourly. 1985. Comparative isolates of Breda virus of calves. Am. J. Vet. Res. 46:1003-1010.*

# MONITORING DRY PERIOD MANAGEMENT

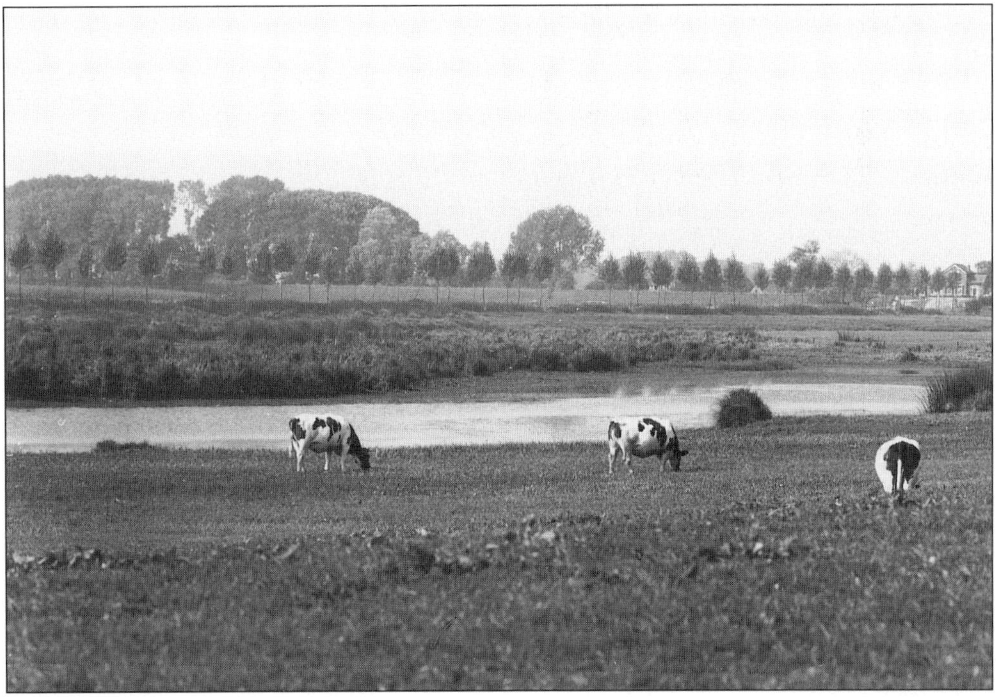

# 3 MONITORING DRY PERIOD MANAGEMENT

Andy L. Skidmore[1], Kees A. M. Peeters[2], Charles J. Sniffen[3] and Arie Brand[4]

[1] Department of Animal Science, Michigan State University, East Lansing, MI 49924, USA
[2] Large Animal Practice, Oude Almeloseweg 101, 7622 CC, Borne, The Netherlands
[3] W.H. Miner Agricultural Research Institute, P.O. Box 90, Chazy, NY 12921, USA
[4] Department of Herd Health and Reproduction, School of Veterinary Medicine, University of Utrecht, Yalelaan 7, 3584 CL Utrecht, The Netherlands

## 3.1 INTRODUCTION

The dry period is metabolically and endocrinologically a very active time in the productive cycle of the cow. It is actually a preparatory period for the next lactation. Therefore, the dry period cannot be considered in isolation, but as an essential part of whole farm management. However, most dairy farmers consider the dry period as a rest period during which the cow is not productive. As a consequence of this attitude, the cow often does not get the attention she needs (Van Saun, 1991).

During the dry period, metabolic activity in the mammary gland can be divided into 3 phases:

1. The drying off or involution phase during which the udder stops secreting milk and becomes non-lactating. Drying off initiates involution of mammary secretory tissue. It consists of reabsorption of milk and a rapid regression of mammary secretory epithelial cells. This phase, with all its changes, takes 30 days.
2. The second or mid phase is a phase of true rest for the mammary gland. The mammary gland is maintaining itself in a non-productive state. The length of this period is dependent on the total length of the dry period.
3. The third phase, lasting about 3 weeks, is called the regeneration phase or close-up period. In this period the mammary gland regenerates in preparation for the next lactation. Colostrum also is secreted in the mammary gland at this time (Van Saun, 1991).

The dry period is a transition period where the dairy cow must alter her metabolic priorities. In midgestation available nutrients are used for net tissue accretion. Due to rapid growth of the conceptus and colostrogenesis followed by initiation of lactation, reserve tissue is mobilized to meet nutrient demands (Van Saun, 1991). Therefore, this preparation period for the new lactation should be monitored thoroughly within the framework of Herd Health and Production Management (HH & PM) services.

In this chapter various aspects of dry cow management will be discussed as well as strategies to optimize health and milk production in the new lactation period.

## 3.2 STRATEGIES BEFORE AND AT DRYING OFF

In this section, management strategies to optimize drying off cows will be discussed. Monitoring body condition and udder health in the dry period are considered of major significance to future productivity. Therefore, special attention will be paid to monitoring and prevention of mastitis, and body condition scoring and at dry-off.

### Cow handling at dry-off

Dry-off can be very stressful due to ration changes, withdrawal of drinking water, separation of cows from herd mates, introduction into a new group and/or environment, cessation of milking, and late-term pregnancy. High levels of stress at dry-off may cause corticosteroid release which may result in abortion in the last trimester of pregnancy. Therefore, there is a need to handle cows to be dried off very gently, and if possible to dry off cows in familiar groups to reduce the impact of stress.

### Body Condition Scoring

The methods of condition scoring and interpretation of scores are presented in the Appendix (pg 191). Cows in the dry period should be fed to maintain body condition within recommended range and to calve with adequate, but not excessive, body reserves. The recommended BCS for cows during the dry period is 3.50 (3.25 to 3.75). High producing dairy cows must calve with adequate tissue reserves to compensate for negative nutrient balance in early lactation. This will help to meet the energy and protein requirements of peak milk production during early lactation (Gearhart et al., 1990).

### Monitoring udder health

All cows should be examined for clinical and subclinical mastitis at dry-off. Cows with a somatic cell count (SCC) higher than 200,000 cells/ml, at the last 2 milk testing dates before dry-off, should be examined by the California Mastitis Test (CMT) and positive quarters sampled for bacteriological testing. This will provide information about pathogens involved and antibiotic sensitivity. Treatment of cows with subclinical mastitis caused by *Staphylococcus aureus* is more effective and less costly at dry-off than in lactation when milk has to be discarded. Chronically infected cows, should be excluded from treatment and should be culled, depending on parity, number of quarters involved, and SCC level. The curative treatment should be followed by a preventive dry cow antibiotic treatment at dry-off (Chapter 6).

### Total or selective dry cow antibiotic treatment

Involution of the mammary gland is associated with the period of highest susceptibility to new infections as is the regeneration phase in the last 10 days of pregnancy (Van Saun, 1991). A question often asked is whether all cows should be given dry cow antibiotic treatment or only selected cows based on mastitis history and/or parity. It is currently advised to treat all cows with antibiotics at dry-off due to the fact that new infections occur 10 times more often in untreated cows as compared with treated cows. Selective dry treatment is only feasible when cows at risk for infection can be identified. At this point in time there is not sufficient data to be able to do so (Schukken et al., 1993).

### Method of drying off

At the time of dry-off, cows are at various levels of milk production. It is thought that reducing milk production before dry-off may help to dry-off the mammary gland quicker and reduce milk leakage. In the authors experience, on some farms up to 40% of cows may leak milk after the last milking at dry-off. This means that dry cow antibiotics infused to prevent infections leak out. Although lowcring milk production may reduce milk leakage, one should keep in mind that milk leakage should be considered in relation to milking speed and bull selection.

Lowering milk production before dry-off can be achieved by reducing energy intake. This can be accomplished by lowering the amount of concentrates in the diet and feeding low energy forages. This strategy requires a separate group of cows to supply a lower energy diet. In some feeding systems, it may be difficult to form this separate group. Anytime dietary changes are made, they need to be made gradually. This is especially important in cows that are producing > 20 kg of milk per day. Even at dry-off, abrupt dietary changes in high metabolically active cows may create metabolic problems. An example would be grass tetany caused by a sudden restriction of minerals.

Most farmers will dry off their cows abruptly. Others use intermittent milking practices to reduce the level of milk secretion before dry-off. It is recommended that all cows be dried off abruptly because it will minimize total stress and is easier to manage.

### Dry-off protocol

Treating cows at dry-off with antibiotics is a very important activity that requires the utmost hygiene and care. Cows need to be restrained sufficiently to allow adequate control for proper administration of antibiotics. The protocol to administer antibiotics at dry-off consists of:

- milking the cow completely, utilizing proper milking techniques,
- cleaning teats with a clean and dry towel,
- predipping all 4 teats with iodine or other effective teat disinfectant,
- leaving the cow alone for 5 - 10 minutes,
- predip again,
- infuse dry cow antibiotics by introducing the tip only 5 mm into the teat canal,
- post-dip all teats and keep the cow restrained for another hour to facilitate the closing of the teat opening and prevent introduction of bacteria into the exposed teat opening.

Cows should be monitored daily for milk leakage, especially in the first week after drying off and in the last week before calving. They should be monitored for swollen quarters and teat damage during the entire dry period. Treatment for mastitis and injuries should be implemented when problems are observed. Retreatment of a cow that leaks milk in the early dry period always should be considered. The cow should be milked out again before retreating. The environment where dry cows are kept should be clean, dry, and comfortable.

**Other treatments**

At dry-off, the feet should be examined and trimmed if needed. Dry cows should also pass through (formalin) foot baths at least once every 3 weeks for prevention of foot rot. Cows with dermatitis digitalis should be treated with oxytetracycline or lincomycin locally to prevent environmental pollution with antibiotics using footbaths. If foot bathing of the dry cows is not practiced, they form a risk group for infecting lactating cows later on. This may explain why regular treatment of lactating cows is not always successful. Cows must have healthy feet in the postpartum period when they are expected to produce high amounts of milk. Foot diseases such as Dermatitis digitalis and interdigitalis will reduce feed intake and subsequent milk production. Therefore, preventive measures must be taken. Foot diseases also may have a negative effect on estrous behavior (Chapter 5, part 2).

Other treatments may include deworming. The need for deworming should be based on farm history, soil and climatological conditions, pasture management, body condition data, clinical examination, and laboratory analysis of fecal and/or blood samples. In addition, cows should be clipped, especially the udder region, to keep them cleaner, and to avoid heat stress in hot weather.

**Length of the dry-period**

The ideal dry-period length is between 50 - 70 days (Funk et al., 1987; Dias et al., 1982; Enevoldsen and Sorensen, 1992). Shorter periods, especially in 1st and 2nd parity cows, give a lower production in the subsequent lactation. A dry period longer than 70 days reduces milk production per lifetime due to lower production per time unit and may increase body condition further. It also may reduce subsequent milk yield indirectly because of metabolic diseases due to excessive body condition loss during early lactation. In case of abnormally long dry periods, reproductive efficiency should be checked since it may indirectly determine dry period length.

## 3.3 MANAGEMENT DURING THE DRY-PERIOD

**Grouping of dry cows**

An appropriate grouping system for both dry and lactating cows must be based on an understanding of the physiologic basis of an animal's response to its environment as well as the impact of man's manipulation of that environment on the animal's response (Sniffen, 1991). Dry cows should be split into at least an early/mid and late dry group. To do this, it is important to have accurate breeding dates and to monitor how long cows are in the close-up group. The late or "close-up" group would comprise those cows that are close to the expected calving date, within 2 - 4 weeks. The early/mid dry group should consist of other cows, recognizing that those cows which have just been dried off might need more critical observation and care. This might be justification to form a third group if possible. Grouping of cows enables the dairy farmer to adequately adapt the ration of dry cows approaching calving to the ration composition of cows in lactation. Special attention needs to be paid to springing heifers because they have a growth as well as a pregnancy requirement. Intake capacity of springing heifers is less on a body weight basis. Therefore, they should be housed and fed separately until they need to be mixed with older dry cows 3 weeks prior to calving. If dry cows and springing heifers are pastured they should be removed from pasture the last 3 weeks before the expected date of calving to control feed intake (Sniffen, 1991).

### Housing of dry Cows

During the dry period, cows can either be housed or pastured. Preference must be given to housing dry cows for better control of the diet. If possible an exercise yard should be made available. Stalls should be kept dry and clean and the size should be adequate for the largest cow in the herd to easily enter and leave. An easy way to measure the size a stall needs to be is to turn the cows out on a new field of tall grass and measure the length and width of the area pressed down in the grass where the cow has laid. Dry cows must be clean. Dirty dry cows can be caused by loose feces due to an unbalanced ration, by a ration composed of low quality feedstuffs or by diseases. However, dirty cows also can be an indication of uncomfortable stalls. Presence of clean dry cows with an optimal BCS is a sign of good nutrition and housing management in the dry period.

### Vaccinations

When neonatal enteric disease occurs in calves in epidemic proportions, it is generally the result of poor sanitation and suboptimal management. Under these conditions, several etiologic agents are usually found, especially *E. coli*, Rota and Corona virus, *Cryptosporidia*, Coccidia and Salmonella (Hjerpe, 1992). Dry cows may be vaccinated against *E. coli*, Rota and Corona viruses to enhance colostral antibodies against these pathogens. The vaccines should be administered according to label.

### Dry cow nutrition

The primary objective of dry cow nutrition is to optimize milk yield, reproduction and health in the subsequent lactation by starting to control negative energy balance and mineral metabolism in the dry period. Poor nutritional management during the dry period may result in fatty liver and milk fever and their associated diseases.

Based on nutrient requirements, dry cows should be divided into an early/mid, and a close-up group. This provides an opportunity to formulate a high fiber/low energy dense ration for early/mid dry cows and a close-up ration that is more energy dense with less fiber. The more energy dense close-up ration is to prepare for the lactating cow diet and compensate for decreasing feed intake and higher metabolic demands during this time. Nutrient requirements for the dry period are presented in Table 1 (Van Saun, 1991).

Early/mid dry cow rations should contain at least 50% neutral detergent fiber (NDF) on a dry matter basis, with 75% of the total fiber coming from coarsely chopped forage or long-stem hay. Rations containing 50 - 55% NDF are best. A high forage (> 85%) content of the early/mid dry cow ration is thought to be beneficial to maintain maximum rumen volume and motility. Due to a higher chewing activity, more saliva is produced. The saliva will buffer the rumen and help maintain a higher rumen pH which will allow rumen wall lesions to recover from high grain rations during lactation (Van Saun, 1991).

The influence of diet during the close-up period, the first 3 week postpartum, or a combination of the two periods on subsequent health, milk production, and reproductive performance tend to be neglected by nutritionists and dairy producers (Grummer, 1995).

The close-up or transition period which starts about 3 weeks before the expected date of calving is characterized by many endocrine and physiologic process changes that prepare the cow for calving and influence subsequent lactation (Grummer, 1995). It is considered as an excellent time to start adapting the cow to a milking cow ration. During the close-up period, dry cows should be on a rising plane of nutrition to compensate for decreasing feed intake, to prevent negative energy balance and subsequent mobilization of adipose tissue, and to meet nutrient requirements of advanced pregnancy (Bertics et al., 1992). Such a ration should contain small amounts of the same forages and concentrates as fed to lactating cows. The majority of this ration also should contain forages with low K and Na content. Increasing the nutrient energy density of the close-up ration can be done by adding high energy feeds such as grains. The change to a higher grain diet in the close-up period must be made very gradually and not be made all at once. Close-up cows should not receive more than 3 - 4 kg of concentrates per day just before calving. The additional grain will not only help the rumen adapt to the higher starch content of the ration in early lactation, but will also provide the nutrients necessary for the growing fetus and other organ changes that are occurring in preparation for lactation. Although nutrient requirements are comparatively low, the composition of the prefreshening diet is as important as how much they eat (Van Saun, 1991).

The crude protein content of the dry cow close-up ration should be 13 - 14% on a dry matter basis (Van Saun, 1991). The increased protein levels should help meet metabolic demands of the fetus in the last few weeks before parturition as well as early lactation. Inadequate protein intake results in mobilization of body protein to meet metabolic demands. This may result in depletion of labile protein reserves (Botts et

*Table 1. Nutrient requirements for dry cows (BW = body weight, DMI = dry matter Intake, CP = crude protein, ADF = acid detergent fiber) (Van Saun, 1991)*

| Nutrient | Early and mid dry period | Close-up period |
|---|---|---|
| DMI, % of BW | 1.9 - 2.1 | 1.6 - 1.8 |
| Crude protein, % DM | 12 - 13 | 13 - 14 |
| Soluble protein, % CP | 40 - 50 | 22 - 28 |
| Degradable protein, % CP | 65 - 70 | 62 - 67 |
| Net energy, Mcal/kg | 1.10 - 1.20 | 1.5 - 1.61 |
| ADF, % DM* | 35 - 40 | 20 - 24 |
| NDF, % DM** | 50 - 65 | 37 - 44 |
| Fat, % DM | 3 - 4 | 3 - 5 |
| Ca, % DM | 0.31 - 0.35 | 0.36 - 0.80 |
| P, % DM | 0.19 - 0.21 | 0.24 - 0.35 |
| K, % DM | 0.65 - 0.75 | 0.70 - 0.80 |
| Mg, % DM*** | 0.18 - 0.20 | 0.25 - 0.28 |
| S, % DM*** | 0.16 - 0.18 | 0.25 - 0.36 |
| Na, % DM | 0.10 - 0.13 | 0.12 - 0.15 |
| Cu, ppm | 10 -15 | 12 - 18 |
| Co, ppm | 0.10 | 0.12 |
| I, ppm | 0.60 | 0.70 |
| Fe, ppm | 50 | 60 |
| Se, ppm | 0.30 | 0.30 |
| N:S ratio | 10 - 13 : 1 | 5 - 12 : 1 |
| Vitamin A, IU/kg | 4,000 | 4,700 |
| Vitamin D, IU/kg | 1,200 | 1,400 |
| Vitamin E, IU/kg | 25 | 30 |

* ADF is a measure of fiber material and is associated with feed digestibility and not feed intake.

** NDF is a measure of total cell wall content and is negatively associated with dry matter intake.

***Increase dietary concentrations to 0.38% when potassium levels exceed 1.1%.

al., 1979), and in lower peak milk yields and productivity. Over-feeding protein results in a very inefficient process. It costs energy to excrete the excess nitrogen. Due to the large amounts of structural carbohydrates in early and mid-dry-period diets, 40 - 50% of the dietary protein should be in the form of soluble protein or non-protein nitrogen sources. In the close-up period this percentage should be reduced to 22 - 28 % (Table 1). The soluble protein sources are rapidly converted to ammonia, an essential nutrient of cellulolytic bacteria. The amount of rumen undegradable intake protein for the close-up period is less well defined. Preliminary results would indicate that additional undegradable protein fed during late gestation may improve body condition at calving, subsequent milk yield, reproductive performance, and result in fewer health disorders (Van Saun, 1991).

Another strategy to adapt close-up cows to the milking ration is to move the close-up dry cows into a lactating group. This is not a recommended practice. A disadvantage is that the ration contains minerals for the lactating cows which may predispose the cow to udder edema and milk fever. The diet is not designed to meet the nutrient needs of the dry cow. There are also many additional management demands placed on farm employees to try and manage 2 very distinct physiologic animals in one physical group. The close-up dry cows are often neglected and do not receive the special care they need to prepare them for calving and lactation. This strategy is a short cut for poor management.

Dry cows must be monitored and provided with sufficient amounts of minerals and vitamins. Mineral elements that have been shown to be essential for cows generally are divided into macrominerals such as: calcium, magnesium, phosphorus, sodium, chlorine, potassium, and sulfur and trace minerals which include cobalt, copper, zinc, iodine, iron, manganese, molybdenum, and selenium. These mineral elements are used as structural components of body organs and tissues, as components of metalloenzymes, and as co-factors in enzyme and hormone systems. Some minerals also serve as constituents of body fluids and are involved in the maintenance of osmotic pressure, acid-base balance, membrane-permeability, and nerve transmission.

With regard to macrominerals potassium (K) levels should not exceed 0.8% of dry matter. If K levels in the ration exceed 1.1% of dry matter, then the upper levels of S, Mg and Ca in Table 1 are recommended to offset the elevated K. The addition of anionic salts to the close-up cow diet has been used successfully in many cases to help offset the negative impacts of elevated K levels. The key starts with high quality low K forage to enhance dry matter intake and to keep the minerals under control. If K levels can be kept at 0.8% of dry matter or less than the lower levels of Ca, Mg and S are recommended. However, it is often difficult to find forages with K levels low enough to maintain ration K levels lower than 0.8% of dry matter. Fresh water should be provided ad libitum at all times (Van Saun, 1991).

In conclusion it can be stated that the different phases of the dry cow period need different levels of nutrition and care to meet respective metabolic challenges during the dry period and subsequent lactation as is recommended by NRC (1989).

## 3.4 PHYSIOLOGICAL CHANGES IN THE DRY- AND ESPECIALLY THE CLOSE-UP PERIOD

During the last three months of gestation, which includes the dry period, there is a relatively increased growth rate of the conceptus (Bell et al., 1995). They found that in Holstein cows, the wet weight of the fetus increased from about 10 kg at day 190 to about 40 kg at day 270 of gestation, and the wet weight of the gravid uterus from about 25 kg to about 80 kg in the same period. Fetal dry matter concentration increased from 180 g/kg wet weight at day 190 to 260 g/kg at day 270 of gestation.

In the close-up period, feed intake is often reduced. The most severe depression in feed intake, takes place just before or at the day of calving when the cow needs energy

*Figure 1. Depression of dry matter intake around calving (Adapted from Bertics et al., 1992)*

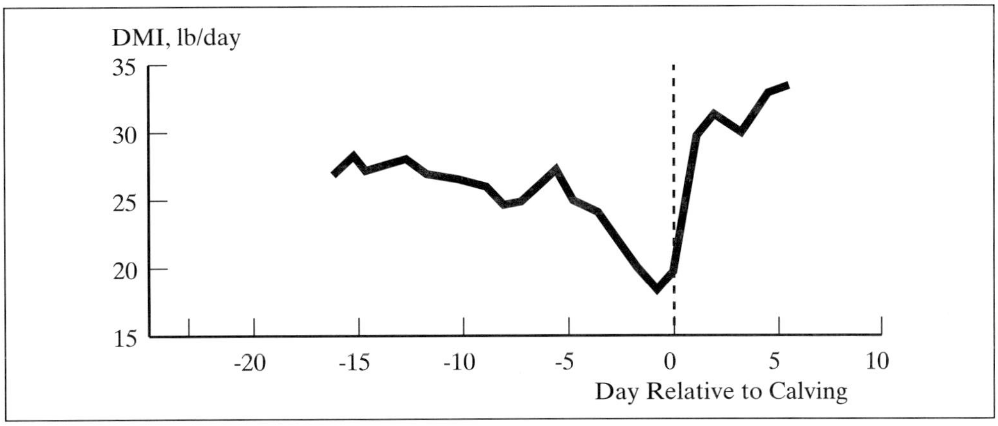


to expel the fetus and increases milk production (Figure 1).

The extent of that depression, varying from 28 to 40%, depends on the energy content of the close-up diet (Bertics et al., 1992; Vazquez-Anon et al., 1994; Studer et al., 1993; Grummer, 1995).

Brydl, 1994 found that rumination time decreased from an average of 500 minutes/day (10 days before parturition) to less of 100 minutes/day at day of calving (Figure 2).

Plasma NEFA (non-esterified fatty acids) concentrations, which are indicative of increasing lipolytic activity, normally increase until completion of calving, and decrease

*Figure 2. Depression of rumination around calving (Adapted from Brydl, 1995)*

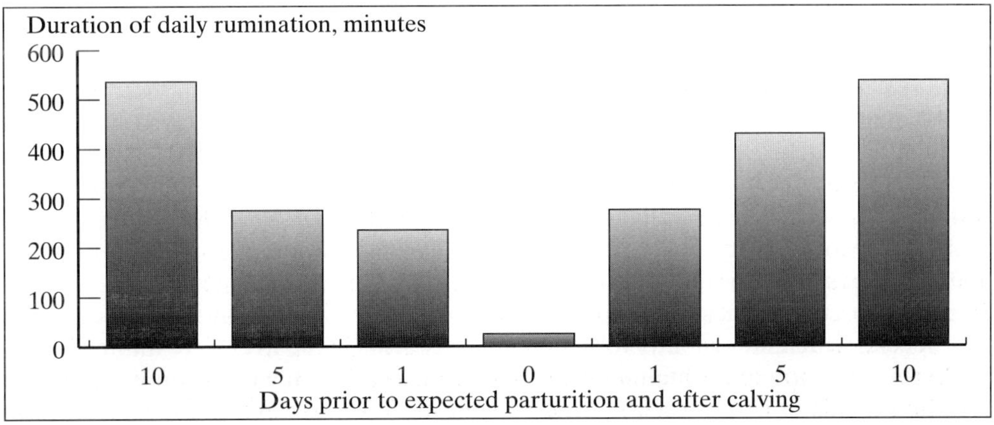

after calving. After calving plasma NEFA levels remain higher than before calving (Grummer, 1995; Studer et al., 1993).

Besides changes in the uterus and in dry matter intake, a progressive reduction of the ruminal mucosa takes place when a energy-poor ration is fed. After changing to a high energy diet, intensive proliferation processes begin. This means that the ruminal mucosa undergoes reductive and proliferative processes in the dry period, depending on the type of feed provided (Dirksen et al., 1985; Dirksen et al., 1992).

One might think that the decrease in dry matter intake could be due to an expanding uterus into the abdomen which may interfer with rumen fill. However, it is doubtful if rumen capacity becomes a sole limiting factor before calving because Bertics et al., (1992) showed that a decrease in dry matter intake of 28% before calving can be overcome by force feeding via rumen cannulas. Therefore, physical rumen fill is not the sole reason for the reduced intake before calving but certainly does influence it. In this respect it has been hypothesized that endocrine factors, such as changes in blood estrogen or estrogen:progesterone ratio, are involved as well in a decreased feed intake around calving (Grummer et al., 1990).

This all means that in the close-up period, requirements of the fetus and associated membranes and the subsequent demands of lactation increase as feed intake decreases. The decrease in feed intake leads to a negative nutrient balance in the close-up period which is a critical factor in influencing the development of a fatty liver (Grummer, 1995).

## 3.5 DISEASE AND DISEASE PREVENTION IN THE CLOSE-UP PERIOD

**Fatty liver syndrome –** Fatty liver is a metabolic disorder of excessive fat accumulation in the liver during periods of negative energy balance. This in contrast to fat being deposited in adipose tissue during positive energy balance. The most common period of negative energy balance is the periparturient period starting two weeks before parturition (Bertics et al., 1992). This happens as a consequence of insufficient gluconeogenesis and energy intake. However, the relative magnitude of the negative energy balance in the dry period is small compared to that encountered during the 1st week postpartum (Grummer, 1995).

In the cow with a negative energy balance, fat is mobilized from adipose tissue stores, leading to increased blood concentrations of NEFA. The NEFA are taken up by the liver and can be oxidized to ketone bodies or carbon dioxide or can be esterified to triacylglycerols (TG) (Top et al., 1995). Fatty liver occurs when the rate of liver TG synthesis exceeds the rate of liver TG disappearance through hydrolysis and export as part of very low density lipoproteins (VLDL) (Vazquez-Anon et al., 1994; Grummer, 1993). Adipose tissue is the predominant site for lipogenesis in ruminants whereas the liver is the predominant site for lipogenesis in birds and humans. It has been suggested that species with limited ability to synthesize fatty acids in the liver have limited ability to secrete lipoproteins containing triacylglycerol from the liver (Pullen et al., 1990). During periods of excessive fatty acid mobilization from adipose tissue, insufficient lipoprotein synthesis may lead to hepatic accumulation of TG, i.e., development of fatty liver (Bertics et al., 1992; Studer et al., 1993; Top et al., 1995). It has been suggested that protein nutrition may influence VLDL rate of synthesis and affect TG export from the liver. Estrogen, specifically estrone of placental origin, which is elevated in late gestation also has been implicated in the development of fatty liver (Grummer et al., 1990), as has depressed feed intake prepartum (Bertics et al., 1992). A fatty liver is a compromised liver and will not respond to metabolic challenges as it should, resulting in impaired health, fertility and milk production (Gerloff et al., 1986a).

Nutrient requirements for pregnancy accelerate with the growth of the fetus (Bell et al., 1992). Cows may experience negative energy balance in the dry period if energy intake is less than demands for maintenance, fetal growth, and organ metabolic changes in preparation for lactation. Any kind of stress will aggravate the situation. Stressors that lower feed intake can stimulate release of fatty acids into the blood and be converted to storage fat in the liver. Hormonal changes around parturition, especially estrogen increases and progesterone decreases, trigger a dramatic rise in NEFA's which potentiate TG deposition in the liver. This is further enhanced by adrenaline and noradrenaline release and hypophagia during calving. Important by-products of fat metabolism for energy are ketones. Any situation that results in fat mobilization can lead to fatty liver and ketosis (Grummer, 1995).

Almost all cows will have an increase in liver fat the day after calving, but the major rise occurs between 2 weeks before and 1 day after calving. There usually are slight increases in liver fat after this periparturient period, but they are minor compared with what occurs just before and during calving (Bertics et al., 1992; Studer et al., 1993). Once deposited in the liver, fat content does not diminish until after the cow returns to positive energy balance and is gaining weight. This typically occurs 5 - 12 weeks after calving. Even at this time of positive energy balance, fat in the liver persists because of the slow rate of removal from the liver (Kleppe et al., 1988; Pullen et al., 1990). During lactation, the mammary gland becomes a deposit for fat being synthesized into milk fat and protects the liver form fat accumulations (Emery, 1993).

**Diagnosis of fatty liver** –Guidelines and test procedures to diagnose fatty liver in cows are described by Herdt (1988). In short to diagnose fatty liver in individual cows, biopsies are taken with a Tru-Cut biopsy instrument (Tru-cut@, Travenol lab., Deerfield, Illinois, USA) via a stab incision over the 10th intercostal space at the level of the greater trochanter and the biopsy needle is directed towards the left elbow joint. Samples collected with this instrument usually weigh 15 - 30 mg and can be divided into 2 or 3 subsamples that can be tested. Samples are plunged beneath the surface of the test liquid and observed for flotation. The exact specific gravity of the liquids used in clinical tests can be varied to meet the needs of the clinician. A convenient and meaningful clinical test can be performed using water and solutions of copper sulfate with specific gravities of 1.025 and 1.055. Liver samples that float in all 3 liquids have fat concentrations in excess of 35%. Those that sink in water, but float in the other 2 liquids have levels greater than 25%, but less than 35% fat. Samples that float only in the solution of 1.055 specific gravity have levels greater than 13% but less than 25% fat.

*Figure 3. Distribution of plasma Non-estrified Fatty Acid Concentrations (Herdt, 1996, with permission)*

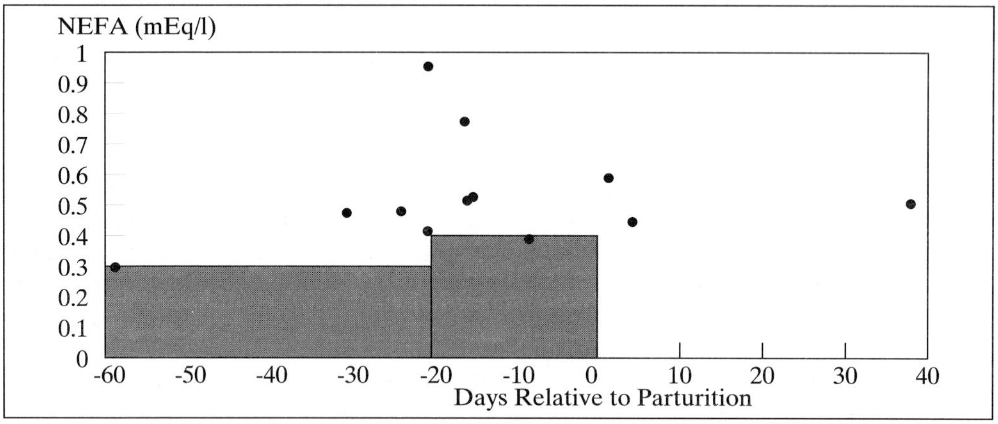


These liver fat concentrations are expressed on the basis of wet weight.

Clinical interpretation of liver fat concentration is not a straight forward process. Cows with hepatic lipid concentrations exceeding 35% essentially have no histologically normal liver tissue and will be clinically ill. Such animals have a very poor prognosis. Cows with liver fat concentrations of 25 - 35% often, but not always, show clinical signs. Whether or not animals in this category become clinically affected probably depends on the severity of concurrent diseases. There is probably an interaction between stress and liver fat concentration that determines whether or not disease will develop. Animals with liver fat concentrations of 13 - 25% often do not exhibit clinical signs but are at increased risk for disease, death, and culling compared to cows with less than 13% liver fat. Liver fat concentrations of less than 13% are clinically insignificant (Herdt, 1988).

An alternative method for the diagnosis of fatty liver at a herd level, is to determine prepartum NEFA, BHBA and glucose in blood plasma. These parameters are strongly correlated with liver TG at day 1 postpartum (Studer et al., 1993). The NEFA concentrations can be plotted against days relative to parturition as presented in figure 3. The shaded areas in Figure 3 represent goal values. Herds should be evaluated for the number of points outside of the shaded areas (Herdt, 1996).

**Ketosis –** Ketosis is a metabolic disorder of the periparturient period and is interrelated with fatty liver. Clinical signs include diminished appetite, decreased milk production, loss of weight, hypoglycemia, hyperketonemia and sometimes nervous signs. In dairy cows, ketosis has been classified into four categories (Kronfeld, 1980):

1. Primary underfeeding ketosis occurs when not enough feed is consumed to meet requirements and body reserves are utilized resulting in ketonemia.
2. Secondary underfeeding ketosis occurs when other diseases cause a reduction in feed intake and nutrient demands are not met.

3. Alimentary feeding ketosis is a result of high intake of ketogenic precursors in fermented feed.
4. Spontaneous feeding ketosis which is due to an insufficiency of lipogenic nutrients relative to glucogenic nutrients.

Susceptibility to ketosis is greatest during high milk production when there is maximal utilization of glucose by the mammary gland.

**Interrelationship between fatty liver and ketosis** – Common to the occurrence of both disorders are elevated plasma NEFA concentrations, fat infiltration into the liver, and negative energy balance. Ketosis is caused by an inadequate supply of glucose to meet metabolic demands. When the diet and glycogenesis are insufficient to meet the demand for glucose, fat is mobilized to provide glycerol as a glucose precursor and meet energy demands to other tissues. Fat mobilization may result in excessive fatty acid uptake by the liver and production of ketones. Excessive fat accumulation in the liver compromises glycogenesis. If this results in enhanced levels of circulating ketones it may diminish appetite and feed intake. Glucose output by the liver then is reduced even more. The low glucose output will decrease insulin secretion and result in increased lipid mobilization creating a vicious cycle of events (Veenhuizen et al., 1991).

**Prevention of fatty liver and ketosis** – The goal is to keep the energy gap in late pregnancy and early lactation as small as possible by maximizing energy intake, in order to reduce fatty acid mobilization from adipose tissue, and prevent excessive depletion of hepatic glycogen (Grummer, 1995).

Strategies for reduction of fatty acid mobilization and prevention of excessive hepatic glycogen depletion can be achieved by minimizing TG deposition in the liver and/or maximizing hepatic glycogen levels. More specifically, strategies must be implemented that will minimize fatty acid mobilization from adipose tissue, decrease esterification of fatty acids in the liver, and increase export of TG as VLDL.
This all can be achieved in various ways.

1. Maintaining maximum dry matter intake prior to calving. This is very critical in minimizing negative energy balance. Bertics et al., (1992) evaluated the effects of prepartum intake depression on the development of fatty liver. Half of the cows were force-fed feed refusals via rumen cannulae. The force-fed cows were maintained at a DMI level equivalent to what was recorded 21 to 17 days before the expected calving date. Feed intake of control cows (non-force-fed) decreased 28% over the final 17 day pre-partum. Liver triglycerides increased 227% in the control cows and only 75% in the force-fed cows during the same time period. Plasma glucose concentrations were also higher for the force-fed cows. This illustrates the importance of dry matter intake on the incidence of this metabolic disease. Another tool to minimize negative energy balance is to increase the energy density of the close-up diet by providing grains. This should start about 2 to 3 weeks before expected date of calving. The amount fed should be increased gradually up to a maximum of 3 kg/cow/at the day of calving.

2. Elimination of stressors around calving. Stressors that may interfere with dry matter intake in the periparturient period will predispose the cow to metabolic disease. Therefore, sudden changes in diet ingredients, especially less palatable ingredients (supplemental fats, rendered protein sources, and anionic salts), should be used with care. New feed ingredients should be introduced gradually. Proper feedbunk management can help minimize dry matter intake challenges.
3. Proper housing management. Higher plasma NEFA's have been associated with close-up cows and early postpartum cows housed in competitive groups versus individual box stalls (Gerloff et al., 1986). Environmental and group changes also will create stress on the cow. If dry cows are kept at a separate facility and are introduced into a new environment, they may go off feed for a while. Therefore, transitions should be made well in advance of calving, not 2 or 3 days before calving when they are predisposed to going off feed.
4. Stimulation of ruminal mucosa proliferation before calving by concentrate feeding. To stimulate proliferation, it is necessary to commence energy rich feeding as early as 4 weeks prepartum. The adaptation of ruminal mucosa to a high energy diet during which the papillae reach maximum length takes about 4 to 6 weeks. Increasing the size of the papillae increases the surface area of the rumen and increases the absorptive capacity for rumen volatile fatty acids. In this way the mucosal adaptation plays a major role in the regulation and stabilization of rumen pH and subsequently, the energy supply for milk production. (Dirksen et al., 1985; Dirksen et al., 1992; Weiss, 1994). Therefore, emphasis has to be put on prepartum diet formulation.
5. Drenching cows with propylene glycol (especially cows wtith a BCS of 4 or more) during the last 7 - 10 days before calving may reduce fatty liver and ketosis but is very labor intensive. Propylene glycol is converted to propionic acid in the rumen which is converted to glucose by the liver and causes the cow to have an insulin response. Insulin reduces fat mobilization from storage depots and consequently reduces liver fat accumulation (Grummer et al., 1994; Studer et al., 1993).
6. Optimization of the close-up ration for protein. Labile protein reserves in the cow are limited relative to lipid reserves. Underfeeding protein in late pregnancy may cause depletion of maternal labile protein reserves (Botts et al., 1979), leading to compromised lactation, health, and reproduction (Curtis et al., 1985; Van Saun, 1991). Increased CP levels in close-up diets may increase milk production through extra absorbable amino acids (Grummer, 1995). Feeding more than 12 to 13% protein in the close-up period was correlated with decreased risk of retained placenta and primary ketosis (Curtis et al., 1985). According to Grummer (1995), increasing dietary undegradable intake protein (UIP) may enhance utilization of mobilized lipid by extra-hepatic tissues. This all may explain why diets with crude protein levels higher than recommended by NRC and undegradable protein supplementation prepartum, have a positive response on performance postpartum (Van Saun, 1993).

Body condition and/or changes in body condition are good indicators of energy balance. Body condition must be managed during the dry period and lactation to minimize its effects in the periparturient period. Overconditioned cows eat less after calving and are more susceptible to ketosis. A cow with a body condition score of 3.5 or less, probably is going to have a greater appetite and fewer metabolic problems after calving. Feeding for a targeted body condition at drying off should begin at mid-lactation or earlier and must be continued through the post-partum risk period.

**Milk fever and prevention of milk fever** – Milk fever or parturient paresis is a metabolic disease occurring just before, at, or just after calving in high producing cows. Milk fever is due to the high Ca drain from blood to milk without a satisfactory compensatory mechanism of Ca resorption from the intestines and/or bones or reabsorption from the kidneys, to keep the concentrations of calcium in blood within physiologic range. In the prepartum period, the cow starts producing colostrum which contains about 2.3 g Ca/kg. A cow producing just 10 liters of colostrum will then lose 23 g of calcium in a single milking. This is about nine times as much Ca as is present in the entire plasma pool of the cow. Calcium lost from the plasma pool must be replaced by Ca absorbed from the reticulo-rumen and small intestines and from bones (Goff, 1992). This is influenced by vitamin D. Dietary vitamin D2 and D3 are absorbed through the small intestines and transported to the liver where they are converted into 25 hydroxy vitamin D. The latter is then transported to the kidney and under the influence of parathyroid hormone (PTH) converted to 1,25 dihydroxy vitamin D, which is the active form of vitamin D. A decrease in plasma Ca causes the parathyroid glands to secrete PTH. PTH rapidly increases renal Ca reabsorption from the glomerular filtrate. If the perturbation in plasma Ca is small, the plasma Ca can be returned to normal and PTH secretion will return to baseline. If the Ca drain from the extracellular pool is large, continued PTH secretion stimulates the kidney toward production of 1,25 dihydroxy vitamin D (1,25 $(OH)_2$ vitamin D). The production of Ca binding proteins is stimulated by 1,25 $(OH)_2$ vitamin D and carries Ca across the intestinal and reticulo-rumen epithelial cells. Under normal conditions this all acts to increase the entry of Ca into the extracellular Ca pool (Goff, 1992). However, in a alkalinic blood state the kidney is less responsive to PTH which causes a time lag before mechanisms can compensate for the sudden demand for Ca. At the same time, dry matter intake around parturition is decreasing resulting in lower Ca intake from the diet. During the time lag, Ca concentrations can decrease further and result in parturient paresis.

In the dry period most of the diets fed are based on forages that are high in cation content; particular K+. These fixed cations tend to keep the cow in a state of mild metabolic alkalosis, as evidenced by the relatively high urine pH of cows fed such diets (Goff, 1992). Studies in rats (Beck and Webster, 1976) and dogs (Burnell, 1971) indicate that bone and perhaps renal tissues, are refactory to the effects of PTH in the alkaline metabolic state, and the stimulatory effects of PTH are enhanced during metabolic acidosis. In the cow, plasma 1,25$(OH)_2$ vitamin D response to hypocalcemia was significantly reduced when fed a high cation diet (Goff et al., 1991). It is suggested that the kidneys then become temporally refractory to stimulation by PTH. Bone Ca resorption, which also requires stimulation by PTH, was also reduced in cows fed the high cation diet, suggesting that bone tissues were also refactory to stimulation by PTH. Addition of anions to the diet restored the ability of these tissues to respond to

PTH, preventing development of severe hypocalcemia (Goff et al., 1991; Goff, 1992).

Taken together, data suggest that the underlying cause of milk fever is an inability of cow tissues to respond adequately to PTH. This causes poor production of $1{,}25(OH)_2$ vitamin D and reduces Ca absorption and resorption from bone stores. The presumption is that metabolic alkalosis somehow disrupts the integrity of PTH receptors on target tissues. Anionic diets may work by increasing target tissue responsiveness to PTH, which permits the cow to successfully adapt to the Ca stress associated with the onset of lactation (Goff, 1992). Therefore, dietary Ca is not as much the causative factor in milk fever as is the metabolic status of the cow at parturition which causes a reduced or enhanced sensitivity of the target tissues to Ca regulating hormones (Horst and Reinhardt, 1983; Block, 1994). In addition dietary acidity or alkalinity can be considered as being more important than Ca intake in controlling milk fever (Oetzel, 1991). For more detailed information see Block, (1994) and Goff, (1992).

**Cation-anion balance** – Controlled studies have established that alkalogenic diets tend to cause milk fever, whereas acidogenic diets tend to prevent it. They have also showed that feeding anionic salts has benefits in preventing milk fever and hypocalcemia (Block, 1984; Oetzel, 1993). (Oetzel et al., 1988; Gaynor et al., 1989; Dishington, 1975; Goff et al., 1991; Leclerc and Goff, 1989). To quantitate the relationship between cations and anions in a diet the following dietary cation-anion difference (DCAD) equation can be used. DCAD has been defined as milliequivalents (mEq) of [(Na+K)-(Cl+($SO_4$)], per 100g dry matter. One equivalent weight is equal to the molecular weight divided by the charge.

The DCAD has a direct influence on blood acid-base metabolism (Block, 1994). It can be used to predict whether a diet will evoke an acidogenic or alkalogenic response. The equation is therefore a good estimate for the prediction of milk fever. The cations of significance are Na and K and the anions are Cl and ($SO_4$). Ca and Mg do not enter the equation because of their relatively low absorption rates (30 to 60%). The recommended DCAD is -10 to -15 Meq per 100 grams of ration DM.

**Prevention strategies** – Prevention strategies are based on the knowledge of the pathogenesis of milk fever. Prevention can be based on:

1. manipulation of the diet by:
   *) lowering the Ca level in the diet,
   *) changing the anion-cation balance.
2. administration of pharmacological doses of vitamin D3 or its metabolites.

**Lowering the calcium level in the diet.** Feeding very low calcium and phosphorus diets prepartum (33 to 42 g Ca/d and 20 to 26 g P/d, NRC, 1989) and high-calcium diets after parturition will reduce the incidence of milk fever (Oetzel, 1993; Goff, 1992). Restriction of calcium intake during the prepartum period prevents the cow's active intestinal calcium absorption and bone calcium resorption mechanisms from becoming quiescent and unable to respond to a sudden Ca outflow as is the case with high Ca intakes during the dry period (Goff, 1992). Calcium intake during the prepartum period can be restricted by feeding forages low in Ca such as corn silage. However, even this approach limits Ca intake to no less than about 50 gm/d. A more stringent Ca restriction is usually not possible without disturbing the balance of other nutrients (Oetzel, 1993). Prepartum diets high in phosphorus (> 80 g PO4/day instead of 20 to 26 g P/day, NRC ,1989) also increase the incidence of milk fever and hypocalcemia in general. Increased dietary phosphorus intake increases the level of phosphorus in blood, which has a direct inhibitory effect on the renal enzymes that catalyze production of 1,25$(OH)_2$ vitamin D3. This reduced production of 1,25$(OH)_2$ vitamin D3 further reduces intestinal absorption mechanisms (Goff, 1992).

**Administration of pharmacological doses of vitamin D3 or its metabolites.** Feeding high doses of vitamin D (250,000 IU/d) for 3 - 5 days prepartum will prevent milk fever. However, repeated treatments necessitated by inaccurate prediction of parturition may lead to toxicity (Block, 1994).

**Manipulating the cation-anion difference in the diet.** The incidence of milk fever appears to be dependent on the metabolic state of the cow in the dry period. Diets fed to prepartum cows are commonly alkalogenic and have a dietary cation-anion difference of about +50 to +300 or more mEq/kg on a dry matter basis. Alkalogenic diets tend to cause milk fever, whereas acidogenic diets tend to prevent it (Oetzel 1993). For prevention of milk fever, dry cows must receive an acidogenic diet (ie a diet with a negative DCAD). A negatively balanced ration varying from -10 to -20 mEq is usually adequate. Acidogenic diets increase receptivity to parathyroid hormone by increasing the amount of 1,25 Dihydroxy vitamin D3, followed by an increase of intestinal Ca absorption and bone Ca resorption mechanisms so that there is a more immediate amplified response to the plasma Ca drop at the beginning of lactation (Oetzel, 1991; Oetzel 1993).

A negative DCAD can be achieved by calculating the DCAD of the diet and adding anionic salts such as $MgSO_4$, $CaSO_4$, $(NH_4)_2SO_4$, $NH_4Cl$, and $CaCl_2$ in moderate amounts to the diet. A better response to a negative DCAD diet occurs when dietary concentrations of Ca reach 1.5 to 2.0% on a dry matter basis (Block, 1994). Therefore, high dietary Ca with low DCAD may be necessary to prevent milk fever. In contrast, milk production and dry matter intake were significantly increased by a higher DCAD in early and midlactation but remained unaffected in late lactation (Delaquise and Block, 1995). The recommended DCAD for lactating cows should be high (+200 to +400 Meq/100 grams of DM) at the beginning of lactation and decrease progressively throughout lactation (Block, 1994).

**Calculation of DCAD** – Balancing the anion-cations in the diet is a relatively new method to prevent milk fever and to improve health and production. To calculate DCAD in mEq/100 g of diet dry matter the percentages of anions and cations in the diet dry matter must be multiplied by a factor (Table 2). A total of 150 to 250 grams of a combination of ammonium chloride, ammonium sulfate, calcium chloride, calcium sulfate and magnesium sulfate are needed per cow per day depending on the concentration of K and Na in the ration fed (Beede, 1992). Increasing the concentration of sulfur above 0.4% is not recommended because of interference with Se and reduction of performance (Beede, 1992). This causes a problem when feeding forages high in K.

*Table 2. Characteristics of anions and cations used in calculating DCAD (Adapted from Oetzel, 1993)*

| Element | Molecular weight (g) | Valence (charge) | Equivalent weight (g) | Factor to convert from % to mEq/kg diet |
|---|---|---|---|---|
| Sodium | 23.0 | 1.0 | 23.0 | 434.98 |
| Potassium | 39.1 | 1.0 | 39.1 | 255.74 |
| Chlorine | 35.5 | 1.0 | 35.5 | 282.06 |
| Sulfur | 32.1 | 2.0 | 16.0 | 623.75 |
| Calcium | 40.1 | 2.0 | 20.0 | 499.00 |
| Magnesium | 24.3 | 2.0 | 12.2 | 822.64 |
| Phosphorus | 31.0 | 1.8 | 17.2 | 581.14 |

*Key factors in a systematic approach to anionic salt supplementation*

* Optimize feeding management before using anionic salts (Oetzel, 1993).
* Obtain an actual analysis of macrominerals in all feeds to be used in the dry cow diet. Besides potassium and sodium, chloride and sulfur determinations should always be included since they are key factors in calculating DCAD (Chase, 1992).
* If possible select forages for dry cows that are low in potassium (Oetzel, 1993).
* Keep track of variation in mineral contents of different feeds and of the same forage from different fields of the same farm,
* Balance dietary Mg and Sulfur at 0.3% on a dry matter basis. Add dietary Chlorine to lower the dietary cation-anion difference to -15 mEq/kg on a dry matter basis. Check dietary non-protein nitrogen and degradable protein intake. These should not exceed 0.5% and 70% of crude protein respectively. If either protein measure is too high, reduce the amount of ammonium salts and/or change the degradable protein content appropriately (Oetzel, 1993).
* Account for the mineral content of water that is consumed (Chase, 1992).
* Add dietary Ca to a daily intake of 150 g and dietary P to 55 gram (Oetzel, 1993).
* Anionic salts have the disadvantage that their palatability is low which may reduce dry matter intake in prepartum cows. Calcium chloride is the least and magnesium sulfate the most palatable anionic salt. A decrease in DMI will influence the energy balance of the cow and subsequently the health status, and therefore would appear to be counterproductive (Chase, 1992). Salts can be added to the ration via a premix. Adding salts directly to a Total Mixed Ration(TMR) which is thoroughly mixed, is preferable from both a palatability and toxicity viewpoint. Dry matter intake should also be monitored when feeding anionic salts (Chase, 1992; Oetzel, 1993).
* Supplementation of the diet with anionic salts should start 10 to 7 days before expected calving date and stop 1 - 3 days after calving.
* In herds with a low milk fever incidence anionic salts may be considered for their potential to improve milk production and reproduction (Oetzel, 1993).

Instead of a systematic approach, a standard daily dose can be offered to dry cows. Examples of recommended standard doses are: 113.5 grams of magnesium sulfate plus 113.5 grams of ammonium chloride or 113,5 grams of magnesium sulfate plus 56.75 grams of ammonium chloride plus 56.75 grams of ammonium sulfate. One always should realize that this dosing system does not properly allow for the existing mineral content of the prepartum diet (Oetzel, 1993).

### Measuring urine pH

As already stated feeding anionic salts requires that the DCAD status of the feed ingredients in the diet must be known. However, in practice it is difficult to get the feed ingredients analysed every time the forages in the diet change. A useful tool is to measure urine pH. The target pH is 5.5 to 6.5 (Beede et al., 1992).

**Associations of DCAD/calcium status and peripartum disorders –** Incorporation of anionic salts in diets of close-up cows increases Ca serum concentrations, reduces incidence of clinical milk fever, subclinical hypocalcemia (Oetzel et al., 1988; Beede et al., 1992), and retained placenta (Oetzel et al., 1988). It also may increase milk yield (Wang et al., 1991) and reproductive performance in the subsequent lactation (Block, 1984; Beede et al., 1992). Hypocalcemic cows (< 8 mg/dl total calcium serum concentration) appeared to be at 4.8 times (Massey et al., 1993) or even 7.35 times (Beede et al., 1992) greater risk of developing left displaced abomasum. Hypocalcemia is also associated with impaired ruminal contractions (Huber et al., 1981), lethargy, inappetence in early lactation (Beede et al., 1992), slowed uterine involution (Oetzel et al., 1988) and prolapsed uteri (Risco et al., 1984). It is thought that subclinical hypocalcemia may have a greater impact than clinical milk fever on the profitability of dairies (Oetzel, 1993).

To minimize the incidence of milk fever, the best strategy is to feed low levels of calcium in the dry period and maximize dry matter intake, especially in the peripartum period. Forages with low K contents (< 1%) should be harvested and fed to dry cows. Supplementation with anionic salts may be particularly beneficial if the array of feed ingredients available does not allow formulation of a diet very low in Ca. However, feeding management of prepartum cows should be optimized before supplementation with anionic salts is initiated (Oetzel, 1993).

### Udder edema and prevention

Acute udder edema occurs in heifers and in high producing dairy cows but is more severe in heifers. It starts a few weeks before calving and can continue up to 3 weeks into lactation. Edema is a condition characterized by an excessive accumulation of lymphatic fluid in interstitial spaces. Visible accumulation sites include the udder, navel and brisket regions, and in exceptional cases the thighs and vulva (Tucker et al., 1992). Udder edema may interfere with milk production, milk let-down, and machine attachment during milking. The teats tend to strut outward so that milking can be more difficult. There can be physical damage, such as cracking of the skin on the teats and harm to suspensory ligaments, leading to broken down udders. Severe mammary enlargement makes walking and laying down difficult and causes discomfort to the cow.

The exact cause of udder edema is not known. Several factors including inheritance, circulatory disturbances, and diet have been implicated in edema (Lema et al., 1992). Genetic factors may play a certain role because some cows tend to have edema annually regardless of feeding programs. However, heritability of edema is low, so selecting against it would be a slow process. A long dry period and an older age at 1st calving may increase the incidence of edema. Serum and urine chemical data do not differ significantly between cows with and without udder edema (Vestweber et al., 1989). There is no clear relationship between concentrate intake, dietary protein content, and the incidence of udder edema (Lema et al., 1992). The common belief that feeding grain causes udder edema may be caused by the practice of salt supplementation in the grain mixture (Nestor et al., 1988). Supplementation of diets with either an excess of 136 g NaCl or 272 g $KHCO_3$ resulted in significantly more severe udder edema in first calf heifers than in control animals. Addition of both salts resulted in less edema than when each salt was fed individually (Nestor et al., 1988).

The prevention of udder edema lies in avoiding excess salt during the close-up period. Another approach consists of feeding anionic salts to prevent milk fever which may also help to prevent udder edema. However this has to be studied in more detail. Provision of moderate exercise along with good care before calving is also indicated. Diuretic treatment can reduce severity and duration of edema. Udder supports may be helpful to protect ligaments from breaking down. In severe cases, one can start milking before calving.

## EPILOGUE

Characterizing the dry period as a resting phase between lactations and emphasizing it as a period of lowest nutritional requirements for the cows has given producers the wrong impression of the critical role of the dry cow. Required nutrient amounts for the dry cow are the sum of maintenance, pregnancy, and reserve replenishment needs with additional requirements for growth during the first two pregnancies (Van Saun, 1991). The most important period in the dry period is the transition between late pregnancy and early lactation. In this period an enormous metabolic challenge to the high-yielding dairy cow occurs (Bell. 1995a). Proper management of the late pregnant dry cow period should be portrayed to dairy producers as an investment in the future; an investment targeted towards achievement of maximal lactational and reproductive performance in the next lactation (Beede et al., 1992). At this time not enough is understood about the effects of feed intake during the dry period on subsequent milk yield and the incidence of fatty liver, milk fever and udder edema. These relationships are still under investigation at the time of this writing.

## APPENDIX: BODY CONDITION SCORING AND INTERPRETATION

### METHODOLOGY

Body condition scoring is a subjective method for estimating the quantity of subcutaneous fat in specific anatomical regions on a live animal. Actual body condition scores (BCS) and changes in scores over time enable the farmer and his advisors to estimate the impact of various management practices, especially the efficiency of nutrition, on health, reproduction, and milk production performance (Edmonson et al., 1989). Scoring body condition enables farmers to estimate and compare body condition in various production groups and how much body tissue is lipolized during the transition period from late gestation to early lactation. Therefore, body condition scoring is an important tool in daily cow management.

Body condition is scored on a scale of 1 - 5 (Wildman et al., 1982; Edmonson et al., 1989; Ferguson et al., 1994). For every whole unit loss in BCS, about 56 kg of body tissue are lost in a mature Holstein cow (Otto et al., 1991). In dairy cattle, a change in BCS is related to both live weight change and change in body tissue reserves (Gearhart et al., 1990). A score of 1 indicates severe underconditioning and a score of 5 is assigned to very obese cows. Quarter and half scores, sometimes expressed as pluses and minuses, can be added to refine the scoring system. The system of Wildman is based upon palpating relevant parts of the back and rump of the cow, to determine the amount of fat tissue covering these areas. The systems of Edmonson and Ferguson visually appraise the same relevant parts.

In scoring body condition, particular attention is given to tissue covering the vertebral spinous processes and transverse processes of the lumbar vertebrae, tuber coxae (hooks), tuber ischii (pins), and tissue depressions between the backbone and the hook and pin bones. In addition, the slope between hook and pin bones and the hollowness between tailhead and pin bones are evaluated (Figure 4). All these areas must be considered for each cow. Using 1 or 2 areas alone can be misleading. For accurate scoring, cows must be standing. Frame size, breed, stage of lactation, milk production level, and health status must be ignored for accurate scoring. Consideration of these factors should be reserved to help interpret what the scores mean.

**Score 1** – The individual spinous processes (SP) are scarcely covered with tissue giving the backbone the appearance of a saw with distinct teeth. The individual transverse processes (TP) of the short ribs are very prominent and more than half their length is visible. The fingers can be put between and under the short ribs that form a shelf. The concave transition between the spinous to the transverse processes has a sharp angular shape. The hooks and pins are sharp with almost no tissue covering. The body line between the hooks and the pins through the thurl (which is the area around the hip joint), is "V" shaped. There are deep depressions between the backbone and the pins and the backbone and the hooks. This gives the whole rump or thurl area, a hollow appearance. The area between the tail head and pins is deeply sunken and

*Figure 4. Drawings of body conformation at different body condition scores*

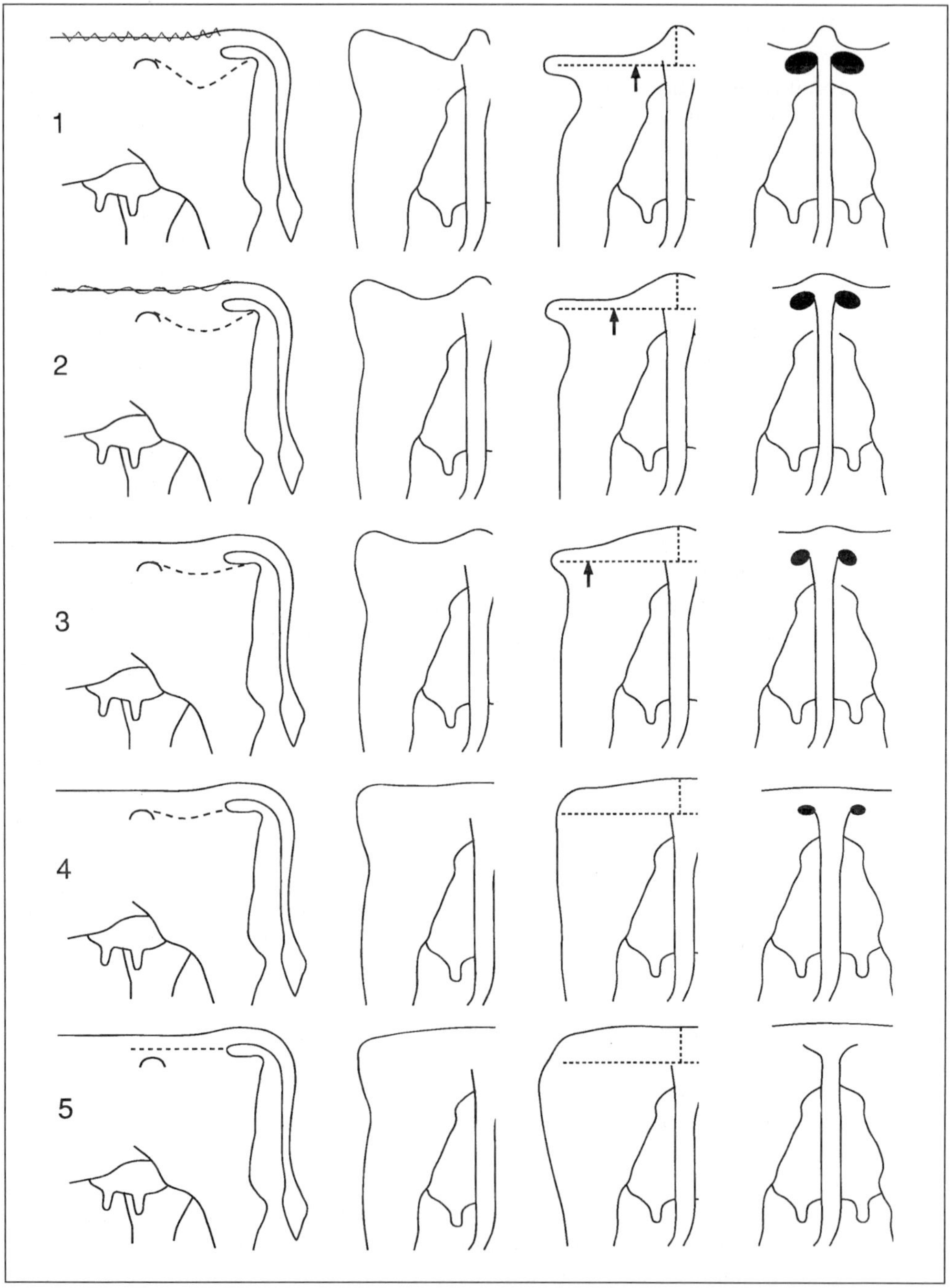

"V" shaped with folds of skin in the depression. The tail head and tail ligaments are prominent.

**Score 2** – The individual spinous processes are still prominently visible but feel more blunt by palpation. The saw appearance of the backbone is much less visible. The individual transverse processes of the short ribs can be felt easily and half of their length is now visible. The short ribs still have a rather distinct and overhanging shelf effect. The transition between the spinous and transverse processes shows an obvious concave but not angular depression. The hook and pin bones are still prominent. The body line between the hooks and the pins through the thurl is concave but is less "V" shaped. The thurl area between the backbone, hooks, and pin bones are still sunken although some tissue covering is present. The area below the tail head and between the pin bones is depressed forming a "U" shaped cavity under the tail with the tail ligament still well palpable.

**Score 3** – The spinous processes of the backbone appear as a rounded ridge but individual processes can still be seen. The individual spinous processes and transverse processes can be felt by applying slight pressure. Less than a quarter of the transverse processes is visible. The transition from the spinous processes to the transverse processes of the short ribs shows a smooth concave curve. The over-hanging shelf effect of the short ribs is hardly noticeable. The hook and pin bones are visible but more rounded and smooth. The thurl area between the backbone and the hook and pin bones is slightly depressed. The area between the tail head and pins is shallow with less distinct ligaments.

**Score 4** – The spinous processes of the backbone are not visible anymore and are rounded and smooth. The individual spinous processes and transverse processes of the short ribs are rounded and distinguishable only by firm palpation. The transition from the spinous to the transverse processes are nearly flat. There is no overhanging shelf effect visible. The hooks and pins are rounded and the span between the backbone and hook and pin bones is flat. The area around the tail head and the pin bones is rounded, with clear evidence of fat deposition. The sacral ligaments are not palpable.

**Score 5** – The bone structure of the backbone, short ribs, and hook and pin bone region is not apparent. The backbone ridge is slightly convex. Subcutaneous fat deposits are very evident. The whole back area can be compared with a rounded table top. The tail head appears buried in fatty tissue.

In summary, it can be stated that score 1 represents cows that are emaciated with a skinny and bony appearance. A high-producing, early lactation cow should have a score not lower than 2.5. A cow with a score of 2 or lower in early lactation indicates a shortage in dry matter/energy intake at an earlier stage. A milking cow in good condition is represented by score 3. Dry cows should score a 3.25 to 3.5. Score 4 represents an overconditioned cow; a potential problem cow at calving if dry and a potential inefficient milk producer if milking. At calving, a cow that scores 4 will have lower dry matter intake and lose more body condition. A score of 5 makes a cow a prime candidate for fat cow syndrome.

## FREQUENCY OF SCORING

BC scoring should be performed every 4 weeks for dry cows and every 3 to 6 weeks after calving depending on the stage of lactation. Young stock should be scored at regular intervals of 2 months or less and every time they are handled. Condition can change very rapidly around puberty. Therefore, this time period should be monitored carefully. Pregnant heifers from about 2 months before parturition can be scored at the same time as dry cows.

BCS should be recorded on a recording sheet as presented in Table 4. This offers the opportunity to follow condition scores of individual cows over time. Individual scores can be averaged and compared across time as presented in Table 3. BCS of individual cows during the dry period should be put on the examination list within the frame work of a herd fertility program (Chapter 1, part 2 and Chapter 5, part 2). This enables the herd health practitioner to compare the current BCS of lactating cows with their score during the dry period. Clinical findings then can be related with changes in body condition.

## EVALUATION OF BODY CONDITION SCORES

During every programmed farm visit, available data on BCS should be evaluated together with the farmer. This may include reviewing and interpretation of rolling condition scores of individual cows (Table 3) or groups of cows (Table 4).

A scatter plot of individual scores (Figure 5) highlights cows with extreme scores and presents the acceptable ranges around the target scores. Factors that might be responsible for extreme values have to be examined and discussed with the farmer. Examples of factors involved with low scores are: diseases such as, retained placenta, severe cases of lameness, metabolic disturbances, and twin pregnancies. Factors connected with extreme high body condition scores are: low milk production in combination with a high plane of nutrition, unbalanced rations high in energy and low in protein, subclinical mastitis, etc.

*Table 3. Sheet for recording rolling condition scores (DIM = days in milk)*

| Cow number | BCS at Dry-off | BCS at Calving | 1st BCS/ DIM | 2nd BCS/ DIM | 3rd BCS/ DIM |
|---|---|---|---|---|---|
| 1 | 4,0 | 4.0 | 3.5/20 | 3.0/41 | 3.0/69 |
| 26 | 3.75 | 3.75 | 3.5/18 | 3.0/39 | 3.0/67 |
| 39 | 3.0 | 3.0 | 2.5/17 | 1.7/38 | 2.0/66 |
| 1 | 3.75 | 3.75 | 3.5/12 | 3.0/33 | 3.0/61 |

*Table 4. Rolling group averages of condition scores*

| | Date 1 | Date 2 | Date 3 | Preset target |
|---|---|---|---|---|
| Dry cows | 4.0 | 3.8 | 3.5 | 3.25 - 3.75 |
| < 60 days | 2.2 | 2.2 | 2.7 | 2.50 - 3.25 |
| 60 - 120 days | 2.5 | 3.2 | 2.8 | 2.50 - 3.00 |
| 121 - 210 days | 2.9 | 2.4 | 3.4 | 2.75 - 3.25 |
| > 210 days | 3.8 | 3.5 | 3.5 | 3.00 - 3.50 |

## RECOMMENDED CONDITION SCORES IN VARIOUS PRODUCTION PERIODS

### Dry Period

Cows with more extreme condition scores at calving are at a higher risk for increased health problems, reproductive disorders, and lower peak and lactation yields (Fronk et al., 1980). Cows that calve with low condition scores (less than 3.0) received inadequate energy during late lactation and/or during the dry period. Such cows may

*Figure 5. Scatter plot of condition scores of individual cows. (Figures indicate number of cows with the same score)*

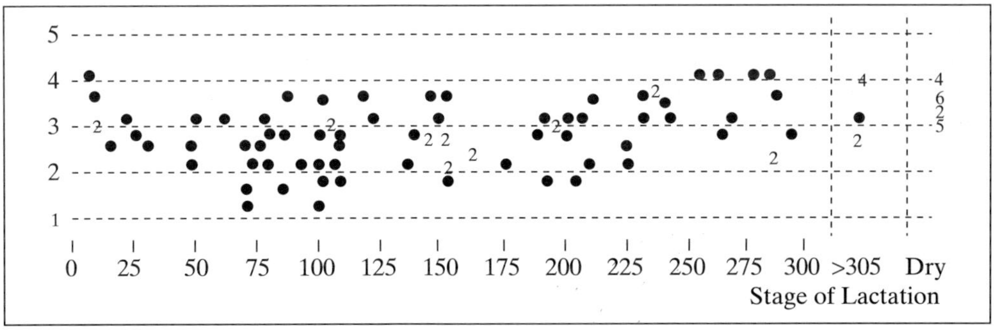

show a suboptimal peak yield with a good persistency. They also will be at risk of lower reproductive efficiency. Additional energy intake may be necessary to achieve maximum milk production in thin cows. One has to realize that body condition can not be easily, nor rapidly adjusted during a normal dry period length. During this period, an increase of 0.5 in BCS is the maximum that can be reasonably achieved.

Cows that calve with a BCS higher than 3.5 indicate that energy intakes were too high during late lactation and/or the dry period. In contrast to thin cows, fat cows calve with sufficient body tissue reserves "to milk some fat off her back" during the period of negative energy balance. They may show a high peak yield and a suboptimal persistency. Generally, an overconditioned cow is at increased risk for calving problems, reduced feed intake, more severe condition loss, and a complex of metabolic, digestive, reproductive, and infectious diseases (Gearhart et al., 1990). Overconditioned cows often have a history of diseases in the previous lactation such as mastitis or infertility and are often dried off early resulting in extended dry period lengths which may result in a vicious cycle. Most of these problems can be avoided in the future if cows are fed balanced late-lactation and dry-cow rations. It is not advisable to reduce body weight during the dry period. This will lead to mobilization of fat from body tissues, deposition of fat in the liver, and all the associated metabolic problems.

Moderate extremes (3.0 to 3.25 or 3.75 to 4.0) in body condition at calving are not necessarily a big problem if nutritional management after calving is optimal. If cows are fed properly after calving, total milk yields are independent of BCS at calving (Ruegg, 1991). Thus, it is important for the dairy farmer to strike a balance between allowing cows to be too fat or too thin at calving and also to monitor body condition changes after calving in order to feed them properly (Perkins et al., 1987).

## Early Lactation

It is recommended that cows in early lactation should not lose more than 0.75 unit of condition score. The target score in this period is between 2.5 and 3.0. Cows that lose 1.0 or more BCS are at increased risk of metabolic problems and reproductive inefficiency. High producing cows under excellent management may drop a full condition score without any problems. After about 4 weeks of lactation, cows should not lose any more condition. At this point in time, dry matter intake should have increased to a level to meet metabolic demands. In other words, BCS should not decrease after 4 weeks. In healthy cows it will take about another 8 weeks (12 weeks postpartum) before BCS will start to increase under normal feeding regimes and adequate nutrient balance.

The greatest challenge in early lactation is to maximize dry matter intake so that body condition changes and negative energy balance will be minimized. The amount and rate of body condition loss is more important than the score at any given time. Ideally, a cow should not lose more than 0.75 of a score over the first thirty days of lactation (Ruegg, 1991). Cows that have lost more than 1 condition score and are not producing to their potential, are not receiving or utilizing enough energy or are experiencing increased incidence of metabolic problems. Feeding management must then be evaluated along with dry matter and water intakes. This might include nutrient balance in the diets along with feeding strategy, and quality of feedstuffs fed.

If BCS change is less than 0.5 units in the first 4 weeks of lactation, cows may not be producing to their potential, nutrient balance and feeding management should be evaluated.

### Mid-Lactation

By 12 weeks post-partum, cows should begin to replete body tissue reserves. At this time a gradual increase in BCS should be observed. The target score level is between 2.75 and 3.25. If BCS is observed not to increase at this time, then cows are receiving inadequate energy and causes should be investigated. If BCS is greater than 3.5, energy intake needs to be reduced to avoid overconditioning and subsequent fat cow problems.

### Late Lactation

During late lactation, BCS should be approaching 3.5 (the recommended BCS at dry-off). This is the most economical time to replete body tissue reserves because metabolic demands are the lowest. The energy demands of milk production are lower while the metabolic demands of the developing fetus are not yet elevated. At this time, dry matter intake is economically sufficient to provide adequate energy.

Cows should not be allowed to become overconditioned nor should they be denied the opportunity to adequately replete body tissue reserves. Either condition will influence productivity in the next lactation.

In high-producing herds and those milked 3 times daily or utilizing bovine somatotropin, a change in grouping strategy may be required to properly manage body condition. Reformulation of rations also may be required.

In summary, research and field data suggest that the degree of changes in body condition after calving influence health, reproduction, and productivity in dairy cows more than the BCS at calving (Ruegg, 1991). Current body condition scores reflect previous energy balance, whereas changes in body condition reflect current energy balance. Rapid loss of body condition after calving may be associated with a higher incidence of fatty liver, impaired fertility, and other health problems.

## REFERENCES

*Beck, N. and S.K. Webster. 1976. Effects of acute metabolic acidosis on parathyroid hormone action and Ca mobilization. Am. J. Physiol. 230:127-131.*

*Beede, D.K., C.A. Risco, G.A. Donovan, C. Wang, L.F. Archbald, and W.K. Sanches. 1992. Nutritional management of the late pregnant dry cow particular reference to dietary cation-anion difference and calcium supplementation. The Bovine Procedings. No 24, pp. 51-55.*

*Bell, A.W., M.B. Rymph, R. Slepetis, W.A. House, and R.A. Ehrhardt. 1992. Net nutrition requirements for conceptus growth in Holstein cows - Implications for dry cow feeding. Cornell Nutrition Conference for Feed Manufacturers. October 13-15, Rochester, NY. pp. 102-109.*

*Bell, A.W., R. Slepetis, and R.A. Ehrhardt. 1995. Growth and accretion of energy and protein in the gravid uterus during late pregnancy in Holstein cows. J. Dairy Sci. 78:1954-1961.*

*Bell, A.W. 1995a. Regulation of organic nutrient metabolism during transition from late pregnancy to early lactation. J. Anim. Sci. 73:2804-2819.*

*Bertics, S.J., R.R. Grummer, C. Cadorniga-Valino, and E.E. Stoddard. 1992. Effect of prepartum dry matter intake on liver triglyceride concentration and early lactation. J. Dairy Sci. 75:1914-1922.*

*Block, E. 1984. Manipulating dietary anions and cations for prepartum dairy cows to reduce incidence of milk fever. J. Dairy Sci. 67:2939-2948.*

*Block, E. 1994. Manipulation of dietary cation-anion difference on nutritionally related production diseases, productivity, and metabolic responses of dairy cows. J. Dairy Sci. 77:1437-1450.*

*Botts, R.L., R.W. Hemken, and L.S. Bull. 1979. Protein reserves in the lactating cow. J. Dairy Sci. 62:433-440.*

*Burnell, J.M. 1971. Changes in bone sodium and carbonate in metabolic acidosis and alkalosis in the dog. J. Clin. Invest. 50:327-332.*

*Brydl, E. 1995. Prevention of metabolic disorders of dairy cowsby multi-phase feeding strategy during the peripartal period. Hung. Vet. J. 50:718-720.*

*Chase, L.E. 1992. Cation-anion balance in dairy rations; Practical considerations. Proc. Cornell Nutr. Conf. pp. 160-167.*

*Curtis, C.R., H,N. Erb, C.J. Sniffen, R.D. Smith and, D.S. Kronfeld. 1985. Path analysis of dry period nutrition, postpartum metabolic and reproductive disorders, and mastitis in Holstein cows. J. Dairy Sci. 68:2347-2360.*

*Delaquise, A.M. and E Block. 1995. Dietary cation-anion difference, acid-base status, mineral metabolism, renal function, and milk production of lactating cows. J. Dairy Sci. 78:2259-2284.*

*Dias, F.M., and F.R. Allaire. 1982. Dry period to maximize milk production over two consecutive lactations. J. Dairy Sci. 65:135-146.*

*Dirksen, G.U., H.G. Liebich, and E. Mayer. 1985. Adaptive changes of the ruminal ucosa and their functional and clinical significance. The bovine practitioner. 20:116-120.*

*Dirksen, G., F. Ahrens, J. Schön, E. Mayer, and H.G. Liebich. 1992. Vorbereitungsfütte rung der trockensthehenden Kuh im hinblick auf Ernährungszustand und Status von Pansenflora bei der Kalbung. Berl. Munch. Tierarztl. Wschr. 105:1-5.*

*Dishington, I.W. 1975. Prevention of milk fever by dietary salt supplements. Acta Vet. Scand. 16:503-512.*

*Edmonson, A.J., I.J. Lean, L.D. Weaver, T. Farver, and G. Webster. 1989. A body condition scoring chart for Holstein dairy cows. J. Dairy Sci. 72:68-79.*

*Emery, R.S., 1993. Energy needs of dry cows. Proc. Tri-State Dairy Nutr. Conf., Fort Wayne, IN. pp. 35-43.*

*Enevolsen, C. and J.T. Sorensen. 1992. Effects of dry period length on clinical mastitis and other major clinical health disorders. J. Dairy Sci. 75:1007-1014.*

*Ferguson, J.D., J.D. Gallagen, and N. Thomsen. 1994. Principal descriptors of body condition score in Holstein cows. J. Dairy Sci. 77:2695-2703.*

*Fronk, T.J., L.H. Schultz, and A.R. Hardie. 1980. Effect of dry period over-conditioning on subsequent metabolic disorders and performance of dairy cows. J. Dairy Sci. 63:1080-1090.*

*Funk, D.A., A.E. Freeman, and P.J. Berger. 1987. Effects of previous days open, previous days dry, and present days open on lactation yield. J. Dairy Sci. 70:2366-2373.*

*Gaynor, P.J., F.J. Meuller, J.K. Miller, N.Ramsy, J.P. Goff, and R.L. Horst. 1989. Parturient hypocalcemia in Jersey cows fed alfalfa haylage-based diets with different cation-anion ratios. J. Dairy Sci. 72:2525-2531.*

*Gearhart, M.A., C.R. Curtis, H.N. Erb, R.D. Smith, C.J. Sniffen, L.E. Chase, and M.D. Cooper. 1990. Relationships of changes in condition score to cow health in Holsteins. J. Dairy Sci. 73:3132-3140.*

*Gerloff, B.J., T.H. Herdt, W.W. Wells, J.S. Leisman, and R.S. Emery. 1986. Inositol and lipidosis. I. Effect of inositol supplementation and time from parturition on liver and serum lipids in dairy cattle. J. Anim. Sci. 62:1682-1692.*

*Gerloff, B.J., T.H. Herdt, and R.S. Emery. 1986a. The relationship of hepatic lipidosis to health and performance in dairy cattle. J. Am. Vet. Med. Ass. 188:845-850.*

*Goff, J.P., R.L. Horst, F.J. Neuller, J.K. Miller, G.A. Kiss, and H.H. Dowlen. 1991. Addition of chloride to a prepartal diet high in cations increases 1,25-dihydroxyvitamin D response to hypocalcemia preventing milk fever. J. Dairy Sci. 74:3863-3874.*

*Goff, J.P. 1992. Cation-anion difference of diets and its influence on milk fever and sub sequent lactation: the good and the bad news. Proc. Cornell Nutr. Conf. pp. 148-159.*

*Grummer, R.R., S.J. Bertics, D.W. Lacount, J.A. Snow, M.R. Dentine, and R.H. Stauffacher. 1990. Estrogen induction of fatty liver in dairy cattle. J. Dairy Sci. 73:1537-1543.*

*Grummer, R.R. 1993. Etiology of lipid-related metabolic disorders in periparturient dairy cows. J. Dairy Sci. 76:3882-3896.*

*Grummer, R.R., J.C. Winkler, S.J. Bertics, and V.A. Studer. 1994. Effect of propylene glycol dosage during feed restriction on metabolites in blood of prepartum Holstein heifers. J. Dairy Sci. 77:3618-3623.*

*Grummer, R.R. 1995. Impact of changes in organic nutrient metabolism on feeding the transition dairy cow. J. Anim. Sci. 73:2820-2833.*

*Herdt, T.H. 1988. Fatty liver in dairy cows. The Vet. Clin. of North Amer.: Food Anim. Pract. 4:269-287.*

*Herdt, T.H. 1996. personal communication*

*Hjerpe, C.A. 1992. Vaccines and vaccination programs. IN: Large Dairy Herd Management. Van Horn, H.H. and C.J. Wilcox (eds.). pp. 538-555.*

*Horst, R.L. and T.A. Reinhardt. 1983. Vitamin D metabolism in ruminants and its relevance to the periparturient cow. J. Dairy Sci. 66:661-679.*

*Huber, T.L., R.C. Wilson, A.J. Stattelman, and D.D. Goetsch. 1981. Am. J. Vet. Res. 42:1488-1490.*

*Kleppe, B.B., R.J. Aiello, R.R. Grummer, and L.E. Armentano. 1988. Triglyceride accu mulation and very low density lipoprotein secretion by rat and goat hepatocytes in vitro. J. Dairy Sci. 71:1813-1822.*

*Kronfeld, D.S. 1980. Metabolic disorders. In:Bovine Medicine and Surgery. Ed. H.E. Amstutz. Am. Vet. Public., Inc. Santa Barbara. Vol.I., pp. 537-614.*

*Leclerc, H., and E. Block. 1989. Effects of reducing dietary cation-anion balance for pre partum dairy cows with specific reference to hypocalcemic parturient paresis. Can. J. Anim. Sci. 69:4411-4423.*

*Lema, M., W.B. Tucker, M. Aslam, I.S. Shin, P. Le Ruyet, and G.D. Adams. 1992. Influence of calcium chloride fed prepartum on severity of edema and lactational performance of dairy heifers. J. Dairy Sci. 75:2388-2393.*

*Massey, C.D., C. Wang, G.A. Donovan, and D.K. Beede. 1993. Hypocalcemia at parturi tion as a risk factor for left displacement of the abdomen in dairy cows. JAVMA 203:852-853.*

*Nestor, K.E., R.W. Hemken, and R.J. Harmon. 1988. Influence of sodium and potassium bicarbonate on udder edema and selected blood parameters. J. Dairy Sci. 71:366-372.*

*Otto, K.L., J.D. Ferguson, D.G. Fox, and C.J. Sniffen. 1991. Relationship between body condition score and composition of ninth to eleventh rib tissue in Holstein dairy cows. J. Dairy Sci. 74:852-859.*

*Oetzel, G.R., J.D. Olson, C.R. Curtis, and M.J. Fettman. 1988. Ammonium chloride and ammonium sulfate for prevention of parturient paresis in dairy cows. J. Dairy Sci. 71: 3302-3309.*

*Oetzel, G.R. 1991. Meta analysis of nutritional risk factors for milk fever in dairy cattle. J. Dairy Sci. 74:3900-3912.*

*Oetzel, G.R. 1993. Use of anionic salts for prevention of milk fever in dairy cattle. Comp. Cont. Educ. 15:1138-1146.*

*Perkins, B.L., R.D. Smith, and C.J. Sniffen. 1987. Trouble shooting your herd with the body condition scoring system. Fact Sheet, Cooperative Extension Service, Cornell Univ., New York State. p. 151.*

*Pullen, D.L., J.S. Liesman, and R.S. Emery. 1990. A species comparison of liver slice synthesis and secretion of triacylglycerol from non-esterified fatty acid in media. J. Anim. Sci. 68:1395-1399.*

*Risco, C.A., J.P. Reynolds, and D. Hird. 1984. Uterine prolapse and hypocalcemia in dairy cows. JAVMA 185:1517-1520.*

*Ruegg, P.L. 1991. Body condition scoring in dairy cows: Relationships with production, reproduction, nutrition, and health. Comp. Cont. Educ. 13:1309-1313.*

*Schukken, Y.H., F.J. Grommers, J. van Vliet, and D. van de Geer. 1993. A randomized blind trial on dry cow antibiotic treatment in a low SSC herd. J. Dairy Sci. 76:2925-2930.*

*Sniffen, C.J., 1991. Grouping management and physical facilities. IN: Dairy Nutrition Management. The Vet. Clin. of North Amer: Food Anim. Pract. Sniffen, C.J. and T.H. Herd (eds.). 7:465-471.*

*Studer, V.A., R.R. Grummer, S.J. Bertics, and C.K. Reynolds. 1993. Effect of prepartum propylene glycol administration on periparturient fatty liver in dairy cows. J. Dairy Sci. 76:2931-2939.*

*Top, A. M. van den, T. Wensing, M.J.H. Geelen, G.H. Wentink, A.T. Van't Klooster, and A.C. Beynen. 1995. Time trends of plasma lipids and enzymes synthesizing hepatic triaglycerol during postpartum development of fatty liver in dairy cows. J. Dairy Sci. 78: 2208-2220.*

*Tucker, W.B., Z. Xin, and R.W. Hemken. 1991. Influence of calcium chloride on systemic acid-base status and calcium metabolism in dairy heifers. J. Dairy Sci. 74:1401-1407.*

*Tucker, W.B., G.D. Adams, M. Lema, M. Aslam, I.S. Shin, P.Le Ruyet, and L. Weeks. 1992. Evaluation of a system for rating edema in dairy cattle. J. Dairy Sci. 75:2382-2387.*

*Van Saun, R.J., 1991. Dry cow nutrition. IN: Dairy Nutrition Management. The Vet.Clin. of North Amer: Food Anim. Pract. C.J. Sniffen and T.H. Herd (eds.). 7:599-620.*

*Vazquez-Anon, M., S. Bertics, M. Luck, and R.R. Grummer. 1994. Prepartum liver try glyceride and plasma metabolites in dairy cows. J. Dairy Sci. 77:1521-1528.*

*Veenhuizen, J.J., J.K. Drackley, M.J. Richard, T.P. Sanderson, L.D. Miller, and J.W. Young. 1991. Metabolic changes in blood and liver during development and the treatment of experimental fatty liver and ketosis in cows. J. Dairy Sci. 74:4238-4253.*

*Vestweber, J.G.E., F.K. Al-Ani, and D.E. Johnson. 1989. Udder edema in cattle: Effects of diuretics on serum and urine electrolytes. Amer. J. Vet. Res. 50:1323-1328.*

*Wang, C., D.K. Beede, G.A. Donovan, L.F. Archibald, M.A. DeLorenzo, and W.K. Sanchez. 1991. Effects of dietary negative cation-anion difference and high calcium content prepartum on calcium metabolism, health, lactational, and reproductive performance of Holstein cows. J. Dairy Sci. 74(Suppl. 1):275 (Abstract)*

*Weiss, B. 1994. Untersuchungen über Beziehungen zwischen der Azidität des Panseninhaltes und dem proliferationszustand der Pansenschleimhaut beim Rind. Berl. Munch. Tierarztl. Wschr. 107:73-78.*

*Wildman, E.E., G.M. Jones, P.E. Wagner, and R.L. Bowman. 1982. A dairy cow body condition scoring system and its relationship to selected production characteristics. J. Dairy Sci. 38:495-500.*

# MONITORING MILK PRODUCTION

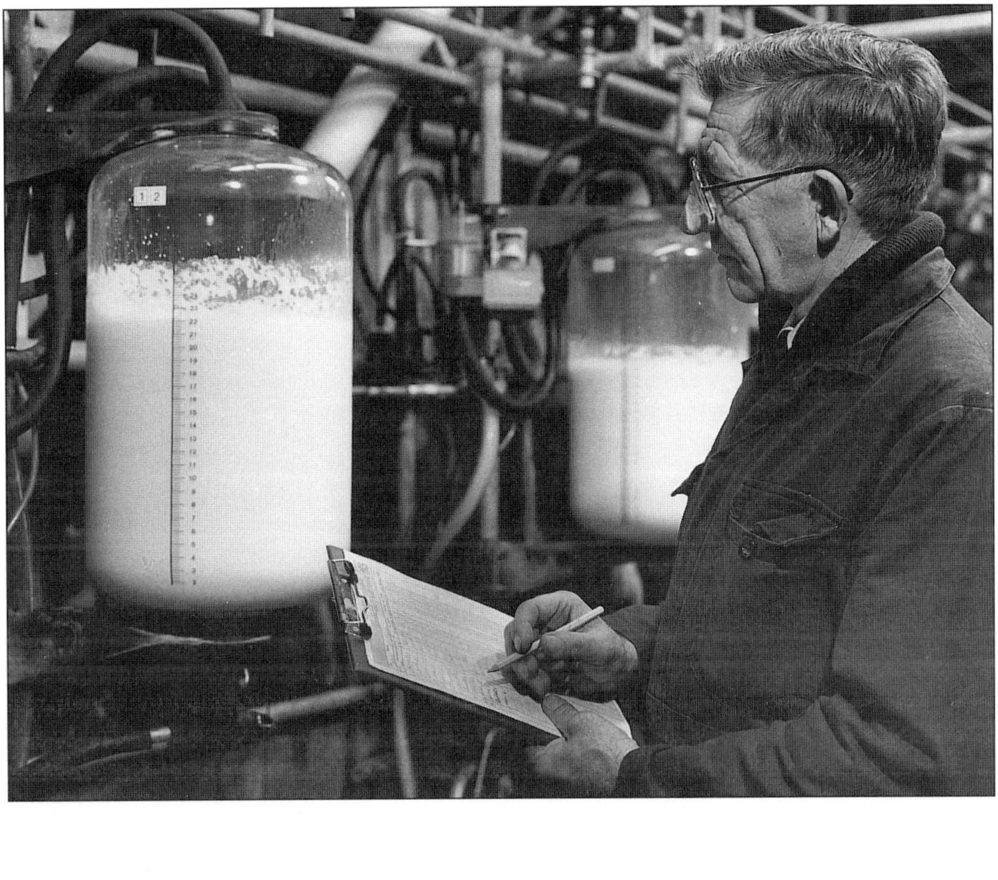

# 4.1 MONITORING MILK PRODUCTION: OPTIMIZING RUMEN DIGESTION IN THE DAIRY COW

Michael F. Hutjens[1], Thomas R. Overton[1] and Arie Brand[2]

[1] Department of Animal Sciences, University of Illinois, Urbana, IL 61801, USA
[2] Department of Herd Health and Reproduction, School of Veterinary Medicine, University of Utrecht, Yalelaan 7, 3485 CL Utrecht, The Netherlands

## 4.1.1 INTRODUCTION

Nutrition plays a paramount role in animal health and production, and hence represents a core element in the dairy farm operation. Veterinary curricula commonly address nutrition in a monodisciplinary setting or related to nutritional or metabolic disorders. Interrelationships between nutrition and other operational management functions of the dairy farm are hardly addressed. For the Herd Health and Production Management (HH & PM) practitioner and farm advisor it is of substantial relevance, that he/she has sufficient background of applied nutrition to elucidate nutritional causes of diseases, and to advise the farmer about measurements related to the interactions between nutrition and health, or between nutrition and (re)production. In case of complex problems the practitioner can always consult the local nutritionist or extension service.

Ruminants such as dairy cows are unique in that they have a "dual" digestive system: microbial fermentation and digestion in the rumen and intestinal digestion similar to other mammals. The reticulo-rumen area (referred to as the rumen in this chapter) of the digestive tract is a dynamic environment. It is an anaerobic, warm, and constantly mixing (contractions every 30 to 60 seconds) fermentation vat which supports a microbial population. Rumen microbes have the ability to ferment and digest fiber, convert non-protein nitrogen (NPN) to high quality protein, and synthesize essential vitamins. The goal of the nutritionist is to manage the rumen of the dairy cow to maximize yield of microbial protein and volatile fatty acids (VFA) and other nutrients from feed offered, reduce metabolic disorders, and produce large quantities of milk with desirable components. At the same time nutrient losses such as Nitrogen should be reduced. In addition the dairy cow should be fed rations which allow passage of microbial protein, undegraded feed protein and amino acids (AA), and undegraded starch and fatty acids from the rumen to the lower digestive tract for further digestion and absorption. Thus, dairy cows require the absorption of large amounts of nutrients from the rumen and intestine to meet their nutrient requirements and minimize the losses of nutrients such as nitrogen, and of body tissue during early lactation.

These goals can be achieved by:
1. Maintaining the rumen pH and microbial balance.
2. Optimizing fiber digestibility and fermentation.
3. Stimulating dry matter intake.
4. Avoiding rumen-based metabolic disorders.
5. Feeding rumen additives to assist rumen fermentation if needed.

In this Chapter some practical issues and tools about feeding dairy cows in general or optimizing rumen digestion in particular are addressed.

## 4.1.2 NUTRIENT DYNAMICS IN THE RUMEN

### Carbohydrate Metabolism

On average, carbohydrates (CHO) contribute 70 to 80% of the diet dry matter while protein, fat, and minerals make up the remaining portion. Carbohydrates are the primary energy substrate for rumen microbes. Two CHO categories occur in feeds: non-structural CHO (sugar and starch) and structural CHO (cellulose, hemicellulose, and pectin). Lignin is not a CHO, but is grouped with structural CHO analytically. Sugars are found in the cells of growing plants and in feeds such as molasses or whey. Starch is the storage form of energy in cereal grains and roots. Structural CHO provides rigidity and strength to the plant. Various CHO fractions are summarized in Table 1.

Nonstructural and structural CHO are digested (converted from complex structures to simple sugars) and fermented to VFA by rumen microbes (Table 2). These VFA provide 60 to 80% of the energy required by the cow. Fat, CHO not degraded in the rumen, and protein provide the remaining energy. When the production and ratios of

*Table 1. Carbohydrate categories, type, rumen digestive rate and extent of digestion, and VFA produced from microbial digestion (Adapted from Chandler, 1978, and Sniffen, 1988)*

| Category of CHO | Type | Rumen Rate | Digestion Extent (%) | VFA[A] |
|---|---|---|---|---|
| Nonstructural | Sugars | Very Fast | 100 | Prop |
| | Starches | Fast | 70 - 90 | Prop |
| Structural | Lignin | Very Slow | 0 | None |
| | Cellulose | Slow | 30 - 50 | Acet-Buty |
| | Hemicellulose | Moderate | 70 | Acet-Prop |
| | Pectin | Fast | 70 - 90 | Acet-Prop |

[A] Prop = propionate, Acet = acetate, Buty = butyrate

*Table 2. Characteristics of microbial groups (Adapted from Sniffen, 1988)*

| Class | Substrate Preference | Nitrogen Needs | Main VFA Produced | pH Range | Time to Double (h) |
|---|---|---|---|---|---|
| Fiber dig bacteria | Cellulose Hemicellulose | Ammonia | Acetate Butyrate | 6.0 - 6.8 | 8 - 10 |
| Starch and sugar dig bacteria | Starch Sugar | Ammonia Amino acids | Prop Lactate | 5.5 - 6.0 | 1 - 2 |
| Protozoa | Starch Sugar | Amino acids | | 6.2 - 7.0 | 15 - 24 |

individual VFA are altered, yield and components of milk change. Ruminal degradation of CHO varies depending on maturity of forages, source of CHO (nonstructural or structural) and processing such as grinding of grain or chopping of forages. VFA are absorbed from the rumen into the bloodstream and transported to the liver, mammary gland, adipose depots, and other tissues.

**Protein and Nitrogen Metabolism**

Protein is essential for maintenance, growth, reproduction, and milk production. The protein requirement of a dairy cow is the sum of amino acids (AA) needed for each of these biological functions. The AA are supplied by the intestinal digestion of microbial protein and feed protein that escapes microbial degradation in the rumen. Approximately 60 to 70 % of dietary protein is degraded by microbes to peptides, AA, or ammonia which are used by the microbes as nitrogen sources (Table 2). Rumen microbes incorporate ammonia into microbial protein. Unincorporated ammonia is absorbed across the rumen wall, passed into blood, converted to urea in the liver, and recycled in saliva or excreted in urine and milk (Figure 1).

Herds having average milk urea nitrogen (MUN) concentrations over 18 mg/dl may indicate rumen protein inefficiency due to excess ammonia in the rumen and/or a deficiency of rumen available energy which limits microbial growth. Three categories of protein can be used to describe the fate of dietary protein in the rumen and define protein requirements of the dairy cow (Tables 3 and 4).

Soluble intake protein (SIP) is the fraction of feed protein that is rapidly degraded in the rumen. Urea or casein are examples of feeds that are quickly degraded to ammonia, peptides, or AA which could be used by rumen microbes. New York and Pennsylvania (NY-PA) researchers have developed a rumen model system which predicts microbial protein yield based on protein sources, rumen fermentable carbohydrate,

*Figure 1. Schematic summary of nitrogen utilization in the rumen by high producing dairy cows (Linn et al., 1994)*

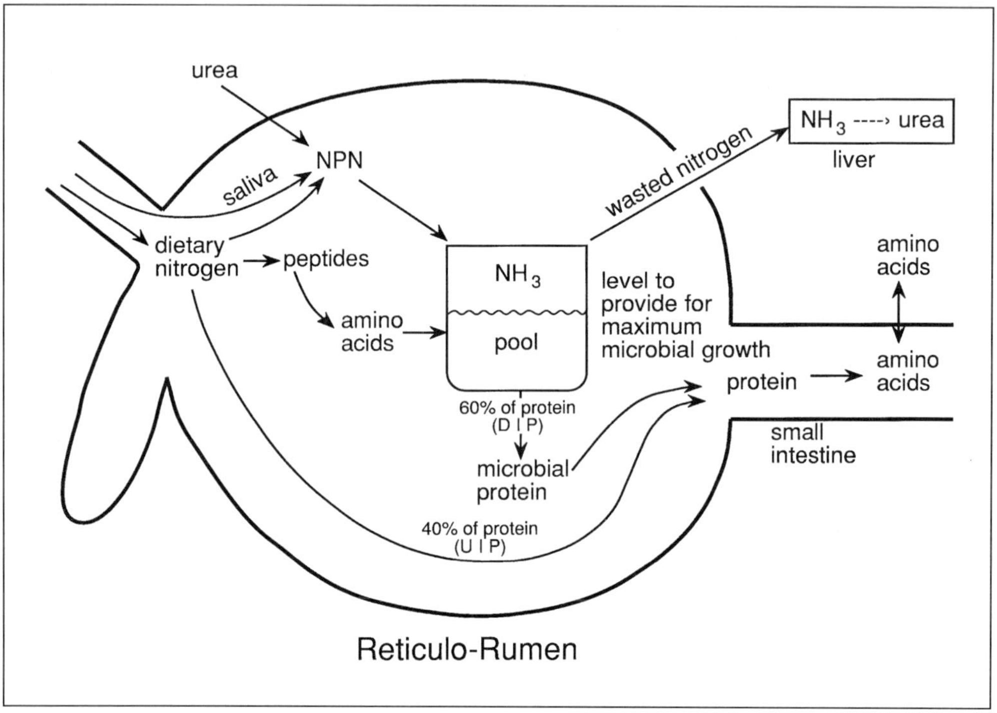


rumen turnover, and rumen pH (Fox et al., 1992; Russell et al., 1992; Sniffen et al., 1992). In the NY-PA model, SIP is referred to as the A fraction (Table 3).

Degradable intake protein (DIP) is the fraction of feed protein that can be degraded in the rumen (includes SIP and more slowly degraded sources). About half of ration DIP should be in the form of SIP (Table 4). In the NY-PA model, the intermediate rate of degraded protein or B1; the slower sources of degraded feed protein or B2; and the A fraction are included in DIP (Table 3). Other terms used in the field to describe DIP include rumen available nitrogen or protein. The ration must contain sufficient DIP to provide 3 to 5 mg/dl ammonia in rumen fluid for optimal synthesis of microbial protein.

Undegraded intake protein (UIP) is the portion of feed protein that is not degraded in the rumen and remains intact as it passes to the lower tract. UIP includes the portion available for lower gut digestion and absorption (also called escape protein or bypass protein) and the portion that is not digested and excreted in feces (also called bound protein, heat damaged protein, acid detergent fiber insoluble nitrogen, or ADF-N). In the NY-PA model, available UIP is referred to as the B3 fraction and unavailable UIP portion is the C fraction. As computer models continue to refine prediction of

*Table 3. Nutrient level in common dairy cow feedstuffs (Adapted from Linn et al., 1994)*

| Feedstuff | Protein | | | Carbohydrate | | | | | Fat (%) |
|---|---|---|---|---|---|---|---|---|---|
| | SIP | DIP | UIP | NFC | ADF | NDF | fNDF | eNDF | |
| | | | | (%) | | | (%NDF) | | |
| | A | A+B1+B2 | B3 | | | | | | |
| | | (% CP) | | | | | | | |
| **Legume/grass** | | | | | | | | | |
| Hay | 30 | 70 | 30 | 25 | 35 | 46 | 100 | 92 | 3 |
| Silage, long | 35 | 76 | 24 | 25 | 35 | 46 | 100 | 70 | 3 |
| Silage, fine | 35 | 76 | 24 | 25 | 35 | 46 | 100 | 30 | 3 |
| Corn silage | 50 | 70 | 30 | 36 | 26 | 48 | 100 | 65 | 3 |
| Barley | 20 | 75 | 25 | 56 | 7 | 26 | 0 | 50 | 2 |
| Blood meal | 5 | 30 | 70 | 6 | 0 | 0 | 0 | 0 | 1 |
| **Corn, shelled** | | | | | | | | | |
| Dry, rolled | 12 | 40 | 60 | 75 | 3 | 9 | 0 | 70 | 4 |
| Dry, ground | 25 | 50 | 50 | 75 | 3 | 9 | 0 | 20 | 4 |
| High moisture | 45 | 60 | 40 | 75 | 3 | 9 | 0 | 40 | 4 |
| Corn gluten feed | 50 | 70 | 30 | 19 | 10 | 45 | 0 | 33 | 2 |
| Fish meal | 12 | 20 | 80 | 2 | 0 | 0 | 0 | 0 | 10 |
| Soybean meal (44) | 20 | 72 | 28 | 29 | 10 | 12 | 0 | 10 | 1 |
| **Soybean seed** | | | | | | | | | |
| Raw | 40 | 80 | 20 | 20 | 10 | 13 | 0 | 50 | 19 |
| Heated | 10 | 52 | 48 | 20 | 10 | 13 | 0 | 50 | 19 |
| Urea | 100 | 0 | 0 | 0 | 0 | 0 | 0 | 0 | 0 |

SIP = Soluble intake protein; the A fraction in NY-PA model
DIP = Degradable intake protein; A+B1+B2 fractions in NY-PA model
UIP = Undegradable intake protein; the B3 fraction in the NY-PA model
NFC = Non-fiber carbohydrate
ADF = Acid detergent fiber
NDF = Neutral detergent fiber
fNDF = NDF derived from forages expressed as percentage of total NDF
eNDF = NDF contributes to cause cud chewing expressed as percent of total NDF

microbial and cow protein requirements and laboratory techniques evolve that can distinguish various fractions, additional protein fractions may be defined.

The nutritionist's goal for AA nutrition is to maximize rumen synthesis of the

*Table 4. Nutrient levels in dry and lactating cow rations for optimal rumen function (Hutjens, 1994)*

| Nutrient | Dry Cow | | Lactating Cows | | | |
|---|---|---|---|---|---|---|
| | Early | Close | Fresh | Early | Mid | Late |
| DMI (kg) | 13 | 11 | 18 | 22 | 20 | 18 |
| Crude Protein (% DM) | 13 | 15 | 19 | 18 | 16 | 14 |
| UIP (% CP) | 30 | 35 | 40 | 38 | 36 | 32 |
| DIP (% CP) | 70 | 65 | 60 | 62 | 64 | 68 |
| SIP (% CP)* | 35 | 32 | 30 | 31 | 32 | 34 |
| TDN (% DM) | 56 | 60 | 75 | 77 | 75 | 67 |
| NE L (mcal/kg DM) | 1.27 | 1.50 | 1.65 | 1.72 | 1.65 | 1.54 |
| Fat (% DM) | 2 | 3 | 5 | 6 | 5 | 3 |
| ADF (% DM) | 35 | 30 | 21 | 19 | 21 | 24 |
| NDF (% DM) | 50 | 45 | 30 | 28 | 31 | 33 |
| NFC (% DM) | 30 | 32 | 38 | 40 | 37 | 34 |
| Effective NDF (% DM) | NA | NA | 23 | 21 | 23 | 25 |
| Forage NDF (% DM) | NA | NA | 23 | 21 | 23 | 25 |

NA = No value available. * SIP is fraction of DIP
TDN = total digestible nutrients, NE L = netto energy for lactation

microbial AA (50 to 70% of total protein required) and complement the microbially produced AA with a balanced source of UIP containing the needed AA to meet the cows's AA requirement. Table 4 lists the ration protein guidelines for meeting the requirements of high producing cows.

### Fat Metabolism

Fat is present at modest levels (2 to 3 percent) in diets fed to early lactation cows or to close-up cows with a maximum of 150 g to avoid palatability effects. When cows are in negative energy balance, supplemental fat can increase energy content of the diet by increasing total fat levels up to 6% of the diet dry matter if DMI is not decreased. Fatty acid (FA) composition and rumen inertness are important characteristics of fats and oils that can impact the rumen environment and dry matter intake. Dietary fat and oil are consumed either as triglycerides (three FA attached to a glycerol molecule) or as free FA. Rumen microbes hydrolyze triglycerides to FA and glycerol (used by rumen microbes as a minor source of energy). The FA in feeds can be classified as: 1) saturated (containing no double bonds) or unsaturated (containing carbon to carbon double bonds such as oleic acid, an 18 carbon FA with one double bond), and 2) short to medium chain (contains < 16 carbon atoms) or long chain (contains 16 or more carbon atoms) FA. Rumen microbes partially hydrogenate unsaturated FA forming more saturated FA with similar carbon length. Unsaturated FA, such as those in soybeans or fish meal, can interfere negatively with rumen fermentation, depress rumen pH, and lower fiber digestibility. Unsaturated FA can be toxic to fiber digesting bacteria and coat fiber particles, thereby reducing bacterial attachment and fiber digestion. To minimize negative effects, one of the following amounts of fat containing feeds can be fed (not additive):

* Added fat from oilseeds should be limited to 400 to 500 g per cow per day. Feed oilseeds whole (cotton and sunflower seed) or coarsely processed (soybean and canola seeds) to minimize exposing rumen microbes to high levels of unsaturated fatty acids.
* Limit fish oil to 50 to 60 g per cow per day.
* Restrict extracted or free oil (such as corn or soy oil) to 200 to 250 g per cow per day.
* Blend fat with other feeds and avoid slug feeding (large amounts eaten per meal) of fat sources.

Animal fat (tallow and grease) is higher in saturated FA making these fat sources more desirable for use in dairy cow rations. Rumen inert fats do not affect rumen fermentation because the FA are partially hydrogenated prior to feeding (harder fat), made into calcium salts, or encapsulated or protected. Rumen inert fats are more expensive compared to animal and oilseed sources and are acceptable sources of fat for use in dairy cow rations.

### Minerals and vitamins

Minerals are needed by rumen microbes for growth and should be mixed and fed with forages and concentrates. Water soluble B vitamins can be synthesized by rumen microbes to meet the requirements of the dairy cow. Cobalt is needed for rumen microbial synthesis of B-12. Sulfur is needed by rumen microbes to synthesize sulfur-containing AA with a desired ratio of nitrogen to sulfur in the diet of 10 to 12:1. See for more details Chapter 3.

## 4.1.3 OPTIMIZING RUMEN DIGESTION

### Volatile fatty acid production

End products of microbial fermentation are VFA which are absorbed from the rumen and serve as a main source of energy for the dairy cow. The primary VFA is acetate which is a two carbon VFA and represents (55 to 70%) of the total production of VFA. Acetate or acetic acid (acid in vinegar) is produced from the digestion of structural carbohydrates and is a major energy source (Table 1). Acetate is used by the mammary gland to synthesize fatty acids for milk fat. Propionate or propionic acid is a three carbon VFA produced from starch, sugar, and pectin digesting bacteria. The level of propionate varies from 15 to 30 percent of the total VFA production. Lactic acid, produced in the rumen, is another propionate precursor. The liver uses propionate to synthesize glucose through gluconeogenesis, thus sparing AA. Synthesizing glucose from the carbon skeletons of AA is metabolically expensive because the nitrogen must be captured in the form of urea and excreted, which requires energy. Glucose is used to synthesize milk lactose. The third major VFA is butyrate or butyric acid, a four carbon VFA produced from the breakdown of structural CHO and sugars that contribute 5 to 15 percent of the VFA produced. Butyrate is used as an energy source by tissue and for milk fat synthesis. Other VFA are produced in the rumen (valerate, iso-valerate, and iso-butyrate), but the amounts are small compared to the three major VFA. The ratio of acetate to propionate (A:P) in rumen fluid (for example, 60% acetate: 20% propionate or 3:1) can indicate characteristics of the overall rumen fermentation. Under optimal conditions, the A:P ratio should be greater than 2.2 to 1. Production of propionic acid is energetically efficient and provides needed glucose precursors for high producing cows. High levels of acetate relative to propionate are indicative of rations high in fiber and low in starch. High levels of propionate relative to acetate may indicate reduced fiber digestion and acidosis. Analysis of VFA in the field is not routinely available, but would be a useful tool to evaluate rumen fermentation and digestion (Garrett et al., 1995).

**Rumen pH effects**

The pH of fluids in the body is critical to normal chemical and health conditions of the cow. In the rumen, the pH can vary from 5.5 to 6.8 with an optimal level of 6.0 to 6.3. Growth of fiber digesting bacteria is favored with pH from 6.0 to 6.8 while growth of starch digesting bacteria is favored by a pH from 5.5 to 6 (Table 2). Thus, the rumen must maintain a pH near 6.0 for optimal growth of both bacteria populations resulting in favorable yields and proportions of individual VFA. Rumenocentesis is a technique used in the field to determine rumen pH and VFA concentrations from intact cows. A 13 cm, 16 gauge needle is inserted through the rumen wall into the ventral rumen and rumen fluid is aspirated. The pH is measured immediately after collecting. In thirty cows, pH in needle samples averaged 5.9 compared to 6.2 for samples collected via a cannula while A:P ratios were 2.48 and 2.46, respectively (Garrett et al., 1995).

Factors which influence rumen pH are discussed below (Davis and Clark, 1981).

*1. Forage to concentrate ratio* – High forage rations favor pH over 6 and stimulate higher rates of saliva secretion. Saliva contains bicarbonate which buffers the rumen and increases acetate production. The main CHO in forage (cellulose and hemicellulose) are not fermented as rapidly by the rumen microbes as CHO in concentrates (starch and sugar). High rumen pH favors acetate production, a high A:P ratio (over 3), and higher milk fat percentage. Feeding excessive amounts of concentrate increases propionate production, decreases pH (under 6), reduces feed intake, reduce microbial nutrient production, and leads to milk fat depression (milk protein percentage increases while milk fat percentage decreases).

*2. Physical form of feeds* – Grinding, pelleting, chopping, or over mixing in mixer wagons change the size of the feed particle. If forage particle size is too short (cows consume less than 2 to 3 kg of particles over 25 to 40 mm), a forage mat in the rumen is not maintained, fiber digestion is decreased, and rumen pH is lowered. Saliva production also is reduced due to less cud chewing time. Cows typically spend over 500 minutes of chewing time per day or 25 to 33 minutes of chew time per kg of dry matter. At any time 60 percent of the cows will be chewing their cuds when resting. If concentrates are finely ground, starch is exposed to increased microbial fermentation. Rumen pH decreases and production of propionate and lactate increases, which lowers milk fat percentage, increases milk protein percentage, and lowers milk yield. Steam flaking, pelleting, or grinding cereal grains will disrupt starch granules and increase their rumen availability and potential to support growth of rumen microbes, but also may increase the risk of rumen acidosis.

*3. Feed intake* – As feed intake increases, especially when rations contain large amounts of fermentable CHO, rumen pH can decrease because more substrate is available for microbial use, increasing acid production (negative effect). The amount of saliva produced per unit of dry matter can also decline (negative effect). High quality proteins and undegraded nonstructural CHO can benefit from greater feed intake as solid fractions pass from the rumen faster, reducing the length of time they are exposed to microbial degradation and fermentation. Higher rates of feed passage also move (wash out) microbes out of the rumen increasing the efficiency of microbial protein synthesis.

*4. Moisture content of the ration* – Wet feeds can reduce rumen pH because less saliva is needed to wet the feed for swallowing. Silage require less chewing because forage particle size has been reduced by mechanically chopping. Silage can have a pH below 4, further increasing acid load. Adding sodium bicarbonate to corn silage to raise the pH of the silage above 5 increased feed intake (Erdman, 1988). If the moisture of the total ration exceeds 50 percent, dry matter intake can be reduced (NRC, 1989).

*5. Feeding unsaturated fats and oils* – Unsaturated FA, such as FA in vegetable and fish oils, can reduce fiber digestibility, be toxic to fiber-digesting bacteria, and coat the fiber particles reducing fiber digestion. Processing of oilseeds (such as grinding or extruding) can rupture the cell wall of the seed and release the oil into the rumen. Feeding whole oilseeds can reduce this risk. Limit oil from oilseeds to 400 to 500 g per cow per day (200 to 250 g if the oil is added as extracted free oil).

*6. Method of feeding* – Feeding total mixed rations (TMR) or complete rations stabilizes rumen pH, provides DIP and fermentable CHO at the same time, increases dry matter intake, and minimizes feed selection. If concentrates are fed separately, limit the amount to 2 to 3 kg per meal, avoid large amounts that contain high starch levels, and minimize feeding of finely processed grains.

These factors illustrate the dynamic state of the rumen environment. Changing one feed can lead to several rumen changes. For example, feeding more corn silage decreases forage particle size, increases fermentable CHO, lowers feed pH, and increases ration moisture.

### Fiber relationships

Dairy cows have the ability to convert feeds containing large amounts of fiber to nutrients which can be utilized. Fiber is classified and used in feed formulation in the following systems.

Crude fiber (CF) is the oldest method and is the residue of a feed that is resistant to successive boiling with dilute acid and alkali treatment. It is not an accurate measure of total fiber or cell walls because some lignin and hemicellulose are not recovered in the analysis. Feed tags list CF as the fiber value.

Acid detergent fiber (ADF) consists of cellulose, lignin, lignified nitrogen compounds (such as heat-damaged proteins), and insoluble ash, but does not include hemicellulose. Therefore, ADF does not represent the total fiber content of a feed. The analytical procedure for ADF is an accurate and rapid method to measure fiber content. Equations using ADF can predict the net energy for lactation (NE L) content of forages (Adams, 1975).

Legumes: NE L (Mcal/kg DM) = [1.044 – (0.0123 x %ADF)] x 2.2

Grasses: NE L (Mcal/kg DM) = [1.085 – (0.0150 x %ADF)] x 2.2

Corn silage: NE L (Mcal/kg DM) = [1.044 – (0.0132 x %ADF)] X 2.2

Neutral detergent fiber (NDF) has become the fiber analysis of choice and consists of ADF plus hemicellulose (total cell wall content). NDF is correlated to feed intake and chewing time (Mertens, 1992). Forage NDF (fNDF) refers to the percentage or amount of NDF in a dairy ration derived from forage sources (hay, silage, and fresh forage). It is used as an index of rumination and forage mat formation in the rumen. No adjustments are made for length of particles and type of forage (Table 3). For example, 10 kg of legume silage DM containing 40 percent NDF would provide 4 kg of fNDF.

Effective NDF (eNDF) refers to the proportion of NDF from all feeds (forages and concentrates) that contributes to the forage mat and rumination (Sniffen, 1988). Feed particle size is measured as a percent of the total that remains on sieves with 1.18 mm aperture. The NDF fiber in feed particles over 1.18 mm contributes to chewing activity and is assigned an eNDF percentage which is multiplied by the percentage of NDF and amount of dry matter fed (Table 3). For example, a legume silage (from the example above) would have 2.4 kg of effective NDF (10 kg of legume silage dry matter times 40 percent NDF times 60 percent eNDF). Coarsely chopped hay silage has higher values (70 percent eNDF) while finely chopped hay silage could be as low as 30 % eNDF.

Two fiber requirements are needed for optimum rumen function: chemical fiber concentration (measured as the percentage ADF and NDF in the total ration dry matter) and physical fiber length (measured as eNDF or fNDF). Guidelines for high producing cows are listed in Table 4.

*Table 5. Estimated dry matter intake at 7 to 12 weeks postpartum (NRC, 1989)*

| Milk Yield (kg 4% FCM) | Body Weight (kg) 400 | 500 | 600 | 700 |
|---|---|---|---|---|
| | DMI (kg/day) | | | |
| 20 | 14.5 | 15.9 | 17.2 | 18.2 |
| 30 | 17.7 | 18.5 | 20.9 | 22.3 |
| 40 | 21.8 | 23.2 | 24.1 | 25.0 |
| 50 | NA | NA | 32.3 | 33.3 |

NA = no value available

## Dry matter intake

Maximum dry matter intake (DMI) is critical for maximum microbial yield of protein and VFA. Table 5 lists the expected DMI that should be reached 6 to 12 weeks postpartum. An equation to predict DMI is listed below (Chase, 1993).

DMI (kg/day) = (.018 X body wt in kg) + (kg of 4% FCM X .305)

An example is illustrated with a cow weighing 600 kg and producing 30 kg of milk containing 4% milk fat.
DMI (kg/day) = (.018 X 600 kg) + (30 kg X .305) = (10.8 kg) + (9.2 kg) = 20.0 kg/day.

Table 5 lists 20.9 kg for this size of cow and level of milk production (which is similar, but not exact).

Cows in early lactation do not consume the amounts listed in Table 5. Dairy managers must adjust feeding rates of concentrates to avoid rumen acidosis and problems in fresh cows due to lower DMI (Table 6). Each additional kilogram of DMI can

*Table 6. Estimated dry matter intake after calving for 545 kg first lactation cows and 635 kg mature cows (Adapted from Kertz et al., 1991)*

| Week Postpartum | First Calf Heifer | Mature Cow |
|---|---|---|
| | kg DMI/cow/day | |
| 1 | 14 | 16 |
| 2 | 16 | 19 |
| 3 | 17 | 21 |
| 4 | 18 | 22 |
| 5 | 19 | 24 |

support 2 to 2.5 kg more milk yield (NRC, 1989). Several causes for lower DMI post-partum can occur:
* Feeding high levels of fat (over 5 percent of ration DM) can increase circulating levels of non-esterified fatty acids (NEFA) from dietary fat. Mobilized body fat also raises NEFA. Cows attempt to reduce circulating fat (NEFA) levels by eating less (Grummer, 1993).
* A poor dry cow transition diet can slow rumen microbial adaptation and decrease rumen fermentation and absorption.
* Metabolic disorders (milk fever, ketosis, displaced abomasum, or acidosis) and other diseases such as, lameness and gastro-intestinal diseases can add stress and lower DMI postpartum.

Dairy cows reduce DMI for the following reasons (Mertens, 1987):
1. Physical fill of the digestive tract (examples are low quality forage, higher forage diets, and rations high in total NDF). These forages are all higher in NDF and lower in digestibility. This will slow the rate of passage and remain in the rumen longer.
2. Chemical feedback signals within the cow (examples are high levels of VFA or NEFA in blood, low rumen pH, and/or elevated blood urea or ammonia levels).
3. Environmental factors not related to ration nutrient characteristics (examples are empty feed bunks, moldy feed, secondary feed bunk fermentation, and heat stress).

The following guidelines for optimizing DMI are listed below (Hutjens, 1994):
* Forage quality should exceed 1.32 megacalories of NEL per kg of dry matter.
* Ration ADF levels should range from 19 to 21%.
* Ration NDF levels should range from 28 to 31%.
* Dairy cows should consume 1.2 percent of their body weight as total NDF or 0.9 percent of their body weight as forage NDF.
* Non-fiber carbohydrate (NFC) levels should range from 36 to 40%. NFC is calculated using the following formula (all values expressed on a 100% DM basis):

  $$NFC = 100 - (\%\ CP + \%\ NDF + \%\ Fat + \%\ Ash)$$

* Feeding TMR avoids feed selectivity.
* Ration DM should range between 50 and 65% when feeding fermented feeds.
* Limit fat levels in the ration DM to 6 percent (5% for fresh cows).
* Avoid over conditioned dry cows because fat cows consume less feed postpartum (3.2 to 3.7 body condition score on a five point scale).
* Avoid empty feed bunks by feeding for a 4% daily feed weigh back.
* Feed a transition ration to dry cows 14 to 21 days prepartum to increase nutrient intake, adapt the rumen microbial population, and increase the size of rumen papillae for increased absorption.
* Increasing feeding frequency and/or pushing up feed.

## 4.1.4 RUMEN BASED METABOLIC DISORDERS

### Rumen acidosis

(Sub)clinical rumen acidosis (RA) is a common nutritional problem postpartum in dairy cows (Nordlund, 1995). Rumen pH declines below 5.9 and remains low for several hours (Figure 2). Two groups of cows are at risk of acidosis:

1. Periparturient cows (0 to 20 days postpartum) being adapted to high energy-high concentrate lactation rations are at risk because the rumen papillae need time to elongate (see Chapter 3), microbial population needs to adapt, and lower dry matter intake near calving can result in depressed forage intake.
2. Cows 45 to 120 days postpartum are at risk of ration formulation error and feed delivery problems (lack of fiber level or form, excessive starch, or feed selectivity).

Production of individual VFA shifts because acetate remains constant while propionate production increases resulting in less than 50% acetate and greater than 30 % propionate with A:P ratios below 2.2:1. Milk fat test can be an indicator of RA. Milk from individual cows has a milk protein percentage test greater than 0.4 percentage unit higher than milk fat test (cows with a 2.7% milk fat test and a 3.2% milk protein test for example).

RA can damage rumen papillae, alter sensitive laminae in the hoof, and reduce dry matter intake. If the hoof surface is not smooth or has ridges, RA occurred several weeks to several months earlier (Nordlund, 1995).

*Figure 2. Effect of pH on the growth yield of fiber and starch degrading bacteria (Davis and Clark, 1981)*

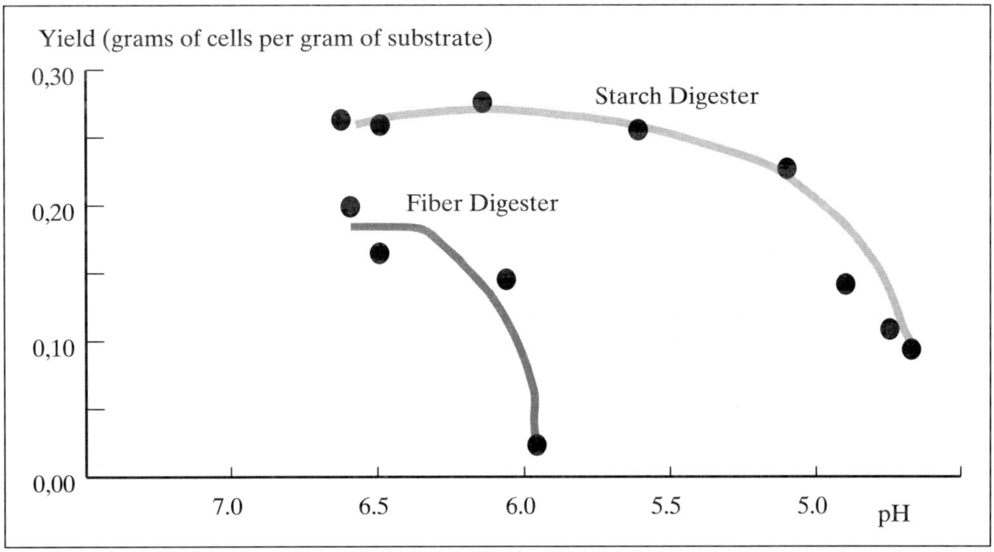

Diagnostic procedures for RA are:
1. Conduct a physical examination to rule out other causes of decreased DM intake.
2. Evaluate the prepartum ration for rumen adaptability.
3. Calculate the rate and method that concentrates are increased postpartum.
4. Consider forage quality (moldiness, availability, coarseness, dustiness, or sorting) which can limit forage intake.
5. Observe cud chewing and ruminating time (over 60% of the cows should be ruminating while resting).
6. Check body condition to determine if cows are thin or heavy.
7. Evaluate manure to see if it is loose or runny (one possible indication of a fiber shortage).
8. Conduct rumenocentesis on six or more cows per group if indicated.
9. Evaluate milk fat and milk protein percentages.
10. Offer sodium bicarbonate and observe if conditions improve.
11. Provide hay ad libitum and watch which cows consume it.

Preventive actions consist of:
1. Implement a transition diet for dry cows 14 to 21 days prepartum.
2. Limit the rate of increasing concentrate feeding postpartum at 0.5 kg per day.
3. Avoid metabolic disorders in fresh cows.
4. Add or increase the amount of long forage in the ration.
5. Control forage and concentrate selectivity and variation.
6. Add a buffer to the ration.

**Displaced Abomasum**

Displaced abomasum (DA) or twisted stomach occurs in 5% of dairy cows in the U.S. 90% of the DA's are diagnosed one week prepartum to three weeks postpartum. A left side displacement (LDA) occurs in about 90% of the cases as the abomasum migrates from the lower right side of the cow to the left side. A right side displacement (RDA) has a twist or torsion on the right side which can restrict blood and nutrient flow and is more serious than an LDA. A combination of factors can lead to formation of DA. The etiology and pathogenesis are still unclear. Displacement of the abomasum is predominantly seen in dairy herds with above-average milk yield, and in cows between the age of 4 to 7 years, which are in the first month after calving and are suffering from ketosis (Geishauser, 1995). Other risk factors include feeding rations low in fiber which may lead to gas formation, and hypocalcemia (Massey et al., 1993) (total blood calcium below 8 mg/dl) which may reduce rumen tone and contractions.

Treatment for DA consists of surgery to sew the abomasum in place and allow scar tissue to form. Casting (rolling the cow on her back from right to left several times) with a diagnosed LDA may allow the LDA to correct itself. If the animal is not valuable, culling is another option (Schmidt et al., 1988).

Some diagnostic signs of cows with DA consist of:
1. off-feed and refuse to eat normal amounts.
2. dilated abomasum with fluid and gases.
3. presence of pinging sounds that can be heard with a stethoscope (snapping the rumen wall causing a hollow steel band sound).
4. the LDA may be seen high on the left side of the animal.
5. secondary ketosis is a common observation.
6. fecal material becomes pasty and dry.

Preventive actions that might be taken include:
1. Gradually shifting of dry cows to a higher energy ration.
2. Limiting feeding of concentrate prior to calving (referred to as lead feeding in the U.S.). Concentrates should be fed from 3 weeks prepartum, starting at a low level up to a maximum of 3 kg just before calving.
3. Stabilizing the rumen with adequate long fiber (2 kg over 40 mm).
4. Avoiding over conditioning of cows (can reduce feed intake postpartum).
5. Drenching cows with propylene glycol (200 to 454 g per day for seven days prepartum) can minimize ketosis and formation of fatty liver.
6. Increasing concentrate gradually after calving (0.5 kg per day).
7. Providing sufficient exercise opportunities for cows.

## Bloat

Bloat is a non-infectious disorder characterized by gaseous distension of the rumen and reticulum observed on the left side of the cow. If the disorder is not treated, death can occur. Two common types of bloat occur; legume and feedlot (grain) bloat. Legume or pasture bloat is linked to substances in feeds which form a stable foam or interfere with nerve reflexes that accompany belching. A lack of coarse forages needed to stimulate eructation also can contribute to bloat. Excessive consumption of feed can cause rumen compaction and limit eructation of gases. Feedlot bloat is usually seen in fattening cattle that are on high concentrate diets. Administration of anti-foaming agents (such as vegetable oil or detergents) can reduce foam formation. Passing a tube down the esophagus into the rumen can release gas above the rumen contents. A rumenotomy (the body and rumen wall are punctured on the left side slightly forward and down from the hipbone) can be performed if the animal is severely bloated. A trocar and cannula is recommended so gas can escape and liquid does not drain internally causing peritonitis (Schmidt et al., 1988).

Diagnostic signs consist of:
1. Excessive accumulation of gas is seen as a bulging on the left side of animal.
2. Labored breathing, frequent urination, and defecation is observed with acute bloat.

Preventive actions might include:
1. Reducing the level of legume in the diet or pasture.
2. Feeding dry hay or feed prior to pasturing can lower succulent pasture intake and

maintain normal rumen function.

3. Supplementing the diet with poloxaline, a non-ionic surfactant, to prevent bloat, or with
4. Monensin, an ionophore, which is used as a bloat preventive in some countries, is administered per os as a slow-release capsule.

## 4.1.5 RUMEN ADDITIVES

Rumen additives can improve rumen environment for fermentation and digestion. Each additive should be evaluated using the criteria: response, research, and return, before incorporation in the ration (Hutjens, 1991):

* Response is the anticipated change the additive should provide (for example, higher milk yield, less ketosis, lower feed costs, or change in milk components).
* Research refers to published data that has been collected in an unbiased manner, statistically analyzed, and reported in peer reviewed technical journals.
* Return reflects the potential profitability the user may obtain. As a guideline, additives should return greater than two times their cost. For example, if an additive cost $0.10 per day, the farmer must recover $0.20 or more in higher milk yield, lower feed or health costs, and/or improved reproductive efficiency.

### Rumen Buffers

Chemically, buffers are a combination of a weak acid and its salt that resist changes in pH or hydrogen ion concentration in the rumen. To function properly, a rumen buffer must be water soluble (calcium carbonate is not) and its equivalence point (pKa) near the physiologic pH of the rumen. Sodium bicarbonate (pKa of 6.25) meets these requirements and would be classified as a rumen buffer. Magnesium oxide would not be classified as a buffer, but is an alkalinizing or neutralizing agent which increases the pH of the rumen fluid.

Sodium bicarbonate (bicarb) is widely used as a rumen buffer. In 24 controlled research studies, the response to adding 150 g of bicarb was one kg of increased milk production with an economic benefit to cost ratio of 2.3 to 1 (Downer and Cummings, 1987). Sodium sesquicarbonate contains a mixture of sodium bicarbonate and sodium carbonate (an alkalinizing agent). Six published studies reported an increase of 1.6 kg of milk and 0.23 percentage point increase in milk fat (Hutjens, 1991). Trona is the naturally-occurring mined form of sodium sesquicarbonate which contains 10 percent inert material (Hutjens, 1991). Magnesium oxide (mag ox) is added as an alkalinizing agent and contains 54 percent magnesium (Hutjens, 1991). One guideline is to combine 2 to 3 parts sodium bicarbonate or sodium sesquicarbonate to one part magnesium oxide in a buffer pack. Calcium carbonate (limestone or $CaCO_3$) has little buffering action in the rumen. Sodium bentonite, a clay mineral, is used as a pellet binder and added to some buffer packs. It can prevent milk fat depression, change rate of passage in the rumen (it swells in the rumen), and adsorb minerals, ammonia, and some mycotoxin.

*Table 7. Feeding recommendations of additives for lactating cows (Hutjens, 1991)*

| Product | Amounts (g/day) |
|---|---|
| Sodium bicarbonate | 110 – 225 |
| Sodium sesquicarbonate | 110 – 225 |
| Magnesium oxide | 50 – 90 |
| Sodium bentonite | 110 – 454 |
| Calcium carbonate | 115 – 180 |
| Potassium carbonate | 270 – 410 |

Potassium carbonate also has been used as a buffer when higher levels of potassium are needed (under heat stress condition) but is more expensive than sodium bicarbonate. Suggested levels of buffers and alkalinizers are listed in Table 7.

The following conditions favor a positive buffer response (Erdman, 1988; Hutjens, 1991):

1. Feeding high-corn, silage-based forage diets (over 60% of the forage dry matter from corn silage).
2. Feeding wet rations (over 50% moisture) due to fermented feeds (not pasture or green chop).
3. Feeding low fiber rations (below 19% ADF or 25% NDF).
4. Feeding rations with little or no hay (less than two kg/day) or silage chopped too finely (less than 2 kg forage DM particles > 40 mm).
5. High concentrate intake (over 2.5% of the cow's body weight).
6. Feeding large quantities of concentrate per meal (over 3 kg).
7. Feeding finely processed concentrates (such as pelleting).
8. Feeding high-moisture grain (especially over 30% moisture).
9. Feeding concentrates high in starch content (such as barley and corn).
10. Cows producing milk with a low fat test.
11. Cows experiencing heat stress.

**Yeast culture**

Yeast culture (YC) is a live culture of yeast (a fungus) and the media on which it was grown. It is dried to preserve the fermenting capacity of the yeast. Milk responses to YC are variable. In a Wisconsin field study with 11 herds and 585 cows, milk yield was increased 0.9 kg by feeding YC compared to control cows, herd response ranged from +2.3 to -1.0 kg per cow per day, and benefit to cost ratio was 1.6:1 (Shaver and Garrett, 1995). Feeding YC may stabilize the rumen environment, increase the number of cellulolytic bacteria, and decrease concentrations of lactic acid in the rumen (Hutjens, 1991). Adding YC to transition rations (three week prepartum to 5 weeks postpartum) might be beneficial.

### Bacterial direct-fed microbials

Bacterial direct fed microbials (BDFM) or probiotics are microorganisms that have been selected for their ability to assist in maintaining bacterial balance in the host animal's digestive tract during stress or disease situations, especially in monogastric animals. The roles of BDFM include the production of products that destroy undesirable microbes, produce beneficial enzymes, detoxify harmful metabolites, and/or lower the oxidation/reduction potential in the digestive tract. Several forms of BDFM are available including powders, boluses, pastes, and liquids containing a wide group of selected organisms (bacillus, streptococcus, pediococccus, lactobacillus, and others). Optimum microbial types and combinations, efficiency, time to administer, and economic response must be defined before routinely recommending the feeding of BDFM to ruminants (Hutjens, 1991).

### Niacin

Niacin is a generic term for nicotinic acid, nicotinamide, and other compounds that have similar biological activity. The major function of niacin is its role as a coenzyme (NAD+/NADP+ system) in biological reactions with lipids, protein, and CHO (Hutjens, 1991). Rumen microbes can synthesize niacin, but niacin could be limiting in early lactation because of ration changes, reduced feed intake, and slow rumen adaptation. The primary benefits of niacin include reducing ketosis, slowing fat mobilization, and lowering risk of fatty liver. Niacin can increase DMI by lowering blood ketone bodies, increasing microbial synthesis, enhancing propionate production, and increasing protozoa numbers (Hutjens, 1991). Niacin is fed at 6 g per day starting three weeks prepartum and 6 to 12 g for 100 days postpartum (when peak dry matter intake occurs). Cows which should be considered for niacin supplementation include high producing cows (over 9000 kg annually), cows experiencing negative energy balance, ketosis-prone cows, and fat cows (with a body condition score over 3 on a 1 to 5 scale).

## REFERENCES


*Adams, R.S. 1975. Equations and conversions using by the Penn State Forage Testing Service. Mimeo 1C:9:75.*

*Chandler, P.T. 1978. Roughage and Fiber. In: Large Dairy Herd Management. Univ. Presses of FL. Gainesville. pp. 354-370.*

*Chase, L.E. 1993. Developing nutrition programs for high producing dairy herds. J. Dairy Sci. 76:3287-3293.*

*Davis, C.L., and J.H. Clark. 1981. Managing the rumen. IL Dairy Report. pp.8-16.*

*Downer, J.V, and K.R. Cummings. 1985. A ten year review of lactation studies. J. Dairy Sci. 68 (Suppl 1):191.*

*Erdman, R.A. 1988. Dietary buffering requirements of lactating dairy cows. J. Dairy Sci. 71:3246-3266.*

*Fox, D.G., C.J. Sniffen, J.D. O'Connor, J.B. Russell, and, P.J. Van Soest. 1992. A net carbohydrate and protein system for evaluating cattle diets; III. Cattle requirements and diet adequacy. J. Anim. Sci. 70:3578-3596.*

*Garrett, E.F., M.N. Pereira, L.E. Armentano, K.V. Nordlund, and G.R. Oetzel. 1995. Comparison of pH and VFA concentration of rumen fluid from dairy cows collected through a rumen canula vs rumenocentesis. J. Dairy Sci. 78(Suppl. 1):299.*

*Geishauser, T. 1995. Abomasal displacement in the bovine - a review on character, occur rence, etiology and pathogenesis. J. Vet. Med. A. 42:229-251.*

*Grummer, R.R. 1993. Etiology of lipid-related metabolic disorders in periparturient dairy cows. J. Dairy Sci. 76:3882-3896.*

*Hutjens, M.F. 1985. Metabolic disorders in dairy cattle. Energy Fats NFIA Proc. pp.1-9.*

*Hutjens, M.F. 1991. Feed additives. Vet. Clinics North Am.: Food Animal Practice. 7:2:525-540.*

*Hutjens, M.F. 1994. Practical approaches to feeding the high producing cow. East. Can. Nutr. Conf. Proc. pp. 101-110.*

*Kertz, A.F., L.F. Reutzel, and G.M. Thomson. 1991. Dry matter intake from parturition to mid-lactation. J. Dairy Sci. 74:2290-2295.*

*Linn, J.G., M.F. Hutjens, R. Shaver, D.E. Otterby, W.T. Howard, and L.H. Kilmer. 1994. Feeding the dairy herd. N.C. Reg. Pub. 346. pp.6-12.*

*Massey, C.D., C. Wang, A. Donovan, and D.K. Beede. 1993. Hypocalcemia at parturition as a risk factorfor left displacement of the abomasum in dairy cows. j. Am. Vet. Med. Ass. 203:852-853.*

*Mertens, D.R. 1987. Predicting intake and digestibility using mathematical models of ruminal function. J. Anim. Sci. 64:1548-1558.*

*Mertens, D.R. 1992. Nonstructural and structural carbohydrates. In: Large Dairy Herd Management. Eds. H.H. Van Horn and C.J. Wilcox. Management Services ADSA, Champaign, IL. pp. 219-235.*

*Nordlund, K. 1995. Questions and answers regarding rumenocentesis and the diagnosis of herd-based subacute rumen acidosis. Four State Dairy Nutrition Seminar. La Crosse, WI. p.88-99.*

*National Research Council. 1989. Nutrient requirement of dairy cattle, 6th rev. ed. National Academy of Sciences. Washington, D.C. pp.138.*

*Russell, J.B., J.D. O'Connor, D.G. Fox, P.J. Van Soest, and C.J. Sniffen. 1992. A net carbo hydrate and protein system for evaluating cattle diets; I. Ruminal fermentation. J. Anim Sci. 70:3551-3561.*

*Schmidt, G.H., L.D. Van Vleck, and M.F. Hutjens. 1988. Principles of Dairy Science, 2nd ed. Prentice Hall. Englewood Cliffs, NJ. pp. 350-363.*

*Shaver, R.D., and J.E. Garrett. 1995. Lactation responses to dietary yeast culture on commercial dairies. Abstracts Midwest ADSA. pp. 54.*

*Sniffen, C.J. 1988. Balancing rations for carbohydrates for dairy cattle. In: The Application of Nutrition in Dairy Practice. Ed: E.J. Robb. Vet. Learning Syst. Co. Inc. pp. 25-35.*

*Sniffen, C.J., J.D. O'Connor, P.J. Van Soest, D.G. Fox, and, J.B. Russell. 1992. A net car bohydrate and protein system for evaluating cattle diets: II. Carbohydrate and protein availability.J. Anim. Sci. 70:3562-3577.*

# 4.2 MONITORING MILK PRODUCTION: DEFINING PRESET TARGETS AND EXECUTION

Andy. L. Skidmore[1], Arie Brand[2] and Charles J. Sniffen[3]

[1] Department of Animal Science, Michigan State University, East Lansing, MI 48824-1225, USA
[2] Department of Herd Health and Reproduction, School of Veterinary Medicine, University of Utrecht, Yalelaan 7, 3584 CL Utrecht, The Netherlands
[3] W.H. Miner Agricultural Research Institute, P.O. Box 90, Chazy, NY 12921, USA

## 4.2.1 INTRODUCTION

Milk production has to be monitored intensively, because more than 85% of the income on dairy farms is earned from the sale of milk. To monitor and manage milk production, milk yield and composition data are needed as well as nutrition, health, and reproductive data. These data are used by:

1. the farmer to monitor milk production and related operational management functions and to make management decisions,
2. milk processors to monitor milk quality and to pay the farmer for milk sold,
3. dairy herd improvement associations (DHIA) to supply management information to the farmer and for genetic improvement purposes,
4. veterinary practitioners and farm advisors to monitor milk production and diagnose problems with milk production and other related operational management functions.

Important operational management functions that influence milk production are: forage production, nutrition, health care, reproduction including breeding policy, and replacement rearing. Nutrition is the most important of these and should be focused on economically optimizing milk production. Nutrition also influences reproductive performance and immune status of a dairy herd. This means that milk production is the product of good management of interrelated operational management functions. For that reason, monitoring milk production plays a key role in Herd Health and Production Management (HH & PM) services.

This chapter will focus on:

1. defining objectives for a HH & PM program for milk production and,
2. a description of how such a program can be executed.

*Figure 1. Herd Health and Production Management Protocol for milk production*

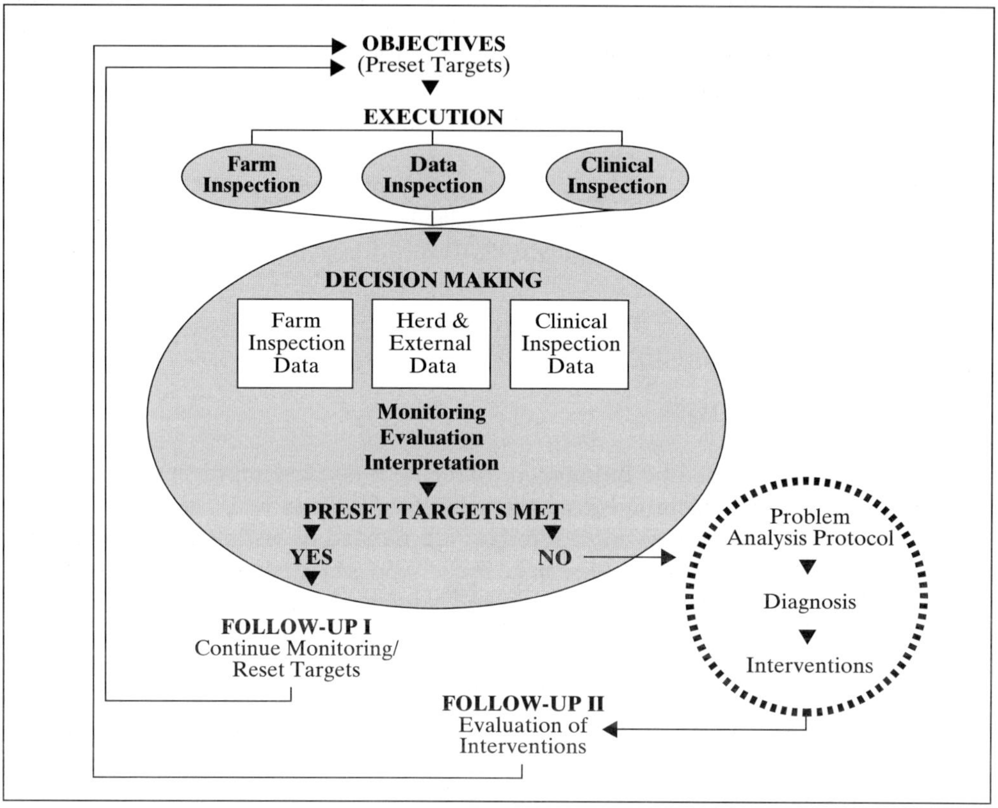


## 4.2.2 PROTOCOL

A HH & PM program for milk production should be focused on continuous monitoring of its performance. This makes it possible to detect, analyze, and adjust deficiencies in actual managerial practices at an early stage before becoming a problem. Once a problem is diagnosed then a problem solving protocol should be followed. The protocols used are presented in Figure 1, which have been described in detail in Chapter 1, part 1.

## 4.2.3 DEFINING PRESET TARGETS

The first step in monitoring milk production is defining preset targets in cooperation with the farmer. The time needed to reach these targets must be discussed and agreed upon as well. To set targets, actual performance indices must be known from either DHIA or on-farm computers. Sometimes actual performance is not known and an inventory of actual performance has to be completed. Preset targets must have an economic basis. Therefore, the economic impact has to be estimated as best as possible. Examples of preset targets for milk production are:

- Increasing milk production per cow per year,
- Filling the milk quota with high producing cows,
- Decreasing the cost of producing milk,
- Improving milk quality,
- Improving or optimizing milk protein/fat ratio
- Taking advantage of milk prices, pasture, or climatic conditions by shifting the calving pattern.

### 4.2.4 EXECUTION

**Materials**

To monitor milk production, the following materials are needed:

- A farm diary for recording daily events on health, reproduction, and general management, for example changes in feed bunk or grassland management or changes in ration composition,
- Milk production reports. Reports, used in many countries, are:
  - Milk testing and milk analysis reports from a Dairy Herd Improvement Association (DHIA) or equivalent organizations. Herds should be tested at 3 - 4 weekly intervals by official employees of these organizations. During a test day, kg of milk produced by individual cows are measured and a composite milk sample for analysis of milk of each lactating cow in the herd is collected.
  - The receipt from the milk processing factory. For payment a sample from the bulk milk tank is taken by an employee of the milk processing factory at every milk delivery or less frequently depending on the processor.
  - The weekly review of protein, fat, and somatic cell count analyses of bulk milk tank deliveries. Collected milk samples are analyzed by milk quality control stations. Analyses normally include protein, fat, lactose, total bacteria, somatic cell count, cleanliness, antibiotic residues, freezing point, etc. However, there are differences between countries and regions.
- Nutritional guidelines (National Research Council (NRC), 1989),
- Feed analyses,
- Relevant laboratory results of blood, milk, urine, and fecal samples,
- A grassland management calendar,
- A 12-monthly list of performance indices,
- Instruments for moisture testing of feedstuffs (scale and microwave),
- Instruments to weigh feeds that are provided (spring scales, mixer wagons with scales).

Other materials may include:
- A farm or external computer with computer software to calculate and analyze relevant performance indices and rations. They also offer the possibility to produce overviews and statistical analyses of data.
- Equipment for automatic measurement of milk produced per cow per milking, concentrate consumption per cow per day, walking activity, electrical conductivity, and milk temperature.

**Methods**

Monitoring milk production performance involves on-going efforts in a quality control monitoring system to detect positive or negative trends in milk production performance and possibly related risk factors. This system includes 3 activities:
* Data inspection
* Farm inspection
* Clinical inspection.

## 4.2.5 DATA INSPECTION

The data inspection part of the farm visit by a HH & PM practitioner or farm advisor should include:
- Evaluation of farmer compliance with data collection. Daily events should be scrupulously recorded by the farmer in a farm diary or other form and kept up-to-date. The currency and completeness of data recording should be checked. It reflects the involvement of the farmer in a HH & PM service and is the heart of the service. With regard to milk production it should include data on all diseases, treatments, and vaccinations of both cows and young stock, reproductive data, and data on management practices such as results of milking machine function evaluations, dates of replacement of liners, changes in diets, purchase and culling of young stock and/or cows. The practitioner or farm advisor must record his (consultative) diagnoses and treatments in the farm diary her/himself. In addition, availability of information from external organizations should be checked.
- An assessment of current herd milk production performance including any complaints or problems from the farmer. A prerequisite for a preliminary assessment and evaluation of available raw data recorded in the farm diary, and herd milk production performance indices, is that the most recent reports are available together with up-to-date records in a farm diary. If the HH & PM practitioner and/or farm advisor are aware of actual performance, then special attention can be paid to certain problem areas during the farm visit.

Data collected by the farmer, HH & PM practitioner (clinical data), or farm advisor can be processed either manually or on-line with an external computer at the veterinary office or elsewhere. Data processing of milk recording and milk analysis is mostly done by DHIA, milk factories, or milk quality control stations.

## 4.2.6 FARM INSPECTION

Generally a farm inspection is directed at an examination of management practices and farm conditions that may contribute to health and production inefficiencies. For a farm inspection related to milk production, the following aspects will be considered:

- Physical facilities
- Feeding systems
- Grouping strategies
- Barn climatic conditions
- Cow comfort
- Daily chore schedule
- Feed bunk management
  * Feed quality
  * Feed analysis
  * Feed palatability
  * Feed stability
  * Feed distribution
  * Particle size and feed mixing
  * Feeding frequency
  * Pushing up feed
  * Total mixed rations
  * Sequence of feeding ration ingredients
  * Feed refusals
  * Bunk scoring system
- Ration balancing and formulating
  * Ration balancing
  * Ration formulation
- Feeding behavior
  * Meal size
  * Number of meals eaten and length of meals
  * Number of rumination bouts and rumination time
  * Water intake
  * Water accessibility
  * Water quality

**Physical facilities**

All physical facilities should be designed and used to aid in farm management as efficiently as possible, and in optimizing cow comfort. The physical facility (stanchion, tie-stall barn, or loose housing system) in which cows are housed, milked, and fed will impact milk production. Therefore, the first step in a farm inspection is to examine and evaluate the quality of housing facilities. In this respect barns and other buildings should be examined in relation to one another. Cows and equipment should be able to be moved from one building to the next efficiently. Young stock should be housed separately from the rest of the herd. One building should not interfere with the ventilation of another. All animal traffic areas should be clean and non-slippery. This will provide adequate footing for cows to show signs of estrus and to move to the feed bunk, waterers, resting areas, and the parlor.

There should be equipment for weighing and mixing tested feeds even if a mixer wagon is not present. The scales of the mixer wagon should be calibrated regularly. Weighing individual feeds, mixing them, and delivering a mix to a group of animals is very important. For this purpose a drive through alley is needed. If computer feeders are used, then there should be no more than 25 - 35 cows per unit. This is dependent on the milk production level, barn lay-out, and cow accessibility. Storage systems for forage and commodities should be evaluated for slopes, cleanliness, and weather loss.

There should be adequate handling and treatment facilities. One person should be able to sort, separate, and restrain any animal on the farm. Self-locking head gates at the manger work well for breeding, herd health checks and treatment. If self-locking head gates are installed at the manger, they should be installed for the entire length of the manger or not at all. In addition, there should be enough light to read a newspaper in any part of the facility between the hours of 5:00 a.m. and 9:00 p.m.

A properly designed and maintained milking system is essential for high quality milk production. Milking machine function should be checked regularly and liners should be replaced after 1,500 milkings or according to manufacturer's recommendations. The milking parlor should be clean and dry in between milkings.

**Feeding systems**

There needs to be adequate bunk space for cows to be able to eat. For high producing lactating cows, this is about 60 cm per cow (minimum). Access to the bunk should be evaluated regularly. If access to feed or water is denied, then dry matter intake will be reduced and/or abnormal "slug" feeding behavior will result. "Slug" feeding is the rapid consumption of abnormally large quantities of feed at reduced frequency during the day. This behavior can result in large changes in rumen pH and cause digestive problems. Both abnormal feeding behavior and reduced dry matter and/or water intake will result in lower milk production.

Feed bunks that are elevated about 45 cm or more above the level of cows feet will reduce available bunk space for less dominant cows and increase feed wastage due to tossing of feed. A socially dominant cow will control about 1 - 2 m of bunk with her head when the bunk is elevated to 45 cm or higher and less dominant cows will stand back and wait for their turn or not even try to eat. If many cows are observed with a lot of feed on their backs from feed tossing behavior, then much feed is being wasted.

The physical condition of the feed bunk needs to be evaluated. If the feed bunk is rough and pitted from years of use, cows will only eat to within 2 - 3 cm of the feed bunk bottom unless they are forced to eat more. The reason for this is that feed is caught in the cracks and pits in the feed bunk and spoils. Cows will avoid eating any feed near the spoiled feed if at all possible. Cows will eat better and more from a smooth and clean surface.

During every farm visit, the condition of all waterers should be evaluated. All waterers in operation should be clean and maintained. Waterers that do not function properly or are dirty may reduce water intake. Waterers including water troughs should also be inspected dayly by the farmer for the build-up of algae, feed particles, manure, and other contaminants. Watering devices need to be properly located near feed, or return alley from the milking parlor. There should be .3 m of accessible water trough perimeter for every 10 cows. This would insure that every cow can access water when she wants it. The major indicator of water accessibility problems is the congregation of cows around the waterer at any time. If this is occurring, then access to water is limited. No dominant cow should be able to control water availability by denying access to a less dominant cow. In stanchion barns or tie-stall barns, where each cow has her own specific location, there should be a waterer for every cow. If not, a dominant cow will limit access to water of the less dominant cow next to her.

The temperature of the water should be measured regularly. Water is most palatable if it is between 15 - 27°C. In hot climates the waterers should be located in a shaded area. The source of water should be noted and the water evaluated for quality.

If cows are on pasture at any time during the year, which animals are pastured and when they are pastured must be identified. This is important in case the diet has to supplemented with forages and/or concentrates. Intake of concentrates only can be monitored and managed if provided exclusively in the barn. Pasture quality, distance to waterers must be evaluated as well. Milk production per day is a good indicator of good or poor pasture management. However, this is only possible when all just mentioned factors are taken into account.

Cows in stanchion facilities should be fed immediately after milking to encourage them to stand until the teat sphincter has closed (about 0,5 hour). This will help to minimize the incidence of mastitis. Cows tend to want to eat after being milked and provision of fresh feed will not only preventing them lying down but will encourage greater feed intake as well.

## Grouping strategies

The grouping strategy of cows on the farm should be examined. Splitting the herd into strings can reduce feed costs by providing less expensive rations for low producers and late lactation cows, while challenging just-fresh and top cows. Variance of requirements in a dairy herd is greater than for any other class of livestock. Ideally, each cow on the farm should be fed individually to meet her unique nutritional needs, but this is seldom practical. Therefore, the grouping of cows with similar requirements is an efficient alternative. The challenge is to group cows on a biological basis that will allow for top productive efficiency with a good return on investment.

The question now becomes, on what biological basis should cows be grouped. Many different production or biological indicators have been and are used today. Williams and Oltenacu (1992) compared 7 different strategies and found that grouping systems, based on nutrient concentrations, were most effective in return over feed costs. The nutrient concentration strategy accounted for nutrients needed for milk yield, pregnancy, maintenance, and other physiological functions. The method based only on test day milk yield was least effective, especially under a system using 3 production groups.

Milking cows should be divided into 3 or more groups provided the herd is large enough. With 2 groups, the transition between groups can be too drastic and impacts milk production. However, the marginal return or benefit above 2 groups declines with each additional group (Pecsok et al., 1992). These grouping strategies assume even calving throughout the year. An argument could be made for one group if the herd calves predominantly at one time of the year. This would still fit the biological principle of uniformity in nutrient requirements within a group. Group sizes should be no larger than what can get through the milking parlor in 1.5 hours.

First lactation cows maintained in a separate group will give substantially more milk than those grouped with mature cows, even when fed the same rations. The competition with mature cows is not advantageous for the younger cows. The difference in production is proportional to the difference in size between young and mature cows (Phelps, 1992).

Grouping should decrease within group variation and increase across-group variation. Knowledge of on-farm variance requires increased frequency of measurement. All input parameters of feeding systems need to be monitored. Some need to be monitored daily such as dry matter intake, some weekly such as moisture content of forages or milk composition, and some less frequently such as milk yield, body condition, or body weight. The collected information must be used. Contingency plans and response systems must be established for rapid reaction to performance indices that are outside preset targets. The ultimate goal is to increase the accuracy of feeding (Sniffen et al., 1993).

**Barn climatic conditions**

The ventilation system maintains the climatic conditions in the barn and must be adequate to prevent drafts and to maintain good air quality. Good air quality will help optimize health by reducing exposure of cows to pathogens, noxious gases, dust, and drafts. It also will increase cow comfort and minimize stress. For proper ventilation, ceiling and wall surfaces should be smooth and allow inlet air to enter and mix properly, especially during cold weather. Obstructions such as beams, ceiling joists, hay bales, open windows, open hay chutes, doors that are ajar, and cracks in the wall produce dead air spots. Drafts and high humidity affect good air movement. All these factors should be inspected regularly, especially air inlets.

Some indicators of potential ventilation challenges are: ammonia smell in the facility at any time (especially in the winter), cobwebs in the rafters, water stains on wooden rafters, and frost on the inside of the roof in the winter. The best way to evaluate air flow is by using smoke emitters and air quality by measuring the concentration of $CO_2$ and $NH_3$.

A proper ventilation system will avoid high humidity in winter and heat build-up in summer. Heat stress causes a cow to eat less, thus lowering milk production. Cows can produce 1.5 - 2.2 liters of moisture per day by respiration alone. Cooling devices such as fans and misters will help alleviate heat stress when properly installed and located.

Cooling systems need to be activated when following conditions exist (Bray and Bucklin, 1996):

- If the cows' rectal temperatures get above 102.5 degrees F. (39.1°C)
- If respiration rates are over 80 per minute,
- If dry matter intake and milk production drops 10% in hot weather.

These parameters can easily be be measured by locking-up 10 cows on a hot day and calculating how many are above set targets.

The first step in cooling cows is to block solar radiation by providing shade. This can be done with trees, but trees usually die quickly with cows around them. An alternative is to use a portable shade cloth. It is usually 3.6 m from the ground with 4.6

square meters/cow provided. Permanent shade structures also can be used. These are about 5 m high with a dirt floor oriented in a north-south position so the cows can chase the shade outside the roof and the sun can dry out the dirt floor.

A sprinkling and fan system can be installed in covered areas or barns were excess water can be collected. An adequate water supply and power to run the fans are essential. The cooling system is only effective if it results in increased feed intake and milk yield. Therefore, the system must be near feed and water. If the above criteria can not be met then other cooling methods should be considered. The following principles apply to 15 minute sprinkler-fan cooling cycles:

- Sprinkle cows for a short period of time, from 0.5 to 3 minutes, apply 125 mm of water per cycle; enough time to soak cows to the skin but before water runs onto the udder.
- Blow forced air onto the cows with fans to evaporatively cool them. The fans should run at least 12 to 14.5 minutes. The fans also can run continuously.
- Use evaporative cooling in freestall barns, feeding barns, shade structures, holding areas and under shade cloth or any covered area with a concrete floor.

Sprinkling without fans or fans without sprinklers will not result in an effective evaporative cooling system in hot humid climates.

Another cooling system is high pressure foggers. They are more expensive and should only be used in tall (3.7 m or higher), open sided and ridge vented barns. These systems cool the air instead of the cooling the cow. Water is applied to the air where it vaporizes absorbing the heat and transferring it away from the cow's environment with air movement.

### Cow comfort

Every day cows are subjected to a number of management and environmental conditions that make cows comfortable or uncomfortable. These factors can not always be measured objectively and are therefore interpreted in a subjective way. Some indicators of potential freestall comfort problems are:

* *Overcrowding* – Overcrowding, with regard to the number of cows per manger headlock and per stall, should be less than 15% in a high producing group of cows. Overcrowding can lead to stress and lowered milk production. The impact of overcrowding due to a shortage of manger headlocks can be modified by feed bunk management.

* *Injuries* – Injuries may occur to hips, necks, shoulders, hocks and knees. If more than 5 to 10% of cows are affected, a search for causal factors should be performed. Improper stall size and maintenance may create inadequate lunge space resulting in difficulties lying down and rising. Improper stall design may result in cows being injured from hitting stall dividers when attempting to lie down or get up.

* *Bedding conditions* – The nature of the stall surface (wood, concrete, clay, rubber), and the amount of bedding present should be considered. A resilient bed that is flat to lie upon is critical in maintaining cow comfort and minimizing injuries. Stalls should be clean and dry. If cows are dirty or have dirty udders, tails, switches and hind quarters, the "wet elbow" test should be done by putting a cloth covered elbow on the

stall surface. If the cloth is wet, the stall is too wet and the cow might be exposed to disease causing organisms, especially mastitis pathogens every time she lies down.

* *Social dominance* – Social dominance of certain cows may disturb the comfort of others. Timid cows will submit to more dominant cows and participate in less productive activities when challenged. The location of greatest social interaction is at the waterers and to a lesser extent at the feedbunk. This is because there are much fewer waterers than there are locations to eat and rest. Facility design can intensify or minimize the effect of social dominance. Facilities must be designed such that less dominant cows are accommodated.

* *Facility design* – Orientation of stalls, size and number of traffic lanes, and grouping within stalls in stanchion or tie stall barns can impact access to food, water, and resting locations and thus, influence dry matter and water intake, and resting behavior. In barns with stalls that face head to head, timid cows may be reluctant to use a stall across from a more dominant cow. She will at least "ask permission" to use the stall. When the facility is overcrowded, this behavior can be accentuated. The timid cows will resort to resting in the traffic lanes. In stanchion and tie stall barns, timid cows will often allow a dominant cow next to them to eat their feed. This is especially true when concentrates are fed separately. If water bowls are shared, the timid cow must get permission from the dominant cow when she wants to drink.

* *Walking behavior* – If traffic lanes do not have flat surfaces, are narrow or slippery, unconfident walking behavior will occur resulting in suboptimal feed intake and/or poor estrous expression. Lameness problems may also result.

* *Behavior of caretakers* – Cows have a inquisitive nature. On farms were cows are treated well by caretakers, cows will approach and be friendly toward farm employees when unaccompanied by visitors. In contrast, on farms were cows are not handled in a friendly way, they will scatter or shy away when a farm employee enters the pen. This is a sign of stress that may affect milk production negatively

* *Ectoparasites* – Large fly populations can have a significant impact on cow comfort, animal productivity, and farm profitability. House flies (*Musca domestica*) breed in manure, spoiled feed, decaying silage, hay, and straw, feed, bedding and other organic material. The blood feeding stable flies (*Stomoxys calcitrans*) choose many of the same areas for breeding as house flies but do not breed in straight manure (Merrill, 1995). The primary control method of fly breeding sites is sanitation. Insecticides are only a supplement and not a replacement for a good sanitation program. Insecticide sprays come as residual surface sprays or knockdown sprays. Overuse of insecticides may induce fly resistance. Insecticides may also kill fly parasites such as wasps. During the farm inspection, potential fly breeding sites should be identified and cleaned up. In this respect, dairy fly control should be focused on calf rearing sites, maternity pens, wet bedding material and feed residues in feed bunks, and manure around water troughs. Feed based breeding sites are often overlooked. Cleaning up after silo filling is just as important as removing manure and used bedding (Rufledt, 1995; Merrill, 1995).

* *other indicators of potential freestall comfort problems are* – presence of dehorned and horned cows in freestalls, percent of cows that will not use stalls or are lying in traffic lanes, percent of cows that are dirty, ratio between cows observed standing and

cows using stalls, and abnormal walking gaits (Roenfeldt, 1995).

## Daily chore schedule

Daily chores may remove cows fron feed. Therefore, a time chart of all management events that remove cows from the bunk should be filled in and evaluated. Events such as time in the holding area for milking, time cows are pushed away from the feed bunk for cleaning of animal traffic areas, cleaning or bedding of stalls, reproductive examinations, switching groups for milking, regrouping of cows, time in exercise lot, or any other activity that removes the cow from sources of feed and water should be monitored regularly (Table 1).

*Table 1. Time chart of daily chores for each group of cows*

| | Group "high cows" | Group "1st lactation" |
|---|---|---|
| 4:30 a.m. | Push-up feed | Push-up feed |
| 5:00 a.m. | Milking, clean traffic | |
| 5:30 a.m. | Milking, clean traffic | |
| 6:00 a.m. | | |
| 6:30 a.m. | | Milking, clean traffic |
| 7:00 a.m. | | |
| 7:30 a.m. | | Milking, clean traffic |
| 8:00 a.m. | | |
| 8:30 a.m. | Feeding cows, exercise | |
| 9:00 a.m. | | |
| 9:30 a.m. | | |
| 10:00 a.m. | | Feeding cows, exercise |
| 10:30 a.m. | | |
| 11:00 a.m. | | |
| 11:30 a.m. | | |
| 12:00 noon | | |
| 12:30 p.m. | | |
| 1:00 p.m. | Push-up feed | |
| 1:30 p.m. | Bedding cows | |
| 2:00 p.m. | | |
| 2:30 p.m. | | Push-up feed |
| 3:00 p.m. | | |
| 3:30 p.m. | | Bedding cows |
| 4:00 p.m. | | |
| 4:30 p.m. | Feeding cows | |
| 5:00 p.m. | | |
| 5:30 p.m. | Milking, clean traffic | |
| 6:00 p.m. | Milking, clean traffic | |
| 6:30 p.m. | | Feeding cows |
| 7:00 p.m. | | |
| 7:30 p.m. | | |
| 8:00 p.m. | | Milking, clean traffic |
| 8:30 p.m. | Push-up feed | |
| 9:00 p.m. | | Milking, clean traffic |
| 9:30 p.m. | | |
| 10:00 p.m. | | |
| 10:30 p.m. | | |
| 11:00 p.m. | Push-up feed | Push-up feed |
| 11:30 p.m. | | |
| midnight | | |

Circle those chores that remove cows from sources of feed and water

## Feed bunk management

Computers, technological innovations, nutritionists, and animal scientists have advanced the science of feeding dairy cows. Even with all this knowledge and technology, the art of feeding remains important. Some farmers are much more successful than others in feeding dairy cattle while using the same technology. In many cases, the rations look good on paper and the producer indicates that everything was mixed properly. The difference in production levels may then be due to bunk management. Bunk management is crucial to efficient production of milk and is just as important as feeding a well designed and balanced ration. Bunk management includes all of the following feed related factors. The basic principle is to get cows to eat all that they can and not a bite more. Consistency in all factors is the key to consistent high production. The appendix contains many rules of thumb for feeding cows (Mahana, 1993).

* **Feed quality**

Feed quality is very important to monitor. It has a direct impact on milk production. Changes in feed quality will change the balance of nutrients and may change feed stability and palatability. Any changes in quality must be compensated for or corrected to maintain high levels of milk production. Remember "Garbage in and garbage out". Aspects of feed quality to monitor are dry matter content, chemical analysis results, palatability, stability, mold, and appearance.

A dry matter analysis of each ensiled forage should be done on a weekly basis. Weekly variation in quality of ensiled forages can be large, especially in uncovered storage structures. Dietary imbalances caused by changes in dry matter content are more likely to occur where forages are measured by weight and not volume. If changes are not detected and weights not appropriately adjusted, the diet will be unbalanced nutritionally and lower milk production and/or metabolic or digestive problems may occur.

Dry matter analysis is best done on the farm rather than through external laboratories because of the frequency and timeliness of results. Oetzel et al., (1993) evaluated 3 on-farm methods for testing dry matter: (1) sequential drying in a microwave oven, (2) commercial on-farm forced-air drying instrument, and (3) a commercial electronic moisture tester. The 3 methods were compared to a commercial laboratory drying oven as the standard.

The microwave oven method provided the most accurate and repeatable results but it also required the most operator skill and time. The microwave method could be used on any feed ingredient and does not require calibration.

The commercial on-farm forced-air method did not require constant operator attention but total time was longer than other methods. This method required much less operator skill than the microwave oven method.

The electronic moisture tester gave results comparable to the other methods for alfalfa silage and the best for high moisture shelled corn but significantly underestimated the dry matter of corn silage relative to the drying oven. This may be a result of inaccuracies in the conversion tables provided with the instrument. The electronic moisture tester has the advantage of least operator skill and time required.

The choice of which method to use on-farm depends on the feed ingredients to be tested and the relative priority the operator places on ease of use, time required for analysis, repeatability, and accuracy.

A chemical analysis of feed ingredients such as grass, alfalfa or corn silage should be done whenever there is any change. Several samples should be taken to know what kind of variation is in the feed. Stored feeds, such as forages, should be evaluated just before they are fed instead of just after harvest. An analysis of fresh feed going into storage is useful to estimate feed quality and better manage feed inventories. If changes in nutrient content are not detected, the diet fed will not be nutritionally balanced and the same problems listed above may occur.

* **Feed palatability**

Feed palatability is very important, especially when feeding commodities or introducing something new into the diet. When a new less palatable ingredient is introduced, it must be done gradually starting with small amounts that are increased every second day. The farmer/nutritionist has to use his/her own judgment and experience to know how much and how fast for each unpalatable ingredient being added, or the cows will immediately refuse to eat and metabolic and digestive problems may result. Commodities such as animal proteins, animal and inert fats, and anionic salts are not very palatable. Always evaluate what ingredients are being fed and their respective palatability.

* **Feed stability**

Secondary fermentation is a process by which feed begins to ferment again after it is removed from storage. This is usually the result of incomplete fermentation when the feed was put into storage. Contact with air will start aerobic fermentation of what substrate is left and heats up real fast. If fermentation was complete then there would be very little substrate left to ferment when air came in contact with the feed. Mold could still grow or other organisms but they take longer to heat up. Fermented or wet feeds are more likely to be unstable and spoil or undergo secondary fermentation. In the heat of summer it will occur much quicker than in the cold of winter. The way to evaluate if secondary fermentation occurs is to measure how long it takes the feed to heat up after it is removed from storage. The longer it takes, the more stable the feed is. The temperature, 20 to 30 cm inside the stack also can be measured with a special device. Climatic conditions will alter this fermentation rate. The way to manage a feed where secondary fermentation is a problem is to increase the frequency of feeding. This results in feed staying in the feed bunk for shorter periods of time and not getting a chance to ferment again. Cows prefer not to eat feed that is hot and fermenting again. Harvesting and storage protocols should be reviewed to prevent this from happening.

* **Feed distribution**

To evaluate how well feed is distributed in the feed bunk only requires observation of the feed bunk when there is feed present. To take full advantage of all the bunk space available, feed must be distributed for the full length of the feed bunk.

This may seem like a trivial matter, but it is very often ignored and is very critical when bunk space already may be a limitation. Unequal feed distribution may cause fighting among cows and thus stress which may affect milk production.

* **Particle size and feed mixing**

The particle size of all feed ingredients must always be evaluated in storage as well as in the feed bunk. Once forage is cut by the harvester, it may go through several machines, including a self-unloading wagon, blower, silo unloader, TMR mixer and conveyor before arriving at the animal. Each of these machines can shorten particle length (Schuler, 1995). 40 to 50% of the forage should be at least 5 cm long to insure good rumen function and digestion. The long particle length helps in the formation of a rumen mat to catch smaller particles for more complete digestion and stimulates cud chewing and saliva flow for the maintenance of an optimal rumen pH (Shaver, 1995). Fifteen to 20% (weight basis) of the particles in TMR's should be more than 5 cm long. TMR's that are too fine may result from overmixing with an auger mixer for longer than 5 minutes. With mixers that are used for hay processing, hay should be processed first, then the other ingredients should be added, followed by mixing. With mixers that must run while adding ingredients, the hay silage should be added last.

Forage or ration physical form also can be too coarse. This will result in: 1) mold formation due to improper packing and fermentation in the storage bunk, thus,reducing the feeding value, and 2) separation of coarse particles in the feed bunk, enabling selective feed consumption. An increase in the incidence of displaced abomasums can therefore be an indication that either the feed in the feed bunk is to fine or too coarse (Shaver, 1995).

There are several ways to evaluate how well a feed is mixed. A quick, easy way is to look for some easily identified concentrate that is not a large percentage of the diet, such as a pellet or fuzzy cottonseed and evaluate if it is evenly distributed in the feed bunk. Another way is to take a sample of the feed at opposite ends of the feed bunk and analyze it for micromineral content. If the feed is well mixed, the mineral content should be similar at both ends of the feed bunk.

* **Feeding frequency**

The frequency of feed delivery is very important to evaluate. Every time feed is delivered, it stimulates the cow to eat again. But with each feeding, it costs money to run the equipment and pay the labor. When feeding a very limited number of times during the day (once a day or less), the feed bunk becomes a feed storage area and must be managed in a manner that will encourage more dry matter intake. The feed must also be very stable and remain fresh (not spoil) for the time it is in the bunk. Spoiled feed is not very palatable, reduces effective bunk space, leads to "slug" feeding, and cows do not like to eat it anymore than a person would. Therefore, the more times a cow can be stimulated to eat, it will not only increase dry matter intake but help to maintain a more consistent rumen pH which results in a healthier rumen and better digestion of the feed.

* **Pushing-up feed**

A management strategy to encourage more dry matter intake and minimize the frequency of feeding is to push feed up in the feed bunk many times during the day. Some farmers will even spray a thin coating of molasses on the feed to encourage feed intake when they push-up the feed. However, molasses is rich in potassium and in sugars, which can be an disadvantage in certain herds. When there is only a small amount of feed left in the bunk (3 cm or less across the bottom of the bunk), and the feed is pushed into piles, then cows will consume 50% more of what is left. Cows like to push feed around with their noses and will eat more if they do not have to lick it off of the feed bunk floor. If the bunk floor surface is rough or has cracks and holes where feed gets caught and spoils, avoidance of eating the last amount of feed is amplified. Pushing the last little amount of feed into piles will help manage around this problem until the manger can be repaired.

* **Total mixed rations**

With regard to the feeding system, one should inspect if a true totally mixed ration (TMR) is fed. If a true TMR is fed, it will include all the feed ingredients that the cows will consume. If some ingredients are fed separately, it is not a true TMR. Even when a TMR is fed, cows may selectively eat what they want. This may result in digestive and metabolic problems. However, these problems occur more frequently when ingredients are fed separately.

* **Sequence of feeding ration ingredients**

If a TMR is not fed, the sequence of ration ingredient delivery to cows will influence rumen function and milk production. This is very important in feeding systems that feed ration ingredients separately. Long stem hay or hay crop silage always should be fed first. If the hay crop silage is high in crude and soluble protein (> 18% of dry matter and > 45% of crude protein, respectively), corn silage should be fed first, immediately followed by hay crop silage. This will result in greater utilization of the forage nitrogen. Hay or hay crop silage will provide more buffering capacity to the rumen and help to form a fiber mat that will increase retention time of corn silage and concentrate. This also facilitates a more complete digestion of smaller particle sized feed ingredients. The higher levels of fiber in the hay or lucerne or their silages will also stimulate rumination and salivation increasing its buffering capacity. The hay or hay crop silage also has a higher buffering capacity itself and helps to protect the rumen from pH insults that may result from concentrate or corn silage feeding.

* **Feed refusals**

Feed refusal from the lactating cows should be evaluated. In high producing herds, cows should be fed for a >2% refusal. The refusals should always resemble the feed that is fed to the cows. If the percentage of refusals is lower or higher than the reference value, the situation needs to be evaluated. There may be many causes of deviations. Less than 2% refusals may be due to not enough feed being offered. A high refusal percentage may be caused by cows sorting feeds and picking out what they want to eat.

If cows are sorting, it is usually due to moldy or off-flavor ingredients. In other instances forage particle size is too long, allowing the cows to easily sort the ingredients. If sorting of feed is happening, look for metabolic or digestive problems and/or investigate why they are not eating particular parts of the ration.

* **Bunk scoring system**

Good bunk management requires many subjective and less measurable skills like good observation and intuition. For many producers, good bunk management is by intuition, learned from experience and practice. One way to remove some of the subjectivity and increase observational skills would be to implement a bunk scoring system. The bunk can be scored on a numeric scale (0 to 5) on a regular basis (Table 2). The results can be used to help determine how much feed and how often feed should be offered to a pen of cows.

A feed bunk can be scored at any time but is most meaningful if the bunk is scored every morning before the first feeding of the day.

A bunk score of "0" for longer than one hour a day is evidence that "empty bunk syndrome" is occurring. Empty bunk syndrome, also known as agroceriosis, is when no feed is present in the feed bunk when there should be feed almost 24 hours a day. This syndrome frequently occurs at night when no one is observing the cows. It is particularly important in hot weather when cows will consume up to 60% of their diet at night. Often this can be diagnosed when making emergency farm calls late at night. Another way to diagnose this syndrome is to set up a video camera and clock for the night, reviewing the tape in the morning. Proper use of a bunk scoring system will help to minimize the incidence of this syndrome.

If the bunk scores a "o" at least one hour before the next scheduled feeding, the amount of feed delivered to that pen could be increased by 3 - 5%; 0 - 1% if a bunk

*Table 2. Five point bunk scoring system (Skidmore, unpublished)*

| Score | Description |
|---|---|
| 0 | No feed remaining in bunk. |
| 1 | Scattered feed present, only pieces of corn cob from corn silage present, or only stems from picked over hay present. Most of bottom of bunk is exposed. |
| 2 | Thin (less than 2 cm) layer of feed across bottom of bunk. The feed looks the same as when delivered. |
| 3 | Five to eight cm of feed across bottom of bunk, 25 - 50% of previous feeding. |
| 4 | More than 50% of previous feeding remaining in the bunk and feed thoroughly disturbed. |
| 5 | Feed virtually untouched. |

scores a "1", and no change is needed if a bunk scores a "2". If a bunk scores a "3" or above, the cause needs to be investigated and rations adjusted accordingly.

The uniformity of feed consumption along the feed bunk should be observed when scoring bunks. Large amounts of feed left in some parts of the feed bunk, while in other parts the feed is totally consumed, may indicate several problems. It could indicate areas of:

- poor bunk surface,
- poor environment along the feed bunk,
- poor or inconvenient access to the feed bunk, or
- a spot of poor feed quality, mixing, or distribution if it was an occasional occurrence.

Bunk scores should be recorded in the farm diary so that trends can be noted and appropriate adjustments made. If the amount of feed delivered every day is also recorded, trends in dry matter intake could be observed. Erratic feed delivery leads to erratic feed intake which leads to erratic production and metabolic problems.

## Balancing and formulating dairy rations

Milk yield and milk composition are, to a large extent, dependent on nutritional management. An important part of nutritional management is feed intake. As mentioned earlier, feed intake is influenced by several factors such as quality and palatability of feedstuffs, feeding strategies, climatic conditions in the barn (temperature and the presence of ammonia), changing weather conditions, weight and age of cows, changes in days in milk, grouping of cows, diseases, etc. Therefore, many dairy farmers need support in their nutritional management in order to reach optimal milk production performance economically. This and the next paragraphs are adapted from a dairy management manual of the Cooperative Extension service, Kansas State University: "Feeding dairy cows" (1990).

### * Ration balancing

An important tool for nutritional management is ration balancing. Ration balancing has to be followed by ration formulation and evaluation.

Dairy rations are balanced by calculating the amount of grain mix needed to supplement the nutrients that are not supplied by forages. It is not feasible to balance a ration for each cow in the herd, and it is not recommended to balance one ration for an entire herd. Rations should be balanced for groups of cows with similar nutritional requirements. Nutritional requirements for cows of different milk production levels are provided by the National Research Council in the USA (Update, 1989) and by comparable organizations in other countries.

Although several computer programs are commercially available the following procedures are suggested for balancing the ration for a herd split into two production groups with average body weights of 600 kg which are producing 27 kg of 3.5% milk fat and 18 kg of 4.0% milk fat. The calculations for balancing the rations for the higher producing group are as follows:

### Step 1. Determining nutrient requirements.

Nutrient requirements are affected by (1) maintenance (body size), (2) milk, milk fat, and milk protein production, and (3) body weight gain. The nutrient allowance for pregnancy is not significant until the last two months of gestation when cows are normally dry. When determining the requirements for milk production, always balance for a higher level of production than the group is averaging. If the herd is grouped by production, the level of production of the high group should be estimated about 7 kg more than the group average. The requirements for production should be about 2.5 kg above average for the low-producing group. If the herd is not grouped, then the production requirements should be estimated at about 30% above the average production. Growth requirements can be estimated by increasing the nutrient allowance for maintenance by 20% for first lactation cows and 10% for second. A typical herd will need about 15% added to the maintenance allowance for growth.

Nutrient requirements for maintenance, maintenance plus pregnancy, milk production at various milk fat percentages, and weight gain are given by the National Research Council (NRC) and shown in an abbreviated way in Table 3. To determine the requirement, select the maintenance requirement which corresponds to the average body size of the cows and the production requirement corresponding to the milk fat percentage of the group. The production requirement is then multiplied by the kg of milk. In this example, the production requirements would be multiplied by 34 (7 kg above group average).

### Step 2. Determining forage intake

Dairy cows should be fed all the forage they will consume. However, there are limits as to how much forage dairy cows can eat. Normally, the maximum consumption of high quality forage dry matter will be about 2.5% of body weight when no grain is fed. Somewhat less consumption can be expected from lower quality forages. An average herd will consume about 1.8 % of body weight as forage dry matter when enough grain is fed to meet requirements. When a herd is split, the high producing cows will probably consume about 1.6% of their body weight as forage dry matter, the mid lactation cows about 1.7% and the lower producing cows will consume about 2% of body weight. This means a group of high producing cows weighing 600 kg would eat 9.5 kg of dry matter from forage while the lower producers would average 12 kg.

### Step 3. Calculate nutrients from forages

Calculate the nutrients supplied from forages by multiplying the kg of forage by the content of nutrients from a forage analysis.

### Step 4. Determine nutrients required in grain mix

Subtract the nutrients supplied by the forages (Step 3) from the nutrient requirements (Step 1).

*Table 3. Daily nutrients requirements of dairy cows (Appendix Table 3, NRC-1989)*

| Live weight (kg) | Energy NEL (Mcal) | Total crude Protein (g) | Ca (g) | P (g) | Vitamin A (1000 IU) | Vitamin D (1000 IU) |
|---|---|---|---|---|---|---|
| **Maintenance mature lactating cows** | | | | | | |
| 400 | 7.16 | 318 | 16 | 11 | 30 | 12 |
| 450 | 7.82 | 341 | 18 | 13 | 34 | 14 |
| 500 | 8.46 | 364 | 20 | 14 | 38 | 15 |
| 550 | 9.09 | 386 | 22 | 16 | 42 | 17 |
| 600 | 9.70 | 406 | 24 | 17 | 46 | 18 |
| 650 | 10.30 | 428 | 26 | 19 | 49 | 20 |
| 700 | 10.89 | 449 | 28 | 20 | 53 | 21 |
| 750 | 11.47 | 468 | 30 | 21 | 57 | 23 |
| 800 | 12.03 | 486 | 32 | 23 | 61 | 24 |
| **Maintenance plus last 2 months of gestation of mature dry cows** | | | | | | |
| 400 | 9.30 | 875 | 26 | 16 | 30 | 12 |
| 450 | 10.18 | 928 | 30 | 18 | 34 | 14 |
| 500 | 11.00 | 978 | 33 | 20 | 38 | 15 |
| 550 | 11.81 | 1027 | 36 | 22 | 42 | 17 |
| 600 | 12.61 | 1074 | 39 | 24 | 46 | 18 |
| 658 | 13.39 | 1120 | 43 | 26 | 49 | 20 |
| 700 | 14.15 | 1161 | 46 | 28 | 53 | 21 |
| 750 | 14.90 | 1209 | 49 | 30 | 57 | 23 |
| 800 | 15.64 | 1254 | 53 | 32 | 61 | 24 |
| **Milk production-nutrients/kg of milk of different fat percentages** | | | | | | |
| **Milk fat %** | | | | | | |
| 3.0 | 0.64 | 78 | 2.73 | 1.68 | – | – |
| 3.5 | 0.69 | 84 | 2.97 | 1.83 | – | – |
| 4.0 | 0.74 | 90 | 3.21 | 1.98 | – | – |
| 4.5 | 0.78 | 96 | 3.45 | 2.13 | – | – |
| 5.0 | 0.83 | 101 | 3.69 | 2.28 | – | – |
| 5.5 | 0.88 | 107 | 3.93 | 2.43 | – | – |
| **Live weigth change during lactation-nutirents/kg of weight change** | | | | | | |
| Weight loss | –4.92 | –320 | – | – | – | – |
| Weight gain | 5.12 | 320 | – | – | – | – |

NOTE: Nel = Net energy for lactation

**Step 5. Determine the kg of grain mix needed**

Divide the energy required from the grain mix by its energy content. Most grain mixes will contain about 1.67 Mcal/kg of NEL on an as fed basis.

**Step 6. Determine protein percentage of grain mix**

Divide the kg of protein needed in the grain mix by the kg of grain mix required.

**Step 7. Determine calcium and phosphorus percentage of grain mix**

Divide kg of calcium and phosphorus required in grain mix by the kg of grain mix required. Similar calculations would be made for the lower producing group.

* **Ration formulation**

One has to realize that at least 5 rations can be distinguished: (1) the calculated ration, (2) the ration that the farmer mixes, (3) the ration that the cows actually consume, (4) the ration or proportion of the ration that is digested and, (5) those nutrients that are absorbed. The last "ration" is the most important one and therefore rations have to be balanced in such a way that the most optimal absorption rates from the digestive tract can be obtained.

After determining the protein, calcium and phosphorus percentages needed (Table 4), the grain mixture can be formulated by using Pearson's Square as follows:

**Step 1.** Write the desired percentage of the nutrient in the center of the square.

**Step 2.** Write the nutrient content, as a percentage, of the grain and supplement in the upper and lower left corners of the square respectively.

**Step 3.** Subtract diagonally across the square, the smaller value from the larger so that the number is always positive, and place the results in the diagonal corner on the right side. The value in the upper right corner corresponds to the parts of the ingredient at the upper left corner and likewise for the lower corners of the square. In the first example, 26 parts of shelled corn and 9 parts of soybean meal will result in a mixture containing 18% protein.

**Step 4.** To convert to percentage, divide the parts of the ingredient by total parts of both ingredients and multiply by 100.
Example: 9 / (26 + 9) x 100 = 25.7% soybean meal.

**Step 5.** Multiply the percentage of the ingredient by the size of the batch to obtain the total kg of that ingredient in the batch.
Example: 25.7% x 912 kg = 234 kg soybean meal.

*Table 4. Balancing dairy rations. Group of 600 kg cows, gaining 454 g per day and producing 34 kg milk with 3.5% milk fat and consuming 4.5 kg alfalfa hay and 16.3 kg corn silage*

| **Step 1** | | **(kg)** | **NEL (Mcal)** | **Protein (g)** | **Ca (kg)** | **P (kg)** |
|---|---|---|---|---|---|---|
| Maintenance* | | 600 | 9.7 | 406 | 24 | 17 |
| Production | | 34(3.5%) | 23.46 | 2856 | 101 | 62 |
| Weight gain | | | 2.32 | 145 | — | — |
| **Total requirements** | | | **35.48** | **3407** | **125** | **79** |
| **Step 2 and 3** | **(kg)** | **D.M (kg)** | **NEL (Mcal)** | **Protein (g)** | **Ca (g)** | **P (g)** |
| Nutrients from Forages | | | | | | |
| Alfalfa** | 4.5 | 4.0 | 5.58 | 694 | 30 | 9 |
| Corn silage | 16.3 | 5.3 | 8.50 | 417 | 14 | 11 |
| **Total** | **20.8** | **9.3** | **14.08** | **1111** | **45** | **20** |
| *Average* | | | *1.51* | *11.9%* | *0.48 %* | *0.21 %* |
| **Step 4 (Step 1 – Step 3)** | | | **NEL (Mcal)** | **Protein (g)** | **Ca (g)** | **P (g)** |
| Nutrients required in Grain mix | | | 21.4 | 2296 | 80 | 58 |

**Step 5** – Grain needed for energy = 21.4 Mcal/1.67 Mcal/kg = 12.8 kg grain*.* Based on a grain mix that is made up of primarily ground shell corn, soybean meal and mineral. If other commodities are used in the grain mix, other rules have to be used.

**Step 6** – Percent protein required in grain = 2.3 kg/12.8 kg * 100 = 18 % protein

**Step 7** – Percent calcium required in grain = 0.080 kg /12.8 kg * 100 = 0.63 % calcium

**Step 8** – Percent phosphorus required in grain = 0.058 kg/12.8 kg * 100 = 0.45 % phosphorus

* The maintenance requirement has been increased by 15% for growth of young cows.

** The calcium content of alfalfa has been reduced by 40% due to low availability.

**Example Calculations – Protein percent = 18**

Shelled corn 9% protein — 26 parts shelled corn

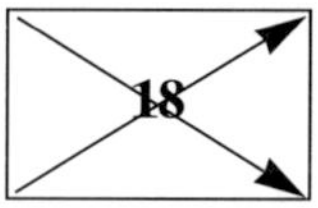


Soybean meal 44% protein — 9 parts Soybean meal

Soybean meal = 9 / (26 + 9) x 100 = 25.7%

**Calcium percent = 0.63**

Grain Mix (0.03% Ca) — 22.37 Parts Grain Mix

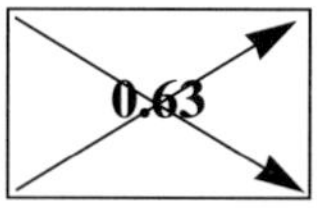


Dicalcium Phosphate (23% Ca) — 0.60 parts Dicalcium Phosphate

Dicalcium Phosphate % = .60 / (22.37 + 0.60) x 100 = 2.6%

**Feeding behavior**

Nutritionists always have emphasized that if dry matter intake could be increased, milk production and profitability would increase proportionately. To increase dry matter intake, it is very important to know and understand the feeding behavior of cows. It is as important as feeding a well designed and balanced ration.

Cows are creatures of habit, very curious and social. Changes in behavior will affect dry matter intake. Facilities will modify cow behavior due to the design or state of repair or how people manage and work in the facility. Farm management must be evaluated relative to its impact on normal feeding behavior of cows.

Several behavioral traits that influence dry matter intake and milk production have been identified and characterized (Dado et al., 1994). They are summarized in Table 5. The cows were housed in tie stalls to facilitate data collection so there was no competition for feed. The same traits may be manifested a little differently in a loose housing situation. Because there was no competition the behavioral traits identified could be considered ideal because the cows had the ultimate opportunity to express their behavior. The ration consisted of 29% alfalfa silage, 29% corn silage, and concentrate for a TMR composition of 51% DM, 17% CP, 31% NDF, .8 %Ca .5% P.

* **Meal size**

Cows must be offered enough time to be able to eat enough for optimal milk production. It is very important to note that cows only eat about 1.8 - 2.5 kg of dry matter every time they eat. Larger meals were observed to be consumed after milking and

*Table 5. Summary statistics for milk production and feeding behavior of 6 primiparous and 6 multiparous lactating Holstein cows measured continuously for 10 days in early lactation (Dado et al., 1994)*

| Variable | Primiparous | Multiparous | All cows |
|---|---|---|---|
| Milk production (kg/d)[a] | 28.7 | 37.5 | 33.1 |
| Dry matter intake (kg/d)[a] | 20.0 | 24.8 | 22.8 |
| Meal size (kg of dry matter) | 1.8 | 2.5 | 2.2 |
| Eating bouts (day) | 11.3 | 10.8 | 11.0 |
| Eating bout length (minutes) | 25.9 | 31.1 | 28.8 |
| Eating time (minutes/day) | 284 | 314 | 301 |
| Ruminating bouts (day) | 15.4 | 12.9 | 14.0 |
| Ruminating bout length (minutes)[a] | 29.7 | 36.0 | 33.3 |
| Ruminating time (minutes/day) | 453 | 460 | 457 |
| Ruminating chew (day) | 29,645 | 28,946 | 29,295 |
| Water intake (L/day)[a] | 63.2 | 89.5 | 77.6 |
| Drinking bouts (day) | 13.0 | 14.9 | 14.0 |
| Drinking bout size (L) | 5.4 | 7.2 | 6.4 |
| Drinking time (minutes/day) | 17.7 | 19.1 | 18.5 |

[a] Means differ between parities ($P < .05$)

allocation of fresh feed. It is not surprising that more mature and higher producing cows will eat more at every meal but, because they did not eat any longer, they had to eat faster. This has very important ramifications in regards to how cows are fed. If higher producing cows eat faster, they are at greater risk of digestive upsets if the ration is not properly mixed or balanced.

* **Number of meals eaten and length of meals**

Just as important is the fact that cows will eat about 11 times every day and only for about 30 minutes each time. This is independent of parity, milk production, and dry matter intake levels. The physical facility and every management activity on the farm must accommodate this behavior. About 21%, or 300 minutes, of the cow's day is spent eating. The facility and management procedures must be examined to evaluate if cows are being allowed to express their normal feeding behavior. This can be examined by evaluating bunk access, bunk space, bunk scores, schedule of daily chores that interfere with feeding behavior, etc.

Milk production is correlated positively with dry matter and water intake (Dado et al., 1994). When cows experience a prolonged period (greater than 2 hours) without feed, the number of meals during the day will be fewer and the amount eaten at each meal will be greater. This abnormal feeding behavior, also known as "slug" feeding, is especially manifested in the first meal after a prolonged absence from feed and will magnify any potential problems with acidosis or other associated metabolic problems.

* **Number of rumination bouts and rumination times**

It is important to note that cows will ruminate about 14 different periods every day. This is independent of parity, milk production, and dry matter intake. The more mature and higher producing cows did ruminate longer every time they ruminated but total time was not different. This would indicate that they ruminate more material per day in the same time as lower producing cows because they are eating more each day. Cows prefer to ruminate lying down. The facility must be comfortable with enough space for cows to lie down and ruminate. Cows spend about 32% of their day ruminating. Eating and ruminating together account for over 50% of a cows day. The facilities and management procedures must be evaluated for their compliance to normal cow behavior to maximize milk production. For example, cow comfort, overcrowding, stall maintenance, feet and leg injuries, time chart of daily chores, etc. must be evaluated.

## Water

Water is a very essential nutrient both for life and milk production. Water makes up about 87% of milk composition yet it is often the most neglected nutrient on dairy farms. Access, availability, quality, and cleanliness of water should always be evaluated.

* **Water intake**

Cows that drink more water also eat more dry matter and produce more milk. The expected daily water intake for different classes of dairy cattle is shown in Table 6.

*Table 6. Drinking water requirements of dairy cattle (Adapted from: Adams, R.S., 1986. Water quality for dairy cattle. Pennsylvania State University)*

| Livestock class | Age or production | Liters |
|---|---|---|
| Holstein calves | 1 month | 4.9 - 7.6 |
| | 2 months | 5.7 - 9.1 |
| | 3 months | 7.9 - 10.6 |
| | 4 months | 11.4 - 13.2 |
| | 5 months | 14.4 - 17.4 |
| Holstein heifers | 15 - 18 months | 22.3 - 26.9 |
| | 18 - 24 months | 27.6 - 36.3 |
| Jersey cows | 13.6 kg milk/day | 49.2 - 58.7 |
| Ayrshire, Brown Swiss and Holstein cows | 13.6 kg milk/day | 54.9 - 64.3 |
| | 22.7 kg milk/day | 90.8 - 102.2 |
| | 36.4 kg milk/day | 143.8 - 159.0 |
| | 45.4 kg milk/day | 181.7 - 196.8 |
| Dry cows | pregnant 6 - 9 months | 34.0 - 49.2 |

Even a small limitation in water intake will decrease dry matter intake by .5 - 1.0 kg daily which could limit peak milk production by 1.0 - 2.5 kg (Grant, 1993).

Water consumption can be estimated with the following equation (Murphy et al., 1983; Murphy, 1992):

*Water intake (kg/d) = 15.99 + 1.58 * dry matter intake (kg/d) + 0.90 * milk production (kg/d + 0.05 * sodium intake (g/d) + 1.20 * weekly minimum temperature (°C).*

It is very important to note that cows will drink about 14 times every day, independent of milk production level, dry matter intake level, or parity (Dado and Allen, 1994). It is also important to note that the length of time for each drink is very short, about 1.3 minutes. Cows prefer to eat, drink, eat, drink in an alternating pattern (Nocek and Braund, 1985). They also like to drink immediately after being milked.

If cows are deprived of water or water is not available in sufficient quantity or quality, cows will loose body weight and dry matter intake and milk production will decrease (Little et al., 1984). Therefore, it is important to pay attention to factors that have been shown to influence drinking behavior. They include eating pattern, water temperature, the way water is provided (trough or water bowl), flow rate into water bowls, animal dominance if bowls are shared, and stray voltage (Murphy, 1992; Grant, 1993). Important environmental factors modulating water consumption of dairy cattle are DMI, nature of the diet, milk production, temperature and humidity. High environmental temperatures increase and a high humidity decrease water intake. The latter is due to a decrease in evaporation (Murphy, 1992).

* **Water accessibility**

Lactating dairy cows require 2.2 - 2.5 kg of water per kg of milk produced (Grant, 1993). Water needs to be accessible to all cows when they need a drink. There can be many different causes for a problem with water accessibility:

1. Not enough waterers for the cow population. There should be at least one waterer per 20 cows (Grant, 1993),
2. Inappropriate location of waterers,
3. Inadequate size of waterers,
4. Inadequate recovery capacity of the water system due to low water pressure,
5. Inadequate water quality.

The major indicator of water accessibility problems is manifested when cows congregate around the waterer. Any one or more of the reasons listed above could be the cause. The times and conditions when cows congregate around the waterer need to be identified and corrected. In hot weather when water consumption goes up, it is often very beneficial to place a water tub in the alley where the cows return from milking. This will take the pressure off the water system in the barn area. Some milk producers in the USA are putting water troughs in milk parlors so the cows may drink as they are being milked.

Water pressure can be evaluated by measuring how long it takes to fill a 7.5 liter bucket during peak water usage times (usually around milking). If it takes longer than 20 seconds, something needs to be done to improve water pressure in the system.

* **Water quality**

Providing insufficient water or water of poor quality to dairy cattle can limit milk production and growth and can cause health problems. Improving water quality may not have the same impact that improving forage quality will have, but it will boost production and profit.

Cows are sensitive to poor water quality (Table 7). Water quality problems can occur with wells and springs, especially when associated with poor environmental management. Cows allowed to drink from surface water sources such as ponds and creeks are potentially at risk for bacteria and cropland runoff containing chemicals. Often it is best to fence-off these areas for better cattle health. Most water problems come from bacteria, acidity, or excessive sulfates and nitrates .

High water levels of sulfate (> 2500 mg of sulfate/liter) may induce decreased feed and water consumption and induce diuresis (Wheet and Hunter, 1971). High magnesium levels may cause diarrhea and increase dietary requirements for selenium, vitamin E, and copper. It also may change the dietary cation anion difference (DCAD) in the

*Table 7. Analysis of water supplies (Adapted from: Adams, R.S. 1986. Water quality for dairy cattle. Pennsylvania State University)*

| Item | Ave. (ppm) | Expected (ppm) | Possible cattle problems if |
|---|---|---|---|
| pH | 7.0 | 6.8 - 7.5 | < 5.5; > 8.5 |
| Dissolved solids | 368 | < 500 | > 3,000 |
| Total alkalinity | 141 | 0 - 400 | > 5,000 |
| Sulfate | 35.5 | 0 - 250 | > 2,000 |
| Fluoride | 0.23 | 0 - 12 | > 2.4 |
| Calcium | 60.4 | 0 - 43 | > 500 |
| Magnesium | 13.9 | 0 - 29 | > 125 |
| Iron | 0.8 | 0 - 0.3 | > 0.3 (taste) |
| Manganese | 0.3 | 0 - 0.05 | > 0.05 (taste) |
| Copper | 0.1 | 0 - 0.6 | > 0.6 - 1.0 |
| Arsenic | | 0 - 0.05 | > 0.2 |
| Cadmium | – | 0 - 0.01 | > 0.05 |
| Mercury | – | 0 - 0.005 | > 0.01 |
| Lead | – | 0 - 0.05 | > 0.10 |
| Nitrate as NO3 | 33.8 | 0 - 10 | > 100 |
| Nitrate as NO2 | 0.28 | 0 - 0.1 | > 4.0 to 10.0 |
| Hydrogen sulfide | – | 0 - 2 | > 0.1 (taste) |
| Barium | – | 0 - 1 | > 10 (health) |
| Zinc | – | 0 - 5 | > 25 |
| Total bacteria/100 ml | 336,000 | < 200 | > 1,000,000 |

dry cow diets. Water with high iron levels may increase the need for dietary copper. Nitrates (> 40 ppm) in water and certain forages may be toxic for cattle. When they are converted to nitrites by rumen microorganisms. Nitrites convert hemoglobin into methemoglobin which may lead to respiratory distress and asphyxation (Harris and Amstutz, 1980). Water with pH less than 5.5 may increase problems related to mild acidosis such as: reduced milk yield, depressed fat content, low daily gains, and off-feed problems (Grant, 1993). High calcium levels in the water may interfere with levels of calcium in the diet of the dry cow and create metabolic problems such as milk fever (Van Saun, 1991).

## 4.2.7 CLINICAL INSPECTION

The clinical inspection performed by the HH & PM practitioner is directed at identifying animal risk factors in the field of health, nutrition, reproduction, etc., that directly or indirectly influence milk production. A clinical inspection starts with examining the disease data recorded in the farm diary. What is the incidence of milk fever, retained placenta, feet/leg problems, metabolic diseases, etc. since the last farm visit? One has to realize that clinical cases only form the tip of the iceberg, which means that subclinical cases may have a much greater impact on milk production. The next step in clinical inspection consists of observing the incidence of nasal, ocular, and oral discharge, alertness of cows, eating or ruminating activity, etc. From behind the cows, the haircoat is examined for the presence of parasitic infections and other abnormal skin conditions, cleanliness of cows, dampness of the haircoat, and average hair depth. Cows are examined for abnormal vaginal discharge, rumen fill, lameness, extreme body condition, fecal consistency, etc. The mammary glands are examined for broken ligaments, teat lesions, milk leaking, etc. The weight of cows in the various production groups is estimated and body condition is scored. Appropriate biological samples should be taken for disease monitoring and metabolic profile tests. Diseased individual cows should be, physically examined and blood, urine, milk, and/or feces samples taken for laboratory examination if indicated. Diseased cows will be treated instantly.

### Gross examination of feces

The gross appearance of fresh feces is not only an indicator of disease of the digestive tract, but can provide valuable clues on the nutritional status of cows in a herd (Skidmore, 1990). Representative samples need to be obtained from cows on each different ration to be evaluated. Only fresh, undisturbed piles of feces should be evaluated. Caution must be taken because several different rations or nutritional groups can be within the same physical group. Any way of selectively feeding cows in a group such as computer of magnetic feeders, feed offered in the parlor, or other ways constitutes a different ration even though the bunk space may be shared.

The consistency of fresh feces is dependent on water and fiber content, type of feed, and passage rate. Normal bovine feces is of a medium porridge-like consistency.

A moderate thickening leads to the passage of fecal discs of a more solid consistency and very high fiber diets or severe dehydration causes the formation of firm balls of feces arranged in facets inside the rectum, the surfaces of which are dark and coated with mucus. The feces of cows with displaced abomasum are often pasty in appearance. Sticky and tenacious manure is commonly seen in the obstruction of the forestomachs (vagus indigestion and chronic peritonitis).

A scale of 1 to 5 can be used to score fecal consistency and evaluate nutritional management when no disease is present or concurrent at the time of evaluation (Skidmore, 1990).

**Score 1.** A score of 1 represents very liquid feces that has the consistency of pea soup. In the absence of disease, this may indicate that there is too much degradable protein or starch in the diet. The excess protein is being digested and urea is being excreted not only in the urine but is recycled into the hind gut. The excess urea in the hind gut creates an osmotic gradient and draws water into the gut creating diarrhea. Excessive feeding of some minerals, such as potassium, can also create an osmotic gradient causing diarrhea.

**Score 2.** A fecal score of 2 means that feces is runny and does not form a nice pile. This score is typical of what might be seen from cows that are grazing lush pasture. It indicative of a low fiber diet with a relatively high amount of degradable protein. Cows consuming low fiber diets may have greater dry matter intake which can result in a faster rate of passage. The increased rate of passage will increase rumen escape of starch (Ireland-Perry and Stallings, 1993) and of degradable protein to the hind gut where it may be fermented. Fecal matter will have a higher content of water when excessive fermentation in the hind gut occurs. It also may lead to loss of starch and nitrogen in feces.

**Score 3.** A score of 3 has a porridge-like consistency and has a plopping sound as it hits the ground or the floor. Another way to evaluate a condition score of 3 is to stick the toe of your boot into the pile and see if it will stick to the end of your boot. This is indicative that the protein and water balance are in line.

**Score 4.** A score of 4 is a moderate thickening of the feces. It is dry enough that it will not stick to your boot, but yet does not bounce off either. This would be typical of what is seen with many dry cow and heifer rations consisting of predominately hay and no or very low amounts of grain. Cows consuming high fiber diets will have lower starch intake and also potentially slower rumen passage rates, leading to greater diet digestibility and reduced losses of starch and other potentially digestible materials to the lower tract and feces (Ireland-Perry and Stallings, 1993).

**Score 5.** A score of 5 represents firm fecal balls. This would indicate a diet consisting of only straw or extreme dehydration if there is no pathology in the gastrointestinal tract.

Both fecal scores of 4 and 5 indicate high fiber diets connected with a potentially longer rumen retention time and thus a slower passage rate. These scores also may indicate that there is not enough degradable intake protein (DIP) or soluble intake protein (SIP) in the ration creating poor fiber digestion.

*Figure 2. Chart to facilitate recording of feces scores*

Date ____________________ Farm ______________________________

______________________________

| Score | Ration 1 "high cows" | Ration 2 "dry cows" | Ration 3 | Ration 4 |
|---|---|---|---|---|
| 5 | | | | |
| 4 | I | III | | |
| 3 | III | IIII | | |
| 2 | IIII | | | |
| 1 | | | | |

Scored by: ______________________________________________

It is recommended that feces have a score of about 3 for all lactating cows, dry cows and heifers. Typically dry cows and heifers will score about a 4 because they are being fed a lower quality feed, but if they are scoring a 4, then their nutritional needs are probably not being met for what is currently recommended that dry cows and heifers be fed. Early lactation cows should score a low 3 to insure adequate nutrition to reach potential peak milk yields. Dry cows and heifers should score a high 3 to achieve their nutrient requirements without over-feeding protein.

A feces consistency scoring chart is presented in Figure 2. When examining a fecal pile, simply put a slash mark in the appropriate cell. The chart will provide a visual representation of the distribution and central tendency of fecal scores for each ration.

**Particles and their size in feces**

The proportion of large plant particles in feces is dependent on the duration and thoroughness of rumination and the rate of passage of ingesta through the fore-stomach. The length of time the digesta is in the post-ruminal digestive tract seems to have no appreciable influence on particle size. Large particles in feces indicates failure in rumination and/or accelerated passage of ingesta through the forestomachs. In some cattle with acute traumatic reticuloperitonitis, the feces may contain small 2 - 3 cm sized chunks of undigested plant fibers which presumably have escaped the cellulose digestive processes of the forestomachs. The presence of grain in the feces is associated with the ingestion of large quantities of grain, failure in rumination, and/or accelerated passage of ingesta through the forestomachs.

Examining fecal samples for particles and particle size requires close examination.

The quantity and quality of the grain must be examined. Corn kernel shells must be distinguished from whole or partial kernels of corn. Corn from silage must also be distinguished from corn grain to properly diagnose the source of the problem. The size of the corn particle and how hard it is will help distinguish between the two. The corn silage kernels will usually be whole kernels that should smash between thumb and finger. Ground kernels are easily missed in the feces and require close inspection.

Forage particle size in the feces should not exceed 0.7 cm in length. To assess forage particle size, fecal samples must be washed to visualize them. This can be done by putting the sample in several layers of cheese cloth or an old milk filter (sock filter works best) or an old nylon stocking and running a hose through it until the water comes out clear. If an excessive amount of larger particles are present, there is a problem with rumination and/or accelerated passage of ingesta through the forestomachs.

An excessive amount of large fecal forage particles may indicate too finely chopped forage causing accelerated passage of ingesta. It also may support a diagnosis of "slug" feeding causing incomplete digestion or inadequate rumen degradable intake protein (DIP) necessary to support the fiber digesting microbes in the rumen resulting in incomplete fiber digestion.

Processing, particle size, and moisture level of grains included in the diet will impact digestion and must be considered when evaluating why they are present in feces. If processing, particle size, and moisture level of the grains in the diet are appropriate, it may indicate disruptive feeding behavior and/or rumen mat integrity has been compromised.

**Amount of feces**

In adult cattle, the passage of ingesta through the digestive tract takes 1.5 - 4 days. Mature cattle generally pass some feces every 0.5 - 2 hours, amounting to a total or 30 - 50 kg/day in 10 - 24 portions.

**Color of feces**

The color of feces is influenced by: the nature of the feed, concentration of bile, and passage rate through the digestive tract. The feces of adult cattle on fresh green forage are dark olive green and on a hay ration they are more brown olive. The ingestion of large amounts of grain produces gray olive feces. A retardation of passage causes the color to darken and the manure becomes ball-shaped and dark brown with a shining surface due to a coating of mucus. Diarrheic feces tends to be more pale than normal because of higher water content and lower concentration of bile.

Hemorrhage into the digestive tract, depending on the amount, location, and rate of passage will result in feces which varies in color from chocolate brown to blackish-tarry (melena). Hemorrhage in the abomasum and small intestine usually causes black, tarry feces. Hemorrhage in the rectum usually causes a red-brown discoloration distributed throughout the manure or red streaks of frank blood adhering to the fecal particles (dysentery).

## Odor of feces

Fresh bovine feces is not normally malodorous. Objectionable odors are usually due to putrefaction or excessive starch fermentation in the large intestine. The feces in cattle with salmonellosis can be fetid.

## EPILOGUE

There are many factors that influence milk yield. None of these factors are independent but are all interrelated. A good understanding of those interactions will help to understand the complexity of milk production management. These factors must be constantly monitored and evaluated to economically optimize milk production. Monitoring and analyzing milk production can best be accomplished within the framework of a HH & PM program. Data recording and analysis, as well as a farm and clinical inspection, are fundamental to such a program. It is the task of the HH & PM practitioner and farm advisor to become knowledgeable and persistent detectives to manipulate milk production in the most profitable manner. To be successful, potential risk factors have to be known and skills to analyze data must be present.

The factors listed in this chapter are not meant to be complete but a fundamental base. New factors and technology are being discovered all the time.

*For references see part 3 of this Chapter.*

# APPENDIX

## RULES OF THUMB FOR FEEDING

The following nutritional thumbrules for early-lactation cows used by feed manufacturers, consultants and extension personnel across the United States of America are adapted from Mahana (1993).

Anticipating nutritional problems will be more important as we set our goals for ever higher production. Thumbrules certainly will not replace the specific nutritional advice given by competent nutritionists, but they can act as a "yardstick" to help us track areas of potential concern.

**Abbreviations used in feeding**

| | | | |
|---|---|---|---|
| ADF | Acid detergent fiber | Mcal | megacalories |
| BUN | blood urea nitrogen | MUN | milk urea nitrogen |
| BW | body weight | NDF | neutral detergent fiber |
| Ca | calcium | NE – l | net energy of lactation |
| cfu | colony forming units | NFC | nonfiber carbohydrate |
| DIM | days in milk | P | phosphorus |
| DIP | degradable intake protein | pH | acidity |
| DM | dry matter | ppm | parts per million |
| DMI | dry matter intake | SIP | soluble intake protein |
| FCM | fat corrected milk | TCL | theoretical length of cut |
| IU | international units | TMR | total mixed ration |
| | | UIP | undegradable intake protein |

**How much cows should eat...**

A. Cows should reach **maximum** daily dry matter intakes (DMI) no later than 10 weeks after calving.
B. Cows should be eating at least 4% of their body weight (BW) per day at peak intake. Example: 1350 lbs (612 kg) cow x 4% = 54 lbs (24.5 kg) dry matter intake per day. (1 lb = 454 g).
C. Cows milked three times per day will eat about 5 to 6% more dry matter per day than if milked two times.
D. With proper feeding, estimate dry matter intake in pounds as:

**DMI (lbs.) = A * .02 * (lbs. of BW) + .3 (lbs. FCM/day) + B (lbs. gain day),**

where A (days in milk adjustment) = 1.0 - .2 * [(80-DIM)/80], FCM (4% fat corrected milk) = (lbs. milk * .4) + (lbs. milk * % fat)* 15, and B (gain adjustment) = 1.0 if cow is gaining weight and 0 if losing weight.

**Example:**
**DMI for a 1350 - pound (612 kg) cow milking 100 pounds (45 kg) of 3,6% milk, 70 days in milk and losing weight =**

**1.0 – .2 [(80-70)/80] * .02(1350) + .3[(100*.4)/[(100*.036)*15] + 0 = .975 * 27 + 28.2 + 0 = 54.5 pounds (24.8 kg) DMI per day.**

- For every 2 pounds (0.91 kg) of expected milk production, cows should eat at least 1 pound (0.45 kg) of dry matter. Eating less than this causes excessive body condition loss and cows are more prone to metabolic disorders.
- Cows usually will eat after milking so have fresh feed available in the feed bunk or manger immediately to encourage higher DMI. High-producing cows will eat up to 12 meals per day each averaging 23 minutes. Adapt your feeding program to the eating behavior of your cows.
- If possible, provide separate milking/feeding string for heifers. First-calf heifers will spend 10 to 15% more time eating when housed separately from older cows.
- The best total ration dry matter is between 50 and 75%. Wetter or drier rations limit consumption. If silage is fed heavily, expect dry matter intake to decline 0.02% of body weight for every 1% increase in total ration moisture above 50%. This is due to wetter feeds fermenting longer raising acid levels and protein degradation products. Example: 60% moisture ration (40% dry matter) - 50% upper limit = 10 x 0.02% x 1350 lbs. (612 kg) cow = 2.7 lbs. (1.2 kg) less DMI/day causing up to a 5 to 6 lbs. (2.3 to 3.1 kg) drop in daily milk.
- If using a TMR mixer with weigh scales, check silage moistures on a routine weekly basis with a microwave/gram scale to ensure weighing in the proper amount of silage dry matter. Provide a chart in the feed room as to how much silage to add, depending on silage moisture levels. Silage moisture changes can alter the forage:grain ratio of the ration causing cows to go off-feed and lowered fat test.
  If intakes are below normal, begin by checking the nonfiber carbohydrate (NFC) and fiber length levels in the ration. Also, check water intake and whether feed is moldy.
- Expect cows to reduce dry matter consumption about 3.3% for every 2.2°F rise in temperature over 75°F (24°C). Cows begin to experience heat stress when temperature exceeds 80°F (27°C), relative humidity exceeds 80% or the two added together exceed 140.
- Provide clean water within 15 m of the feed bunk. Expect cows to drink about 1.9 liters for each pound of milk. Periodically check waterers for stray voltage. If water tests indicate high bacterial counts, consider water chlorination.
- Consider feed bunk/manger design. Cows spend more time eating, waste less feed and produce more saliva to buffer the rumen when forced to eat in a grazing-like, head-down position.
- Feed at least 60% of the ration at night during hot weather.
- Silage pH (acidity) should be less than 4.2 for corn or cereal silages and less than 5.0 for legume silages. Silages with higher pH (less acid) are more prone to excessive spoilage and poor bunk life.

- Feeds with mold counts in excess of 10,000 colony forming units (cfu) per gram may cause digestive upsets. Counts are of little use unless the individual molds are identified. Mold growth does not automatically indicate mycotoxins are present. Test for mycotoxins if dangerous mold populations have been identified in the feed.
- Feed should be available to cows at least 20 hours per day. Try to manage so it takes less than 3 hours total per day to feed cows.
- Provide each cow 60 to 75 cm of bunk space. Sweep feed bunks or mangers clean daily, especially during hot weather.
- Encourage eating by sweeping up feed, routinely getting cows up to eat and providing periods of light during evening hours.
- Income over feed costs is a more important profitability measure than simply monitoring feed costs per hundred weight (45.36 kg) of milk.

**Look at peaks...**

- Cows should peak in milk at 5 to 7 weeks.
- First-calf heifers should peak within 25% of older cows.
- For each extra 1 pound of milk at peak, a cow will produce 200 to 225 pounds (91 to 103 kg) more milk for the entire lactation.
- If cows are not peaking as expected, check protein. If cows are peaking well but not persistent, check energy.
- After peak milk, heifers will drop about 0.2% milk per day, and older cows will drop about 0.3% milk per day (or 3% every 10 days). High-genetic-potential cows tend to peak higher, reach that peak later and show more persistency.
- Summit milk (average of highest two milk yields during first three DHI tests) should be within 5 pounds (2.3 kg) of the average milk yield of all cows fresh less than 100 days. Greater differences indicate problems with maintaining early-lactation production.
- Milk protein:fat ratios should be near 0.90 for Brown Swiss and Milking Shorthorns, 0.85 to 0.88 for Holsteins and Ayrshires and near 0.80 for Guernseys and Jerseys. Higher values could indicate fat test problems. Lower values could mean protein test problems from too much fat or too little total or undegraded protein in the ration.
- When feeding to improve milk components, milk fat will respond the most, protein will change much less and lactose hardly will change at all.
- To maximize protein test, rumen bacterial growth must provide adequate protein/aminoacid production to the small intestine. Watch protein ration levels, degradable intake protein (DIP); soluble intake protein (SIP); undegradable intake protein (UIP) and rumen fermentable carbohydrates (NFC) . This also will help reduce protein test problems associated with supplementing fat.
- To boost fat test, maximize forage intakes and the digestibility of forages by harvesting at proper maturities. The better the quality of forages the larger portion of the ration they will be able to provide. Also watch "effective fiber" so cud chewing is maintained to buffer the rumen.

- To improve fat test, balance the types of carbohydrates and their degradation rates. For example: Barley is more quickly fermented in the rumen than corn. Monitoring ration fiber levels and feed sequencing can help offset potential rumen acidosis problems with rapidly degraded grains or commodity feeds.
- To maintain fat test through the heat of the summer, encourage forage intakes by keeping feed fresh in the feed bunk, feeding more during evenings and considering additives such as direct-fed microbials and yeast cultures which can improve forage intake and digestibility. Buffers also can compensate for reduced buffering from lowered forage intake during hot weather.

**Target protein levels…**

- Provide 18 to 19% crude protein in the total ration. Excess protein is costly, will not significantly raise protein test and may reduce breeding efficiency.
- Provide 60 to 65% degradable intake protein (DIP) in the entire ration.
- Provide soluble intake protein (SIP) levels to equal about half (30 to 32%) of the DIP levels. This ensures readily available nitrogen for rumen bacterial growth.
- Provide undegraded (bypass) intake protein (UIP), levels of 35 to 40% in the total ration. The upper range is suggested if feeding supplemental fat. Fat is not metabolized in the rumen, thus reducing nutrients for microbial growth. To make up for less microbial protein flow to the intestines, higher levels of bypass protein are required.
- Blood urea nitrogen (BUN) levels exceeding 25 mg % or milk urea nitrogen (MUN) levels over 20 mg %) may indicate improper ration formulation for degradable and undegradable protein. Conception may be affected.
- In corn silage or corn-based rations, restrict corn by-product feeds as a source of undegraded protein. Consider meat and bone meal, blood meal, heat-treated soybean products or dried brewers' grains to provide potentially limiting amino acids such as lysine and methionine. Commercial "blends" of protein sources attempt to prevent amino acid deficiencies.
- For cows milking more than 75 pounds (34 kg) of 4% fat corrected milk per day (79 pounds (36 kg), 3.7%), consider providing 1 pound (0.45 kg) of protein from an animal or marine source to lower the risk of amino acid and peptide deficiencies.
- Silage with nitrate levels up to 4,000 ppm nitrate-nitrogen should be diluted with other low-nitrate feeds to achieve 1,000 ppm or less concentration in the total ration available to cattle.

**Fiber for rumen health…**

- Forage dry matter consumption should be near 2% of the cow's body weight (BW). Example: 1,350 pound (612 kg) cow x 2% = 27 pounds (12.2 kg) dry matter from forages.
- Provide at least 19 to 21% acid detergent fiber (ADF) in the total ration. Levels at 17% are adequate for high-corn silage-based rations or herds using total mixed

rations.

- Provide at least 28 to 30% neutral detergent fiber (NDF) levels in the total ration.
- Make sure that forages provide at least 21% NDF in the total ration DM. Boost this to 24% if corn silage makes up more than one-fourth of total forage dry matter. **Example: If forages in the ration average 44% NDF, then 21%/44% = 47.7% of the total ration DM should come from forages.**
- Forage NDF should be about 0.9% of body weight. Example: 1350 pound (612 kg) cow x 0.9 = 12.15 pounds (5.5 kg) of ration NDF supplied by forages.
- Make sure that 65 to 75% of the total ration NDF is supplied by forages.
- The maximum pounds of total ration NDF should be about 1.25% of BW. Example: 1350 pound (612) kg cow x 1.25% = 16.8 pounds (7.6 kg) NDF. 16.8 pounds (7.6 kg)/total DMI is upper % NDF in the ration. 16.8 (7.6 kg) NDF/ 54 pounds (24.5 kg) typical DMI = 31% upper limit for % NDF in the total ration. Exceeding these NDF levels may result in lower dry matter consumption.
- Provide at least 5 pounds (2.3 kg) of fiber per day (by weight) that is more than 1-1/2 inches (2.5 - 1.25 cm) long. Underfeeding of "effective" fiber can cause off-feed and milk fat test problems.
- Rumen pH should be above 6.0. A lower pH (more acid) could limit fiber digestion and protein synthesis, and the potential for acidosis could cause reduced feed intake.
- Fiber particles should be long enough to stimulate 15 minutes of cud-chewing time per pound (0.45 kg) of dry matter. This will provide a cow eating 50 pounds (22.8 kg) of dry matter with 35 to 40 gallons (132 to 151 liters) of saliva production to buffer the rumen environment.
- Silages should be chopped at 3/8 to 1/2 inch (.95 to 1.3 cm) theoretical length of cut (TLC), to ensure that 15 to 20% of the silage particles are more than 1 - 1/2 inches long. Finer-chopped silage do pack better in storage structures, but high-silage-based rations need adequate particle length to stimulate rumen buffering from cud chewing.
- Sodium bicarbonate, or its buffer equivalent, should be added at 0.75% of the total ration dry matter, especially in high-corn-silage or high-moisture-corn rations. Example: 50 pounds (22.7 kg) dry matter x 0.75% = 0.170 kg.

**To meet energy needs...**

- Energy density of your top cow ration should be up to 1.7 megacalories (Mcal) net energy of lactation (NEL) per kg of dry matter in rations containing no added fat, up to 0.80 Mcal NEL for rations with added fat and up to 0.82 Mcal NEL for rations adding ruminally inert (bypass) fat.
- If you're lead feeding, cows should be eating 6 to 8 pounds (2.7 to 3.6 kg) of grain at calving. Boost grain 1 to 2 pounds (0.45 to 0.91 kg) per day, from three days after freshening until you have reached desired grain levels.
- Don't feed more than 5 to 7 pounds (2.3 to 3.2 kg) of grain at any feeding. This reduces the changes in rumen acidity and prevents off-feed problems.
- At less than 40 pounds (18.2 kg) milk, grain intake for Holsteins and Brown Swiss should be about 0.45 kg grain (as fed) per 4 pounds (1.8 kg) milk, between 40 and

70 pounds (18.2 to 31.8 kg) it should be near 0.45 kg grain for each 3 pounds (1.4 kg) milk and above 31.8 kg it should be about 0.5 kg grain for each 2.5 pounds (1.1 kg) milk. Higher-solids breeds should receive about 0.45 kg grain per 3 pounds (1.4 kg) milk (up to 30 pounds (13.6) kg milk), 0.45 kg grain per 2.5 pounds (1.1 kg) milk 31 to 60 pounds (13.6 to 27.3 kg) and 0.45 kg grain per 2 pounds (.91 kg) milk (over 61 pounds (27.3 kg)).

- Grain intake should not exceed 60% of ration dry matter.
- If too much corn passes undigested into the manure, check grain level, extent of processing and harvest maturity (harvest corn silage at 1/2 to 2/3 milkline). Also check levels of DIP and SIP protein (important to rumen bacteria) and amount of fiber intake that's more than 1 - 1/2 inches (2.5 to 1.25 cm) long (important for the rumen mat).
- Provide nonfiber carbohydrate (NFC) levels of 35 to 42% in the total ration. NFC (by difference) = 100 - (% crude protein + % NDF + % fat + % ash). Providing excess sugars and easily fermented carbohydrates can result in acidosis and fat test problems.
- Provide between 30 to 40% starch in the total ration.
- Manure pH levels should not be less than 6.0. Lower pH (more acid) means excess starch is escaping the rumen and being fermented in the small intestines.
- Consider feeding added fat to cows milking more than 75 pounds (34.1 kg) of 4% FCM milk per day (79 pounds (35.9 kg), 3.7%). As production rises, it becomes more difficult for cows to physically consume enough feed to meet energy requirements. Older cows generally will respond better than 2-year-olds. Fat levels in excess of 5 to 6% of the ration are not recommended during the first five weeks of lactation. Supplement the first 1/4 pound (0.1 kg) in the transition ration, up to 1 pound (0.45 kg) at freshening and, if needed, additional fat after five weeks in milk.
- Limit total fat to no more than 7-1/2% % of the ration dry matter. Example: 4 pounds (1.8 kg) total fat in the ration per 55 pounds (25 kg) typical DMI = 7.2%. Too much fat interferes with fiber digestion and lowers fat test.
- Provide the same amount of fat in the ration as pounds of milk fat produced. Example: 100 pounds (45.4 kg) milk per day x 4% fat = 4 pounds (1.8 kg) milk fat and 4 pounds (1.8 kg) total fat in the ration.
- Provide one-third of fat in ration from normal ration feeds, one-third from oilseeds or fats and on-third from rumen inert (bypass) fats. Example: If 4 pounds (1.8 kg) of fat are to be provided in the ration, about 4 pounds (1.8 kg) x 33% = 1.3 pounds (0.6 kg) of fat should be from oilseeds such as whole cottonseed or soybeans. If soybeans are 20% fat, then 1.3 pounds (0.6 kg) / 20% = 6.5 pounds (3.0 kg) whole soybeans in the ration. Any additional fat should be provided by commercially available inert sources because they bypass the rumen.
- Boost calcium to 1% and magnesium to 0.3% of ration dry matter when feeding supplemental fat. Fats bind with calcium reducing calcium and magnesium availability.

**If feeding a TMR...**

- Total mixed rations (TMR's) conservatively can result in 2 pounds (0.91 kg) more fat-corrected milk per day for older cows and up to 4 pounds (1.8 kg) more milk for heifers from improved feed consumption and utilization. This will vary, depending upon the feeding program before switching to a TMR.
- A "poor man's TMR" consisting of blending forages and multiple feedings of grain (3 to 4x per day) can approximate the benefits of a TMR mixer. However, it is not quite as efficient or precise and may not allow for using or masking of more unpalatable commodity feeds.
- TMR mixers generally pay for themselves in 12 to 18 months through more milk, lower feed costs and improved animal digestive health.
- TMR's are only as good as the quality of the individual feed components. Forage quality and feed bunk life still are critically important.
- Base mixer capacity on 60 to 70% of the struck level capacity with a minimum requirement of 2.5 cubic feet (0.067 cubic m) per cow, assuming two feedings per day. Recommended mixing time is 3 to 6 minutes. Have magnets at feed-outs. Accurate scales are a must, and silage moistures should be monitored weekly. Several manufacturers have mixers with knives that permit the use of unchopped, long-stemmed hay.
- using a single-group TMR system in herds above 20,000 pounds (9100 kg) of milk may offer advantages in feeding simplicity, labor, cow movement and production potential but will result in more costly use of specialty ingredients and has the potential to overcondition some cows.
- Having two milking groups and a single dry group is workable for most herds. This also can be easily adapted to a tie stall barn by the use of a mechanized feed cart.
- To prevent digestive upsets, there should be no more than a 15% change in nutrient density between TMR groups. Early-lactation cows will rebound from off-feed problems and re-establish production much more quickly and easily than mid- to late-lactation cows.
- Cows moved to a new TMR group in later lactation usually drop in milk more than cows moved in early lactation. A workable system proven overseas challenges all cows for 45 days to establish milk potential. High-potential cows are maintained in the high group, and low cows are shifted to a lower TMR group.
- The range of cows within a TMR group should not exceed 20 to 25 pounds (9 to 11.4 kg) of 4% fat-corrected milk (22 to 27 pounds 10 to 12.3 kg), 3.7%).
- Balance TMR groups for milk production 30% above the actual average of a one-group system. 20% for a two-group system and 10% for a three-group system. This will challenge fresh cows and allow for replacing lost body condition in late-lactation cows.
- The use of electronic, computer grain feeders has advantages, especially for one- or two-group systems. However, cow requirements must be updated continually, and feeders must be serviced and monitored routinely for accuracy.
- When making TMR group changes, move as many cows at one time as possible, over-

feed slightly on move day and move at night when activity is lowest to reduce stress.

- With more than one TMR grouping, do not move cows solely based on production. Also, take into account body condition score, age and breeding status. High-producing cows and 2 year-olds may need to stay longer in the high string to allow for growth and replenishing of lost body reserves.
- If TMR rations are balanced correctly for fiber and energy, move fresh cows directly into the high group. A "transition" or "close-up" dry cow ration can assist in making this period of ration and environmental changes less stressful.
- University research shows no benefit of feeding haylage-based rations more than once a day… if the feed remains fresh in the feed bunk and crowded feed bunks are not an issue. If corn silage comprises more than 30% of the forage, rations should be fed two times per day, especially during hot, humid weather. Use of research proven silage additives can improve bunklife and palatability. Pushing up the TMR ration to cows three to four times per day also can help encourage consumption.
- Offer the TMR up to a 5 to 10% refusal. Less refusal is acceptable if eating behavior is normal and the refusal looks similar to the original TMR mix. Bunk sweepings should be analyzed and then reblended as a base mix for other milking groups or heifers. Watch mixing time when reblending as overmixing can reduce feed particle size.
- Don't overpredict a group's dry matter intake when starting to feed a TMR. This will cause lower than required nutrient density in the ration. Start balancing a TMR with intakes set 5% lower than estimated and raise feeding levels to a point of 5% refusal.
- In TMR herds with poor housing or environment, raise energy density for the ration (with better forages or fats, not more grain) to near 1.8 Mcal NEL per pound (0.45 kg) of ration dry matter to adjust for lowered intakes (3.5% of body weight). Reduce NFC to 30% and NDF to 25% in the total ration.
- If beginning a TMR with commodity feeds, evaluate more than cost. Consider handling and storage, variability, palatability and the loss of feed manufacturer's technical advice.
- Cows should freshen with body condition scores of 3+ or 4- (1, skinny: 5, fat). This should prevent metabolic problems from occurring after calving. Second-lactation "burn out" or "sophomore slump" often is due to a lack of condition on high-producing, first-calf heifers.
- Cows should not lose more than 1 body condition score (1 - 5 system) or more than 2 pounds (0.91 kg) per day during early lactation to reduce ketosis and breeding problems. One point of body condition score equates to about 56 kg of weight.
- 1 pound (0.45 kg) of body weight loss provides enough energy for about 6 to 7 pounds (2.7 to 3.2 kg) of milk but only enough protein for 3 to 4 pounds (1.4 to 1.8 kg) of milk.
- It requires 2.3 Mcal of net energy of lactation (NEL)(or 2.5 pounds (1.1 kg) shelled corn dry matter) to replace 1 pound (0.45 kg) of body weight loss. Use the tall end of the lactation to replace lost body condition. The cow is most efficient at replacing weight while still milking and is less prone to fatty liver problems that can

occur when trying to condition a diverse group of dry cows.

- If necessary, you can supplement grain during the dry period to improve condition of individual cows that are dried off when underconditioned. In larger dairies, two dry lots may be justified to separate cows with different needs.

**Minerals and vitamins...**

- Provide **at least** 3,960 international units (IU) of vitamin A per kg of ration dry matter daily. Example: 54 pounds (24.5 kg) DMI x 3,960 IU per kg = 97,020 IU per day.
- Provide **at least** 990 IU of vitamin D per kg of dry matter daily. Example: 54 pounds (24.5 kg) DMI x 990 IU per kg = 24,255 IU per day.

  Provide at least 15 IU of vitamin E per kg of dry matter daily. Example: 54 pounds (24.5 kg) DMI x 15 IU per kg = 368 IU per day. Many consultants supplement vitamin E at levels up to 500 IU per day to fresh cows and 1,000 IU per day to dry cows. Higher dry cow supplementation may help prevent some of the 20% of new mastitis infections that occur during the dry period.
- Provide 0.3 parts per million (ppm) of selenium in the ration dry matter. Parts per million can be converted to % by moving the decimal point four places to the left. Example: 54 pounds (24.5 kg) DMI x 908,000 mg/kg x 0.00003% = 7.4 mg selenium/day.
- Watch elevated potassium levels of over 1.0% in the total ration of dry cows fed grass-based rations due to binding of magnesium (tetany) and calcium mobilization interference causing milk fever, retained placenta and downer cow problems at calving.
- Provide elevated levels of potassium (1.5%), sodium (0.5%) and magnesium (0.35 %) in the ration during heat stress.
- Provide a nitrogen to sulfur ratio of 11-13.1 in the ration to meet rumen bacterial needs.
- Force-feed 1 ounce (28 grams) of trace-mineralized salt for maintenance and 28 grams of salt for every 30 pounds (13.6 kg) of milk to meet chloride requirements.
- For early-lactation cows, consider 25% of the mineral supplementation in the form of chelates, especially copper, cobalt, manganese and zinc (zinc methionine).
- For milk-fever-prone herds, limit dry cow calcium to less than 80 to 100 grams per day (0.5 to 0.7% of ration DM) and limit phosphorus to less than 45 grams per day (0.3 to 0.35% of ration DM). Hold the Ca:P ratio to less than 2:1 without exceeding phosphorus limits.
- For herds with milk fever problems that are unable to avoid feeding high-calcium dry cow rations, adjust the dry cow ration-anion balance to provide a negative level of milliequivalents (sodium + potassium - chlorine) per 100 grams of ration dry matter. Anionic salts such as ammonium chloride, ammonium sulfate and magnesium sulfate can be supplemented to keep dry rations high in anions like chloride, sulfur and potassium. Milking rations should strive for a positive 30 to 40 milliequivalent level.

# 4.3 MONITORING MILK PRODUCTION: DECISION MAKING AND FOLLOW-UP

Andy L. Skidmore[1], Arie Brand[2] and Charles J. Sniffen[3]

[1] Department of Animal Science, Michigan State University, East Lansing, MI 48824, USA
[2] Department of Herd Health and Reproduction, School of Veterinary Medicine, University of Utrecht, Yalelaan 7, 3584 CL Utrecht, The Netherlands
[3] W. H. Miner Agricultural Research Institute, P.O. Box 90, Chazy, NY 12921, USA

## 4.3.1 INTRODUCTION

Milk production forms the economic "heart" of a dairy farm. 80 to 90% of farm income results from milk sales. Veterinary practitioners and farm advisors must keep this in mind when they visit a dairy farm and make recommendations. In addition, one must realize that milk production is predominately regulated by three operational management functions: reproduction, health care and last but not least nutrition. They can be considered as "flywheels" of milk production. Reproduction offers the farmer the possibility to optimize the calving interval in relation to milk production and to improve the genetic make-up of his herd. Health care is the foundation whereupon optimal milk production is based. Nutrition delivers the daily "fuel" needed to live and to produce and takes a key role in milk production. All three "flywheels" need the daily attention of the farmer and therefore must be part of a veterinary herd health and production management (HH & PM) program, because they directly influence milk production and thus farm income.

Milk yield and milk composition can be indicators of either optimal or suboptimal conditions in nutrition, health care and even reproduction. For example abnormal fluctuations in rolling milk performance indices, may reflect responses to changes in management practices in any of these areas and/or changes in environmental conditions. For that reason milk production performance has to be monitored and evaluated continuously in order to optimize milk production and to make adequate decisions at proper times if indicated. Against this background, we shall discuss:

1. How milk production data can be monitored within a HH & PM program,
2. How information generated by the monitoring system can be interpreted to optimize milk production and related operational management functions.

## 4.3.2 MILK RECORDING AND MILK ANALYSIS

In many countries milk production and milk composition is monitored by Dairy Herd Improvement Associations (DHIA). For that purpose the kilograms of milk produced by individual cows are measured and composite milk samples of all lactating cows in the herd are collected by employees of DHIA at regular intervals. In addition a sample from the bulk milk tank is taken by an employee of the milk processing factory at every milk delivery. The collected milk samples are analyzed by milk quality control stations. The analysis normally includes protein, fat and lactose content, somatic cell and bacterial count, cleanliness, antibiotic residues, and freezing point. Other milk components such as: urea, acetone, antibodies against Leptospira, BHV1, Bovine Leukosis Virus, and many others can be assayed in milk. Milk has the advantage that it can be collected easily and at low costs within the framework of milk recording. This means that the importance of milk for not only monitoring production but also health will increase in the near future.

Milk recording and analyses data are used by: 1) milk factories to monitor milk quality and to pay the farmer for delivered milk, 2) dairy herd improvement associations to select bulls based on the milk production performance of their daughters, and 3) to monitor milk production performance, udder health, milking hygiene, metabolic diseases and last but not least nutrition, by farmers, HH & PM practitioners, and farm advisors.

Results of analyses of milk at the milk quality control stations are transferred by mail or electronically to: 1) the farmer, 2) Dairy Herd Improvement Associations, and 3) milk factories. Further processing of data is done by these organizations or by the milk quality control station itself.

## 4.3.3 DECISION MAKING BASED ON MONITORING, EVALUATION AND ANALYSIS OF MILK PRODUCTION AND RELATED DATA

The process of decision making in the operational management function of milk production, described in this chapter, reveals ongoing efforts directed at assessing and evaluating the milk production status of a given dairy herd and factors that influence milk production performance.

For decision making data are required. These include raw milk production data and clinical and farm inspection data. These have to be processed into performance indices and summarized into tables and graphs. As in other operational management functions, evaluation of milk production performance involves the comparison of actual performance indices with preset targets. Before concentrating on an example farm, the various sources of information that have to be included in the decision making process will be discussed.

### Sources of information

Decision making within the HH & PM protocol is based on interpretation of information derived from monitoring and evaluation of:

- herd and individual cow data collected by the farmer, which are retrospective in nature,

- actual clinical, and farm inspection data collected by the HH & PM practitioner and farm advisor during their farm visit,
- herd and individual cow data collected by external organizations (DHIA and others). This information is presented as:
  - milk testing (recording and analysis) reports,
  - milk receipts of the milk processing factory,
  - feed analysis reports.

As stated earlier many data have to be processed, summarized into tables and graphs. Examples of such data manipulation include:
- lactation curves/tables,
- a twelve-monthly list, or
- herd summary reports.

**Herd data collected by the farmer**

Herd data recorded in a farm diary by the farmer have already been discussed in part 2 of this Chapter. They may include clinical events such as the number and percentage of cows that experienced metabolic disease, displaced abomasum, off-feed syndromes, sudden drop in milk production, mastitis, or lameness. They are all indicators of suboptimal nutrition practices either in the dry and/or the lactation period or in health care that might influence milk production performance. This information must be integrated with the information derived from the clinical and farm inspection activities and from external data sources, such as DHIA. The ultimate goal is to arrive at a herd performance diagnosis in the area of concern.

**Clinical and farm inspection data**

Collection, storing, and processing of clinical and farm inspection data is the task of the HH & PM practitioner and/or farm advisor during or after each farm visit. The information derived from the farm inspection may be quantitative or qualitative. It always should include information on ration composition. The execution of a farm and clinical inspection and the type of information that can be derived from a farm and a clinical inspection have been described in detail in part 2 of this Chapter.

**Herd and cow data collected by external organizations: Milk testing report**

Milk testing reports including data on milk production and milk analyses from DHIA or comparable organizations become available periodically (usually every 3 - 4 weeks). The report lay-out may differ from country to country. These reports should be monitored and evaluated by both dairy farmers, HH & PM practitioners, and farm advisors on a regular basis. Rolling milk production and milk analysis performance indices, especially abnormal fluctuations in these indices, may reflect responses to changes in management practices, for example in nutrition and health care and/or changes in environmental conditions. The overall information may signal rising problems in the herd that need to be examined more closely during the next clinical and farm inspection.

## Milk Yield at Herd, Group, and Cow Level

Milk production performance data and indices can be summarized at the herd, group, and individual cow level. The main performance indices that should be examined during every farm visit are the most current and rolling averages of:
- milk yield,
- the herd standard cow (HSC) and other rolling indices,
- protein and fat percentage,
- somatic cell counts.

### Milk yield

The average milk yield per cow per day gives a general impression of the milk production level of the herd. However, the average yield is constantly influenced by herd factors such as days in milk (DIM), season of calving, and the parity of each cow, and irregularly by management factors and farm conditions such as changes in ration composition, dry matter intake, feed quality, grassland management, weather conditions, inconsistent milking intervals, etc. To differentiate between herd factors and management and farm condition factors, a standardized milk production calculation should be used. An example of a standardized milk yield calculation is the Standard Cow (SC) or Herd Standard Cow (HSC) index.

### Herd Standard Cow index

The SC calculation used in the Netherlands, adjusts actual milk yields of individual cows for DIM, parity and season of calving to a standard cow. This standard cow is 8 years old, calved in February, and is in the 2nd month of lactation. The corrected milk yield of every cow is then averaged across the entire herd to create a HSC index. This index indicates the potential production capacity of the herd if all cows were 8 years old, calved in February, and were in the 2nd month of lactation. By calculating the indexes, performance of individual cows, groups of cows or the herd as a whole, can be compared over time. The comparison is independent of parity, stage of lactation, or season of calving. This also can be done across herds. This means that farm management and farm conditions that influence milk yield performance can be assessed because deviations are no longer due to those common factors that have been adjusted for. In other words deviations in a HSC or Group Standard Cow (GSC) index must be caused by farm management factors such as ration composition, dry matter intake, feed quality, grassland management, weather conditions, inconsistent milking intervals, etc. Besides the Netherlands, some other countries already have developed standardized milk yield calculation indexes. An internationally accepted standard milk yield calculation index has not yet been developed.

*Table 1. HSC (Herd Standard Cow) and GSC (Group Standard Cow) values on a milk testing day*

| | | | | |
|---|---|---|---|---|
| # cows/1st parity cows | | = | 63/31 | |
| # dry cows | | = | 11 | |
| Average kgs milk per day | | = | 23.6 | |
| HSC kgs milk per day | | = | 37.0 | |
| | | | | |
| Cow parity 2+: | GSC | = | 36.6 | (n = 51) |
| 0 - 60 days: | GSC | = | 33.3 | (n = 9) |
| 61 - 120 days: | GSC | = | 38.0 | (n = 13) |
| 121 - 260 days: | GSC | = | 37.0 | (n = 29) |
| | | | | |
| Cow parity 1: | GSC | = | 37.6 | (n = 29) |
| 0 - 60 days: | GSC | = | 38.0 | (n = 8) |
| 61 - 120 days: | GSC | = | 37.7 | (n = 3) |
| 121 - 260 days: | GSC | = | 37.4 | (n = 18) |

## Monitoring, evaluation and analysis of the HSC index

The HSC index is monitored and compared with rolling values. Rolling values might be provided by the Dairy Herd Improvement Organization or may be produced with the help of specific computer software or just by keeping a 12-monthly list. When the HSC index has decreased by > 2 kg/day, further analysis needs to be performed. Such an analysis can be done at either the group or individual cow level. An example is given in Table 1.

The HSC index can be split into Group Standard Cow (GSC) indexes as presented in Table 1. The GSC index is calculated the same way as HSC except that only the cows in each respective group are averaged together instead of the entire herd. Data in Table 1 indicate that the GSC value of first parity cows is one kg higher than of older parity cows. This might be a sign of an adequate breeding policy and young stock rearing if it is consistent across time.

The group of cows with parity greater than 2 and 0 - 60 days-in-milk has a lower GSC value than first parity cows. This might be due to diseases or managerial factors such as nutrition in the dry period or environmental factors. It is the task of the veterinary herd health practitioner to detect the factors that cause the drop in milk production.

For monitoring milk production at the individual cow level, a frequency distribution of individual Standard Cow Values (SCV) can be used (Table 2). In the interpretation process, attention should be paid to the occurrence of a narrow or a wide distribution of standard cow values around the mean (37) and to the number of cows with a relatively low SC index. A wide distribution is indicative of suboptimal management. Low SC values might be due to diseases observed or not observed by the farmer.

In any case special attention should be paid to these cows during the clinical inspection of the herd.

*Table 2. Frequency distribution of individual standard cow values (SCV) on a milk testing date (Mean HSC = 37.0 kg). * First recording after freshening*

| | | | | | | | |
|---|---|---|---|---|---|---|---|
| | | 372 | | | | | |
| | | 371 | | | | | |
| | | 405 | 370 | | | | |
| | | 397 | 366 | | | | <= cow identification numbers |
| | 393 | 360 | 403 | | | | |
| | 392 | 343 | 396 | | | | |
| | 387 | 337 | 394 | | | | |
| | 384 | 330 | 376 | | | | |
| | 364 | 321 | 369 | | | | |
| | 362 | 315 | 407* | 361 | | | |
| | 354 | 308 | 404 | 357 | | | |
| | 333* | 300 | 401 | 355 | | | |
| | 324 | 283 | 399 | 353 | | | |
| | 319 | 273 | 398 | 347 | 373 | | |
| | 316 | 270 | 395 | 346 | 340 | | |
| | 313 | 260 | 391 | 331 | 338 | | |
| 380* | 378 | 285 | 23 | 390 | 323 | 329 | |
| 352* | 272 | 239 | 107 | 389 | 297 | 264 | |
| 345 | 92 | 225 | 95 | 388* | 133 | 128 | |
| 311 | 44 | 9 | 31 | 386 | 106 | 48 | |

| **SC** | **15** | **20** | **25** | **30** | **35** | **40** | **45** | **50** | **60** | **70** |
|---|---|---|---|---|---|---|---|---|---|---|

## 4.3.4 LACTATION CURVES

Milk production data of individual cows can be listed in a table or in a curve. They are very useful instruments to monitor trends in milk production performance of the herd over time. Lactation curves can be generated with the help of a computer program or manually. With automatic milk measuring devices in the milking parlor, recording milk yield of individual cows can be performed daily. The kgs of milk produced by individual cows on test days over a 4 to 5 month period are listed in Tables 3 and 4 and graphically presented in Figure 1. It offers the possibility to observe what peak yield and persistency is in the first half of lactation. For proper interpretation of lactation curves or tables, one has to correlate information from these curves or tables with management practices and environmental conditions that might be responsible for unwanted trends. Interpretation must be based on an adequate number of cows in order not to derive conclusions that won't be biased by one very good or very poor cow.

*Table 3. Milk yield of individual cows with a good peak yield and a poor persistency (P)*

| Cow | Calving date | Milk yield on test days (kg/day) | | | | | Parity | P |
|---|---|---|---|---|---|---|---|---|
| | | 10 - 24 | 11 - 15 | 12 - 5 | 1 - 5 | 1 - 27 | | |
| 182 | 9 - 28 | 46.5 | 41.9 | 42.0 | 36.6 | 33.0 | 5 | – |
| 33 | 9 - 29 | 43.4 | 33.4 | 38.4 | 32.8 | 30.7 | 7 | – |
| 221 | 9 - 29 | 38.8 | 39.0 | 39.5 | 37.8 | 36.8 | 4 | + |
| 247 | 9 - 30 | 52.5 | 49.8 | 44.1 | 41.0 | 38.7 | 4 | – |
| 43 | 10 - 3 | 29.6 | 38.4 | 34.7 | 30.8 | 28.9 | 6 | – |
| 152 | 10 - 3 | 44.4 | 60.3 | 51.0 | 50.1 | 49.3 | 5 | + |
| 301 | 10 - 26 | dry | 35.5 | 41.4 | 32.9 | 33.6 | 3 | – |
| 11 | 10 - 29 | dry | 37.4 | 46.1 | 41.0 | 37.2 | 8 | – |
| 305 | 11 - 3 | dry | 45.6 | 50.7 | 50.0 | 48.3 | 2 | – |

*Table 4. Milk yield of individual cows with a low peak yield and a good persistency (P)*

| Cow | Calving date | Milk yield on test days (kg/day) | | | | | Parity | P |
|---|---|---|---|---|---|---|---|---|
| | | 11 - 19 | 12 - 17 | 1 - 22 | 2 - 18 | 3 - 17 | | |
| 310 | 10 - 19 | 31.4 | 32.9 | 30.0 | 30.5 | 29.1 | 5 | + |
| 260 | 10 - 19 | 31.8 | 29.8 | 30.2 | 29.5 | 29.2 | 6 | + |
| 355 | 10 - 20 | 28.8 | 30.0 | 26.8 | 24.8 | 23.0 | 4 | – |
| 372 | 10 - 23 | 30.2 | 29.3 | 29.7 | 27.6 | 30.4 | 4 | + |
| 385 | 11 - 4 | 21.9 | 23.2 | 22.7 | 21.1 | 20.8 | 2 | + |
| 340 | 11 - 17 | dry | 32.2 | 29.0 | 28.1 | 26.7 | 3 | – |
| 307 | 11 - 20 | dry | 27.2 | 28.7 | 27.8 | 27.9 | 5 | + |

## 4.3.5 PROTEIN AND FAT CONTENT AT HERD, GROUP, AND COW LEVEL

In addition to milk yield, current protein and fat content, the sum of both, rolling values, and protein to fat ratio at the herd level should be monitored and evaluated against preset targets during every farm visit. Herd or group protein and fat content are very useful parameters to monitor nutrition practices and health performance.

### Herd level

Herd protein and fat content of milk can be obtained from the milk testing report, the milk factory receipt, or the weekly review of bulk tank milk deliveries. Weekly review of bulk tank milk deliveries offers the possibility to use more current and timely

*Figure 1. Lactation curves of cows with a good persistency and a poor persistency*

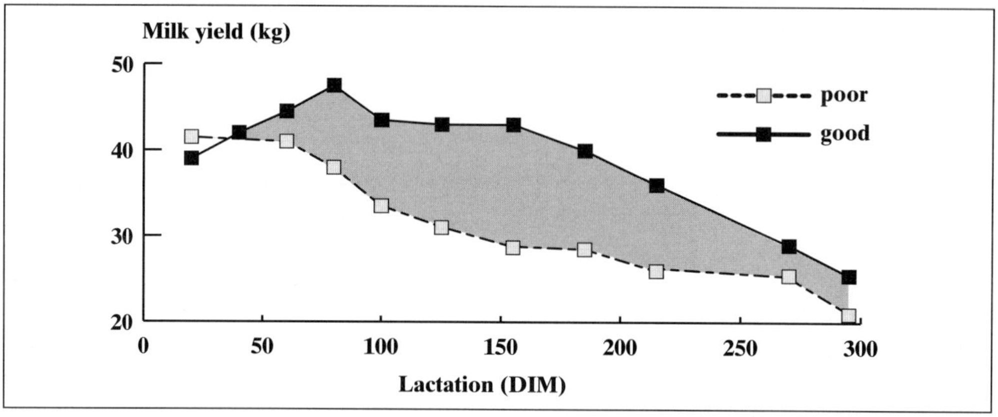


information. If cows are pastured during summertime, protein and fat content will be lower. This is the result of fluctuations in grass growth and quality due to variable weather conditions. In wintertime, cows are fed diets of a more constant quality, thereby reducing fluctuations. Although these changes can only be evaluated in a retrospective way, they enable the farmer to get a better understanding of his management. The lessons learned can be used for future management decisions. Figure 2 demonstrates a series of bi-weekly protein to fat ratios calculated from the milk factory receipts.

An economic optimal protein to fat ratio is dependent on the price of milk protein and fat and of feedstuffs required to reach that ratio. Many factors originating in managerial, climatic and farm conditions may influence this ratio. Special attention

*Figure 2. Overview of the protein to fat ratio of a herd. (* = protein/fat ratio, + = protein content)*

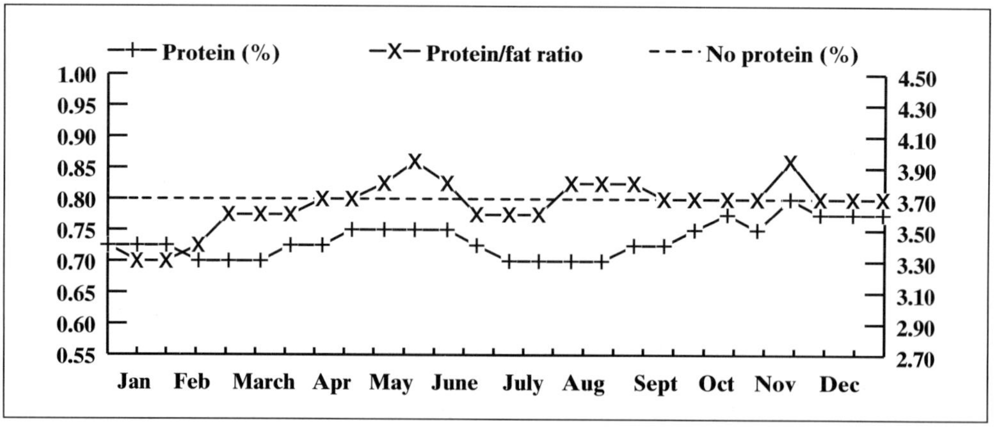

should be paid to energy and fiber content of feedstuffs. Many farms experience a low ratio when cows are pastured and a relatively high ratio when cows are housed (Figure 2). Nongrazing farms may show a more constant ratio over the year.

### Group Level

Protein and fat contents of the whole herd may hide milk production inefficiencies in certain production groups. To evaluate if there is a problem in a group, herd indices should be divided up into group indices and presented as rolling indices, even when the herd indices look normal.

The interpretation follows the same procedure as described for herd indices. Changes in levels and fluctuations most frequently are due to management practices, health status, and genetic make-up of individual cows in the group. As an example, group strategy may influence cow density in different pens where one group may be overcrowded and another group under populated resulting in nutritional challenges for all cows. These nutritional challenges could be manifested as abnormal fat and protein content of milk. Days in milk differences between groups also will manifest itself as differences in fat and protein content of milk.

### Cow Level

Individual cows on test should be evaluated for fat and protein content and somatic cell count in relation to days in milk. Protein and fat content are relevant indicators of metabolic diseases and high somatic cell counts for subclinical mastitis. The number of cows with a fat and protein content lower than a certain threshold level are counted. The cut-off point has to be defined for every breed and country due to different genetics and nutritional practices and must be based on experience for increased risk for metabolic diseases such as: ketosis, milk fat depression, and acidosis. Cows with a protein/fat ratio less than 0.60 and cows with a relatively low protein content should be examined for ketosis. Cows with a relatively low fat percent should be examined for rumen acidosis.

## 4.3.6 MILK FACTORY RECEIPT

The receipt from the milk factory provides information concerning:

- the kgs of milk delivered to the milk factory per delivery and per bi-weekly period,
- fat, protein, and lactose content of milk per delivery and average over a bi-weekly period,
- milk quality parameters such as: bulk milk SCC (BMSCC), total bacterial count from both a raw and preincubated sample, residues of antibiotics including sulfonamides, freezing point, etc. In addition, averages of milk constituents of all milk delivered by other farmers in the region might be presented. If herd fat and/or protein content have decreased, the milk factory receipt can be used in a retrospective

way to pinpoint the time the decrease started. This enables the farmer to relate the change to changes in management practices, especially nutrition, or on-farm conditions. This may help to prevent the problem in the future.

### 4.3.7 THE 12-MONTHLY LIST

From time to time, data from the farm diary, or clinical and farm inspection data have to be processed manually or electronically (VAMPP, Dairy Comp 305) into indices and transferred to a 12-monthly list (Table 5). They are combined with indices provided by DHIA and other organizations. The composition of the list is optional and can be adapted to local circumstances and wishes. On a 12-monthly list, the rolling milk production performance indices and fluctuations in these performance indices can be evaluated over time. This can lead to early diagnosis of impending problems which may be related to nutrition and/or health problems and/or management problems.

### 4.3.8 DECISION MAKING

Decision making is essentially a problem solving process. The first step in decision making is defining if there is a problem and if so, what is the problem. This consists of comparing data and information previously collected with preset targets defined by the farmer. If these targets are not well defined or communicated to the farm advisor or HH & PM practitioner the "wrong" problem may be resolved and no significant progress made. Appropriate definition of problems requires accurate judgment of the data and the information collected or how to get the data and information needed.

A mistake often made is defining the problem in terms of a proposed solution, "need more energy in the ration" rather than a preset target not being achieved, "milk yield is below and body condition loss is greater than preset targets". Another mistake often made is diagnosing a problem in terms of its symptoms, "the cows are too skinny". Problem solving, not elimination of temporary symptoms should be the focus of farmers, farm advisors and HH & PM practitioners. The biggest deficiency from poorly defined problems is that many potential solutions to the "true" problem are not considered.

The most difficult part of decision making is correctly defining what the problem is. Sometimes a more detailed data analysis and diagnostic workup has to be initiated to define what caused the deviation from preset targets. Such an analysis should include nutritional management, especially ration balancing and formulation, feeding strategy and a thorough clinical and farm inspection. The problem analysis protocol outlined in Chapter 1, part 1 and as demonstrated in Chapter 2, part 3 and 4 can help provide a guide on how to diagnose the problem. Problem check lists with potential causal factors are included as an aid to help define the problem. An optimum search to define the problem or cause of the problem continues only until the cost of the search outweighs the value of the added information.

*Table 5. Example of a 12-monthly list with some milk production performance indices and related indices on subsequent milk testing days*

| **Date farm visit** | **5 - 11** | **6 - 18** | **7 - 16** | **8 - 31** | **9 - 28** |
|---|---|---|---|---|---|
| **Date milk testing** | **5 - 7** | **6 - 7** | **7 - 8** | **8 - 20** | **9 - 21** |
| HSC | 43 | 43 | 41 | 41 | 40 |
| Milk yield kg | 28.2 | 27.1 | 27.3 | 28.0 | 25.5 |
| Fat % | 4.12 | 3.83 | 3.86 | 3.79 | 4.43 |
| Protein % | 3.48 | 3.34 | 3.32 | 3.31 | 3.39 |
| DIM | 173 | 182 | 166 | 144 | 135 |
| # in lactation | 47 | 41 | 39 | 43 | 52 |
| # < 100 DIM | 14 | 8 | 10 | 18 | 22 |
| # 1st parity cows | 16 | 16 | 14 | 17 | 24 |
| # dry cows | 8 | 13 | 12 | 10 | 8 |
| **Milk yield kg/day** | | | | | |
| < 61 DIM | 40.1 | 46.3 | 36.2 | 35.7 | 35.6 |
| 61 - 120 DIM | 37.5 | 36.1 | 41.9 | 38.7 | 34.1 |
| 121 - 210 DIM | 31.2 | 28.4 | 29.6 | 28.0 | 29.6 |
| > 210 DIM | 23.3 | 22.7 | 21.7 | 21.3 | 18.8 |
| **Fat %** | | | | | |
| < 61 DIM | 4.46 | 3.47 | 4.17 | 3.60 | 4.79 |
| 61 - 120 DIM | 4.07 | 3.86 | 3.63 | 3.49 | 4.15 |
| 121 - 210 DIM | 3.97 | 3.49 | 3.75 | 4.19 | 4.34 |
| > 210 DIM | 4.45 | 4.27 | 3.97 | 3.77 | 4.97 |
| **Protein %** | | | | | |
| < 61 DIM | 3.46 | 3.10 | 3.23 | 3.13 | 3.31 |
| 61 - 120 DIM | 3.32 | 3.22 | 3.06 | 3.17 | 3.31 |
| 121 - 210 DIM | 3.45 | 3.39 | 3.33 | 3.48 | 3.47 |
| > 210 DIM | 3.77 | 3.64 | 3.59 | 3.54 | 3.91 |
| # fat % < 3.8% | 12 | 18 | 15 | 18 | 7 |
| # protein % < 3.0% | 1 | 2 | 2 | 6 | 3 |
| BMSCC | 242 | 298 | 454 | 100 | 110 |
| # milk fever | | | 1 | 1 | |
| # ketosis | | | | 1 | |
| # displaced abomasum | | | 2 | | |
| # indigestions | 1 | | | | |
| # laminitis | | | | | |

Once the problem has been diagnosed correctly alternative solutions must be identified. An inappropriate amount of search time is often spent seeking alternatives, creating a barrier to effective decision making. As with defining the problem, the optimum search of alternative solutions continues only until the cost of the search outweighs the value of the added information.

Before the best solution can be identified the criteria by which the solutions will be compared must be identified. Such criteria could be: cost to implement, ease of implementation, likelihood of being successful, time required to observe results, potential lost income or milk, amount of labor required to implement, etc. The criteria will have varying importance to the decision maker. The decision maker will have assess the potential consequences of selecting each alternative solution based on each criteria.

Following these steps a logical decision can be reached by the decision maker. The decision maker is the farmer or owner of the business not the farm advisor or HH & PM practitioner. The farm advisor and HH & PM practitioner help the decision maker to define the problem, to evaluate criteria and potential solutions, and may help in evaluating the alternative solutions but they do not make the decisions.

**Example herd**

For the decision making process an example herd is created. This herd consist of 80 lactating cows, 15 dry cows and 50 young stock. The last year's annual milk production was 7000 kg of milk with 3.4% protein and 4.20% fat. The farmer is managing the farm himself. Cows are confined in a free-stall barn during wintertime and pastured in summer. In wintertime a total mixed ration is fed. Nutrients fed are wilted grass silage and corn silage, byproduct feeds (beet pulp and brewers grains) completed with concentrates to meet feeding standards. Milk recording is performed every 4 weeks. The farmer uses a nutritionist to balance and formulate rations at a regular basis. He also participates in a HH & PM service offered by his local practitioner. Daily data recording is done using a farm diary. Data from this diary are entered in a PC and processed by the VAMPP program (Noordhuizen et al., 1984). The preset targets for milk production are defined as follows:

1. an annual milk yield per/cow of 7500 kg,
2. a milk fat content of 4.40%,
3. a milk protein content of 3.40%,
4. a Bulk Milk Somatic Cell Count (BMSCC) of < 150.000 cells/ml, and a predicted calving interval of < 385 days.

The first step in decision making consists of comparing actual milk production performance indices with the preset targets as defined by the farmer. During the last three years information about milk production is stored in the VAMPP database. The indices needed to make the comparison with the preset targets can be retrieved from this database and from the 12-monthly list (Table 5). A retrospective evaluation of the milk production over the last half year reveals that average daily milk production amounts 26 kg. If milk production stays at this level for the rest of the year it can be expected that the target of 7500 kg milk per cow per year will be met. This is not the case with the fat and protein content of milk which are both below the targets of 4.40 and 3.40. The BMSCC is higher than defined in the preset targets. This all means that on short term measures have to be taken to reach the targets in the near future. For this purpose a more detailed data analysis and a diagnostic search has to be initiated to find factors that might be responsible for the deviation from preset targets. Such an analysis should include nutritional management, especially ration balancing and formulation, feeding strategy and a thorough clinical and farm inspection. In case this might not lead to a a diagnosis, the problem analysis protocol should be followed as outlined in Chapter 1, part 1 and as demonstrated in Chapter 2, part 3 and 4. To help to analyse the problem check lists with potential causal factors that might influence protein and fat content of milk in a negative way. For completeness a checklist of factors that might influence milk yield is also presented.

## 4.3.9 CHECKLIST OF FACTORS THAT AFFECT FAT AND PROTEIN LEVELS IN MILK AND MILK YIELD

### Factors Influencing Fat Content

Factors that influence milk fat content are:

- Days in milk (lowest fat percentage at peak lactation and highest at end of lactation). Fat content may be high at the beginning of lactation due to a suboptimal dry matter intake pre- and postcalving, followed by negative energy balance, and mobilization of body fat. Fat content decreases a few weeks after calving. This is caused by an increased intake of concentrates and a changing roughage to concentrate ratio. It may also be due to dilution with increasing milk yields. After peak yield when energy intake and energy output through milk is reaching an equilibrium, the fat content of milk rises again,
- Breed of cows (certain breeds have lower fat content than others; Holsteins vs. Jerseys),
- Rapid changes in ration composition, especially when the ration is inadequate in fiber,
- Feeding effects. Feeding effects on MFC are primarily related to changes in rumen fermentation. Rumen fermentation changes affect the acetate:propionate ratio. which is specifically dependent on the number and activity of cellulolytic microorganisms that ferment fiber. The primary fiber fermentation product by cellulolytic microorganisms is acetate. The primary starch fermentation product is propionate. The ratio between acetate and propionate influences fat content in milk. A wide ratio is responsible for a high fat content and a narrow ratio for a low fat content. The optimum molar ratio of acetate:propionate (A:P) in ruminal content for maintenance of milk fat percent is > 2.5 (Palmquist, 1994). To permit maximum growth and activity of cellulolytic microorganisms, rumen pH must be > 6.2.

  The acetate:propionate ratio is influenced by:

- Fiber quantity in the ration. A very important function of fiber is to let the cow ruminate and produce saliva to buffer the rumen. A rule of thumb is to provide total ration effective neutral detergent fiber (NDF) at 1% of body weight. If forage particle size meets the criteria below, total ration effective NDF can go to 0.8% of body weight. Three-fourths of the dietary NDF should be provided by forage. Dietary fiber is a primary regulator of chewing activity (Palmquist, 1994; Woodford et al., 1986),
- Particle size of forages. Fine particle size reduces ruminal pH, A:P ratio, milk fat percent, and increases plasma glucose and insulin (Grant et al., 1990a). 15 to 20% of the particles in a ration or 20 to 25% of forage particles should be greater than 3.5 cm in length.
- High grain, low forage diets. A low forage to concentrate ratio will depress MFC. These diets are characterized by low fiber, small particle size, and highly fermentable substrate. This will result in a high acid output and inadequate buffering from saliva, thus causing low ruminal pH (Palmquist, 1994).
- Feeding high amounts of concentrates and by-products that are rich in highly degradable starch. High amounts of highly degradable starch will cause milk fat depression and a decrease in short chain fatty acids. The depression of short chain fatty acids may be caused by increased uptake by insulin-stimulated adipose tissue (Sutton et al., 1988), or by specific inhibition of *de novo* synthesis by the high amount of trans-unsaturated fatty acids (Wonsil et al., 1994).
- Dietary fat. Large amounts of unsaturated oils have toxic effects on ruminal cellulolytic bacteria (Palmquist and Jenkins, 1980). This causes lowered ruminal fiber digestion and lower A:P ratio, resulting in a lower fat content in milk. Free unsaturated oils are converted in trans-unsaturated fatty acids which cause depression of milk fat synthesis in the mammary gland (Palmquist, 1994). Products high in unsaturated fats are extruded whole beans, fish meals, and leafy pasture grass.

**Factors influencing milk protein Content**

- Fat content of the diet. A high fat content of the diet may decrease milk protein content (MPC) (Cant et al., 1993a and 1993b), while adding limiting amino acids (Cant et al., 1993b) and undegradable starch to the ration may increase protein content, especially at the start of lactation,
- Acetonemia and hypocalcemia are associated with depressed milk protein (Distl et al., 1989),
- Increased nutrient delivery to mid and late lactation cows increases MPC (Klusemeyer et al., 1990),
- Forage to concentrate ratio in the diet. An increased forage content leads to depressed MPC (Klusemeyer et al., 1991),
- Days in milk of the herd. MPC increases slowly to the end of lactation from approximately post calving (Ng-Kwai-Hang et al., 1982),
- Cow age. After the third lactation a decrease of MPC is observed (Ng-Kwai-Hang et al., 1982),

- Farm management factors. In an observational study on 1,200 Dutch farms, Scholl (1992) found that farms with a high bulk tank milk protein content (BTMPC) differed from low BTMPC farms, among others in the following managerial and herd characteristics:
  - higher energy content of the grass silage fed,
  - use of high protein supplements in lactating cow rations (especially when corn silage diets were fed),
  - higher average adjusted individual daily milk yield,
  - participation in routine herd health veterinary services.

**Factors influencing milk yield:**

- Dry matter intake. (This directly influences milk yield because all the nutrients to produce milk and maintain the cow are contained in the feed she eats. Usually, farmers overestimate the quantities of feed they supply. Dry matter intake is influenced by many factors such as: selection of feedstuffs, changing weather conditions, changes in days in milk, diseases, ration composition, quality of feedstuffs, rate of digestion, rumen passage rate, and their respective interactions. For example, a high fiber or low quality diet has a slow digestion rate as well as a slow rumen passage rate. Therefore, dry matter intake will be low. In contrast, a diet that is lower in fiber or more digestible will increase passage rate and dry matter intake as long as the health of the rumen ecosystem is maintained,
- Feed quality (stability of feed in the feed bunk and palatability of feed ingredients)
- Total mixed ration vs. individual ingredient feeding and how well the feed is mixed,
- Feeding practices such as: frequency, quantity and sequence of feed delivery, and frequency of pushing-up feed,
- Quantity and quality of herbage in pasture,
- Physical facilities,
- Grouping management,
- Climatic conditions (outside and within the barn),
- Cow comfort,
- Management of computer/magnetic feeders,
- Social dominance, in relation to cow density and quantity of headlocks per cow,
- Milking frequency and milking machine/parlor maintenance
- Feed particle size,
- Number of watering devices, location and accessibility, waterer size and refill time, water quality and cleanliness, and cooling devices,
- Lighting intensity,
- Configuration and quantity of freestalls and maintenance of traffic areas with non-slippery surfaces,
- Bunk space per cow, quality of feedbunk bottoms and how long cows are locked up in head locks,
- Feedbunk space per cow, physical access to the feedbunk, time away from the feedbunk, elevated of the feed bunks, and time available to eat a meal,

- Stress due to physical handling of cows,
- Many diseases may impact milk production. Some diseases have a direct impact on milk production where others have a more indirect impact. For example, subclinical mastitis has a direct impact causing a decrease in milk secretion. Lameness has an indirect impact causing a decrease in dry matter intake resulting in lower milk production,
- Calving interval.

**Herd performance diagnosis**

The ultimate goal of the data analysis and clinical and farm inspection is to arrive at a herd performance diagnosis, followed by intervention and follow-up activities. Examples of herd performance diagnoses could be:
- low quality feeds,
- overcrowding and excess competition,
- poor bunk management,
- poor ration composition,
- Inadequate dry cow management,
- diseases, especially metabolic diseases such as fatty liver and ketosis.

It is beyond the scope of this Chapter to discuss in detail the various factors mentioned in the clinical and farm inspection parts. The procedure discussed was aimed to show the reader how to manage decision making.

Finally, the resulting information has to be translated to the farmer by both the veterinarian and/or the farm advisor in concise reports. Reports written by the HH & PM practitioner and farm advisor have to be delivered during or directly after the farm visit. The interval between data generation and feedback of information has to be very short but varies with the type of report.

## 4.3.10 FOLLOW-UP

In the follow-up process, the measures taken and advice given during the last or previous herd visits should be evaluated. If the results obtained are not satisfying, other measures should be considered.

## EPILOGUE

The milk recording and milk analysis report form the skeleton of a milk production monitoring program. At the farm level, the milk testing report is an external database for HH & PM practitioners and agricultural farm advisors to support farm management.

During a farm visit herd daily milk production, fat and protein content, the ratio between them, the average herd somatic cell count and if present the actual and rolling values of the Herd Standard Cow value, should be monitored. Milk yield, and protein and fat content of milk are very useful tools to monitor nutrition. These parameters are also indicators of metabolic diseases such as ketosis and rumen acidosis. The somatic cell count reflects udder health. The same milk production performance indices can be monitored, after proper data processing, for groups based on parity, stage of lactation or body condition. At the individual cow level milk production of fresh cows and cows at the end of lactation can be examined. The number of cows with a daily milk production > 30 kg, > 40 kg, etc., age at first calving, number of cows > 305 or 350 days in lactation, number of cows with a protein content < 3.00% or with a fat content < 3.8%, and number of cows with an individual cell count < 150.000, > 250.000 and/or > 500.000 cells per ml should be calculated (see Chapter 4). Peak yield and persistency of peak yield of individual cows can be visualized with tables or lactation curves. Peak yield and persistency are useful parameters to check management practices. In conclusion it can be stated that milk production performance is the mirror image of nutrition, so the farmer should always use milk performance data to monitor his nutrition practices. In cases of suboptimal milk production or milk composition, the herd health practitioner and farm advisor have to act as detectives to trace causes or risk factors that may be responsible. This can best be done within the framework of a herd health and production management support program. Deficiencies in managerial practices can then be detected at an early stage.

## REFERENCES

*Anonymous. 1990. Feeding dairy cows. Cooperative Extension Service. Kansas State University. Manhattan. Dairy Management Manual. A Western regional dairy Extension Project. 502.00- 502.16.*

*Bray, D.R. and R.Bucklin. 1996. Recommendations for cooling systems for dairy cattle. Cooperative Extension Service. University of Florida, Gainesville. Fact Sheet DS-29.*

*Cant, J.P., E.J. DePeters, and R.J. Baldwin. 1993a. Mammary amino acid utilization in dairy cows fed fat and its relationship to milk protein depression. J. Dairy Sci. 76:762-774.*

*Cant, J.P., E.J. DePeters, and R.J. Baldwin. 1993b. Mammary uptake of energy metabolites in dairy cows fed fat and its relationship to milk protein depression. J. Dairy Sci. 76:2254-2265.*

*Dado, R.G. and M.S. Allen. 1994. Variation in and relationships among feeding, chewing, and drinking variables for lactating dairy cows. J. Dairy Sci. 77:132-144.*

*Distl, O., A. Wurm, A. Glibotic, G. Brem, and H. Krauslich. 1989. Analysis of relations hips between veterinary recorded production diseases and milk production in dairy cows. Livest. Prod. Sci. 23:67-78.*

*Grant, R.J., V.F. Colenbrander, and D.R. Mertens, 1990a. Milk fat depression in dairy cows: Role of particle size of alfalfa hay. J. Dairy Sci. 73:1823-1833.*

*Grant, R.J., V.F. Colenbrander, and D.R. Mertens, 1990b. Milk fat depression in dairy cows: Role of silage particle size. J. Dairy Sci. 73:1834-1850.*

*Grant, R. 1993. Water quality and requirements for dairy cattle. Nebguide. G 93-1138-A. Published by Coop. Ext. Inst. of Agric. Nat. Resources. Univ. of Nebraska.*

*Harris, W.F. and H.E. Amstutz. 1980. Plant and Plant related poisonings. In: Bovine Medicine & Surgery. Ed. H.E. Amstutz. American Veterinary Publ. Santa Barbara, USA. pp. 450-452.*

*Ireland-Perry, R.L. and C.C. Stallings. 1993. Fecal consistency as related to dietary composition in lactating Holstein cows. J. Dairy Sci. 76:1074-1082.*

*Klusemeyer, T.H. , M.R. Cameron, C.C. McGoy, and J.H. Clark. 1990. Effects of feed processing and frequency of feeding on ruminal fermentation, milk production, and milk composition. J. Dairy Sci. 73:3538-3543.*

*Klusemeyer, T.H., G.L. Lynch, J.H. Clark, and D.T. Nelson. 1991. Effects of calcium salts of fatty acids and proportion of forage in diet on ruminal fermentation and nutrient flow to duodenum of cows. J. Dairy Sci. 2220-2232.*

*Little, W., B.F. Sansom, R.Manston, and W.M. Allen. 1984. Importance of water for the health and productivity of the dairy cow. Res. Vet. Sci. 37:283-288.*

*Mahana, B. 1993. 100 updated feeding thumbrules. Hoard's Dairyman. September 25, pages 672,673,686.*

*Merrill, M.S. 1995. Now it is time to plan fly control strategy. Hoard's Dairyman, May 10, pp.392.*

*Murphy, M.R. 1992. Water metabolism of dairy cattle. J. Dairy Sci. 75:326-333.*

*Murphy, M.R., C.L. Davis, and G.C. McCoy, 1983. Factors affecting water consumption by Holstein cows in early lactation. J. Dairy Sci. 66:35-38.*

*Ng-Kwai-Hang, K.F. J.F. Hayes, J.E. Moxley, and J.E. Monardes. 1982. Environmental influences on protein content and composition of bovine milk. J. Dairy Sci. 65:1993- 1998.*

*Nocek, J.E. and D.G. Braund, 1985. Effect of feeding frequency on diurnal dry matter and water consumption, liquid dilution rate, and milk yield in first lactation. J. Dairy Sci. 68:2238-2247.*

*Noordhuizen, J.P.T.M. and J. Buurman. 1984. VAMPP: A veterinary automated management and production control programme for dairy farms. The Vet. Quart. 6:66-72.*

*Oetzel, G.R., F.P. Villalba, W.A. Goodger, and K.V. Nordlund. 1993. A comparison of on farm methods for estimating the dry matter content of feed ingredients. J. Dairy Sci. 76:293-299.*

*Otto, K.L., J.D. Ferguson, D.G. Fox, and C.J. Sniffen, 1991. Relationship between body condition score and composition of ninth to eleventh rib tissue in Holstein dairy cows. J. Dairy Sci. 74:852-859.*

*Palmquist, D., 1994. Effects of feeding on milk composition. Tri-State Dairy Nutrition Conference, Fort Wayne, IN. May 24-25. pp. 85-106.*

*Pecsok, S.R., M.L. McGilliard, R.E. James, T.G. Johnson, and J.B. Holter, 1992. Estimating production benefits through simulation of group and individual feeding of dairy cows. J. Dairy Sci. 75:1604-1615.*

*Phelps, A., 1992. Vastly superior first lactations when heifers fed separately. Feedstuffs (May 11):11.*

*Roenfeldt, S. 1995. Rate your cow's comfort. Dairy herd management. February. pp. 8-10.*

*Rufledt, L. 1995. An integrated approach will limit fly populations. Hoard's Dairyman, June, pp. 438-439.*

*Scholl, D.T. 1992. An epidemiological study of dairy farm managemnet and farm bulk tank milk protein concentration. PhD. thesis, University of Utrecht.*

*Shaver, R.D. 1995. Look in the bunk when there are feeding problems. Hoards Dairyman. pp.798.*

*Schuler, R. 1995. Adjust machines for proper particle size. Hoard's Dairyman, pp. 440*

*Skidmore, A.L., 1990. Gross examination of manure. Animal Science Newsletter, Michigan State University, East Lansing, MI. Vol. II(9):5-6.*

*Sniffen, C.J., R.W. Beverly, C.S. Mooney, M.B. Roe, A.L. Skidmore, and J.R. Black, 1993. Nutrient requirements versus supply in the dairy cow: strategies to account for variability. J. Dairy Sci. 76:3160-3178.*

*Sutton, J.D., I.C. Hart, S.V. Morant, E. Schuller, and A.D. Simmonds, 1988. Feeding frequency for lactation cows: diurnal patterns of hormones and metabolites in peripheral blood in relation to milk-fat concentration. Brit. J. Nutr. 60:265-274.*

*Van Saun, J., 1991. Dry cow nutrition: the key to improving fresh cow performance. The Veterinary Clinics of North America. Dairy Nutrition Management. Sniffen, C.J. and T.H. Herdt (eds.). 7:599-621.*

*Wheet, H.J. and J.E. Hunter. 1971. Drinking of sulfate water by cattle. J. Anim Sci. 32:277-281.*

*Williams, C.B. and P.A. Oltenacu, 1992. Evaluation of criteria used to group lactating cows using a dairy production model. J. Dairy Sci. 75:155-160.*

*Wonsil, B.J., J.H. Herbein, and B.A. Watkins, 1994. Dietary and ruminally derived trans-18:1 fatty acids alter bovine milk lipids. J. Nutr. 124:556-565.*

*Woodford, J.A., N.A. Jorgensen, and G.P. Barrington. 1986. Impact of dietary fiberand physical form on performance of lactating dairy cows. J. Dairy Sci. 69:1035-1047.*

# MONITORING REPRODUCTIVE PERFORMANCE

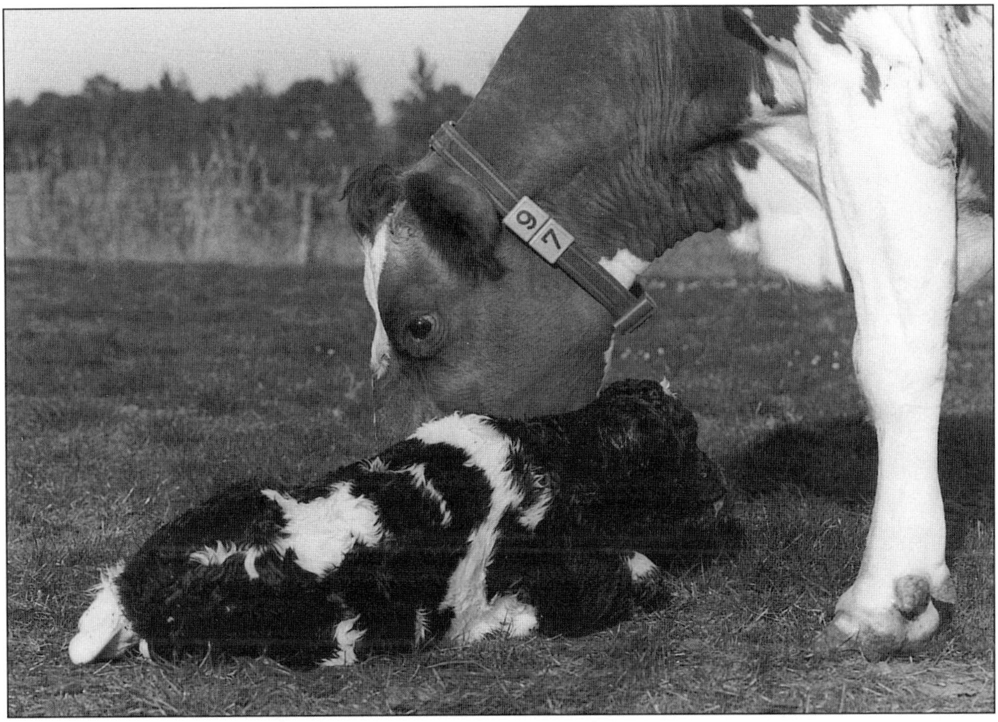

# 5.1 MONITORING REPRODUCTIVE PERFORMANCE: OBJECTIVES, REPRODUCTIVE INDICES AND MATERIALS AND METHODS

Arie Brand[1] and Mark Varner[2]

[1] Department of Herd Health and Reproduction, School of Veterinary Medicine, University of Utrecht, Yaleaan 7, 3584 CL Utrecht, The Netherlands

[2] Department of Animal Sciences, University of Maryland, College Park, MD 20742-2311, USA

## 5.1.1 INTRODUCTION

Herd fertility programs (HFP) have been developed to help farmers and veterinary practitioners monitor and manage dairy reproductive performance. A HFP is not only the cornerstone, but also the stepping stone to an extensive Herd Health and Production Management (HH & PM) service. The levels of activities that play a role in reproductive performance are depicted in Figure 1.

As in other operational management functions, activities related to reproduction

*Figure 1. Levels of reproductive performance activities*

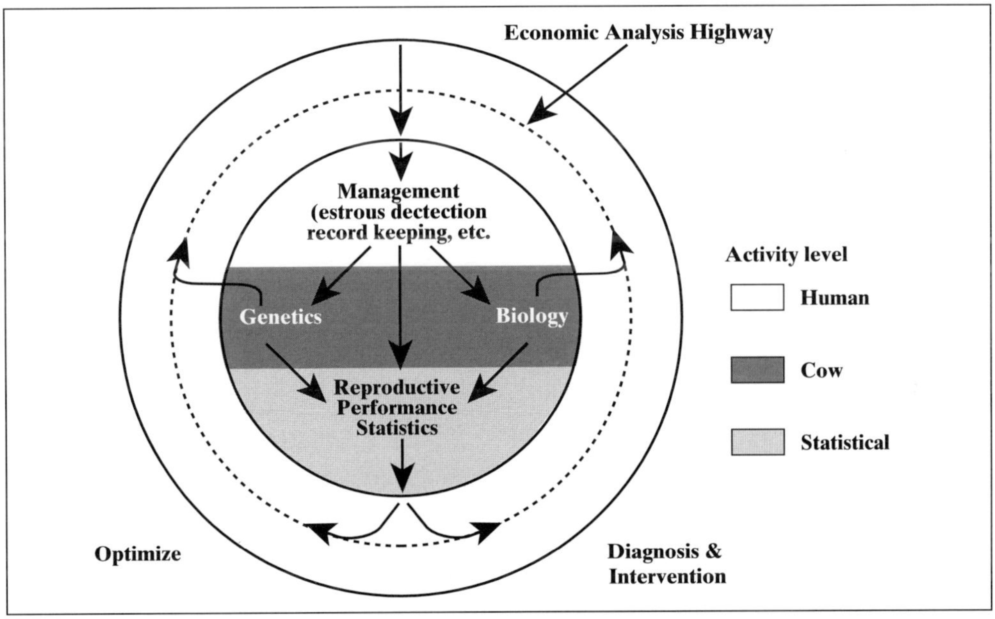

are executed at the human, cow and statistical level. The activities are all interrelated and have to be evaluated by humans using statistics appropriate to an economic framework as indicated in Figure 1. The biological component of reproduction is frequently the only characteristic considered by veterinary practitioners within the framework of a HFP. In contrast, dairy farmers are often heavily focused on genetics for milk production and conformation traits. The bridge between genetics and reproductive biology is formed by management. Management makes up over 90% of reproductive performance, so great attention should be paid to management within a HFP. Further, practitioners who are involved in herd fertility programs should go beyond assessing the biological components of reproduction to give their services added value (Ferry, 1992).

A comprehensive HFP is performed according to a protocol which is centered around accurate, reliable, and up to date record keeping, regularly scheduled farm visits, consultative services and record analysis. These are followed by interpretation of information and recommendations (Chapter 1, part 1), forming the core of a routine herd fertility program.

In this this part of the Chapter the general objectives, primary and secondary reproductive performance indices and a summary of materials and methods, used in a HH & PM protocol, to monitor herd fertility are described.

### 5.1.2 REPRODUCTION PROTOCOL

A protocol to monitor herd fertility consists of four components as described in Chapter 1, part 1 and presented in Figure 2. It includes two sections, one for monitoring reproductive performance in a preventive way and another for problem analysis. In the preventive monitoring section, data are collected routinely to monitor trends in reproductive performance. If an abnormal trend is identified in the decision making process, then archived data is analyzed for problem diagnosis and possible intervention. Details of the protocol are described in Chapter 1, part 1.

### 5.1.3 OBJECTIVES

General objectives for the operational function of reproduction are to:

1. improve the genetic potential of a herd by making use of high quality sires and dams,
2. optimize reproductive performance through managing short calving intervals,
3. minimize management deficiencies and reproductive or health disorders,
4. minimize involuntary reproductive culling of cows to allow for either greater female genetic selection and corrective mating or an increase in herd size.

Goals for reproductive performance are expressed as unique preset targets for individual herds, which are in turn expressed as performance indices.

*Figure 2. Protocol for monitoring herd fertility*

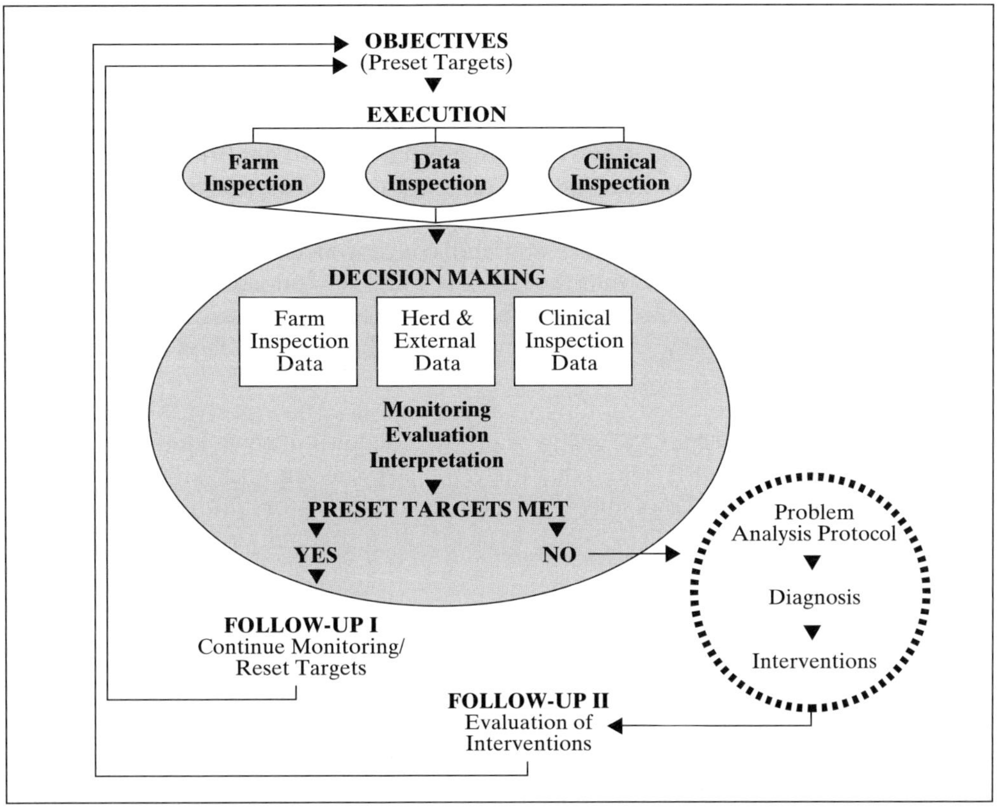


## Definition of primary and secondary reproductive indices

Reproductive indices can be divided into four primary and a number of secondary indices. A set of standardized reproductive performance indices has been proposed for broad use (Fetrow et al., 1990). By using common definitions, comparison and interpretation of reproductive performance indices can be less confusing nationally and internationally. Definitions of reproductive indices, as defined by Fetrow et al. (1990), are presented below.

### Primary indices

### Projected average minimum calving to conception interval or days open

This index provides the best combined estimation of current reproductive performance in a dairy herd. It is an average of days from calving to actual or estimated conception for three groups of cows: pregnant, inseminated, and open. All cows that will be culled are excluded from the calculation.

For pregnant cows the number of days from calving to confirmed conception date is calculated. Cows for which pregnancy has not yet been confirmed comprise two categories: bred cows and open cows. The last category can be split up into two groups of cows: cows bred earlier but known to be open and in cows not yet bred but past their voluntary waiting period. Cows inseminated, but not yet confirmed pregnant are assumed to be pregnant from their last breeding. For open cows, it is assumed that they will conceive 10 days from the current date.

Inclusion of cows with assumed or estimated conception dates allows the use of the word "projected", to designate that the index is what may be expected in the future. The use of the word "minimum" with the index, refers to the fact that the actual reproductive performance of these cows is unknown, and that due to delays in conception, the index is usually higher.

In large herds the projected minimum calving to conception interval should also be defined for relevant cows per age group or production level of cows. Heifers may need a longer period of time until rebred due to their energy need for growth in addition to lactation. High producing cows may need a longer calving interval for biological reasons such as recovery from high demands of lactation or to maintain longevity as a high producing cow.

### Projected average minimum age at first calving for heifers

This index is defined as the average estimated age at calving for pregnant and inseminated heifers in the herd. The projected age at calving for pregnant heifers is calculated by adding the number of days from birth to last insemination date to 280 days as the estimated length of pregnancy. Inseminated heifers without a confirmed pregnancy are assumed to be pregnant from the most recent insemination and the same calculation as for pregnant heifers is done. As with projected minimum calving to conception interval, existing computer programs frequently do not calculate the projected minimum age at first calving properly. They do not include estimated age at calving for both pregnant and inseminated heifers. The programs typically calculate age at calving for primiparous milking cows. By using such a calculation method, the index typically reflects reproductive performance of over one year ago.

### The reproductive culling rate on a yearly basis

This index includes the number of cows culled for reproductive problems, divided by average total number of milking and dry cows present in the herd over a one year period. Calculation of the culling index over shorter time periods has a disadvantage. The time when a cow is culled is usually months after the reproductive problem occurred. With shorter time periods, the culling activity is not included in the same time frame as with the various failed reproductive activities. Accurate records of reasons for culling are critical for this index to have validity and value for interpreting reproductive performance.

## Percentage of abortions per confirmed pregnancy

To define an abortion the stage of pregnancy has to be taken into account. Prior to 42 days of pregnancy, losses are termed early embryonic deaths. After 260 days of gestation, birth of the fetus is termed a premature delivery. Losses between the 42nd and 260th day are the only losses termed abortions (Committee on bovine reproductive nomenclature, 1972).

In practice two types of abortions are included in this index. The first type refers to abortions that are observed and reported by the farmer. The second type comprises cows previously confirmed pregnant by the practitioner and subsequently determined to be open. The index should be calculated separately for both adult pregnant cows and nulliparous pregnant heifers. The numerator is the number of abortions by the given definitions. The denominator is the average number of cows/heifers pregnant during the period under evaluation. This number usually varies over time, so it is estimated by adding the number of pregnant cows at the start of the period studied to the number of pregnant cows at the end of the period studied and dividing by two. The index requires a regular program of rechecks for pregnancy to identify the second type of abortion. Rechecks are typically done infrequently. Regular monitoring is needed to detect problems as they develop. Summaries should therefore be performed monthly or at least quarterly depending on herd size.

The first two primary indices reflect the actual reproductive performance of both cows and heifers at the herd level, respectively. The second two indices reflect reproductive wastage due to infertility at the herd level. All four indices must be taken into consideration in order to get an overall insight in the reproductive performance of a herd. If a reproductive problem arises for one or more primary indices, secondary reproductive performance indices have to be evaluated in order to examine the situation in greater detail. One has to realize that even in situations where the average is acceptable, there might still be a problem with some individual cows.

## Secondary indices

### Calving to first insemination interval

The calving to first insemination interval includes the average days lost by the voluntary and involuntary waiting periods. The voluntary waiting period (VWP) is defined as the time that a dairy producer waits before attempting the first insemination. This may vary between cows on a farm, due to postpartum complications or decisions made by the farmer. An average for the farm should be used. The involuntary waiting period is the extra days between the voluntary waiting period and first insemination. If all cows were having regular estrous cycles and the farmer was observing 100% of estrous periods, then, without the use of prostaglandin-F-2-$\alpha$, the involuntary waiting period would be 10.5 days on an average due to the fact that cows in a group will come into estrous over a twenty-one day period.

### First insemination to conception interval

This index includes the extra days lost from first insemination to actual or assumed conception. With a 100% first service conception rate, the first insemination to conception interval is zero. With lower first insemination conception rates the extra days lost originate from cows that did not conceive after first insemination due to various reasons listed in Chapter 5, part 3.

### The percentage of possible estruses detected

The index of percentage of possible estruses detected includes all reported estruses or breedings in eligible cows, over a given period, divided by the total number of potential estrous cycles in that period and the result is multiplied by 100. Eligible cows are cows past the voluntary waiting period, and they include:

1. cows never bred,
2. cows known to be open and not yet rebred,
3. bred cows not yet known to be pregnant,
4. pregnant cows with days in the period up to the last breeding date,
5. open cows to be culled with days past the voluntary waiting period up to date reported (unless the cow is pregnant in which case she is handled as a pregnant cow), and
6. open cows turned out with a bull, (days past VWP in period up to date when turned with bull).

For each cow in each category, the number of estrous cycle days is determined and summed. This sum is divided by 21 to determine the number of potential normal estrous cycles. Some herds do not record observed estrous periods before the first insemination or from cows on the culling list. This variation in herd estrous recording policy requires that the existing policy must be determined and taken into account when establishing preset targets for this index.

The validity of this index is based on the assumption that cows have normal 21 day estrous cycles. Prostaglandin-F-2-$\alpha$ treatments shorten the estrous cycle, and if more than 10% of the herd is treated, the assumption is no longer valid and the use of this index should be discouraged (Fetrow et al., 1994).

### Number of services per pregnancy for all cows

This index is defined as the number of breedings during the analysis period for all cows inseminated divided by the number of pregnancies confirmed during that same time period.

### Number of services per pregnancy for pregnant cows

The index is sometimes called services per conception, and it is defined as the number of breedings for cows diagnosed pregnant during the test period divided by the number of pregnancies confirmed during that same period. Pregnancy diagnosis by rectal palpation is preferred, though 56-day non-return can be used. The preset target for this index should be increased by about 8% if a non-return rate is used.

**First service conception rate**

This index is calculated for all cows who received their first service during the period of interest. The number of first services that resulted in a pregnancy is divided by the total number of first services during the same time period. It is the most sensitive and reliable index of overall herd fertility. When the voluntary waiting period is short, this index can be lower. First service conception rates for heifers are known to be higher than for lactating cows (Rhaeja et al., 1989). Therefore, separate indexes should be calculated for heifers and cows.

**Setting objectives or preset targets**

Four steps must be taken when directing a HH & PM program for monitoring herd fertility. First, ultimate reproductive performance objectives are established by instituting preset targets. The preset targets have to be determined in conjunction with the farmer, taking into account that historic performance indices are available. If these are not available, the second step consists of calculation of the current primary reproductive indices. Third, current indices are compared to preset targets that the farmer has in mind. If the difference between the current indices and targets is greater than the progress that might be expected in a year's time, then a fourth step is required. This fourth step is to establish interim preset targets that might reasonably be achieved by that herd over a specific time frame.

An example of establishing preset targets is:

1. Projected minimum age at first calving of 25 ± 1 months while the actual age is 27.1 months.
2. A projected (minimum) calving to conception interval of 95 days, in contrast to an existing interval of 112 days.
3. A reproductive culling rate due to fertility problems of < 5% on a herd basis over one years time, while the actual level was 10%.
4. An abortion rate (abortions per confirmed pregnancy) of < 4% while the calculated herd rate was 7%.
5. Average predicted transmitting ability for milk greater than the average for the top 20% of active AI sires, while the actual average was below the average for active AI sires.

In order to interpret reproductive performance indices, the number of cows that produce a given calculated rate (denominator of calculation) should always be provided.

The preset targets may vary from farm to farm depending on the actual level of reproductive performance, the managerial capacity of the farmer and/or unique farm conditions. One has to recognize and to consider that each farm has its own specific factors that can influence reproductive performance specifically.

## 5.1.4 MATERIALS, METHODS, AND EVALUATION SKILLS

A herd fertility program requires that a number of materials or instruments and methods must either be available or they must become available. The way such a program is executed is described in Chapter 5, part 3.

### Materials

1. A record system is required. While there is great variety in effective record keeping systems, key components of successful record keeping systems are:
   - A self-copying farm diary for hand recording of data on reproduction and related activities. The farmer keeps a copy and the practitioner takes a copy back to the clinic for either manual or computer assisted analysis if indicated (see Chapter 1, part 2).
   - A herd fertility chart that lists cows in order of their calving date. This chart is efficient for examining the history of an individual and it provides an overview of the herd at a glance for about 120 cows. Daily and accurate transfer of data from the farm diary and/or individual cow cards to a herd fertility chart or a herd management computer summarization system, if available, is essential (see Chapter 1, part 2).
   - An on-farm personal computer for data processing. This enables communication between farm data sources.
     The on-farm computer can also provide communication between external informational resources such as, milk recording and testing centers, milk processing company, dairy consultants and practitioners. Hand-held and pen-based computing technologies will allow input of data events, like results of rectal palpation or insemination information, at the time of the event, resulting in reduced manual transfer of recorded data.
   - Sophisticated software which makes it possible to monitor herd performance and provide simultaneous evaluation and analysis from various sources of electronic information to help diagnose causes of decreased or improved herd fertility.
   - A file for both the farmer and the practitioner to store relevant information. Accurate and up-to-date data recording followed by manual or electronic data processing by the farmer, the practitioner and/or an external organization is the heart of an effective HH & PM program to monitor reproductive performance. Examples of such software systems are: VAMPP (Noordhuizen et al., 1984) DairyCHAMP (Udomprasert and Williamson, 1990), DAISY (Esslemont et al., 1991), Dairy Comp 305 (Goodger, 1987).
2. Gynecological instruments, including a speculum, lamp and sterile sampling supplies. In some instances equipment for ultra sound examination and kits for milk progesterone analysis may be useful.
3. Pedometers, pressure sensitive sensors for measuring standing mounts and impedance monitoring devices are currently being used or tested as estrous detection aids. Telemetric electronic data acquisition from these devices can be performed.

The data are collected in an automated milking parlor. Currently, this type of electronic equipment may be rare on dairy farms, but it will become more common in the future (Varner et al., 1994; Devir et al., 1995).

## Methods

The following methods should be employed:

1. Data inspection for content, completeness and actuality,
2. Farm inspection activities directed at risk factors or, rather, categories or clusters of risk factors in the environment that might influence reproductive performance, such as feeding practices, hygiene, housing, and climatic conditions.
3. Clinical inspection activities, including genital palpation. For this purpose a work list of cows to be examined by the practitioner is required. The composition of this list may be flexible, but usually contains the following categories:
   - postpartum and pre-insemination checks,
   - cows with abnormal vaginal discharge,
   - cows not observed in estrus,
   - cows with abnormal estrous or insemination intervals,
   - cows for pregnancy check,
   - cows that aborted or had other abnormalities.
4. Regular farm visits. Frequency of farm visits is usually determined by herd size and/or calving pattern. In herds of 80 to 100 cows a frequency of once in 3 to 4 weeks seems optimal. In cases where the herd fertility program is part of a more extended HH & PM service, the time available for reproduction should be balanced with other components. In general, in a 100 cow herd the average duration of the fertility component should not exceed 1 hour.

## Evaluation skills

Evaluation skills that are needed consist of:

1. Ability to monitor, evaluate and to interpret primary and secondary reproductive performance indices as well as indications from estrous detection aids, especially electronic device (pedometer) readings,
2. Familiarity with automated data processing and veterinary epidemiology concepts and methods (Chapter 1, part 4),
3. Familiarity with interpreting reproductive disorders and knowledge of effective treatments and/or herd reproductive management strategies, such as estrous induction and/or synchronization programs.

## EPILOGUE

A herd fertility program as part of a HH & MP program starts with defining preset targets and identifying materials and methods to reach those preset targets. Milk, reproductive and veterinary data recording by the farmer form an essential element in a herd fertility program. Without data, reproductive performance cannot be evaluated and analyzed. In a journey, one must know where to start, where to go, and the route to get there. In the journey towards optimal reproductive performance, records of existing reproductive performance allow farmers to know where they are starting from. Preset targets allow farmers to know where they are going. The materials and methods of a herd fertility program provide the route. The practitioner can be thought of as the experienced guide helping the farmer during the journey to achieve and maintain optimal reproductive performance.

Reproductive management serves milk production, and hence, farm income. The most efficient milk production period is in the first 4 months of lactation when feed is most efficiently converted to milk and when over 60% of cow's lactational production is produced. In order to make an optimal use of this period the length of the rest of the lactation period must be optimized. Therefore, the execution of a HFP must enable the farmer to reach the highest pregnancy rates for most of the herd within the first 3 to 4 months after calving. With short calving intervals more offspring is produced that allows a dairy herd to grow or for a farmer to selectively breed only the best cows. Another prerequisite is an optimal dry cow management especially with regard to nutrition in the close up period (Chapter 3).

*For references see part 4 of this Chapter.*

# 5.2 MONITORING REPRODUCTIVE PERFORMANCE: EXECUTION

Arie Brand[1] and Mark Varner[2]

[1] Department of Herd Health and Reproduction, School of Veterinary Medicine, University of Utrecht, Yalelaan 7, 3584 CL Utrecht, The Netherlands
[2] Department of Animal Sciences, University of Maryland, College Park, MD 20742-2311, USA

## 5.2.1 INTRODUCTION

The execution of a Herd Fertility Program (HFP) within extended Herd Health and Production Management (HH & PM) services comprises three activities: 1) data inspection, 2) farm inspection, and 3) clinical inspection. All three activities contribute to a practitioner's ability to examine the herd's reproductive management.

Data inspection is directed at assessing the accuracy and quality of data collected by the farmer. It also gives insight into the herd's current reproductive performance.

The farm inspection activity consists of a thorough inspection of management practices and of the cow's environment to detect risk factors that might have an impact upon cow and herd reproductive performance. To do this the practitioner and/or farm advisor have to act as a detective, using all available senses.

The clinical inspection of the herd is focused on reproductive and general health aspects of the cows and young stock. One has to realize that the operational function of reproduction can not be monitored by clinical inspection only. Reproductive performance is interrelated with other operational farm functions such as: nutrition, milk production and health care (see also Chapters 3, 4, 7, 8, and 9) and has to be approached as such. Therefore, the veterinary practitioner must relate clinical reproductive tract findings with findings from other operational management functions

In this part of Chapter 5, the three inspection activities will be described and important elements emphasized.

## 5.2.2 DATA INSPECTION

### Completeness and accuracy of data

The dairy producer is primarily responsible for data collection, followed by the veterinary practitioner and any farm advisors. An important role of the practitioner is to provide regular motivation for the farmer to collect relevant data. A useful mechanism for motivating the farmer is for the practitioner or advisor to provide regular feedback on herd performance with information derived from data collected by the farmer. Reproductive events may be recorded on individual cow cards, on a farm diary, directly on a herd fertility barn sheet or into a farm computer. The use of a management information computer program on dairy farms is still limited but increasing in numbers. The computer program might come from a DHIA organization or from a commercial firm. It is possible that the veterinary practice might be linked with the farmer's computer to provide analytical services. The completeness and accuracy of data records and transfer have to be checked by the practitioner before every farm visit. The data monitoring process depends on the way data is recorded and processed.

### Gathering information for the farm visit

Data inspection should be combined with gathering of information from a farm diary, the herd fertility barn chart, and/or other forms which can be used during the actual farm visit. The raw data recorded in a farm diary provides information about reproductive events of individual cows since the last farm visit. Incidence of abnormal calvings, calves born dead or alive, cows with retained placenta and/or vaginal discharge, abortions, and cows treated for reproductive disorders in between farm visits can be derived easily. The herd fertility barn chart typically has information on cows not yet seen in estrous or not yet inseminated, repeat breeders and on other recorded information such as diseases and culling.

The next step in the data inspection activity is made by reviewing recently processed data and relevant information from the last farm visit(s). This may include evaluation of primary and secondary reproductive indices, information recorded on a 12-month list (Chapter 1, part 2), genital examination results from recent herd visits, relevant laboratory findings, and summary of recommendations made during the last farm visit. Adoption rate of practices recommended during previous farm visits should be determined. Conclusions from this review should be kept in mind during the actual herd visit.

When the farmer is making use of electronic data processing, more information might be available before the farm visit. This will likely be the case when the veterinary practice is linked with the farmer's computer. Customized lists of actual performance figures and other relevant information could then be printed beforehand to facilitate discussions with the farmer after the visit and improve recommended practice adoption.

### Examination list

A list of cows for clinical examination has to be made up just prior to every farm visit. This list typically has cow identification number, most recent calving date, and estrous or breeding dates for all cows that will be examined. The list can be manually or electronically prepared by the farmer, or by the practitioner. Commercial herd management computer programs usually have predefined lists. The practitioner must either adapt him/herself to those lists or aid in developing custom defined lists. An advantage of the practitioner providing the software program to the farmer is that the practitioner can be much more experienced with developing custom lists.

If the list is made up by the farmer, it should be checked for completeness by the practitioner. Often, a few more cows are added for reproductive or other reasons. If the list is generated by the practitioner, she/he should ensure that the latest reproductive events have been included. Not only does the checking process reinforce the importance of the records to the producer, it also ensures more accurate billing. Billing of veterinary services is frequently based on a per cow fee, so accurate records of cow examination are invaluable to producer confidence in bills. Examination lists provided by the practitioner or farm advisor also help increase the value of their service to the producer. The examination list should be self-copying so that both the farmer and the practitioner can have a copy of the list with the added information after the farm visit.

## 5.2.3 FARM INSPECTION

In many cases reproductive inefficiencies have a multifactorial cause, which means that attention should not only be paid to biological cow factors, but also to environmental and/or management factors. For this reason, a farm inspection is an essential part of a herd fertility program. It is aimed at the recognition of factors that have the potential to influence reproductive performance negatively. Each factor may not be limiting reproductive performance now, but it may limit performance in the future. The factors shall be grouped around: management practices, the cow, farm conditions, and nutrition.

### Management practices

#### 1. Estrous detection

Efficient and accurate estrous detection is the most important factor limiting reproduction in most dairy herds (Britt et al., 1986; Senger, 1994). Efficiency defines the proportion of cows seen in estrus of all cows eligible for showing estrus. Accuracy gives the percentage that were correctly identified as being in estrus. In well managed herds, the maximal estrous detection rate was found to be 60% of ovulations when dairy cows are observed two or three times daily. With continuous observation, the detection rate may increase to 95% in the second and later postpartum ovulations (Villa-Godoy, et al., 1990). In another study however, estrus was observed for only 75% of ovulations, even when continuous videotaping was used. Slippery slatted flooring was used in this study, and may account for part of the reduced estrous detection efficiency (Varner, 1994). Failure to observe cows in estrus delays first service, lengthens estrous intervals, and is one of the primary factors lengthening projected average minimum calving to conception interval by increasing the number of days open. It contributes more to lengthy calving intervals than conception failure (Stevenson et al., 1983). In addition, inaccurate estrous detection lowers conception rate. Many cows are inseminated when not in estrus. As many as 1/3rd of dairy herds may have a significant estrous detection accuracy problem. Estrous detection is affected by both cow and management factors:

1. Cow factors affecting estrous detection are:
   a. time after calving.
      – inactivity of ovaries. The time from calving to the first postpartum ovulation can vary greatly due to energy balance, endocrine and uterine dysfunction, and general health (Kyle et al., 1992).
      – ovulation number. Only 10 to 30% of cows express their estrus at their first postpartum ovulation (Fagan and Roche, 1986). The proportion increases with later ovulations, and may be due to prior exposure to progesterone (Kyle et al., 1992).
   b. stage of estrous cycle.
      – high versus low progesterone level. Cows in the high progesterone phase are sexually less active than cows at and around estrus. The number of estrual cows have a larger influence on mounting behavior than the number of preestrual cows (Helmer and Britt, 1985).
2. Management factors affecting estrous detection:
   a. frequency and time of observation.
      – Increasing the number of daily periods of observation increases the rate for detection of a sexually active group. Cows are more sexually active at certain times of day. Those times may differ from farm to farm, depending the farmstead design, time of feeding, and environmental conditions (Hurnik et al., 1975; Esslemont et al., 1985; Varner et al., 1994).
   b. level of milk production.
      – A high level of milk production may influence estrous detection negatively. This most likely caused by a longer lasting influence of negative energy balance. A negative energy balance and a low body condition (Chapter 3) lead to delayed onset of ovarian activity (Hurley et al., 1979; Esslemont et al., 1980; Helmer and Britt, 1985; Larson and Ball, 1992).

Efficient reproductive management depends on the ability to detect estrus. There should be a systematic program for estrous detection. Factors and evaluation criteria of such a program are: times of observation (three times a day minimum), time allotted to observations (20 minutes per time for a herd of 300 cows) and assignment of employees to estrous detection (no other duties at estrous detection times). Employees should be trained in proper methods for: estrous detection, semen handling and artificial insemination. If there is shortage of labor, investment in estrous detection aids should be considered.

As described before, reproduction is a multifactorial biological process. There are other limitations to effective estrous detection than the cow's reproductive physiology. These may include diseases and management and environmental conditions.

Therefore, to further improve estrous detection, attention should be paid to:

* improving health care especially with regard to lameness,
* improving housing, feeding and/or loafing conditions.

In addition to this, estrous synchronization techniques can be implemented.

## 2. Synchronization of estrous

Estrous detection programs can be ineffective due to poor record keeping or inaccurate estrous detection. These same poor management strategies can lead to cows being given estrous synchronization treatments. Synchronization of estrous can not only be a therapy to alleviate problems with estrous detection efficiency, but it can also cause problems. This may happen if pregnant cows are treated with prostaglandin or if cows are treated when not in a proper condition. Therefore, a subjective evaluation of the herd's management ability to handle an estrous synchronization program should be conducted by the practitioner before initiating that program.

Various methods for synchronization of estrus in dairy cattle have been recently reviewed (Odde, 1990; Larson and Ball, 1992; Wenzel et al., 1991; Stevenson, 1994). Prostaglandin-F2α (PGF) was recognized as the most effective method for synchronizing estrus although some cows appear not to respond to PGF or are not observed. This may be due to problems with estrous detection at the herd level or to individual cow problems with giving PGF at an inappropriate time of the estrous cycle. If PGF is prescribed for cows, but the treatment is given by the farmer, then the practitioner should review with the farmer the importance of PGF injection timing to the stage of the estrous cycle and the number of cows to be injected. Sufficient numbers of cows should be synchronized with PGF to allow for formation of a sexually-active-group, facilitating detection of estrus (Britt, 1986). Further, PGF synchronization has been used to facilitate scheduling of estrous during times when frequent observations are possible.

PGF treatment programs have been developed as strategic alternative to continuous estrous detection, especially for herds with less than 100 cows (Ferguson and Galligan, 1993 a and 1993 b) or which are short in labor. Cows that are past the voluntary wait period are injected on a Monday. Observations for estrus are made only on Wednesday and Thursday. Cows in estrus are inseminated. Any cow not observed in estrus is retreated on the next Monday. Any cow that has gone past her voluntary wait period during the previous week is also injected with PGF. Any inseminated cows that come into estrus are reinseminated. Inseminated cows without estrous are examined for pregnancy 35 - 42 days post insemination. Variations on the treatment have been developed, but none appears to be more successful than the others. It has to be stressed that even after estrous synchronization, estrous detection remains important.

## 3. Record keeping

Optimal reproductive performance is based on correct identification of cows, efficient/accurate detection of estrus, and accurate/timely recording of all reproductive events. Inadequate recording of relevant reproductive events by the herdsman such as calving and estrous dates, may result in inseminations being too early or too late in lactation. Timing of corrective therapies are typically based upon reproductive records, and poor records can lead to ineffective therapy or additional problems like abortion. These problems can then lead to a longer calving to conception interval. In addition, deficient record keeping makes actual monitoring, evaluation and analysis of reproductive performance difficult, if not impossible.

### 4. Culling percentage/strategy

A disadvantage of descriptive statistics for reproductive performance is that they usually does not include cows culled for subfertility. Without data on culled cows, the reproductive indices may not reflect actual performance (Gaines, 1989; Fetrow, 1994), and problems with reproductive performance can be underestimated. For example, a herd with relatively poor reproductive performance can still have reproductive indices that are good. If all cows that do not conceive after a second insemination are culled, calving to conception interval could still be acceptable. However, this policy would increase the reproductive wastage rate. Therefore, a high annual culling rate for fertility reasons is indicative of reproduction problems despite an acceptable calving to conception interval (Weaver, 1986). The overall culling percentage and reasons for culling have to be recorded and examined.

Culling strategy should be based on culling cows with low milk production. The overall culling capacity is greatly reduced in herds with fertility problems because of the number of cows that must be sold due to breeding failure and because fewer replacements are born. Additional losses due to reduced genetic progress and extra veterinary costs and semen costs in repeat breeding cows can be substantial (Barth, 1993).

### 5. Choice of sire

Bull choice in relation to ease of calving is of special importance for virgin heifers. All replacement heifers should be mated with AI sires known to be below breed average for calving difficulty. When bulls are used for natural service, a comprehensive breeding soundness examination should be performed. This includes a physical exam, screening for infectious diseases, as well as an evaluation of libido, mating ability, and semen quality.

Bulls vary in conception rate and frequent use of sub-fertile bulls will lower herd reproductive performance (Gwasdauskas et al., 1981). Semen from bulls with low fertility are not released by artificial insemination organizations. The fertility of some natural service bulls (clean-up bulls) is not known. Thus, natural service bulls require a comprehensive breeding soundness examination.

Monitoring bull choice is also important in relation to average transmitting ability. Genetic merit accumulates across time, and wise decisions related to genetics can provide favorable long-term returns on investments. Therefore, farmers should make an intensive use of proven bulls. HH & PM practitioners should be aware of, and able to check, factors responsible for not making use of such bulls. These factors include: 1) price level of semen asked for by AI organizations, 2) reducing expenditures on semen by the farmer, 3) suboptimal estrous detection or failing getting cows pregnant after second or more inseminations, 4) labor saving, especially for getting heifers in calf that are in pasture, and 5) breeding dairy cows with semen from non-dairy breeds to increase value of calf sold as dairy-beef cross. Farmers can make use of a computer-assisted sire selection procedure to ensure an economically sound genetic development program (Weaver, 1992). Linear programming has been used to select a portfolio of bulls that meets the producer's breeding objectives (Galligan et al., 1994).

### 6. Semen handling and insemination techniques

Inferior semen handling and/or poor artificial insemination techniques will lower conception rates. Farmers who inseminate their own cows, and even professional inseminators, may develop bad semen handling and artificial insemination technique habits over time. Retraining is frequently required (Barth, 1993).

Semen should be thawed according to recommendations provided by the bull stud. Variation exists in optimum time and temperature, and using one stud's recommendations on another stud's semen may produce poor results. If a number of straws has to be thawed at one time, straws always should be agitated to prevent them from freezing together. Freezing together can lead to poor thawing rates and sperm death.

Straw retrieval for thawing should be done in the shortest possible time. Also, the frequency with which the canister is raised into the neck of the nitrogen refrigerator should be limited as much as possible. Therefore, an accurate semen inventory should be kept with the nitrogen tank to speed retrieval by reducing the time for searching. At dairies where the farmer or herdsman is inseminating cows, the refrigerator should be monitored regularly for damage and level of liquid nitrogen (Senger, 1992).

Deposition of semen in the uterus results in higher conception rates than deposition in the vagina or cervix (Gwazdauskas et al., 1981). Time of insemination should be based on the am-pm rule. This means that cows seen in estrus for the first time in the morning should be inseminated the same day. Cows observed in estrus in the afternoon or evening should be inseminated the next morning (Gwazdauskas et al., 1981).

## Herd factors

### 7. Herd or group size

The number of open cows has to be taken into account when considering estrous detection. Estrus requires participation of at least 2 cows. Cows approaching estrus or cows in estrus are the most likely cows to participate in estrous mounting activity (Helmer and Britt, 1985). Cows in the middle of their estrous cycle are poor estrous detectors. When more than one cow is in or near estrus, they frequently form a sexually active group (SAG). The presence of a SAG may triple mounting activity (Macmillan, 1992). A small proportion of open cows in a herd may contribute to missed estruses because SAG's are formed infrequently. PGF can be used to synchronize estrous and form a SAG, thus increasing the opportunity for producers with small herds to observe the cows in estrus.

## 8 Age composition of the herd

Conception rate is higher for replacement heifers than for cows (Gwazdauskas et al., 1981; Raheja et al., 1989). Intervals to first service is longer for older cows than first parity cows (Stevenson et al., 1983). Lactating cows often have highest fertility in their second lactation, which then declines with increasing age (Hillers et al., 1984; Lucey et al., 1986). The incidence of retained placenta (van Werven et al., 1992), twin pregnancies, cystic ovarian disease and reproductive diseases increase with age (Nielen et al., 1990; Laporte et al., 1994) and may be a risk factor for lower fertility.

### Cow Factors

## 9. Dystocia-Retained Placenta-Metritis Complex

Delayed uterine involution, defined as a retarded return of the uterus to prepartum size and position, is a major risk factor for poor postpartum reproductive performance (Bonnet et al., 1993). Important risk factors for delayed uterine involution are: abortions, premature birth and stillbirth, multiple births, dystocia, unsanitary conditions at calving, retained placenta, multiparity and metabolic diseases such as milk fever and ketosis (Montes and Pugh, 1993). Many of these risk factors can lead to metritis. Metritis is associated with increased days to first service, decreased 1st service conception rate, increased total services, lengthened calving interval, occurrence of cystic follicles, reduced productivity and culling due to reduced reproductive performance (Thompson et al., 1983; Djemali et al., 1987; Dohoo and Martin, 1984).

## 10. Lameness

Lame cows have reduced mounting activity during estrous. Severe lameness, especially sole ulcer and white line disease (Chapter 7), is associated with longer calving to first insemination and calving to conception intervals (Lucey et al., 1986; Collick et al., 1989; Barkema et al., 1994). Lameness has also been reported to decrease conception rate and increase risk for culling (Collick et al., 1989).

### Farm conditions

## 11. Housing system

The pasture can be regarded as the natural environment for cows. In many countries, cows stay in the fields throughout the year. Housing can impair reproductive performance, especially through suboptimal estrous detection. Estrous detection is much more difficult in tie-stalls than in loose housing systems where freedom of movement exists. Behavioral signs of estrous, such as grouping, mounting, riding and the standing reflex are easier to observe with loose housing. Estrous may also be affected by light intensity in the stall (De Kruif and Brand, 1978). Light intensity should be such that a newspaper can be easily read in every part of the barn.

Another factor that influences estrous behavior is footing surface of the housing area, exercise lot or pasture (Britt et al., 1986). Slippery and muddy surfaces severely inhibit mounting activity. Cows may also be hesitant to mount on slatted floors. Mounting activity is greater on dirt surfaces rather than on concrete floors (Dozier-Vailes and Britt, 1990).

### 12. Climatic conditions

Heat stress during summer months may be responsible for a large increase in early embryonic mortality in lactating dairy cattle (Folman et al., 1979; Wolfenson et al., 1988; Hansen et al., 1992). The detrimental effect of heat stress is less in pregnant replacement heifers than in cows (Folman et al., 1979). Effects of heat stress on animal performance are likely to become even more important in the future if predictions of global warming prove accurate (Hansen et al., 1992). The effects of high temperature and humidity on reproductive performance of dairy cows are:

- delayed onset of puberty, caused by reduced feed intake (Thatcher, 1993),
- reduced duration and intensity of estrus when temperatures are above 27°C. The upper critical temperature (i.e., when hyperthermia occurs) can be as low as 24 - 27°C in lactating cows. Thus, dairy cattle suffer the consequences of heat stress in a variety of climates (Senger, 1994),
- increased incidence of anestrus due to ovulations without associated sexual behavior. Decreased physical activity during heat-stress may be in part responsible for the increased numbers of missing heats during warm months (Hansen et al., 1992),
- a higher incidence of early embryonic death resulting in reduced pregnancy rates in spite of normal fertilization rates. Embryonic survival may be reduced by adverse effects of elevated body temperatures on developing zygotes and embryos (Ealy et al., 1993). Heat stress results in an increase in rectal temperature from 0.5°C to 2.1°C in subtropical and tropical countries (Badinga et al., 1993). Embryos are most sensitive to deleterious effects of maternal heat stress at day 1 of pregnancy. They become more resistant to heat stress effects by day 3 of pregnancy (Ealy et al., 1993; Hansen, 1994). Besides negative effects of heat stress on early embryonic development, periovulatory changes that take place before ovulation are also sensitive to heat stress and can lead to disruption in subsequent embryonic development (Putney et al., 1989),
- more detrimental effects of retained placenta because of more rapid bacterial multiplication,
- reduced birth weights of calves and milk yield of the dam if heat stress occurs during the last trimester of pregnancy (Collier et al., 1982).

## Nutritional Management

Of the many nutritional factors that may be involved in reproductive performance of dairy cows, energy intake and energy balance are considered as the most important ones. Besides nutrition, milk production is thought to influence reproductive performance. However, there is evidence to suggest that energy intake is more closely associated with reproductive performance than milk yield (Grummer, 1993). The influence of some metabolic factors, influencing reestablishment of reproductive activity post calving, will now be discussed in more detail.

## 13. Energy balance

In most cows, energy balance starts to decline before calving when feed intake decreases prepartum (Bertics et al., 1992) and continues after calving (Canfield and Butler, 1991). During early lactation the cow is losing more energy, primarily in milk, than she is able to take in. This net loss of energy is termed negative energy balance (NEB). At least 80% of dairy cows experience a period of NEB, but magnitude and duration are variable among cows (Villa-Godoy et al., 1988).

Declining EB is the most powerful factor in inhibition of ovarian activity postpartum by suppressing pulsatile GnRH and LH secretion. The pulsatile LH secretion, responsible for ovulation, is suppressed until the declining EB nadir is reached. As soon as NEB starts returning towards balance, LH pulse frequency, LH baseline and mean LH significantly increase, while LH pulse amplitude tends to decrease. An increased LH pulse frequency then stimulates first ovulation. The duration of declining EB or days to negative EB nadir after calving is positively related to the duration of postpartum anestrus or the interval from calving to first ovulation (Canfield and Butler, 1990; Zurek et al., 1995). First ovulation normally does not occur earlier than 8 to 24 days after the time NEB reaches the nadir which occurs at about 2 weeks postpartum (Butler et al., 1981; Canfield et al., 1990; Canfield and Butler, 1991; Zurek et al., 1995). A post nadir period, of approximately 2 weeks length, during which the NEB is returning to equilibrium, is apparently required to activate the signaling system to the hypothalamus and to allow time for follicular growth and maturation (Zurek et al., 1995). Cows that move early and quickly towards positive energy balance may experience multiple estrous cycles, prior to the recommended breeding period, and usually have more favorable reproductive performance than cows with an extended period of declining EB (Huszenicza et al., 1987; Butler and Smith, 1989; Ruegg, 1991).

Besides the duration of declining EB after calving, the magnitude of energy deficit and rate of recovery also appear to be important factors in inhibition of ovulation (Butler and Smith, 1989; Zurek et al., 1995). A severe NEB in early lactation may reduce luteal function, expressed as lower progesterone production, during second and third luteal phases (Villa-Godoy et al., 1988; Staples et al., 1990; Ljokjel et al., 1995). Recovery from a NEB is the key factor responsible for initiation of postpartum ovarian cyclicity (Butler and Smith, 1989). Thus the cumulative effect of a NEB, particularly duration of declining period and depth, may determine the resumption of ovarian cyclicity, and reestablishment of a normal LH pulse frequency secretory pattern. This all means, that following the EB nadir, a shift in the hypothalamic-hypophyseal function or gonadotropin secretion occurs. However the exact mode by which postpartum energy balance, and thus the availability of energy substrates, affects this function of the cow is not clear.

To meet energy requirements during NEB in the postpartum cow, fat from fat depots is lipolysed thereby increasing the NEFA concentration in blood (Canfield and Butler, 1990). Plasma fatty acids in blood plasma, are thought to participate in metabolic signalling to the hypothalamus-hypophyseal axis, controlling ovarian function in the postpartum dairy cow (Butler and Canfield, 1989; Canfield and Butler, 1990; 1991),.

Another signal may come from degradative changes in muscle protein (Zurek et al., 1995). Muscle protein is besides fat in fat depots, also a source of energy substrates. Amino acids derived from muscle proteins are used for milk synthesis during early lactation as well as for glucose production (Trenkle, 1981), because the amount of the most important gluconeogenic precursor propionate and glucose (from intestinal resorption) is inadequate to meet the requirements (Zurek et al., 1995). There is virtually no limit on how much fat can be lost without affecting basic vital body functions. However, great limitations are placed on the loss of total protein reserves (25% of body protein for a lactating cow, Botts et al., 1979). Synthetic or degradative changes in muscle protein may change in response to the change in nutritional and endocrinological states that the cow experiences following parturition. Zurek et al. (1995) found that increased mobilization of muscle protein occurred during the first 3 weeks after calving indicating that muscle protein is no longer needed as an essential supplier of energy substrates after that period. Amino acids become then available for glucose generation for reproductive purposes which has been associated with alteration of LH concentrations (Rutter et al., 1983).

During the recovery period from NEB, one member of the large neutral amino acids, tyrosine, increased significantly in absolute values as well as in relative proportions to the large neutral amino acids. Tyrosine also correlated positively with the activity of LHRH-LH pulse generator and LH secretions. Based on these findings, Zurek et al. (1995) concluded that decreased gluconeogenesis from amino acids is associated with duration of recovery from NEB and with increased LH secretion during postpartum anestrus, and that tyrosine is thought to participate in metabolic signaling to the hypothalamus-hypophyseal axis controlling ovarian function in the postpartum cow. Furthermore, it was hypothesized that degradative changes in muscle protein might be the primary source of information about the metabolic status of the cow for the hypothalamus. It was also postulated that the mechanisms by which the dynamic changes in EB (duration of declining EB, magnitude, and rate of recovery) affected the duration of anovulation, might be through differences in ability of cows to mobilize muscle protein.

Another possible mechanism that influences resumption of postpartum ovulation might be a decreased ovarian sensitivity to LH signalling. Decreased ovarian sensitivity may be related to energy status (metabolites) or to circulating levels of insulin (Canfield and Butler, 1991).

As stated earlier the cow tries to compensate for NEB by mobilizing her own body fat and by gluconeogenesis from muscle protein. This compensation from body fat mobilization results in body weight and body condition loss. Body condition reflects the energy balance (EB), and since EB is very difficult to measure in cows, body condition scoring is used to monitor the energy dynamics of the cow (see Chapter 3). Research has shown that excessive tissue mobilization (rather than a high or low body condition score at calving) may be associated with longer days to conception (Ruegg, 1991). Cows losing one or more body condition points on a scale of 1 to 5 from calving to breeding are mostly cows that calve with a body condition score higher than 3.5. These cows have a lower dry matter intake after calving, have a higher fat content in milk (Holter et al., 1990), and have significantly greater days to first observed estrus, days to first service and lower first-service conception rates than cows with either minimal loss or improving body condition scores (Butler and Smith, 1989; Ferguson, 1990; Ruegg, 1991; Ruegg et al., 1992; Ferry, 1992). Further, these cows are more likely to develop cystic ovarian disease and metabolic, reproductive and foot problems after calving (Gearhart et al., 1990). In other words, cows that move more quickly into positive energy balance have more favorable reproductive performance. Fat cows also have lower prepartum feed intake that can lead to health problems (Emery, 1993). A Body Condition Score (BCS) of 3.5 on a five point scale at calving is therefore considered to be an optimum for milk yield, health and fertility.

## 14. Milk production level

Results of observational studies evaluating the relationship between milk production level and reproductive performance are contradictory. This may be due to confounding effects of management factors with possible biological effects (Hillers et al., 1984; Butler and Smith, 1989; Ferguson, 1994). High milk-producing cows are frequently bred later, since farmers believe that these cows take longer to conceive and require more services per conception than low milk-producing cows (Berger et al., 1981). This kind of intentional bias often clouds interpretation of research results. However, according to Butler and Smith, (1989), the studies that include herdmate comparisons have less confounding effects and overall demonstrate significant negative effects of milk yield on conception rate.

Selection for milk yield has increased blood concentrations of somatotropin and prolactin, which are stimulators of lactation and decreased insulin a hormone that is antagonistic to lactation and may be important for normal follicular development. These changes in hormone concentrations promote higher milk yield but may be potentially detrimental to other physiological functions, such as reproduction, if the management is not adequate to meet the metabolic demands of lactation. Timing and magnitude of NEB apparently interact to determine the extent to which NEB alters hypothalamic secretion of GnRH and its effect on gonadotropin secretion and, therefore, ovarian secretion of progesterone, which affects expression of estrus and support the uterus during early pregnancy (Nebel and McGilliard, 1993). High milk production has been reported to be antagonistic to estrus, but not to reestablishment of ovarian function (Harrison et al., 1990). It may be that increased yields of milk are associated with a more severe and extended NEB thereby reducing fertility. Milk yield per se does not need to account for negative impacts of production on reproduction if nutritional practices can compensate for severe negative effects of energy balance (Nebel and McGilliard, 1993; Ferguson, 1994).

## 15. Percent protein in the ration

Crude protein entering the rumen consists of nonprotein and true protein nitrogen. Nonprotein nitrogen is considered degradable crude protein and is usually converted to ammonia. True protein may escape rumen microbial degradation or it may be degraded to form peptides, amino acids, and ammonia. The ammonia is converted to microbial protein, and the amount depends on a variety of factors such as fluid dilution rate, amount and rate of fermentable carbohydrate, and pH. Ammonia that is not converted to microbial protein is absorbed through the rumen wall and is converted at energy cost, to urea by the liver. Ammonia also is formed during glucose synthesis from amino acids and can subsequently contribute to the blood urea pool (Chapter 4, part 1). Blood ammonia concentration may increase if the capacity of the liver to form urea is exceeded.

Increasing the amount of crude protein in dairy cow rations often results in higher milk yield. Many dairy farmers therefore feed their cows more protein than required or recommended according to feeding standards. An extra intake of protein above recommended standards may lead to a lower reproductive performance (Canfield et al, 1990; Elrod and Butler, 1993). Some authors have linked the detrimental effects on fertility to a high degradable fraction of protein in the ration (Folman et al, 1981; Canfield et al, 1990). Excess degradable protein in the ration, over the rumen degradable protein requirement, will increase blood ammonia content. This ammonia is then converted in the liver into urea, which results in elevated urea nitrogen concentrations in plasma, milk, urine and cervical mucus, especially when combined with a low ration energy content. Urea has been demonstrated to lower conception rates via fertilization failure or early degeneration of embryos, when urea nitrogen vaginal mucus concentrations exceeded 100 mg/100ml (Carrol et al., 1988; Blanchard et al., 1990), or when plasma concentrations exceeded 20 mg/100 ml (Ferguson et al., 1988).

Another explanation is given by Elrod and Butler (1993). Feeding an excess of protein, both rumenally degradable protein (Elrod and Butler, 1993) or undegradable protein (Elrod et al., 1993) results in a lowered intrauterine pH in the luteal phase of the estrous cycle. The pH during estrus was not different from cows fed a balanced diet. In addition, high protein diets may be associated with the normal luteal phase rise in ions such as, Na, K, PO4, Mg and Zn and nonalbumin proteins in the reproductive tract. These alterations in the uterine secretory activity might explain the lower first service conception rate (Canfield et al., 1990; Elrod et al., 1993) due to embryonic death and not so much to fertilization failure (Elrod and Butler, 1993).

Although many studies, mentioned before, state that an excess of protein may influence reproductive performance negatively, others cannot confirm this (Howard et al., 1987; Carroll et al., 1988; Figueroa et al., 1992). Effects of dietary protein on reproductive performance are not consistent. Degradability of crude protein is probably as important as total amount of crude protein fed, but few investigators have characterized the undegradable or degradable protein contents of the diets. Altering dietary crude protein, undegradable protein, or both may influence milk yield, dry matter intake, or both. Given the important impact energy balance may have on reproduction, trials to evaluate protein effects on reproduction should also report energy balance data, with sufficient number of cows per treatment so that the reader can attempt to delineate protein versus energy effects on reproductive performance (Grummer, 1993). More research is needed to confirm the preliminary indications that excess of crude protein and/or degradable protein in combination with a certain energy content of the diet has an adverse effect on reproductive performance.

## 5.2.4 CLINICAL INSPECTION

### General inspection

Clinical inspection relevant to reproductive performance starts with a general inspection of the herd. The inspection includes general health aspects such as: an impression of body condition of cows (Chapter 3), condition and shine of the hair coat, rumen fill, signs of lameness and indicators of other diseases, and more specifically alertness of cows related to cows standing and showing signs of estrous. The general inspection of the herd should be followed by a more detailed reproductive inspection of individual cows. This might include the presence of udder edema associated with recent calving, the presence of fresh skin lesions on or near the rump and/or dirty flanks as recent signs of estrus, swelling or lesions of the vulva caused by dystocia, the presence of vaginal discharge of either physiological secretions (cervical mucus or metestrous bleeding) or pathophysiological secretions (pus to watery secretum). The smell and color of vaginal discharge should always be determined.

### Genital tract examination

All cows to be examined should be identified on a list. This list also makes a convenient recording sheet for findings, diagnoses, treatments and/or management advice. The palpation starts with the vulva and pelvic area and proceeds up the reproductive tract to the ovaries. The vulva should be examined for acute (vesicles, pustules, erosions and /or erythema) and for chronic lesions due to dystocia and infectious disease such as ureaplasma (linear rows of cysts). The pelvic area is examined for perivaginal injuries. The cervix is retracted over the floor of the vagina to detect discharge via the vulva of cervical mucus, metestrous blood, urine as an indicator of an urovagina or other abnormalities. In postpartum cows the stage of uterine involution is estimated. One essential criteria is the presence or absence of longitudinal corrugations. By day 20 postpartum, the uterus should be retractable into the pelvic area. The diameter of the cervix and uterine horns is estimated. A well involuted cervix and uterine horns measure 3.5 cm and 2.0 to 2.5 cm respectively in diameter one month after calving. The uterus is further examined for the muscle tone associated with estrus. A high incidence of cows with a tone that have been observed in estrus on the same day by the farmer indicates a good accuracy in estrous detection. The uterus should then be examined for the presence of metritis, pyometra, adhesions and/or

*Table 1. Criteria for estimating duration of pregnancy*

| Diameter amniotic vesicle | Days pregnant | Head length | Days pregnant | Diameter uterine artery | Months pregnant |
|---|---|---|---|---|---|
| 1 finger | 40 | 1 finger | 70 | 3 mm | 3 |
| 2 fingers | 45 | 2 fingers | 80 | 6 mm | 4 |
| 3 fingers | 50 | 3 fingers | 90 | 9 mm | 5 |
| 4 fingers | 55 | 4 fingers | 100 | 12 mm | 6 |
| 5 fingers | 60 | 5 fingers | 110 | 15 mm | 7 |
| width of hand | 65 | width of hand | 120 | 18 mm | 8 |

other abnormalities. Pregnancy diagnosis is based upon criteria listed in Table 1. If pregnant, multiple pregnancies should be diagnosed. The length of pregnancy should be assessed (Table 1) and compared to recorded insemination dates. The proportion of cows found nonpregnant at pregnancy check is a measure of post breeding estrous detection.

The overall size of the ovaries, as well as adhesions affecting the ovaries, are investigated. The presence or absence of a corpus luteum, normal and cystic follicles is determined. Based on the diameter and the consistency of the corpus luteum, the day of the estrous cycle is estimated. The proestrous and metestrous stage may feel similar upon rectal palpation. The palpation of a corpus haemorrhagicum may be discriminated. Just after ovulation, both ovaries are small and difficult to differentiate from true anestrous cows. A second examination about one week later will reveal a definite diagnosis. True anestrus is most often combined with a low body condition score and is more prevalent in first parity cows than in older cows.

At first postpartum check, the location of the corpus luteum and/or a follicle, if present, is recorded as ipsilateral or contralateral to the previously gravid horn. A corpus luteum in the ovary on the non-gravid, and a follicle in the ovary on the previously gravid uterine horn at first postpartum check are both associated with improved reproductive performance (Bonnet et al., 1993). Rectal examination is followed by vaginoscopic inspection if metritis is suspected. Use of ultrasonography is restricted to very specific diagnoses due to the time and costs involved in practice.

When infectious or metabolic diseases are suspected, appropriate samples or swabs may be collected for laboratory analysis. A serologic profile of the herd may give insight into the disease status of the herd, for example BHV-1 and 4, BVD and others. When abortions occur, special sampling tools or culture media may be required. Cervical exudates or scrapings can be cultured for presence of Ureaplasms, *Campylobacter fetus* and *Trichomona fetus*. It can be worthwhile to take milk samples for antibiotic residue testing after treatment. Vaccinations related to reproductive performance are performed according to a vaccination program designed to meet both the farmer's needs and the herd disease status.

The next step consists of body condition scoring of all cows or of cows presented for rectal examination. The body condition score in the dry period or at calving should be listed on the examination list as a reference value and compared with the actual score. A loss in body condition score of > .75 point after calving may help explain fertility problems (Ruegg, 1991).

## Calving care

Calving care should be monitored if the incidence of dystocia, neonatal calf death and disease and cow diseases in the early lactation period is above acceptable levels. The monitoring process is directed at both clinical and farm inspection aspects. The following aspects should be monitored: 1) prepartum breeding policy, nutrition and health care, 2) calving environment, 3) calving management, 4) post calving cow and early calf care.

### Prepartum breeding, nutrition and health care.

Factors that must be monitored are:

1. raising strategy of replacement heifers that fulfills or does not fulfil requirements to help them to reach the proper body size and pelvic development at the time of calving (Chapter 2, part 2),
2. use or non use of bulls for breeding heifers that are listed by AI organizations for ease of calving,
3. proper body condition at calving. Cows should calve with a body condition score of 3.25 to 3.75. Cows with a score of 4 or more generally are slow calvers that need assistance in many cases. This can be associated with a prolonged calving process and the birth of weak or dead calves (Maree, 1986),
4. nutrition in the dry period must be considered as an instrument by excellence to prepare the cow for her next lactation (Chapter 3). Cows and heifers should be moved to a close-up group 2 to 3 weeks before the expected date of calving. During this period attention should be paid to mineral and feed intake, especially to an increasing energy intake. An inadequate mineral balance in the diet will lead to milk fever. A low energy intake in the dry-period and early postpartum will lead to a negative energy balance and subsequently fatty liver disease possibly followed by other metabolic diseases such as ketosis and displaced abomasum in the lactation period. Therefore, the energy content of the diet in the close-up period should be increased. In addition to this, the close-up ration should be balanced for a negative dietary cation-anion difference. This causes a mild acidosis which will increase Ca absorption from the intestines and mobilization of Ca from bone tissue. To balance the ration mineral content of the forage and concentrates in the ration must be known. However, negative dietary cation-anion difference salts may reduce milk fever incidence, even when Ca content in the diet is high (Chapter 3),
5. a planned dry cow vaccination program to prevent scours in the newborn calf caused by *Escherichia coli K 99* and Rota and Corona virus.

## Calving environment

For every 100 cows in the herd, an area with a minimal holding capacity of 5 cows should be permanently set aside for close-up cows and heifers. For cows at term a maternity pen should be available adjacent to the holding pen with the cow in eye contact with her close-up herd mates. This will prevent stress caused by removing cows from herd mates in the holding pen at the time of calving. Dry cows should be moved into the holding pen 2 to 3 weeks before expected calving date (close-up group), or as a last resort, when calving is imminent. The calving area should be under continuous supervision and specific persons assigned to monitor the area, especially on large dairy farms. The maternity pen must be situated in a quiet environment, with the cow in eye contact with the herd, accessible enough to permit regular and easy supervision, equipped with good restraint facilities if needed and have good footing for the cow and good footing areas to get up and down or move around, have dimensions that enables the cow to move freely at the time of calving, and that allows the use of calving aids if necessary. The maternity pen should also be dry, freshly bedded with straw, draft free and well ventilated, and clean. Cows should have access to clean water and fresh and palatable feed. An hygienic environment at the time of birth is a prerequisite for optimal health performance of the new-born calf. For that reason legs and feet, hindquarters, perineum and udder of the dam should then be cleaned. Maternity pens should follow the all in-all-out system with disinfection in between, in order to prevent infections. Ideally, cows should calve in pasture which is clean and dry and which has shade. A study in the U.S. (National Animal Health Monitoring System, 1992) found that pasture resulted in low calf mortality. Obviously, the pasture must have good drainage to minimize mud and allow the cow to get off by herself for calving.

## Calving management

Before calving, individual cow records should be checked for prior risk conditions, such as milk fever or obstetrical problems that may affect the cow at parturition. Sanitary procedures in the maternity area include: keeping the pen clean and well bedded with straw, cleaning the vulva, perineal area, tail and pelvic area before calving.

## Calving assistance and hygiene

Sanitary procedures during calving assistance include: tying the tail to the neck of the cow, supply of clean water in a few clean buckets, lubricant and two obstetrical chains, keeping obstetrical instruments in clean water with disinfectant added. Calving aids should be sterilized between calvings. Farmers should be instructed on how to perform vaginal examinations, with great attention to hygiene and use of proper lubricant. The hands and arms should be washed with soap and water and lubricated. Soap and detergents should not be used as lubricants because they de-fat and remove the natural lubrication from walls of the birth canal. Mineral oils and Vaseline make very good, lasting lubricants (Drost, 1992).

Assistance should be given when indicated after vaginal examination or when there has been no visible progress for two hours after appearance of the amnion bag. Farmers should know how to use extra traction in order to prevent trauma to cow and calf. Extraction in a anterior position can be initiated if a hand can be placed between the head of the calf and the sacrum of the dam and if the shoulder joints are less than 10 cm away (< 5 cm in a recumbent position) from the pelvic inlet. In case of a posterior position the hips of the calf have entered the pelvic cavity if the hocks are > 10 cm out of the vulva. Difficult calvings which the farmer or assistant cannot resolve should be reported to a veterinary practitioner early so that further evaluation and action is performed in time.

The percentage dystocia in heifers should be lower than 15 and in multiparae lower than 8. The percentage of dystocia is dependent on the gender of the calf, the breed, bull choice, position at the time of birth, the body condition of the dam and the parity of the dam. Any calf born as a result of dystocia is much more prone to stillbirth, neonatal mortality and colostrum deprivation (Waltner-Toews et al., 1986). Where increased calf mortality and morbidity occur, calving supervision including the competence of attendants and hygienic conditions should be examined.

**Post calving cow and calf care**

After calving, the date and sex of the calf born should be recorded. Calving complications, such as dystocia, and conditions of significance should be recorded on the health record of the cow. Cows should stay in the maternity pen until the placenta is released (small farms), or should be moved to a separate postparturient pen. The calf should be separated from her/his mother as soon as possible and transported to a clean and dry calf hutch, to prevent transfer of infectious agents. Each cow should be examined daily for signs of fever, depression, mastitis and abnormal uterine discharge. Body condition should be scored and recorded as a reference point for lactation and dry cow nutrition (Weaver, 1992). The cow should be milked in a clean container after disinfection of the teats with a post-milking teat dip. The navel of newborn calves should be disinfected with a 5 percent iodine solution and 1 to 1,5 liters of colostrum should be given as soon as possible after birth.

## EPILOGUE

Herd data collected by the farmer and clinical and farm inspection data collected by the practitioner and/or farm advisor, lead to the creation of three data resources. They form the basis for monitoring, evaluation and analysis of reproductive performance. After the farm visit all activities are directed at integrating the information from these three data resources. Informed decisions can then be made by integrating facts and/or information from the HH & PM activities to optimize herd reproductive performance (see part 3 of this Chapter).

For clinical examinations, rectal palpation skills are needed. However, reproductive performance is not only a function of the reproductive tract and the endocrine system but also of the managerial practices and of environmental conditions. For that reason a farm inspection has to be performed at every farm visit. Without evaluation and analysis of farm inspection data, a HFP is incomplete and conclusions can be misleading.

*For references see part 4 of this Chapter.*

# 5.3 MONITORING REPRODUCTIVE PERFORMANCE: DECISION MAKING AND FOLLOW-UP

Mark Varner[1] and Arie Brand[2]

[1] Department of Animal Science, University of Maryland, College Park MD 20742-2311, USA
[2] Department of Herd Health and Reproduction, School of Veterinary Medicine, University of Utrecht, Yalelaan 7, 3584 CL Utrecht, The Netherlands

## 5.3.1 INTRODUCTION

Decision making plays a key role in Herd Health and Production Management (HH & PM) programs, and that role is especially important in a Herd Fertility Program (HFP). Decision making is based on monitoring and evaluation of data and/or indices and then interpretation of information resulting from the monitoring and evaluation.

Monitoring of data, processing of raw data into performance indices, and evaluation of these indices are drawn from three sources of information. The first source is a database of herd reproductive performance variables collected by the farmer, the HH & PM practitioner and/or external organizations. The second source is a database of information collected by the practitioner and/or farm advisor during the farm inspection. The third data source consists of clinical and/or laboratory findings related to reproductive and health events. The interpretation of information from these three sources enables the practitioner, farm advisor and/or dairy farmer to make decisions about reproductive performance.

The first decision in the process is whether reproductive performance is proceeding as planned. When this is the case, the farmer will be advised to continue with ongoing activities. In cases when a problem arises, an in-depth analysis has to be conducted. This process starts with a problem definition and is followed by a preliminary or final herd performance diagnosis.

The follow-up process in a herd fertility protocol requires that in the case of acceptable reproductive performance, the preset targets may need to be reset to levels reflecting improved goals. In the cases where preset targets are not met, the success of interventions has to be evaluated during subsequent farm visits. This part of Chapter 5 is intended to provide an illustration of decision making and of problem analysis in a herd participating in a HFP with different levels of data availability. This means that the practitioner and/or farm advisor does not have to start from the beginning. An example of decision making in a herd without the use of a HFP can be found in part 4 of this Chapter.

## 5.3.2 DECISION MAKING

Making decisions about the herd's reproductive performance uses three processes: monitoring, evaluation and interpretation (See Figure 1, of part 1 of this Chapter). These processes are used to reach a decision near the end or after the farm visit.

## 5.3.3 MONITORING AND EVALUATION

Monitoring concerns records from the farm diary and the herd fertility chart, as well as individual cow records and processed data from external organizations. Information from past visits, including recommendations given, also has to be monitored. Monitoring can be defined as a process that warns of problems, and/or that recognizes patterns which may provide insight into problem causes. Irrespective of the level of data processing the monitoring process always starts before the beginning of each farm visit.

Routine evaluation of reproductive indices is conducted by comparing them to preset targets. Incidence rates of clinical findings, and some farm inspection observations, are also evaluated if targets are set beforehand. If targets are unavailable, observations should be weighed against the personal experience and opinion of the practitioner or farm advisor.

Interpretation of data and information should be considered in light of factors that control reproduction. These factors originate from biological processes inside the cow and from management practices of the farmer and environmental conditions outside the cow.

The decision making process, as based on monitoring, evaluation and interpretation, will be discussed at three levels of data availability through data processing.

## 5.3.4 DATA PROCESSING

Data processing consists of converting raw data into usable sources of information. Informational sources include performance indices, summaries, tables, graphs, and others. Primary and secondary indices should be calculated on a monthly, seasonal and/or an annual basis. The frequency depends on, the size of the herd, calving pattern, the nature of the index, changes in management, timing of interventions, frequency of herd visits, attitude of the practitioner and/or farm advisor towards data processing and, last but not least, the availability of electronic data processing systems.

Data processing can be done manually or electronically. Manual data processing is laborious, so indices of reproductive performance are rarely calculated that way. Evaluation of reproductive performance is then restricted to inspection of herd fertility charts or individual cow records for detection of crude trends in reproductive performance or information concerning a specific cow.

Data processing more commonly involves computer programs, either at the farm or externally by third party organizations. Many farms have progressed from manual data processing to third party data processing, for example by Dairy Herd Improvement centers (DHI). The processing activity can include reproductive events, body condition scores, milk production data, somatic cell counts, economic data and other types of data. Many organizations are increasing their data storage and processing capabilities to include clinical data and data produced by electronic devices in automated milking parlors. When clinical inspection information is included, the resulting indices of reproductive performance are much more valuable. For example, when results of pregnancy diagnosis by genital examinations are known and included in data processing, non-return rate indices can be replaced with accurate pregnancy rates.

The accuracy of data and information used in monitoring, evaluation and interpretation depends on the farmer providing timely and complete data. If primary and secondary reproductive performance indices are provided by an external organization, the summarization is usually delayed. This delay restricts decision making by delaying interpretation. The veterinary practice might also provide data input and have specialized computer programs (VAMPP, Dairycomp 305, DairyChamp and others, see Chapter 5, part 1). Some computer programs not only reduce data processing delay, but they also increase the value of the information provided. These programs have detailed evaluation and/or analytical capabilities beyond those found in other programs.

On-farm processing has the advantage that the performance indices can be generated quickly and monitored while the client is still mindful of the problem(s). When on-farm processing is used, the veterinary practice or farm advisor can be connected to the farmer's computer by either direct connection or via computer networks. This capability significantly improves the practitioner's access to the performance indices that might be needed for further analysis and decision making.

## Levels of data availability in relation to data processing

The extent of monitoring and evaluation that can be conducted within a herd depends on data availability and the processing systems used. Three sources of data might be available:

1. **herd data:** Calving history (dystocia), calves born (sex, dead or alive), estrous, insemination, pregnancy and culling dates. The data are recorded daily by the farmer on individual cow charts, a herd fertility chart and/or on a farm diary;
2. **farm inspection data:** These data include management factors or events and farm conditions that might be related with reproductive performance. In contrast to herd and clinical data they have a more qualitative character and will be recorded on the farm diary and/or on the report that is send to the farmer at the end of the farm visit;
3. **clinical inspection data:** They involve findings from regular rectal examinations and from a general clinical herd inspection. They are recorded on an examination list during the planned farm visit, once every two to six weeks, depending on the size of the herd.

It has to be stressed that the farmer has primary responsibility for data collection followed by the practitioner. Herd's data play a key role in the decision making process of reproductive performance (Nelson and Redlus, 1989). Without these data, monitoring, evaluation and eventual analysis of reproductive performance is incomplete.

With regard to data processing three levels of data processing can be distinguished:

1. Only herd data is available and no form of data processing is used. The herd fertility program is typically restricted to cow genital reproductive examinations;
2. Herd, farm, and clinical inspection data are available with manual data processing restricted to clinical inspection and farm inspection data,
3. Herd, farm, and clinical inspection data are available with on farm and external detailed data processing, and analysis.

### Monitoring and evaluation at different levels of data availability and processing capability

An example herd is used to demonstrate the value of information availability and processing in diagnosing herd reproductive performance and associated problems. The levels of data processing and availability reflect typical industry practices and likely future practices that will be adopted. The example herd is first described and then information is evaluated using different levels of availability.

### Example Herd Characteristics

The herd has on average 100 Holstein cows and 94 young stock. Last year's annual milk production per cow amounted 9140 kg with 4.40% fat and 3.50% protein. Average daily milk production per cow is 30 kg. Calving interval is 390 days. Labor force consists of the farmer, one hired person and the farmer's spouse. Cows are confined in a free-stall barn all year long, and milked in a double-six herringbone parlor. The farmer and the hired laborer alternate milkings. Automated concentrate feed supply stations are installed. Nutrients fed are wilted grass silage, corn silage, by-product feeds (beet pulp, potatoes, brewer's grains), and concentrates to meet NRC guidelines. Embryo transfer is done at a regular basis. Surplus breeding stock is sold every year. Reproductive data are recorded in a farm diary, on a herd fertility chart and on individual cow records. The main herd health concerns of the farmer are cow fertility and udder health.

### 1. Herd data available with no data processing

The herd does not participate in a milk recording program like DHIA. A herd fertility protocol is not used at this level, even though the practitioner or farm advisor visits the farm on a semi- to regular basis. Preset targets are not defined. The farmer is recording reproductive data on a herd fertility barn chart or individual cow charts. The herd's reproductive data are not processed into indices. Cows for clinical veterinary examination are identified by the farmer and not by the practitioner, who is focusing only on conducting genital exams. Those cows with fertility problems are given appropriate treatments. An evaluation of management practices and/or inspection of farm conditions is not done.

Veterinary herd fertility services at this level consist solely of cow genital examinations, diagnoses and immediate treatments of reproductive tract abnormalities. Although this is a common approach among veterinary practitioners, it offers no possibilities for monitoring, evaluation, and interpretation of reproductive performance at the herd level. The dynamics and interaction of underlying managerial and/or biological processes related to a problem can also not be identified. Therefore, it must be clear that a HFP conducted at the level of "rectal tourism" is not suitable for objective decision making. More clearly, the service offered cannot be considered as a programmed herd fertility service.

## 2. Herd, clinical and farm inspection data available with some manual data processing

As in example 1) the herd does not participate in a milk recording program provided by DHIA. A herd fertility protocol is partially followed and includes recording of data in a farm diary. However, preset targets are not defined. The herd's reproductive data are not processed into performance indices. The incidence of relevant diagnoses from clinical inspections reported on the examination list, are calculated for categories such as proportion of: cows with retained placenta; cows with metritis at postpartum check; cows not seen in estrus but diagnosed with an active corpus luteum; and cows presented for pregnancy examination found pregnant. For other clinical findings the number of cows with a specific diagnosis, for example the number of cows with cystic ovarian follicles, are simply counted. Interpretation of clinical and farm inspection data are conducted on the spot. The prevalence of reproductive findings are recorded on a 12-monthly list and compared with previous prevalences. An example of a 12-monthly list is in Table 1. Only some of the categories in Table 1 are recorded by the farmer at this level.

During a farm visit to the example herd, 18 cows were offered for genital examination in the following categories: postpartum check, not seen in estrus and pregnancy diagnosis. The following findings were made: of the 5 cows examined for postpartum check, 2 cows had experienced dystocia and 1 cow had retained the placenta for 5 days. These 3 cows had also developed vaginal discharge due to uterine infection. Six cows were examined for failure to demonstrate estrus. One cow had pyometra. True anestrus was diagnosed in two first-lactation heifers which had a low body condition score, produced more than 40 kg of milk and had no palpable ovarian structures. The other 3 cows were diagnosed as having active ovaries. Four out of seven cows examined for pregnancy were pregnant, of which 2 out of five after embryo transfer. No abnormalities were found in the nonpregnant cows.

An overall clinical inspection of all cows was conducted after the genital examinations were completed. The inspection revealed that about 10% of the cows were treading on their hind feet while in the feeding fence headlocks. Some cows had periarthritis of the hock. A general impression of body condition for the whole herd was that an acceptable variation in body condition occurred, with only a few very fat and very thin cows. Rumen fill was normal. Feces consistency was scored and fell within normal limits of 2 to 3 on a scale of 1 to 5.

*Table 1. Part of a 12- monthly list on reproduction*

| DATE OF VISIT | 10/01 | 7/02 | 13/03 | 9/04 | May | June |
|---|---|---|---|---|---|---|
| **COWS/YOUNG STOCK** | | | | | | |
| – # COWS MILKING | 80 | 86 | 83 | 85 | – | – |
| – # COWS DRY | 19 | 16 | 20 | 17 | – | – |
| – # YOUNG STOCK PREGNANT | 38 | 35 | 41 | 38 | – | – |
| – # YOUNG STOCK OPEN | 57 | 57 | 48 | 41 | – | – |
| **REPRODUCTION** | | | | | | |
| – # COWS CALVED | 4 | 7 | 7 | 8 | – | – |
| – # RET. PLACENTA | 3 | 0 | 2 | 1 | – | – |
| – # METRITIS | 2 | 1 | 1 | 3 | – | – |
| – # PYOMETRA | 0 | 0 | 0 | 1 | – | – |
| – # NOT SEEN IN ESTRUS | 3 | 2 | 4 | 3 | – | – |
| – # TRUE ANESTRUS | 4 | 1 | 0 | 2 | – | – |
| – # CYSTIC OVARIAN FOLLICLES | 4 | 5 | 1 | 0 | – | – |
| – % PREG/COWS EXAMINED | 3/9 | 3/6 | 5/8 | 4/7 | – | – |
| – # SERVICES/PREGNANCY | 2.0 | 2.1 | 1.9 | 1.8 | – | – |
| – DIM AT 1ST SERVICE | 76 | 69 | 70 | 75 | – | – |
| – DIM AT CONCEPTION | 97 | 90 | 89 | 94 | – | – |
| – # ABORTIONS | 0 | 0 | 0 | 0 | – | – |
| – AGE AT 1ST CALVING | 790 | 710 | 703 | 730 | – | – |
| – # COWS/HEIFERS CULLED/SOLD | 3/0 | 0/0 | 3/0 | 1/9 | – | – |

The farm inspection revealed that high quality feed is available at the feed bunk. Adequate space is provided in both the free stalls and at the feeding fence. The barn is well ventilated and cool. The light intensity in the barn is moderate due to dirty windows in the barn roof. Some parts of the slatted floor in alleyways are uneven.

The results of herd checks at this level may be interpreted either as no problem, as a warning of developing problems or as a strong indication of an existing problem. An existing problem would be indicated in the case of a steady increase in clinical incidence observed on the 12-monthly list. With regard to this example herd, three out of seven cows that were not found pregnant together with 3 cows with active ovaries but not seen in estrus suggest that estrous detection efficiency might be a current problem. No problem was observed in estrous detection efficiency over the previous 12 months. The diagnosis of a current estrous detection efficiency problem is supported by the observation of a significant number of cows treading on their hind feet during genital examination and the farm inspection observation that the slatted floors in the alleyways were uneven. Treading on hind feet is a symptom of lameness. Uneven slatted floors could provide poor footing. Poor footing and lameness are known to be associated with reduced expression of estrus in dairy cows (Chapter 7).

**3) Availability of farmer's, clinical and farm inspection data as in 2) with external data processing**

At this level a Herd Fertility Protocol has been fully implemented for several years. Availability of farmer's, clinical and farm inspection data is as in example 2) with external data processing. Preset targets are defined together with the farmer. The reproductive preset targets of primary reproductive indices and some secondary reproductive indices for this herd are as follows.

Primary Reproductive Indices:

*) a projected average minimum calving to conception interval of 85 ± 10 days. More than 85% of cows that calved receiving a first insemination and at least 90% that were inseminated become pregnant.

*) culling rate due to reproductive failure < 5% (20% of cows culled),

*) abortion rate < 4%,

*) a projected average minimum age at first calving of 24 ± 1 months.

Secondary Reproductive Indices:

*) an interval calving to first insemination < 70 days,

*) an interval first insemination to conception < 10 days.

*) first service conception rate of > 60%,

*) # services per conception of < 1.5.

Reproductive policies:

*) no voluntary waiting period.

Reproductive data are collected and recorded in a farm diary by the farmer. Data recorded are mailed to the veterinary practice just before the next farm visit and processed electronically. Action lists are made up at the veterinary clinic together with relevant reports that should be discussed with the farmer. Due to the time delay in processing, the action lists have to be updated with recent data from the farm diary at the time of the farm visit of the practitioner.

The clinical data and some farm inspection data are processed at the veterinary clinic after the farm visit. Instead of a hand recorded 12-monthly list, as in level 2, a printed 12 monthly list can now be delivered to the farmer by the veterinary clinic. Qualitative farm inspection data are included in the report that is sent to the farmer after the farm visit. As stated earlier another option is that the farmer enters and processes all the data in his PC, supported by his practitioner and/or farm advisor.

The national DHI center provides the example farm with primary and secondary indices of herd reproductive performance as listed in Table 2. They can be calculated over any lenght of period. This particular DHI organization calculated the retrospective interval or days in milk (DIM) from calving to conception and not the projected average minimum interval, that is preferred for evaluation. Also, age at first calving is calculated instead of the preferred projected average minimum age at first calving. The processing of herd data, and relevant clinical and some farm inspection data by external organizations, can provide extensive statistical information.

*Table 2. Primary and some secondary indices of reproductive performance of the example farm over a one year period*

| | Cows | Heifers |
|---|---|---|
| # cows/heifers calved | 73 | 28 |
| # cows/heifers inseminated | 62 | 27 |
| Predicted calving to conception interval (days) | 106 | |
| # cows culled due to reproductive failure | 9 (9%) | |
| # cows aborted | 4 (4%) | |
| Age at first calving (months) | 23.5 | |
| Interval first AI to conception (days) | 29.6 | |
| Interval calving to first AI (days) | 85 | |
| First service conception rate | 54.8 | |
| # services per pregnancy | 1.83 | |

In our example herd at level 3, evaluation of the primary indices of reproductive performance (Table 2) indicates that calving to conception interval was longer, and culling rate due to reproductive failure was higher than preset targets. The abortion rate and age at first calving was within normal limits. Evaluation of the secondary indices of reproductive performance indicate that cows are inseminated later after calving than planned. Further, there are too many days from first insemination to conception but first service conception rate and services per pregnancy are relatively good.

The evaluation results of the clinical and farm inspection findings are the same as level 2). Instead of a general impression of body condition scoring in the herd, like at level 2), body condition is now scored for all individual cows. Evaluation of these data revealed that 6 (11%) of cows from calving through approximately 100 DIM had scores of 2.5 or less. These six cows are first or second parity cows and they have a high milk production level. The anestrus observed in these high producing cows is likely caused by a severe and a long lasting negative energy balance connected with excessive body tissue loss. Low body conditions are indicative for a (prolonged) negative energy balance in the postpartum period which may delay first ovulation and/or estrous expression (Ferguson, 1990).

**Preset targets met?**

After monitoring, evaluation and interpretation of data and information, a decision must now be made if performance is developing as planned. If the performance meets the preset targets for primary indices, no further action is taken. If the actual performance indices deviate from the preset targets an analysis of relevant indices is done to find risk factors (see part 4 of Chapter 5). The criteria used to determine what is acceptable and unacceptable depend upon the types of data available and the insight/experience of the practitioner and/or farm advisor. The best approach is to combine the human insight with a statistically based evaluation of herd performance indices.

If the most actual reproductive performance indices and the clinical and farm inspection findings do not deviate from preset targets, the final step in the protocol consists of continuation of record keeping of relevant reproductive events. If no important recommendations have to be given repeatedly, it could be advised to reset the pre-set targets at a level that can be realistically achieved. In cases where primary indices deviate significantly and/or over a long time period from preset targets, a problem analysis should be initiated.

In the previous paragraphs, evaluation was performed at three levels of data collection and data processing.

At level 1, no preset targets are defined. The herd fertility chart is the only data source available and no data are processed into indices. Therefore, Decision making based on monitoring, evaluation and interpretation of reproductive performance indices is not possible. In this herd decision making has to be done in an intuitive way.

At level 2 no preset targets were defined. The recorded and processed clinical and farm inspection data, but not the herd data, were evaluated by the practitioner after the farm visit. Statistical estimation and analysis of overall reproductive performance is therefore not possible. A final decision concerning reproductive performance can not be made objectively since primary and secondary reproductive performance indices at the herd level are unavailable. In the example herd, the evaluation only suggested an estrous detection problem. The impression of the existence of a problem can be strengthened if the 12-monthly list provides the same trends over a longer period.

At level 3, preset targets are defined and data processing of herd and clinical data allow for evaluation of performance indices. Decision making based on hard facts instead of intuition is now possible. The evaluation of example herd data, revealed that the calving to conception interval which was 106 days, was greater than the preset target of 85 days. The average calving to first insemination interval for the example herd was 85 days which is greater than the preset target of 70 days. The first service to conception interval was also confirmed as being abnormal. This makes the example herd at level 3 substantially abnormal for three reproductive performance indices. This finding was supported by some farm inspection data. Now the decision can be made that the example herd has a problem. Thus, a detailed analysis is required to come to a final problem definition and/or diagnosis.

### 5.3.5 PROBLEM ANALYSIS

Herds participating in a HFP, like the example herd at level 3, have the advantage that additional data are available for problem analysis. Herds without this data are discussed in part 4 of this Chapter.

The first step in analyzing reproductive performance is to determine if herd size is changing. When the goal for herd size is to stay constant, culling and replacement rates must be in balance. An elevated involuntary culling rate or reduced replacement rate can be thought of as risk factors causing an imbalance in rates. Presence of one or both of these risk factors means that cows must be purchased or problem cows must be retained in the herd longer than desirable to prevent herd size from decreasing (Ferguson, 1991).

In cases where problem cows must be retained, reproductive indices may be influenced negatively. Conception rate will be low and services per conception will be high if problem breeders are part of the retained animals. Treating such a herd as a conception failure will not solve its problem (Ferguson, 1991). Control points that determine herd size are projected minimum age of calving for heifers and projected minimum calving to conception interval. In contrast, high involuntary culling rates, due to reproductive problems, may mask the problems since culled cows frequently do not contribute to calculation of reproductive indices.

Problems are analyzed separating relevant indices into their composing elements and searching for factors which may be potential causes for the indices that fall outside acceptable levels. A checklist is used for identification of relevant risk factors for each problem. Diagnoses of causes are then made after consideration of supporting and refuting evidence from these analyses.

For the example herd at level 3, problems were identified for the following primary parameters: calving to conception interval and culling rate due to reproductive failure (Table 2).

**Interval calving to conception**

Before starting analysis, one must recognize that mean calving to conception interval, or the preferred projected minimum calving to conception interval, as an index of reproductive performance is misleading because they do not reflect the distribution of cows in the herd for that index. Herds with an acceptable calving to conception interval can still have reproductive problems in some cows that get pregnant late after calving. This then results in a wide and/or skewed frequency distribution for this index. On the other hand, herds with a high average for calving to conception, or age at first calving, can still have acceptable reproductive performances. The deviation in the index from preset targets is then due to intentional herd breeding policies. Such herds with abnormal averages and acceptable reproductive performance are characterized by having a tight distribution around the average for that index.

Based on these considerations a detailed analysis of the reproductive performance for the example herd starts with an examination of the frequency distribution for calving to conception interval (Figure 1) which was 106 days. The distribution has a wide dispersion, and the herd can be thought of as two groups of cows. One group, consisting of 64 cows (75%) has no reproductive problems and an average days to conception of 85 days. The other 16 (25%) cows with an interval of at least 130 days from calving to conception, are problem cows with an average of 185 days. The frequency distribution of calving to conception intervals for individual cows confirms that there is a problem with calving to conception in at least some cows.

In a search for possible causes, this primary index is analyzed further. Calving to conception interval is broken into its components. Since this herd has no voluntary waiting period, the components are interval from calving to first insemination and interval from first insemination to conception.

### The interval from calving to first insemination

The frequency distribution for calving to first insemination interval is depicted in Figure 2. In the example herd 6.75% of cows were inseminated before 51 days and 39% after 90 days, causing a wide distribution for this index. As with calving to conception interval, only some cows have problems that are reflected in this interval.

*Figure 1. Frequency distribution of the intervals from calving to conception*

<= cow identification numbers

| | | | | | | | | | | |
|---|---|---|---|---|---|---|---|---|---|---|
| | | | 461 | | | | | | | |
| | | | 312 | | | | | | | |
| | | | 309 | | 311 | | | | | |
| | | | 307 | | 310 | | | | | |
| | | | 289 | | 303 | 313 | | | | |
| | | | 284 | 306 | 296 | 302 | | | | |
| | | | 254 | 295 | 291 | 298 | | | | |
| | | | 253 | 294 | 266 | 293 | | | | |
| | | | 247 | 269 | 260 | 292 | | | | |
| | | | 223 | 256 | 224 | 258 | | | | |
| | | | 221 | 239 | 211 | 245 | | | | |
| | | | 214 | 201 | 203 | 238 | | | | |
| | | | 210 | 196 | 202 | 227 | | | | |
| | | | 199 | 190 | 160 | 209 | | 305 | | 301 |
| | | | 196 | 183 | 152 | 207 | | 264 | | 297 |
| | | | 172 | 171 | 144 | 182 | 252 | 237 | 299 | 241 |
| | 7 | | 169 | 143 | 115 | 83 | 229 | 234 | 290 | 138 |
| | 11 | 186 | 136 | 43 | 89 | 78 | 148 | 188 | 249 | 134 |
| % | 2.5 | 1.3 | 22.5 | 16.3 | 20.0 | 17.5 | 3.8 | 6.3 | 3.8 | 6.3 |

10 — 30 — 50 — 70 — 90 — 110 — 130 — 150 — 170 — 190

→ DIM

*Figure 2. Frequency distribution of the intervals from calving to first AI*

<= cow identification numbers

| | | | | | | | | | |
|---|---|---|---|---|---|---|---|---|---|
| | | 284 | | 306 | | | | | |
| | | 264 | | 295 | | 311 | | | |
| | | 254 | | 295 | | 310 | | | |
| | | 253 | | 288 | | 301 | | | |
| | | 252 | | 269 | | 299 | | | |
| | | 247 | | 256 | | 298 | | | |
| | | 237 | | 249 | | 296 | | | |
| | | 224 | | 239 | | 293 | | | |
| | | 223 | | 211 | | 292 | | | |
| | | 221 | | 201 | | 271 | | | |
| | | 214 | | 196 | | 266 | 302 | | |
| | | 213 | | 190 | | 260 | 290 | | |
| | | 210 | | 188 | | 255 | 258 | | |
| | | 209 | | 183 | | 203 | 245 | | |
| | | 205 | 461 | 171 | | 202 | 238 | | |
| | | 199 | 312 | 143 | | 160 | 234 | | |
| | 305 | 196 | 309 | 134 | | 152 | 227 | 297 | |
| | 291 | 172 | 307 | 83 | | 144 | 207 | 241 | |
| 11 | 186 | 169 | 303 | 78 | 313 | 138 | 182 | 229 | 300 |
| 7 | 115 | 136 | 289 | 43 | 308 | 89 | 100 | 148 | 162 |

% 2.2 — 4.5 — 29.2 — 24.7 — 21.3 — 11.2 — 4.5 — 0.0 — 2.2 —

10 — 30 — 50 — 70 — 90 — 110 — 130 — 150 — 170 — 190 -

→ DIM

**Checklist**

The potential risk factors of prolonged intervals from calving to first insemination either at herd or cow level are:

* inefficient estrous detection (Kyle et al., 1992; Senger, 1994),
* a long voluntary waiting period,
* inadequate identification of cows,
* poor maintenance of records,
* restricted or seasonal breeding period, which may be based on seasonal differences in milk price,
* use of heifers and cows as embryo recipients,
* postponement of first insemination in cows with a high milk production, based on perceived increase in fertility for inseminations in later lactation, especially with use of expensive semen in cows with high genetic value,
* inactive ovaries caused by a severe negative energy balance, especially in first parity

cows with high milk production levels (Huszenicza et al., 1987; 1988),
* reproductive tract abnormalities such as metritis and pyometra due to dystocia, and retained placenta (Gwazdauskas et al., 1986; Bonnet et al., 1993),
* ovarian dysfunction such as cystic ovarian follicles (Laporte et al., 1994),
* other diseases with an indirect influence on reproductive performance, such as: metabolic diseases (Miettinen, 1990) and claw disorders (Lucey et al., 1986; Montes and Pugh, 1993; Barkema et al., 1994).

Most of the factors listed can be manipulated through management. This means that management plays an very important role in reproduction. An exception is seasonal milk price which is out of control of a dairy farmer.

Analysis sofar suggested that embryo transfer of cows, a declining energy balance associated with high milk production (especially for first parity heifers), first insemination policy and inadequate estrous detection were the most likely causes for the present situation.

**Interval from first service to conception**

The interval from first service to conception, which is the second component of calving to conception interval, is now analyzed with the help of a frequency distribution (Figure 3). The interval is influence by the conception rate and both estrous detection efficiency and accuracy. For the example herd, the interval was 29 days, which is greater than the preset target of 10 days. Over 35% of the cows have a first service to conception interval greater than 37 days, demonstrating a skewed distribution for this index.

**Checklist**

Potential risk factors of a prolonged interval from first insemination to conception are:
* low conception rate. Conception rate usually improves with time postpartum (Britt, 1975; Ferguson, 1991),
* inaccurate estrous detection (Roche et al., 1992),
* inefficient postbreeding estrous detection,
* ovarian dysfunction like cystic ovarian follicles (Laporte, et al., 1994),
* poor semen quality of bulls used for insemination,
* inaccurate AI procedures (Barth, 1993; DeJarnett, 1994):
  - improper semen handling, such as; thawing procedures and tank maintenance,
  - improper breeding technique; placement of semen in vagina/cervix versus uterine body,
  - wrong timing of insemination either too early or too late at observed estrus (am/pm rule) or at improper predicted estrus (based on palpation criteria or blind insemination based on previous records or on estrous synchronization),
* early embryonic/fetal death, which may be reflected in abnormal estrous intervals (Wilmut et al., 1986; Alexander et al., 1995),
* venereal diseases (Barr and Anderson, 1993),

*Figure 3. Frequency distribution of the intervals from 1-st service to conception*

<= cow identification numbers

| | | | | | | | |
|---|---|---|---|---|---|---|---|
| 199 | 258 | | | | | | |
| 196 | 256 | | | | | | |
| 196 | 254 | 461 | | | | | |
| 190 | 253 | 312 | | | | | |
| 186 | 247 | 311 | | | | | |
| 183 | 245 | 310 | | | | | |
| 182 | 239 | 309 | | | | | |
| 171 | 238 | 307 | | | | | |
| 169 | 227 | 306 | | | | | 305 |
| 162 | 223 | 302 | | | | | 301 |
| 160 | 221 | 300 | | | | | 299 |
| 152 | 214 | 296 | | | | | 297 |
| 144 | 210 | 295 | | | 313 | | 252 |
| 143 | 207 | 294 | 303 | | 308 | | 249 |
| 136 | 205 | 289 | 293 | | 290 | | 241 |
| 89 | 205 | 284 | 292 | | 288 | | 237 |
| 43 | 203 | 269 | 271 | | 234 | 291 | 213 |
| 11 | 202 | 266 | 211 | | 224 | 264 | 138 |
| 7 | 201 | 260 | 83 | 289 | 78 | 188 | 134 |

% 66.3 —— 0.0 – 7.2 —— 1.2 —— 8.4 — 0.0 – 3.6 —— 13.3 ——

0 —— 4 —— 18 —— 26 —— 37 — 48 — 57 —— 71 ——

——► days

* suboptimal energy balance (Ferguson, 1991; Britt, 1994),

* excessive rumen degradable protein together with low energy intake (Canfield et al., 1990; Ferguson, 1991),

* high ambient temperatures (Hansen, 1994),

* a high percentage of cows with a parity of > 3 (Stevenson et al., 1983; Hillers et al., 1984).

Conception rate, estrous detection accuracy, infertility, low semen quality, AI procedures, early embryonic/fetal death, venereal diseases and excessive rumen degradable protein did not appear to be risk factors for prolonged interval from first insemination to conception in the example herd since first service conception rate and services per conception were adequate. The herd did not have a large number of cows in 4th or later parity and high ambient temperatures were not a factor in prolonged interval.

Inefficient postbreeding estrous detection and prolonged negative energy balance were both risk factors for prolonged interval from first insemination to conception for this example herd. The herd, clinical, and farm inspection data confirmed that both risk factors might be causing a problem.

**First service conception rate and services per pregnancy**

First service conception rate is thought to be the most sensitive measure of herd fertility. The first service conception rate for the example herd is 56%, and is at an acceptable level.
Services per pregnancy is another common secondary index of reproductive performance. The average for the example herd is 1.83, which is higher than the preset target of 1.5. but which is still acceptable. The levels for these two indices demonstrate that accuracy of estrous detection is good since high fertility rates could not be obtained if estrous detection is inaccurate.

In total, 29.6 days were lost from first insemination to conception. If every estrus would have resulted in a pregnancy only 1 insemination per pregnancy would have been needed. In reality 1.83 inseminations were performed. These extra inseminations were responsible for .83 times 21 days (length of normal estrous cycle), or 17.4 days loss in calving to conception interval. The remainder of the interval is due to missed estrous cycles. This means that 29.6 minus 17.4 or 12.2 extra days were lost due to unobserved estrus after first insemination, assuming that early embryonic death did not occur. These 12.2 extra days confirm that estrous detection efficiency was a problem for this herd.

A high number of services per pregnancy may also be caused by a few cows that inflate the average in a small herd. This means that culling policy for repeat breeders, either early or late, can have an impact on services per conception.

**Inter-service interval**

Various lines of evidence confirm that estrous detection efficiency is a problem at the example farm. The potential causes are given in part 4 of this Chapter. Inter-service interval is a secondary reproductive performance statistic that is frequently used to determine whether estrous detection is accurate and/or efficient. The frequency distribution of inter-services intervals for pregnant cows in the example herd is depicted in Figure 4, and demonstrates repeat breeding cows at normal and abnormal inter-service intervals.

Inter-service interval analysis is based on the assumption that cows have normal (21 day) estrous cycle lengths. The use of estrous synchronization programs or hormonal therapies for unobserved estrus can change the length of inter-service interval so that it is no longer a "normal" length. Thus, inter-service interval should be used only in herds where no estrous synchronization drugs or hormone therapies are used.

*Figure 4. Frequency distribution of inter-service intervals*

<= cow identification numbers

| | | | | | | | | | |
|---|---|---|---|---|---|---|---|---|---|
| | | | 288 | | | | | | |
| | | | 288 | | | | | | |
| | | | 271 | | | | | | |
| | | | 264 | | | | | | |
| | | | 249 | | | | | | |
| | | | 249 | | | | | | |
| | | | 237 | 313 | | | | | |
| | | | 237 | 313 | | 297 | | | |
| | | | 224 | 308 | | 291 | | | |
| | | | 224 | 308 | | 264 | | | |
| | | | 211 | 303 | | 252 | | | |
| | | | 209 | 301 | | 252 | | | |
| | | | 188 | 301 | | 249 | | | |
| | | | 188 | 297 | | 237 | | | 305 |
| | | | 188 | 293 | | 234 | | | 301 |
| | | | 138 | 292 | | 209 | | | 299 |
| | | 305 | 138 | 291 | | 134 | | 297 | 241 |
| | | 300 | 83 | 290 | 298 | 115 | | 213 | 213 |
| | 134 | 297 | 11 | 290 | 264 | 78 | 297 | 138 | 134 |
| % | 1.6 | 4.9 | 54.1 | | 3.3 | 19.7 | 1.6 | 4.9 | 9.8 |

0 4 18 26 37 48 57 71

→ days

**Percent possible estrous periods detected**

Inefficient detection of estrus is the leading cause of reproductive inefficiency in dairy cows. Many factors can influence estrous expression and detection of estrus.

A checklist with potential risk factors may include:

Cow factors:

* time after calving (Kyle et al., 1992)
  - inactive ovaries,
  - ovulation number,
* reproductive diseases (pyometra, luteinized cysts),
* lameness,

Management factors:

* presence of a sexual active group or number of open cows in the herd or group (MacMillan, 1992),

* frequency and timing of estrous detection,
* inadequate identification of cows,
* inadequate record keeping (Smith and Schmidt, 1987),
* quality of footing surface (Dozier-Vailes and Britt, 1990),
* housing system used (tie stall versus loose housing system),
* nutritional factors influencing the energy balance (Ferguson, 1991; Zurek et al., 1995).

## Culling rate

Reproductive culling rate was not a problem for the example herd. Factors that most often contribute to culling due to reproductive failure are: infertility caused by chronic genital infections and ovarian dysfunction, abortion, and sterility (blocked oviducts).

## Age at first calving

Although age at first calving was no problem in the example herd, a list of potential causes may include the following:

* inactive ovaries due to a negative energy balance at breeding time which might be caused by nutritional inefficiencies,
* poor estrous detection practices,
* poor record keeping (Nelson and Redlus, 1989),
* seasonal breeding (Gwazsdauskas, 1981)
* embryonic loss and abortions (Barr and Anderson, 1993; Alexander et al., 1995),
* natural mating with an infertile bull (Gwasdauskas et al., 1981).

## Abortion rate

Abortion rate was not a problem in the example herd. A checklist of potetial risk factors include:

* viral, bacterial, and protozoal diseases (Barr and Anderson, 1993),
* stress situations in the last trimester of pregnancy,
* insemination of pregnant cows,
* prostaglandin injections in pregnant cows,
* harmfull rectal examinations (Thurmond and Picanso, 1993),
* toxins in feed (Putnam, 1989).

## Herd performance diagnosis

The example herd has some acceptable and some unacceptable reproductive performance indices. Age at first calving meets the preset targets with plenty of replacements available. Abortion rate is low. Pregnancy rate at first breeding is relatively high and the number of services per pregnancy is acceptable. However, the main problem is a relatively long calving to conception interval. This excessive interval is made up of a long interval from calving to first breeding and from first breeding to conception.

An analysis of the distribution of individual calving to conception intervals revealed that the herd can be split in two parts. One has normal reproductive performance and the other has abnormal performance. In the retrospective analysis of the latter group, 4 cows were first parity, 7 were second and 4 were third or later parity cows. A detailed analysis revealed that nearly all these cows experienced some problems such as, a severe and prolonged negative energy balance, reproductive diseases and/or other health problems.

The final conclusion concerning a herd performance diagnosis is that the calving to conception interval was excessive in only a few cows. Since herd data are historical, the extent of problem must be considered for the current situation. Results of the latest farm and clinical inspection provide clues to the current status. The analysis identified the risk factors as embryo transfer of cows, a declining energy balance associated with high milk production (especially for first parity heifers), first insemination policy and inadequate estrous detection were the most likely causes. The latest clinical and farm inspection revealed that these risk factors were currently still present. The finding that estrous detection problems were still apparent were based on the fact that some cows were not pregnant and others were not seen in estrus at the time of the latest genital examination. The clinical evaluation suggested that inefficient estrous detection was especially a problem for cows after first insemination. High milk production may be contributing to problems with estrous detection and conception rate through a prolonged negative energy balance, reproductive disorders and other diseases such as lameness.

### 5.3.6 INTERVENTIONS AND RECOMMENDATIONS

Assessment of results requires translation of the results and analysis into recommendations. These recommendations must be related to actions that will have the desired effects. The first recommendation is to put greater attention on estrous detection. Effective attention will probably have the greatest effect on reproductive performance. To facilitate recognizing the cows needing extra attention, a list of eligible cows should be carried by the heat detector at all times. Another recommendation is greater attention to lameness problems. Reduced lameness should improve estrous detection and could also improve feed intake and reduce the negative energy balance in some cows. Renovations of the barn floor are recommended. The roof windows should be cleaned to improve illumination. However, the farmer should recognize that the high milk production can increase the length of time a cow is in a negative energy balance and lower body condition. To improve the energy balance already in the dry-period, a close-up group should be formed and rations should be balanced and examined for cation-anion difference, together with dry matter intake and feeding strategy (see Chapter 3). This should result in more cows being inseminated before 75 days after calving. A more aggressive prostaglandin therapy approach is recommended for cows with unobserved estrus. Advice for the future would be to use pedometers to aid identifying cows in heat.

A report is written with the results of the analysis, the recommendations given and the interventions employed. The interpreted information always has to be translated into understandable or familiar terms when reported to the farmer. Carefully chosen information can provide an educational opportunity for the practitioner and/or farm advisor to explain what can be obscure to a client and to reinforce recommendations. The date of the next visit is fixed. This report is sent to the farmer as soon as possible after the farm visit. A copy of the report is kept in the file of the herd health practitioner.

### 5.3.7 FOLLOW-UP

Recommendations and control measures should be reviewed during subsequent farm visits. The activity and progress towards implementing the recommendations and control measures should be evaluated. The producer should be informed of this evaluation, both verbally during the farm visit and by a written report. The success of interventions should also be evaluated. Intervention outcome should be communicated to the producer verbally and by written report.

## EPILOGUE

Evaluation of herd reproductive performance must be done on a regular and frequent basis. The sources of data used for evaluation can be thought of as historical and actual. Historical data consists of the herd's database of past information including prior clinical and farm inspections. The actual data consists of the most recent clinical and farm inspection findings, as well as the events recorded in the farm diary but have the disadvantage of being related to only a sub-population of the herd. The historical data set is used to monitor and analyze trends in reproductive performance. Since the data is historical, any trends may or may not be current. Therefore, actual data from the clinical and farm inspections must be used to confirm or refute the trends from historical data. When used judiciously, actual data can have great value to support or refute the trends observed in historical data. When the actual data refutes the trends, it can have even greater value by helping focus the practitioner's clinical and farm inspection on potential problems during the next visit.

The amount of actual data available for analysis is typically much less than the amount of historical data. The differences in the amount of data frequently make practitioners reluctant to place much weight on the actual information derived from clinical inspection and some farm inspection data. However if no attention is paid to historical data or if data from one inspection part is lacking, no monitoring, evaluation and analysis can be done.

Most of the veterinary practitioner's time is devoted to the biological aspects of reproduction, such as disease conditions. Practitioners have to realize that reproduction disorders typically influence only that affected cow or a small part of the herd.

The management factors predisposing a herd to a reproductive disorder such as record keeping, culling, estrous detection and genetics, are then given little attention, while treating the symptoms of the reproductive disorder receive virtually all the attention. Therefore one has to realize that management aspects have a much greater influence on reproductive performance, since they impact the herd as a whole.

In conclusion, a herd fertility program must follow a protocol that is focused upon the unique characteristics of each herd. The protocol establishes a monitoring and evaluation system to monitor reproductive performance in its entirety. Not only can existing problems be studied with the protocol, but the onset of developing problems can be identified. If a herd fertility program is not followed completely, reproductive performance can not be evaluated and analyzed in full depth. One has to realize that the amount of data and information available for decision making for herds participating in a HFP is much greater than for herds without a HFP. Decision making for herds with a HFP is also easier because the practitioner can organize the data and information into various conceptual layers.

*For references see part 4 of this Chapter.*

# 5.4 MONITORING REPRODUCTIVE PERFORMANCE: CASE STUDY ON AN ESTROUS DETECTION PROBLEM

Mark Varner[1] and Arie Brand[2]

[1] Department of Animal Sciences, University of Maryland, College Park, MD 20742-2311, USA
[2] Department of Herd Health and Reproduction, School of Veterinary Medicine, University of Utrecht, Yaleaan 7, 3584 CL Utrecht, The Netherlands

## 5.4.1 INTRODUCTION

Reproductive problems can occur in any herd. Producers that participate in a herd fertility program (HFP) have an advantage, however, when solving the problem. A key component of a HFP is the continuous collection of information, which allows for early evaluation and analysis. In contrast, problems in herds without a HFP will be more difficult to analyze due to absence of key information. Sometimes, the only data source that might be available is DHIA records and/or a manual breeding chart.

A problem solving protocol is used to solve reproductive problems in a herd, regardless of how many data sources are available. Such a protocol consists of farmer's complaint, history taking, an inspection of available data, and the execution of a clinical and a farm inspection. This is then followed by an analysis of available and collected data. Differential diagnoses of dairy herd reproductive problems are then made. Additional clinical and/or laboratory information can sometimes be required to discriminate between possible problems. The herd performance diagnosis is now complete and possible interventions can be considered. An economic analysis of the costs and benefits of each intervention should be conducted. This part of Chapter 5, follows a case-study of a dairy herd reproductive problem caused by ineffective estrous detection.

## 5.4.2 COMPLAINT OF THE FARMER

The farmer contacts his local practitioner concerning reproductive problems with his herd. He is breeding cows by artificial insemination, but he catches a low percentage of the cows in estrus. The farmer is thinking of using a bull for natural breeding and asks for help and opinions.

## 5.4.3 HISTORY TAKING

A history of the farm's reproductive management policies and practices related to the complaint is required. The practitioner should interview the farmer about a number of relevant items. These include information on herd characteristics, nutrition, estrous detection and breeding practices, reproductive performance information, and/or veterinary or herd health policies (see Appendix A). It is the responsibility of the practitioner or farm advisor to determine which questions are important for a particular herd.

Not all answers will be utilized initially to construct a list of possible diagnoses. Those answers may be required later to interpret some subsequent clinical or laboratory analysis, or may serve as a historical basis for analysis of any future problems in this herd. Consequently, the practitioner or farm advisor must be judicious when selecting which questions and have an eye open to the future.

### Results of history taking for the case-study herd

The herd contains 80 cows in milk, 10 dry cows, 5 non-lactating heifers over 24 months of age, 20 heifers between 13 and 24 months of age, and 20 heifers and calves under 12 months of age. All are Holstein cattle. The lactating cows are managed as one group of cows. The producer measures milk production for every cow on a 6 week basis. Average 305-day milk production amounts 6200 kg. Cows and dry cows are pastured in summertime and housed in wintertime. Dry cows are kept in one group which means that no close-up ration is provided. In wintertime, grass silage and hay are the main forage fed. Forages are tested on a regular basis, and records of the analyses are available. A consulting nutritionist formulates rations.

The herd is owned and managed by a husband and wife team who live on the farm. They have 3 children under the age of 10. The wife is responsible for a few farm chores. All of the other work is done by the husband. No one works off the farm in another job. The husband and wife ranked the herd's problem areas from most to least serious as: reproduction, lameness, nutrition, operating costs, milk production and mastitis.

No specific time is dedicated to watching cows for estrus due to a shortage of labor. However, the cows are watched for estrus in: 1) the housing area while the farmer is maintaining the free stalls, and 2) the holding pen before milking. Any one sign of estrus is sufficient to signal for inseminating a cow. No estrous detection aids or methods to anticipate estrous are used, and no specific method is used to help anticipate estrus.

A herd fertility chart is used to record reproductive events. However, only calving and insemination data are recorded. Estrous dates occurring before breeding are not recorded. No voluntary wait period is used. Cows are inseminated when they are observed in estrus. The farmer is not participating in a herd fertility program. Instead, the farmer consults his practitioner for only serious and specific disease problems, such as difficult dystocia, milk fever and displaced abomasum. The farmer would then ask the practitioner to do fertility work on an irregular and infrequent basis. The fertility work would include pregnancy examinations of inseminated cows and clinical examination of infertile cows. Prostaglandin-F-2-$\alpha$ (PGF) is used by the practitioner to treat cows not observed in estrus. Potential for responsiveness to the PGF is via rectal exam by the veterinary practitioner. Cows not observed to be in estrus within 5 days after injection are not retreated with PGF until the practitioner comes to the farm for the next irregular visit. Only 10% of the herd is treated with PGF.

Heifers must be at least 16 months old before being inseminated, and no weight cutoff is used. Estrus is not synchronized in heifers. Pregnancy checks are not done with heifers.

Records on diseases are not kept. However, the farmer estimates that approximately 40% of the cows retain their placenta more than 24 hours. Dystocia is infrequent (less than 6% of births), though the farmer pulls the calf for over 80% of births. Milk fever and ketosis ranked second in disease frequency.

A seasonal calving pattern is applied by aiming most calvings in the spring. No cutoff is used to designate cows without observed estrus for veterinary examination. Cows that will not calve in the desired calving season are culled.

## 5.4.4 INSPECTIONS

### Data inspection

Data inspection involves the review of any relevant reproductive information recorded by the farmer or provided by third party organizations and the processing of relevant data. After processing of recorded data on the herd fertility barn chart the following primary indices of reproductive performance could be calculated: 1) projected minimum calving to conception interval is 185 days; 2) projected minimum age at first calving for heifers is 27 months; 3) reproductive culling rate for fertility, on an annual basis was 40%; and 4) abortion rate per confirmed pregnancy was 2%. Processing of the recorded data from the herd fertility barn chart allowed calculation of the following secondary indices of reproductive performance. Days to first insemination averaged 120, and the first service conception rate was 52%.

### Farm inspection

The farm inspection involves the practitioner or farm advisor focusing his/her attention on the farm site, facilities and managerial practices. The farm inspection is tailored to the complaint of the dairy farmer and the facilities present. Instead of interviewing the farmer, as was done in the history taking section, the practitioner or farm advisor must now be a detective and look everywhere where relevant, using a critical eye.

Not all areas of attention will be appropriate for every farm, but a full inspection should be made. Observations not utilized to construct a list of possible diagnoses may be required later to help interpret some kind of subsequent analysis or in an economic evaluation. As mentioned earlier, the observations also serve as a historical basis for analysis of any future problems.

### Results of farm inspection for the case study herd

Cows are housed in a free stall (cubicle) barn. The bedding consists of dry wood shavings, and an adequate amount is provided. The floor surface of the barn and feeding area is smooth slippery ungrooved concrete. Some gritty material is sprinkled on parts of the floor in the housing and feeding areas, but not on a regular and frequent basis. The cows have 24 hr/day access to an exercise lot with a dirt surface. No foot baths are used.

The feed bunk space was adequate for the herd size. There was insufficient good quality feed remaining in the feed bunk 8 hrs after last feeding. Since the cows are fed twice daily, there was 4 hours until the next feeding. Only a few uneaten corn cobs are present in the bottom of the feed bunk. There was no evidence that the feed bunk was cleaned out on a regular basis, and a few wooden sticks were in the bunk, indicating that some time had gone by since the last cleaning. The feed analyses indicated that moderate to high quality forages were available to feed the cows. The concentrate was properly formulated to complement the forages.

### Clinical inspection

Herd clinical inspection includes a general health evaluation and rectal palpation of all cows on the farm. Since the herd is not participating in a HFP, genital palpation should be conducted on all cows to determine reproductive status of the herd as a whole, which can be regarded as a "snap-shot" of current and past reproductive performance. The number of pregnant cows and heifers and the incidence of various reproductive problems, such as cystic ovarian disease, anestrus, vaginal discharge and pyometra should be determined from clinical examinations and producer records, if available. Body condition scoring should be conducted on all milking and dry cows in the herd (Chapter 3). All cows should be observed for signs of lameness (Chapter 7).

### Results of the clinical inspection for the case study herd

The clinical inspection findings for reproductive status are presented in Table 1. Due to the seasonal calving pattern no voluntary waiting practice was used by the farmer. So no emphasis can be placed on this index, even if conducting the analysis at the right time of the year. A high percentage of cows were open. The seasonal calving pattern accounts for part of the results. The timing of the producer's call came when few cows had calved recently. Preparing a stage of lactation distribution for open cows can be used to clarify what kinds of interventions might be required.

*Table 1. Reproductive status for the herd*

| Cow Status | Number | Heifer Status | Number |
|---|---|---|---|
| Pregnant Dry Cows | 10 | Pregnant over 24 mo | 10 |
| Pregnant Lactating | 30 | Pregnant 13 - 24 mo | 40 |
| Open | 40 | Open | 40 |
| Inseminated < 30 days | 10 | Inseminated < 30 days | 10 |
| Voluntary Wait Period | – | | |

*Table 2. Distribution of open cows by stage of lactation*

| Stage of Lactation | Number of Cows |
|---|---|
| DIM < 60 | 0 |
| DIM 60 - 120 | 10 |
| DIM > 120 | 40 |

*Table 3. Incidence of various reproductive disorders*

| Reproductive Disorder | Incidence (% of milking cows) |
|---|---|
| Cystic Ovarian disease | 8% |
| Anestrus | 0% |
| Pyometra | 15% |
| Vaginal Discharge | 5% |

*Table 4. Body condition score for various groups of cows*

| Cow Group | Average Score | Range |
|---|---|---|
| Early Lactation | 2.0 | 1 - 3 |
| Mid Lactation | 2.2 | 1 - 3 |
| Late Lactation | 2.7 | 1 - 4 |
| Dry | 3.0 | 2 - 4 |

A stage of lactation distribution for open cows is in Table 2. There were no open cows under 60 days postpartum due to seasonal calving. Consequently, there are no cows entering the optimal insemination period, and potential intervention plans do not have to take this class of cows into consideration. Too many cows beyond 120 days in lactation were open. These cows need special attention when designing any intervention plans. An analysis of reproductive disorder incidence is required to help identify a cause for this problem. No open cows were dry.

The prevalence of various reproductive disorders is in Table 3. The incidences of cystic ovarian diease and metritis are normal. The pyometra incidence is high. The incidence of anestrus, based on small and/or inactive ovaries is low. However, no cows were less than 60 days in milk so the risk of an estrous was very low. No firm conclusions concerning the potential of anestrus problems leading to the current situation can be drawn from this incidence. Further observations will be required when cows, susceptible to anestrus, are in the herd.

Body condition scores of cows in different lactation groups are in Table 4. Average and minimum score in the range are too low for all groups. Cows are too thin both at an individual and at a herd level. An examination of ration formulation and feed analyses is required. Lameness was observed in approximately 25% of the milking cows.

## 5.4.5 EVALUATION OF FINDINGS AND CONCLUSIONS

The herd is a seasonal calving herd, with most cows long past early lactation. Fitting into the seasonal calving pattern is the primary reproductive culling criteria. Cow reproductive performance is a serious problem, based on projected minimum calving to conception interval. Since reproductive performance is so poor, too many cows are not bred in time to maintain the seasonal calving pattern. These cows are then culled, which increases the involuntary reproductive culling percentage. Average days to first insemination is unacceptably high, especially when considered in light of the herd's seasonal calving goal. Seasonal calving requires cows to become pregnant during a narrow time frame, soon after calving. The first insemination performance almost precludes the producer from meeting the goal. First service conception rate was acceptable. Heifer reproductive performance is suboptimal, based on projected minimum age at first calving.

Average body condition scores are too low, suggesting that the feeding program needs to be evaluated and that anestrus is a possible cause for the farmer not observing cows in estrus. The ration was formulated to meet nutrient requirements for cows at the level of production and stage of lactation for this herd. Insufficient feed was available for the cows.

No estrus detection aids or estrous expectancy devices are used, making estrous detection difficult. No special times are set aside for detection of estrus, and since labor is in such short supply, not enough time is dedicated to estrous detection. Observation of cows for estrus is done when animals are on non-grooved slippery concrete that is treated with gripping material on an infrequent and irregular basis.

No HFP was being conducted, leading to: no voluntary wait policy, no structured program to identify cows with no observed estrus, and an ineffective PGF therapy program. Too many cows may be assisted with birth, but inadequacy of records makes it difficult to be sure. Retained placenta incidence may be too high, but inadequacy of records makes it difficult to be sure. Pyometra prevalence was too high. Lameness is a producer recognized problem, and this problem is made worse by the lack of regular footbath use and the lack of a hoof care component in the herd fertility program.

PGF use is ineffective when used due to the lack of the follow-up injection 14 days after the first injection in cows not observed in estrus. Further, PGF is not used often enough when considering the severity of the reproductive problem in the herd. Cows are not treated early enough in lactation. The stage of the estrous cycle when cows are treated is determined by genital palpation, but a second treatment for non-responders, 14 days after the first treatment, is not used to catch misclassified cows.

## 5.4.6 DIFFERENTIAL CAUSES LIST

The farmer's complaint for this case-study herd was specific concerning an estrous detection problem. First service conception rates were acceptable, supporting the producer's complaint, thus, factors such as infertility do not need to be considered. The possible causes of an estrous detection problem are in Table 5.

*Table 5. Possible causes of an estrous detection problem*

| | |
|---|---|
| Small herd size | Infrequent use of PGF |
| Poor record keeping | Ineffective use of PGF |
| No participation in a HH & PMP | Negative energy balance |
| Hot weather in breeding season | Poor body condition |
| Observation failures | Lameness |
| Poor footing | Anestrus or inactive ovaries |
| No estrous detection aids used | |

The results of data inspection (history taking), clinical inspection and farm inspection should first be used to eliminate possible causes. Herd size can be eliminated as a cause, since it is large enough to allow sexually active group formation. Moreover, seasonal breeding will facilitate the formation of such groups.

Poor record keeping prevents a dairy farmer from effectively using estrous expectancy charts and estrous detection aids. Both of these tools can be used to improve a farmer's chances of finding a cow in estrus. The poor record keeping system also allowed problem cows to go too far along in lactation before they received veterinary attention. The herd was also not in a veterinary HH & PM program. The lack of timely veterinary care because of poor disease record keeping was made worse by the absence of a routine program for cow reproductive examinations. Further, the lack of consultation and advice provided in a HFP may also be contributing to the estrus detection problem since no voluntary wait policy was established and no mechanism was set up for early problem identification.

Hot weather during the breeding season can reduce estrous detection rates, and this herd's seasonal calving pattern results in a summer breeding season. However, this herd is located in the northern latitudes, and hot weather is not a serious problem during most years.

Observation failure is one likely cause of estrous detection problems in this herd. No one person is taking responsibility for the job. No time is spent observing cows for estrus when no other chores are being done. Observations are not done when cows are in the dirt floored exercise lot, where most estrous behavior is likely to occur.

Poor footing in the housing and feeding areas is another likely cause of estrous detection problems for this herd. Both areas have slippery concrete flooring. Neither area has grooves in the concrete. Sand, or another gritty substance, is not provided on a frequent and routine basis to prevent the cows from slipping.

PGF is used under the supervision of a veterinarian and based on the presence of an active corpus luteum, suggesting that this is not a cause of the problem. Mis-classification of ovarian status when using rectal palpation alone has been demonstrated, however (Pankowsky et al., 1995). Typically, cows not observed to respond to the first injection of PGF are given a second injection 14 days after the first. Any cow misclassified during the examination should be responsive to PGF 14 days after examination. The farmer is not giving this second injection of PGF 14 days after the first, thus allowing some PGF injections to be ineffective. Additionally, less than 10% of the herd is being treated with PGF, even though unobserved estrus is a problem. This low PGF use is likely caused by the herd not participating in a HFP, is preventing the farmer from reducing short-term consequences of the problem while long-term solutions are being established.

Negative energy balance and poor body condition are frequently related, and both can be caused by inadequate nutrition. In this herd, the feeds are tested and rations formulated appropriately, but, insufficient amounts of high quality feed are provided to the cows. Cows are forced to clean up even the larger cobs from the corn silage due to hunger. The farmer desires to have the cows "clean up the feed" rather than clearing out a small amount of discarded feed on a regular basis. Even though feeds are formulated properly, the empty feed bunks are evidence that not enough is fed. This lack of feed availability is a likely cause of the poor body condition in the herd, as evidenced by low body condition scores. Energy balance was not directly measured in this herd, but could be a likely contributing cause.

Lameness can reduce a cow's mobility and ability to find a sexual partner or a sexually active group. Lameness is a problem in this herd, due to inattention to hoof care and lack of a foot bath. Further, cows spend most of their day on concrete, which tends to wear the hooves in a disproportionate manner. Lameness could be contributing to the estrous detection problem for the herd.

Anestrus was not found to be a problem in the herd, but few cows were currently at the most susceptible state for inactive ovaries. Thus it could be a problem if more cows were at risk. A lack of feed is suspected as a problem, which can put cows less than 60 days in milk at greater risk for anestrus. Consequently, a monitoring program for anestrus is needed to examine cows next calving and breeding season for anestrus.

Anestrus was further supported as a cause by the high rate of pyometra. Pyometra can prevent onset of ovarian activity or cause persistent corpus luteum, both of which can lead to anestrus. The high prevalence of pyometra may have been caused by the high incidence of retained placenta and/or assisted births, which then may lead to pyometra. The lack of a herd health program hampered the pyometra problem from coming to the attention of farmer or from being treated in a timely manner.

### 5.4.7 ADDITIONAL CLINICAL ANALYSIS AND INFORMATION

A definite diagnosis frequently requires additional information and/or analysis. However, in this case study the information collected is sufficient to come to a definite diagnosis. A limited amount of additional information will be required in the future to monitor progress towards preset targets. That information will be described in the Intervention and Follow-up sections.

## 5.4.8 DEFINITE DIAGNOSIS

Based on the data, farm, and clinical inspections, it can be concluded that the suboptimal estrous detection rate is caused by a complex of interacting factors:
*) Estrous observation failure,
*) Poor footing in housing and feeding areas,
*) Lameness.

Contributing factors include:
*) Suboptimal nutrition,
*) Poor record keeping,
*) High incidence of retained placenta.

## 5.4.9 RECOMMENDATIONS

A herd fertility program within the framework of an extended HH & PM program, should be started with this herd. As an integral part of that, a voluntary wait period policy, a record keeping system, and a program for identifying veterinary examination candidates should be established and reviewed with the farmer.

Good reproductive performance starts in the dry period before calving and not after calving. Therefore, cows should be grouped in a close-up group 3 to 4 weeks before expected date of calving. The close-up diet should contain forage ingredients of the early lactation diet with the main objective to acclimate cows to lactating rations and minimize the negative energy balance which starts already before calving (Bertics et al., 1992). Furthermore, feeding strategy during the lactation period should be improved. Fresh and palatable feed should be available during 24 hours a day. At least 5% of the ration should be swept up and feed to other animals daily to ensure cows have sufficient access to high quality feed. Cows need to reach a condition score of 3 to 3.5 at the end of lactation and to keep it in the dry period.

An estrous observation program should be established to improve estrous detection efficiency. Availability of labor is extremely limited, so possible interventions should be focused upon one or both of two approaches: making what little time is available most effective, or using a technological solution that can free up labor or does not require additional labor. Approaches that can be used that improve the chances of observing cows in estrus with existing labor are:

- Identification of a time and location when most mounting behavior occurs in the herd. The steps for this are:
  * Draw a facility map and use the map as a part of the farm inspection and place an X where a cow is observed to stand for mounting by another cow. All areas of the facility should be watched, including those areas not watched now (exercise lot). Write the time next to the X. Record only one X per cow per estrus, and make the location and time the first standing mount observed.

  * When the map contains approximately half the number of X's as cows in the milking herd, the map should be examined and the locations where most mounting occurs identified. These spots are termed "hot spots", and they are typically located where the footing is the best and/or in areas where cow traffic comes together or moves in a direction. Examples are an exercise lot or a dirt lane to a pasture.
  * The times should be examined to determine when most mounting occurs. These times are termed "hot times", and they typically occur near sunrise and sunset, during times of herd movement, and sometimes after feeding.
  * Access to the "hot spot" by the herd should be restricted to times near the established "hot times". The designated observer should then open the access to the "hot spot", and do nothing other than observe cow behavior. Typically, the observer can open a gate after milking so the cows are given access to an exercise lot or pasture when the observer is available to watch.
- Estrous detection aids require a small amount of time to apply, but these aids can help identify cows not otherwise observed in estrus. These aids include an estrus expectancy chart, tail-chalk, tail painting or glue-on pressure-sensitive devices. Fertility of inseminations based on the results from estrous detection aids alone are often sub-optimal.

When extra labor is just not available, as with this example herd, some herds may be willing to use technological approaches to improve identification of estrus. Some of these approaches include:

- Estrous synchronization therapies can be used to schedule only certain days of the week or month for observation of estrus. These PGF treatments have been shown to be effective, and the improvement in herd reproductive performance typically more than pays for the cost of the synchronization therapies.
- Ovulation synchronization therapies have been developed to allow producers to schedule insemination of cows at a certain time, with no need for estrous observation. The treatments include a GnRH - PGF - GnRH treatment regime, and are much more expensive that PGF estrous synchronization regimes. Ovulation synchronization programs have been shown to result in acceptable levels of fertility, but the cost-effectiveness of ovulation synchronization therapies have not been evaluated extensively. The example herd, however, has few alternatives, so ovulation synchronization should be considered.
- Electronic devices have been developed to help identify cows in estrus. Commercial devices include computerized pedometers and pressure-sensitive mount detectors. The predicting value for positive identification of estrus has been variable for electronic pedometers, and has limited their adoption in dairy herds. Early results with electronic pressure-sensitive mount detectors indicate that favorable fertility results can be obtained. The cost of these devices have limited their adoption in commercial dairy herds.

## 5.4.10 FOLLOW UP

The follow-up for this case-study herd involves not only evaluation of whether recommendations have been carried out, but it also involves further clinical analysis due to the seasonal calving. Specific steps were recommended to improve the estrous detection program on the farm. Those steps should be reviewed to insure that they are carried out.

Improvements in estrous detection efficiency should occur within one month, and a mechanism to measure estrous detection efficiency should be used. The percentage of possible estruses detected is an appropriate secondary reproductive performance index for this situation. An easy to obtain measure of this index is the percentage of cows examined found pregnant during pregnancy exam. This should be over 80%. If all estrous periods are identified, then open cows should not end up being examined by the practitioner for pregnancy. The effectiveness of PGF therapy should also be evaluated by determining the proportion of cows not inseminated at first PGF injection who did receive a second injection.

Cows in this herd may be at risk for true anestrus, but no cows in the herd were currently in the stage of lactation when greatest risk occurs due to the seasonal calving cycle. A part of the follow up would be to record ovarian activity, as determined by rectal palpation or milk progesterone, during the next seasonal calving cycle. The proportion of cows with inactive ovaries by 30 days post-partum should be determined.

## REFERENCES

*Alexander, B.M., M.S. Johnson, R.O. Guardia, W.L. Van de Graaf, and R.G. Sasser. 1995. Embryonic loss from 30 to 60 days post breeding and the effect of palpation per rectum on pregnancy. Theriogenology. 43:551-556.*

*Badinga, L., W.W. Thatcher, T. Diaz, M. Drost, and D. Wolfenson. 1993. Effect of environmental heat stress on follicular development and steroidgenesis in lactating Holstein cows. Theriogenology 39:797-810.*

*Barkema, H.J., J.D. Westrik, K.A.S. van Keulen, Y.H. Schukken, and A. Brand. 1994. The effects of lameness on reproductive performance, milk production and culling. Prev. Vet. Med. 20:249-260.*

*Barr, B.C. and M.L. Anderson. 1993. Infectious diseases causing bovine abortion and fetal loss. Vet. Clin. North America: Food Animal Practice. 9:343-368.*

*Barth, A.D. 1993. Factors affecting fertility with artificial insemination. Vet. Clin. of North America: Food Animal Practice. 9:275-289.*

*Bertics, S.J., R.R. Grummer, C. Cadorniga-Valino, and E.E. Stoddard. 1992. Effect of prepartum dry matter intake on liver triglyceride concentration and early lactation. J. Dairy Sci. 75:1914-1922.*

*Berger, P.J., R.D. Shanks, A.E. Freeman, and R.C. Laban. 1981. Genetic aspects of milk yield and reproductive performance. J.Dairy Sci. 64:114-125.*

*Blanchard, T., J. Ferguson, L. Love, T. Takeda, B. Henderson, J. Hasler, and W. Chalupa. 1990. Effect of dietary crude-protein type on fertilization and embryo quality in dairy cattle. Am. J. Vet. Res. 51:905-908.*

*Bonnet, B.N., W. Martin, and A. Meek. 1993. Associations of clinical findings, bacteriolo gical and histological results of endometrial biopsy with reproductive performance of postpartum dairy cows. Prev. Vet. Med. 15:205-220.*

*Botts, R.L., R.W. Hemken, and L.S. Bull. 1979. Protein reserves in the lactating dairy cow. J. Dairy Sci. 62:433-440.*

*Britt, J.H. 1975. Early postpartum breeding in dairy cows. J. Dairy Sci. 58:266-271.*

*Britt, J.H., R.G. Scott, J.D. Armstrong, and M.D. Whitacre. 1986. Determinants of estrous behavior in lactating Holstein cows. J. Dairy Sci. 69: 2195-2202.*

*Britt, J.H. 1994. Follicular development and fertility: Potential impacts of negative ener gy balance. Proc. Nat. Reprod. Symp. Ed. E.R. Jordan. Sept. 22-23, Pittsburg. pp. 103-112.*

*Butler, W.R., R.W. Everett, and C.E. Coppock. 1981. The relationship between energy balance, milk production and ovulation in postpartum holstein cows. J. Anim. Sci. 53:742-748.*

*Butler. W.R. and R.W. Canfield. 1989. Interrelationships between energy balance and postpartum reproduction. Proc. Cornell Nutr. Conf. pp.66 Ithaca, NY.*

*Butler, W.R. and Smith, R.D. 1989. Interrelationships between energy balance and post partum reproductive function in dairy cattle. J. Dairy Sci. 72: 767-783.*

*Canfield, R.W. and W.R. Butler. 1990. Energy balance and pulsatile LH secretion in ear ly postpartum dairy cattle. Domest. Anim. Endocrinol. 7:323-330.*

*Canfield R.W., C.J. Sniffen, and W.R. Butler. 1990. Effects of excess degradable protein on postpartum reproduction and energy balance in dairy cattle. J. Dairy Sci. 73:2342-2349.*

*Canfield, R.W. and R.W. Butler. 1991. Energy balance, first ovulation and the effects of naloxone on LH secretion in early postpartum dairy cows. J. Anim. Sci. 69:740-746.*

*Collier, R.J., S.G. Doelger, H.H. Head, W.W. Thatcher, and C.J. Wilcox. 1982. Effects of heat stress during pregnancy on maternal hormone concentrations, calf birth weight and postpartum milk yield of Holstein cows. J. Anim. Sci. 54:309-319.*

*Collick, D.W., W.R. Ward, and H. Dobson. 1989. Associations between types of lameness and fertility. Vet. Rec. 125:103-106.*

*Committee on Bovine Reproductive Nomenclature. 1972. Recommendations for standardizing bovine reproductive terms. Cornell Vet. 62:216.*

*Carroll, D.J., B.A. Barton, G.W. Anderson, and R.D. Smith. 1988. Influence of protein intake and feeding strategy on reproductive performance of dairy cows. J. Dairy Sci. 71;3470-3481.*

*DeJarnette, J.M. 1994. Interactive effects of semen quantity, semenquality and insemination techniques on conception rates of artificially inseminated cattle. Proc. Nat. Reprod. Symp. Ed. E.R. Jordan. Sept. 22-23, Pittsburg. pp. 139-150.*

*Devir, S., J.A. Renkema, R.B.M. Huirne, and A.H. Ipema. 1993. A new dairy control and management system in the automatic milking farm:basic concepts and components. J.dairy Sci. 76:3607-3616.*

*Djemali, M., A.E. Freeman, and P.J. Berger. 1987. Reporting of dystocia scores and effects of dystocia on production, days open, and days dry from DHI data. J. Dairy Sci. 70:2127-2131.*

*Dohoo, I.R. and S.W. Martin. 1984. Disease and culling in Holstein Friesian cows. IV. Effects of disease on production. Prev. Vet. Med. 3:755-770.*

*Dozier-Vailes, L. and J.H. Britt. 1990. Influence of footing-surface on mounting and other sexual behaviors of estrual Holstein cows. J. Anim. Sci. 68:2333-2339.*

*Drost, M. 1992. Management of obstetrics. In: Large dairy herd management. Eds. H.H. Van Horn and C.J. Wilcox. American Dairy Science Association. Campaign, IL. USA. pp.185-192.*

*Ealy, A.D., M. Drost, and P.J. Hansen. 1993. Developmental changes in embryonic resistance to adverse effects of maternal heat stress in cows. J. Dairy Sci. 76:2899-2905.*

*Elrod, C.C. and W.R. Butler. 1993. Reduction of fertility and alteration of uterine pH in heifers fed excess ruminally degradable protein. J. Anim. Sci. 71:694-701.*

*Elrod, C.C., M. Van Amburgh, and W.R. Butler. 1993. Alterations of pH in response to increased dietary protein in cattle are unique to the uterus. J. Anim. Sci. 71:702-706.*

*Emmery, R.S. 1993. Energy needs of dry cows. Tri-state Dairy Nutrition Conference. Fort Wayne May 18-19, USA, pp. 35-43.*

*Esslemont, R.J., J.H. Bailie, and M.J. Cooper. 1985. Fertility management in dairy cattle. Collins, London pp. 84*

*Esslemont, R.J., R.G. Glencross, M.J. Bryant, and G.S. Pope. 1980. A quantitative study of pre-ovulatory behaviour in cattle (British Friesian heifers). Appl. Anim. Ethol. 613-622.*

*Esslemont, R.J., B.R. Wassell, L.M. Grimbleby, T.R. Wassell, J.M. Lamb, S. Horne. 1991. The application of planned animal health and production to dairy farms: DAISY - The dairy information system. Bovine Practitioner 26:28-41.*

*Etherington, W.G., J. Fetrow, B.E. Seguin, W.E. Marsh, L.D. Weaver, C.L. Rawson. 1991. Dairy herd reproductive health management: Evaluating dairy herd reproductive performance - Part II. Comp. Cont. Educ. 13:1491-1502.*

*Fagan, J.G. and J.F. Roche. 1986. Reproductive activity in postpartum dairy cows based on progesterone concentrations in milk or rectal examination. Irish Vet. J. 40:124-131.*

*Ferguson, J.D., T. BLanchard, D.T. Galligan, D.C. Hoshall, and W. Chalupa. 1988. Infertility in dairy cattle fed a high percentage of protein degradable in the rumen. J. Am. Vet. Med. Assoc. 192:659-662.*

*Ferguson, J.D. 1990. Production and reproduction in dairy cows. Proc. Soc. Ontario Vet. Ann. Conf. pp. 165-175.*

*Ferguson, D. 1991. Nutrition and reproduction in dairy cows. Vet. Clinics of North America: Food Animal Practice. 7:487-507.*

*Ferguson, J.D. and J.D. Galligan. 1993a. Prostaglandin synchronization programs in dairy herds - Part I. Comp. on Cont. Educ.15: 646-654.*

*Ferguson, J.D. and J.D. Galligan. 1993b. Prostaglandin synchronization programs in dairy herds - Part II. Comp. Cont. Educ. 15:1127-1130.*

*Ferguson, J.D. 1994. Patterns in fertility in dairy cows. Proceedings National Reproduction Symposium, 22 & 23 September. Ed. E.R. Jordan, Pittsburgh, PA, Texas A & M University, Dallas. pp. 113-120.*

*Ferry, J.W. 1992. Reproductive herd health: going beyond rectal examinations. Comp. Contin. Educ. 14:87-90.*

*Fetrow, J., D. McClary, R. Harman, K. Butcher, L. Weaver, E. Studer, J. Ehrlich, W. Etherington, W. Gutherbock, D. Klingborg, J. Reneau, and N. Williamson. 1990. Calculating selected reproductive indices: recommendations of the American Association of Bovine Practitioners. J. Dairy Sci. 73:78-90.*

*Fetrow, J., S. Stewart, M. Kinsel, and S. Eicker. 1994. Reproduction records and production medicine. Proceedings National Reproduction Symposium, 22 & 23 September. Ed. E.R. Jordan, Pittsburgh, PA, Texas A & M University, Dallas. pp. 75-89.*

*Folman, Y., A. Berman, Z. Herz, M. Kaim, M. Rosenberg, M. Mament, and S. Gordin. 1979. Milk yield and fertility of high-yielding dairy cows in a subtropical climate during summer and winter. J. Dairy Res. 46:343-346.*

*Gaines, J.D. 1989. The role of record analysis in evaluating subfertile dairy herds. Vet Med. 84:353-343.*

*Galligan, D.T. and J.D. Ferguson. 1994. Application of linear programming in bull selec tion for a dairy herd. JAVMA, 206:173-176.*

*Gearhart, M.A., C.R. Curtis, H.N. Erb, R.D. Smith, C.J. Sniffen, L. E. Chase, and M.D. Cooper. 1990. Relationships of changes in condition score to cow health in Holsteins. J. Dairy Sci. 73:3132-3140.*

*Goodger, W.J. 1987. Dairy Comp 305 Program. Vet. Clin. North America. Food Anim. Pract. 3:553-559.*

*Grummer, R.R. 1993. Nutrition and reproduction relationships. Tri-state Dairy Nutrition Conference. Fort Wayne May 18-19, USA, pp. 7-35.*

*Gwazdauskas, F.C., J.A. Lineweaver, and W.E. Vinson. 1981. Rates of conception by artificial insemination of dairy cattle. J. Dairy Sci. 64:358-362.*

*Gwazdauskas, F.C., W.D. Whittier, W.E. Vinson, and R.E. Pearson. 1986. Evaluation of reproductive efficiency of dairy cows with emphasis on time of breeding. J. Dairy Sci. 69:290-302.*

*Hansen, P.J., W.W. Thatcher, and A.D. Ealy. 1992. Methods for reducing heat stress on pregnancy. In: Large dairy herd management. Eds. Van Horn, H.H. and C.J. Wilcox. Management Services American Dairy Association. Champaign, USA. pp 116-126.*

*Hansen, P.J. 1994. Causes and possible solutions to the problem of heat stress in reproductive management of dairy cows. Proc. Nat. Reprod. Symp. Ed. E.R. Jordan. Sept. 22-23, Pittsburg. Texas Agricultural Extension Service, Dallas. pp.161-170.*

*Harrison, R.O., S.P. Ford, J.W Young, A.J. Conley, and A.E. Freeman. 1990. Increased milk production versus reproductive and energy status of high producing dairy cows. J. Dairy Sci.73:2749-2758.*

*Helmer, S.D. and J.H. Britt. 1985. Mounting behavior as affected by stage of estrous cycle in Holstein heifers. J. Dairy Sci. 68:1290-1296.*

*Hillers, J.K., P.L. Senger, R.L. Darlington, and W.N. Fleming 1984. Effects of produc ion, season, age of cow, days dry,and days in milk on conception to first service in large commercial dairy herds. J. Dairy Sci. 67:861-867.*

*Holter, J.B., M.J. Slotnick, H.H. Hayes, C.K. Bozak, E.E. Urban, Jr., and M.L. McGilliard. 1990. Effect of prepartum dietary energy on condition score, postpartum energy, nitrogen partitions, and lactation production responses. J. Dairy Sci. 73:3502-3511.*

*Howard, H.J., E.P. Aalseth, G.D. Adams, L. J. Bush, R.W. McNew, and L.J. Dawson. 1987. Influence of dietary protein on reproductive performance of dairy cows. J.dairy Sci. 70:1563-1571.*

*Hurley, W.L., L.A. Edgerton, D. Olds, and R.W. Hemken. 1979. Estrous behavior and endocrine status of dairy heifers with varied intakes of phosphorus. J. Dairy Sci. 65:1979-1992.*

*Hurnik, J.F., G.J. King, and H.A. Robertson. 1975. Estrous and related behaviour in postpartum Holstein cows. Appl. Anim. Ethol. 2:55-68.*

*Huszenicza, G., L. Molnar, L. Solti, and J. Haraszti. 1987. Postpartal ovarian function in Holstein and Crossbred cows on large scale farms in Hungary. J. Vet. Med. A, 34:249-263.*

*Huszenicza, G., J. Haraszti, L. Molnar, L. Solti, S. Fekete, K. Ekes, and A.C. Jaro. 1988. Some metabolic characteristics of dairy cows with different postpartum ovarian functions. J. Vet. Med. A. 35:506-515.*

*Kyle, S.D., C.J. Calligan, and R.D. Allrich. 1992. Effect of progesterone on the expression of estrus at the first postpartum ovulation in dairy cattle. J. Dairy Sci. 75:1456-1460.*

*Kruif de, A. and A. Brand. 1978. Factors influencing the reproductive capacity of a dairy herd. New Zealand Vet. J. 178:183-189.*

*Laporte, H.M., H. Hogeveen, Y.H. Schukken, and J.P.T.M. Noordhuizen. 1994. Cystic ovarian disease in Dutch dairy cattle, I. Incidence, risk factors and consequences. Livest. Prod. Sci. 38:191-197.*

*Larson, L.L. and P.J.H. Ball. 1992. Regulation of estrous cycles in dairy cattle: A review. Theriogenology. 38:255-267.*

*Ljokjel, K., G. Klemetsdal, E. Prestlokken, and E. Ropstad. 1995. The effect of energy balance on ovarian activity in a herd of Norwegian cattle. Acta Vet. Scand. 36:533-542.*

*Lucey, S., G.J. Rowlands, and A.M. Russell. 1986. The association between lameness and fertility in dairy cows. Vet.Rec. 118:628-631.*

*Macmillan, K.L. 1992. Reproductive management. In: Large dairy herd management. Eds. H.H. Van Horn and C.J. Wilcox. American Dairy Science Association. Champaign, IL, USA. pp. 88-99.*

*Maree, C. 1986. The influence of high level feeding on the duration of parturition and the incidence of dystocia in dairy cows. J. So. Afr. Vet. Ass. 57:151-153.*

*Miettinen, P.V.A. 1990. Metabolic balance and reproductive performance in Finish dairy cows. J. Vet. Med. A. 37:417-424.*

*Montes, A.J. and D.G. Pugh. 1993. Clinical approach to postpartum metritis. Comp. Cont. Educ. 15:1131-1137.*

*Nebel, R.L. and M.L. Mcgilliard. 1993. Interactions of high milk yield and reproductive performances in dairy cows. J. Dairy Sci. 76:3257-3268.*

*Nelson, A.J. and H.W. Redlus. 1989. The key role of records in a Production Medicine Practice. Vet. Clin. North America: Food Animal Practice. 5:517-552.*

*Nielen, M., Y.H. Schukken, D.T. Scholl, H.J. Wilbrink, and A. Brand. 1989. Twinning in dairy cattle: A study of risk factors and effects. Theriogenology. 32:845-864.*

*Noordhuizen, J.P.T.M. and J. Buurman. 1984. VAMPP: a veterinary automated management and production control program for dairy farms. Vet. Quart. 6:66-72.*

*Odde, K.G.. 1990. A review of synchronization of estrus in postpartum cattle. J. Anim. Sci. 68:817-830.*

*Pankowski, J.W., D.M. Galton, N.H. Erb. C.L. Guard, and Y.T. Grohn. 1995. Use of prostaglandin F2a as a postpartum reproductive management tool for lactating dairy cows. J. Dairy Sci. 78:1477-1488.*

*Putnam, M.R. 1989. Toxicologic problems in food animals affecting reproduction. Vet. Clin. of North America: Food Animal Practice. 5:325-344.*

*Putney, D.J., S. Mullins, W.W. Thatcher, M. Drost, and T.S. Gross. 1989. Embryonic development in superovulated dairy cattle exposed to elevated ambient temperatures between the onset of estrus and insemination. Anim. Prod. Sci. 19:31-51.*

*Raheja, K.L., E.B. Burnside, and L.R. Schaeffer. 1989. Heifer fertility and its relations hip with cow fertility and production traits in Holstein dairy cattle. J. Dairy Sci., 72:2665-2678.*

*Roche, J.F., M.A. Crowe, and M.P. Boland. 1992. Postpartum anoestrus in dairy and beef cows. Anim. Reprod. Sci. 28:371-378.*

*Ruegg, P.L. 1991. Body condition scoring in dairy cows: relationships with production, reproduction, nutrition, and health. Comp. Cont. Educ. 13:1309-1313.*

*Ruegg, P.L., W.J. Goodger, C.A. Holmberg, L.D. Weaver, and B.M. Huffman. 1992. Relation among body condition score, serum urea nitrogen and cholesterol concentration and, reproductive performance in high producing Holstein dairy cows in early lactation. Am. J. Vet. Res. 52:10-14.*

*Rutter, L.M., R.D. Randel, G.T. Schelling, and D.W. Forrest. 1983. Effect of abomasal infusion of propionate on the GnRH-induced LH release in prepubertal heifers. J. Anim. Sci. 56:1167-1173.*

*Senger, P.L. 1992. Handling frozen semen. In: Large dairy herd management. Eds. Van Horn, H.H. and C.J. Wilcox. Management Services American Dairy Association. Champaign, USA. pp 110-116.*

*Senger, P.L. 1994. Automated detection of estrus: Can it be a reality. Proceedings National Reproduction Symposium, E.R. Jordan, ed. 22 & 23 September, Pittsburgh, PA. Texas A & M University, Dallas. pp. 1-10.*

*Senger, P.L. 1994. The estrus detection problem: New concepts, technologies, and possibilities. J.Dairy Sci. 77:2745-2753.*

*Smith, T.R. and G.H. Schmidt. 1987. Relationships of use of dairy herd improvement records to herd performance measures. J. Dairy sci. 70:2688-2694.*

*Staples, C.R., W.W. Tatcher, and J.H. Clark. 1990. Relationship between ovarian activity and energy status during the early postpartum period of high producing dairy cows. J. Dairy Sci. 73:938-947.*

*Stevenson, J.S., M.K. Schmidt, and E.P. Call. 1983. Factors affecting reproductive performance of dairy cows first inseminated after five weeks postpartum. J. Dairy Sci. 66:1148-1154.*

*Stevenson, J.S. 1994. Hormonal intervention in the control of fertility in dairy cattle. Proceedings National Reproduction Symposium, E.R. Jordan, ed. 22 & 23 September. Pittsburgh, PA Texas A & M University, Dallas. pp. 11-22.*

*Thatcher, W.W. 1993. Environment and reproduction. In: Reproduction in domestic animals. Editor G.J. King. Elsevier Scientific Publishers. London. pp. 433-457.*

*Thompson, J.R., E.J. Pollack, and C.L. Pellissier. 1983. Interrelationships of parturition problems, production of subsequent lactation and age at first calving. J. Dairy Sci. 66:1119-1127.*

*Thurmond, M.C. and J.P. Picanso. 1993. Fetal loss associated with palpation per rectum to diagnose pregnancy in cows. J. Am. Vet. Med. Ass. 203:432-435.*

*Trenkle, A. 1981. Endocrine regulation of energy metabolism in ruminants. Fed. Proc. 40:2538-2550.*

*Udomprasert, P. and N.B. Williamson. 1990. A computerized recording system for dairy herds. Vet. Rec. 127:256-262.*

*Varner, M.A., K. Maatje, M. Nielen, and W. Rossing. 1994. Changes in dairy cow pedometer readings with different number of cows in estrus. Dairy Systems for the 21st Century, Proceedings of the Third International Dairy Housing Conference. 2-5 February 1994. Orlando, FL. Am. Soc. Ag. Engineers. St. Joseph, MO, USA. pp.103.*

*Villa-Godoy, A., T.L. Hughes, R.S. Emery, L.T. Chapin, and R.L. Fogwell. 1988. Association between energy balance and luteal function in lactating dairy cows. J. Dairy Sci. 71:1063-1072.*

*Villa-Godoy, A., T.L. Hughes, R.S. Emery, E.P. Stanisiewski, and R.L. Fogwell. 1990. Influence of energy balance and body condition on estrus and estrous cycles in Holstein heifers. J. Dairy Sci. 73:2759-2765.*

*Waltner-Toews, D., S.W. Martin, and A.H. Meek. 1986. Dairy calf management, morbidity, and mortality in Ontario Holstein herds. IV. Association of management with mortality. Prev. Vet. Med. 4:159-171.*

*Weaver, L.D. 1986. Evaluation of reproductive performance in dairy herds. Comp. Cont. Educ. 8:247-254.*

*Weaver, L.D. 1992 Reproductive health programs. In: Large dairy herd management. Eds. Van Horn, H.H. and C.J. Wilcox. Management Services American Dairy Association. Champaign, USA. pp. 99-109.*

*Wenzel, J.G.W.. 1991. A review of prostaglandin F products and their use in dairy repro ductive herd health programs. Vet. Bull. 61:433*

*Werven, T. van, Y.H. Schukken, J. Lloyd, A. Brand, R. Heeringa, and M. Shea. 1992. The effects of duration of retained placenta on reproduction, milk production, postpartum disease and culling rate. Theriogenology 37:1191-1203.*

*Wilmut, I., D.I. Sales, and C.J. Ashworth. 1986. Maternal and embryonic factors associa ted with prenatal loss in mammels. J.Reprod. Fert. 76:851-864.*

*Wolfenson, D., I. Flamenbaum, and A. Berman. 1988. Hyperthermia and body energy store effects on estrous behavior, conception rate, and corpus luteum function in dairy cows. J. Dairy Sci. 71:3497-3504.*

*Zurek, E., G.R. Foxtroft, and J.J. Kennely. 1995. Metabolic status and interval to first ovulation in postpartum dairy cows. J.Dairy Sci. 78:1909-1920.*

# MONITORING UDDER HEALTH

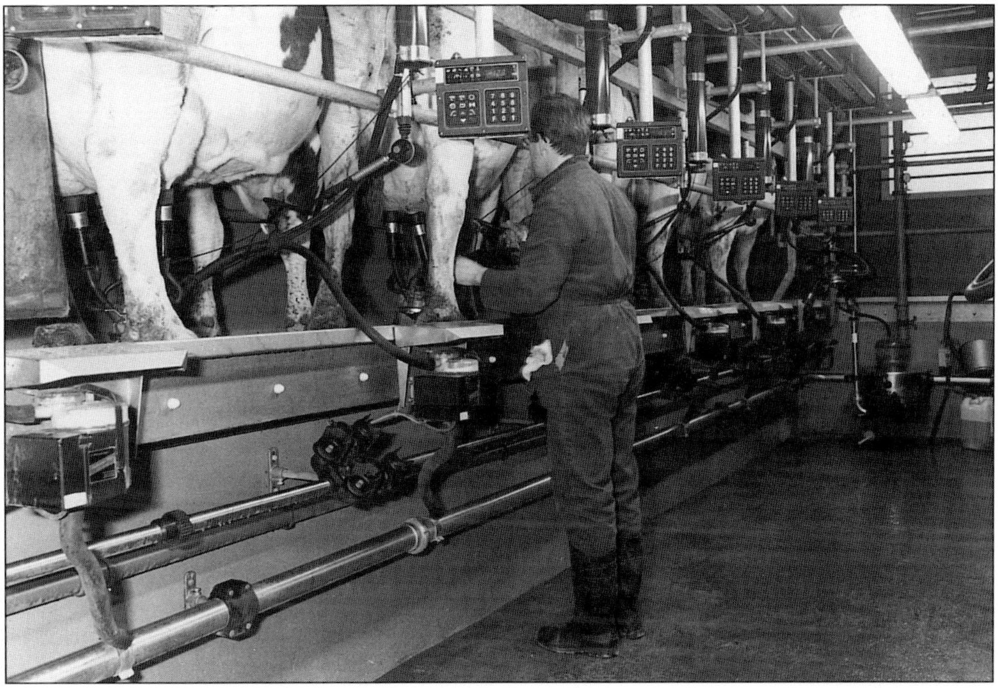

# 6.1 MONITORING UDDER HEALTH: OBJECTIVES, MATERIALS AND METHODS

Ynte H. Schukken and Wim D. J. Kremer

Department of Herd Health and Reproduction, School of Veterinary Medicine, University of Utrecht, Yalelaan 7, 3485 CL Utrecht, The Netherlands

## 6.1.1 INTRODUCTION

Mastitis is probably the most important health disorder on dairy farms. This is caused by a high incidence of clinical mastitis and a high prevalence of subclinical mastitis. Milk production loss in combination with treatment costs and culling due to mastitis constitute the major costs of mastitis (Dijkhuizen, 1977). Additionally, mastitis causes the quality of the milk to decrease. This means that either farmers produce less milk, or the milk industry obtains a suboptimal product. To this end, the dairy industry faces worldwide penalty programs trying to increase the nutritional quality of milk (Schukken et al., 1992). The most important way to continuously produce milk of good quality is to keep the udder health situation in the herd under tight control.

Clinical mastitis can be defined as 'a farmer observed abnormality on either the milk and/or the udder'. Clinical mastitis then, is an observable disease. Cows are visibly sick, or the milk is visibly abnormal. The incidence of clinical mastitis ranges from 0 to more than 200 cases per 100 cows per year. In most European studies the median incidence is around 20 - 25 cases per 100 cows per year (Wilesmith, 1986; Schukken et al., 1989). Clinical mastitis occurs in all dairy herds. Even well-managed herds, as judged by somatic cell count level and a high level of milk production, may be suffering from a high incidence of clinical mastitis (Schukken et al., 1991; Erskine et al., 1988; Hogan et al., 1989). Clinical mastitis is mostly caused by bacteria. The most important are *S.aureus, E. coli*, and Streptococci (*S. uberis, S. dysgalactia*).

Subclinical mastitis is often defined as the presence of a microorganism in combination with an elevated somatic cell count (SCC) of the milk. Subclinical mastitis is a costly disease in the majority of herds. Various SCC cut-off points for the definition of subclinical mastitis on quarter and cow level have been proposed. Most recent research seems to agree at a cut-off point at about 200,000 cells/ml. (Reneau, 1986; Dohoo and Leslie, 1991). Several researchers have shown a log-linear relation between the somatic cell count of milk and milk production of the cow. The production decreases linearly with an increase in the log (SCC) (Tyler et al., 1989). Subclinical mastitis is mostly caused by *S.aureus* and *S.agalactiae* and to a lesser extent by other streptococci.

Subclinical mastitis is both a problem at cow and herd level. When the bulk milk somatic cell count levels exceed regulatory criteria the dairy industry imposes a fine on the farmer, or completely rejects to process the milk. In recent years, these regulatory limits for bulk milk somatic cell counts (BMSCC) have been considerably tightened.

The European Community has a regulatory limit of 400,000 cells/ml., Ontario, Canada has a limit of 500,000 as of 1995, and in 1993, USA introduced a federal limit of 750,000 cells per ml. (Schukken et al., 1992).

The clinical mastitis problems, the subclinical mastitis problems, and the problems regarding milk quality require monitoring and control of the udder health situation in a herd. The objective of this Chapter is to describe an udder health program integrated in a herd health and production management (HH & PM) program.

## 6.1.2 PATHOBIOLOGY

Before discussing the HH & PM approach to udder health, we shortly introduce the patterns of infection that are seen in bovine mastitis. Mastitis is a multifactorial disease problem. It is a classical example of the interaction of micro organisms, host factors and environment.

### Dynamics of infection

When evaluating data on udder infections, it is important to realize that cows live in an environment with a high exposure to infection. An udder infection itself (including the host response, i.e. rise in cell count, conductivity, body temperature etc.) should therefore not be considered as a pathologic process. Only when the infection is not cured by the host-defence mechanisms it becomes a patho-physiologic problem. Single measurements will not be able to distinguish between infection with subsequent self cure, and infection that is not cured by the defence mechanisms. Repeated measurements in time make it possible to distinguish between these two processes. When evaluating the prevalence of infection, a time component should always be included. This can be two or more SCC measurements, repeated bacteriological cultures, or a combination of these two. Intervention with the host-defence mechanisms should only be undertaken when evidence of failure of the system (i.e. clinical symptoms and/or long term high SCC) is present .

### Epidemiology of infection

Two distinct patterns in the epidemiology of mastitis can be recognized. The first pattern is a contagious disease pattern where transfer of microorganisms from cow to cow is essential to propagate the disease. The second pattern is a pattern of opportunistic microorganisms. Host factors and environmental factors put an animal at risk. A wide range of microorganisms can then enter the mammary gland and cause disease. In Table 1, infection patterns from seven intensively monitored dairy herds are shown. These were herds with a low BMSCC, but still all major pathogens were present. The difference in infection pattern between the contagious and environmental pathogens is clear from these data (Lam, 1996). Coliform infections result specifically in isolated

*Table 1. Total number of intramammary infections with major pathogens in seven dairy herds with low bulk milk somatic cell count, during a period of 20 months*

| | Number* | Clinical mastitis Isolated† | Acute-chronic∫ | | Chronic§ | | Subclinical chronic≈ |
|---|---|---|---|---|---|---|---|
| *E. coli* | 105 | 89 | 6 | (14) | 4 | (4) | 6 |
| *S. aureus* | 171 | 21 | 18 | (6) | 23 | (33) | 109 |
| *S. dysgalactiae* | 80 | 31 | 10 | (6) | 11 | (15) | 28 |
| *S. uberis* | 79 | 28 | 10 | (2) | 11 | (21) | 30 |

* Total number of intramammary infections.

† Isolated cases of clinical mastitis. Pathogens were only cultured from the sample collected from the case of clinical mastitis.

∫ Acute cases of clinical mastitis, which developped into chronic mastitis. The number of clinical flair-ups after the initial clinical case is presented between brackets.

§ Clinical mastitis cases which occurred in the course of a chronic intramammary infection. The total number of clinical flair-ups is presented between brackets.

≈ Subclinical mastitis cases (no clinical signs).

clinical cases (85%), wheras *S.aureus* infections result mostly in chronic subclinical cases (64%). Environmental streptococci show a pattern in between these two. From these data it can be concluded that coliform mastitis is mostly not contagious, whereas *S.aureus* has opportunities to spread between cows.

**1. Contagious disease pattern:**

This pattern involves the transmission of disease from a carrier to a susceptible host. It involves mainly the spread of two major pathogens: *S.agalactiae* and *S.aureus* (Natzke, 1981; Lam, 1996). Other epidemic contagious disease outbreaks have been reported, and involve *Nocardia* spp, *Mycoplasma* etc. Contagious diseases only remain endemic when the mean number of susceptible individuals infected by an infected individual is equal to one or larger than one (Anderson, 1991; Becker, 1989). This implies, that reduction of the number of new infections is the major goal of prevention programs. Typically, herds with high BMSCC show a pattern of contagious disease problems.

**2. Opportunistic disease patterns:**

This involves an interaction of microorganism, host factors and the environment. When solving herd problems, this epidemiologic triangle should be kept in mind. Typically, herds with a high incidence of clinical mastitis and an acceptable or low BMSCC show a pattern of opportunistic disease problems.

### Microorganisms

The most important micro organisms involved are the coliforms and the environmental streptococci (Smith et al., 1985). Microorganism related factors (serum resistance, antigen determinants) are related to the severity of clinical mastitis. However, a problem solving approach only based on microorganism reduction is likely to fail. Most cow-, management-, and environmental risk factors will remain. It is likely that another microorganism will fill the niche that is created by expelling one specific species.

### Host factors

Several host factors are important in determining the outcome of an infection. Infection may result in either rapid elimination of the microorganims, acute clinical symptoms of inflammation, or in chronic infection with high SCC and/or episodes of clinical disease. Actually, most infections result in very few clinical signs (Smith et al., 1985). Host parameters like peripheral blood leukocyte count, blood leukocyte activity, and presence of antibodies have predictive value with regard to outcome of intramammary infection (Lohuis et al., 1990; Kremer et al., 1993).

### Environmental factors

Several factors in the environment affect the exposure of a cow to mastitis pathogens. Sources of environmental exposure are manure, bedding, feedstuff, dirt, mud and water. An example of this is *E. coli*, this microorganism is present in the environment of the cow. Several studies have indeed linked the cleanliness of the barn, and the colony count in the bedding with the incidence of clinical mastitis (e.g. Bramley and Neave, 1975).

## 6.1.3 COMPONENTS OF AN UDDER HEALTH PROGRAM: THE PROTOCOL

The general protocol for monitoring and control udder health is shown in Figure 1. This protocol applies to all parts of a HH & PM program, but will be specified for the udder health situation.

## 6.1.4 OBJECTIVES

Objectives are defined as performance indices and for individual farms expressed as preset targets. They can be divided in primary and secondary indices or preset targets. The most important objectives of an Udder Health Program are summarized in the primary preset targets. We suggest that the primary targets for udder health are:

*Figure 1. Herd Health and Production Management Protocol*

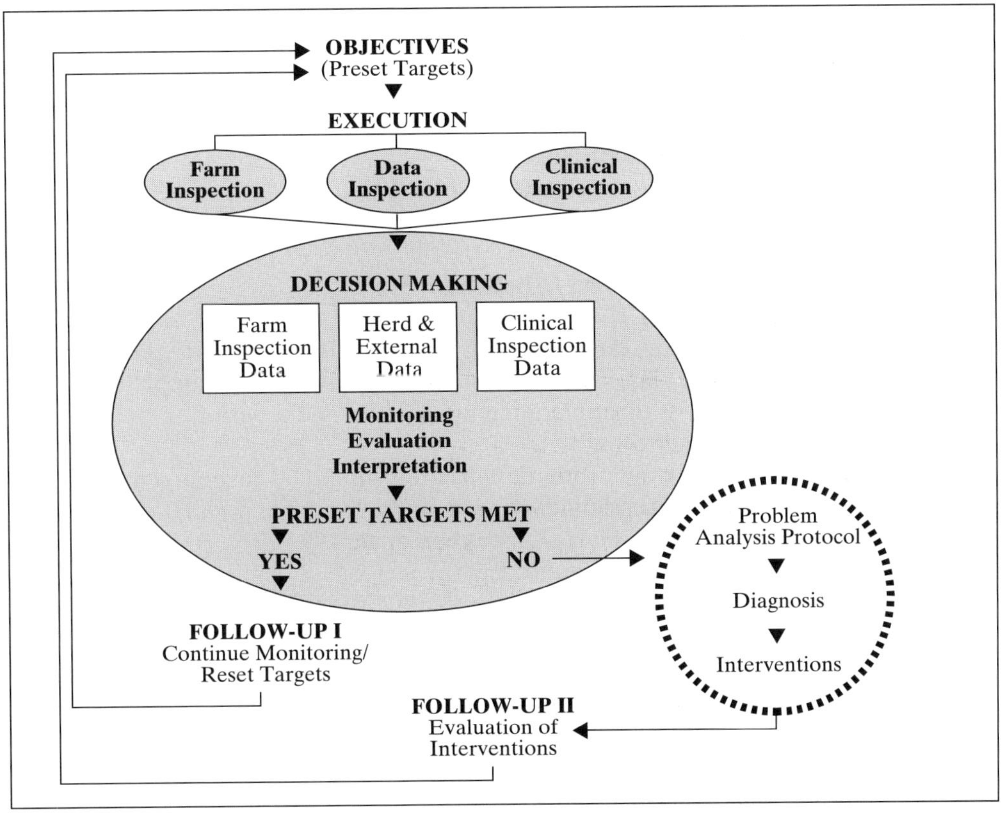


*Figure 2. The required mean annual BMSCC at various penalty levels*

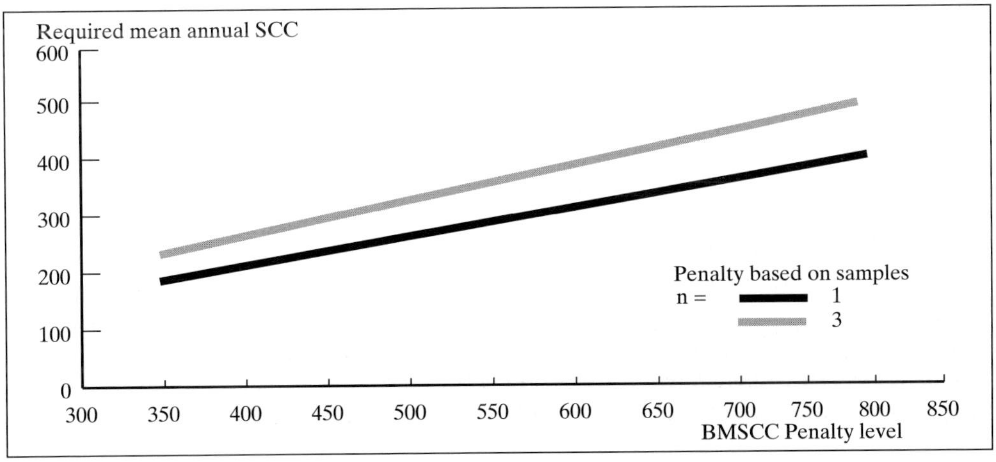

1. Bulk Milk Somatic Cell Count: < 250.000 cells/ml,
2. Incidence of clinical mastitis: < 25 cases/100 cows per year,
3. Number of cases of mastitis per affected cow: < 1.4, and
4. Number of culls due to mastitis or other udder health problems: < 5% (as a proportion of all cows in the herd).

Examples of secondary preset targets are:
1. % cows above SCC cut-off limit (e.g. 200.000): < 20%,
2. Risk of 'new infection': < 10%
3. Elimination ('cure') risk: > 30%, and
4. Contribution of highest SCC cows to bulk milk SCC.

To be able to evaluate short term and long term effects, the primary preset targets may be calculated for three time periods. A short term effect, for example the last 12 weeks, a long term effect, for example an annual mean, and a period in between, for example the mean of the last 6 months.

The objective for the bulk milk somatic cell count should be an annual mean below 200,000 - 250,000 cells/ml. This estimate is based on the available population data from European and North-American Herds (Schukken et al., 1992). The BMSCC seems to follow a Log-Normal distribution, indicating an increasing standard deviation with increasing mean. This is reflected in the large variability of BMSCC within one herd. To ensure that a herd remains below a penalty level of 400,000 - 500,000 cells per ml., the objective for the annual mean BMSCC should be below 200,000 - 250,000 respectively. The relation between the penalty level and the objective of the annual mean is shown in Figure 2. The required mean depends strongly on the number of observations that are used to decide on a penalty.

Herd BMSCC performance may be monitored using a graphical description of BMSCC performance. For example, in the current Dutch penalty program a herd is penalized when any individual BMSCC score is over 400,000 cells/ml. To prevent such a penalty, the advised annual performance goal is a mean BMSCC of 200,000 cells/ml or less. The Ontario penalty is based on three BMSCC counts and a penalty level of 500,000. The performance goal is then approximately 300,000 cells/ml or less.

Economical arguments may play an important role in deciding the level of acceptable cell count levels. The somatic cell count level of a cow has a direct relation to production loss. There is a log-linear relation between SCC and milk production loss. As a rule of thumb, every natural log-step increase above a natural log value of the SCC over 5.0 will cause a milk loss of approximately 1 kg per day (Tyler et al., 1989). For example, a cow with a somatic cell count of 750,000 cells (Ln 750 = 6.6) has an estimated milk loss of about 6.6 - 5.0 = 1.6 kg per day. An estimate of milk production loss can also be obtained from the BMSCC. Every 100,000 cells increase above 150,000 is associated with a production loss in the herd of 1.5% (see also Table 10, part 2). A BMSCC of 350,000 is then associated with a production loss of approximately 3%.
The incidence of clinical mastitis varies widely between herds. Therefore it is difficult to define a general objective. A realistic objective should be defined in accordance

*Table 2. Reported annual incidence of clinical mastitis*

| Reference | Incidence of Clinical mastitis | Standard Deviation | Reported Mean BMSCC |
|---|---|---|---|
| Bartlett et al., (1986) | 25% | – | – |
| Dohoo et al., (1983) | 17.5% | – | 210,000 |
| Wilesmith et al., (1986) | 28.2% | – | 320,000 |
| Erskine et al., I (1988) | 51% | 3.2% | 120,000 |
| Erskine et al., II (1988) | 35% | 1.3% | 800,000 |
| Schukken et al., (1989) | 18.3% | 8.7% | 150,000 |

with the herd manager. To give some ideas about population values, the incidences of some surveys are summarized in Table 2. It appears that the mean incidence is approximately 25 - 30 cases per 100 cows per year.

Again economic arguments should be considered when determining a realistic goal. Cost of disease prevention must be weighed against cost of disease occurrence. The average case of clinical mastitis is associated with a production loss of approximately 350 kg milk. When treatment costs and labour are included, the estimated loss per clinical case amounts to ± $125 (Bartlett et al., 1991).

A similar argument holds for culling due to mastitis. However, few data are currently available to support the definition of an achievable objective. Fetrow (1988) summarized the existing literature and reported an annual mean culling for mastitis of 2.9% of the lactations, or 15.1% of all culls. A general advice based on these data may be < 5% of the cows are culled annually because of mastitis reasons, this would be < 15% of the culled cows that are culled due to mastitis reasons. Economically, an unplanned cull is estimated at a loss of about $ 750.

When the primary indices parameters signal a problem, more analyses of existing data may give information as to the source and the cause of the problem. Secondary performance indices should then be analyzed. Further possibilities for analyses or graphical displays and the definitions of secondary performance indices are presented in Table 3. Performance goals of some of these indices have been discussed by Dohoo and Morris (1993). Their recommendations are based on the 25th percentile of the population of herds from Prince Edward Island. The percentage of cows above 200.000 cells/ml. should not exceed 20%, the infection risk should not exceed 10% per four weeks, and elimination risk should exceed 30%. A high contribution of a cow or a few cows to the bulk milk SCC may indicate a cow instead of a herd problem. These secondary measures will yield additional information to interpret the data with regard to the presence of an udder health problem.

## 6.1.5 MATERIAL AND METHODS

### Materials

1. A record system is required. While there is great variety in effective record keeping systems, key components of successful record keeping systems are:
   - A self-copying farm diary for hand recording of data on clinical mastitis, dry treatment, culling, preventive measures and related activities. Both farmer and practitioner keep a copy.
   - A herd mastitis chart that lists cows in order of their mastitis date. This chart is efficient for examining the history of an individual and it provides an overview of the herd's udder health performance at a glance. Regular and accurate transfer of data from the farm diary and/or individual cow cards to a herd mastitis chart or a herd management computer summarization system, if available, is essential.
   - An on-farm personal computer for data processing. This instrument enables communication between and among on-farm data sources. An on-farm computer with modem can also provide communication between external informational resources such as, milk recording centers, milk processors, dairy consultants and veterinary practitioners.
   - Software that makes it possible to monitor herd performance.
   - A file for both the farmer and the practitioner to store relevant information.

   Accurate and up-to-date data recording followed by manual or electronic data processing by the farmer, the veterinary practitioner and/or an external organization is the heart of an effective herd health and production management program.

2. Milk recording, with inclusion of somatic cell count information is essential to monitor and evaluate udder health. Presentation systems have been discussed by Reneau (1986) and Dohoo and Leslie (1991). Further information on processing of individual cell counts will be presented in part 2 of this Chapter.

3. Sampling material such as a CMT panel, CMT fluid, cotton, alcohol, sterile sampling tubes and waterproof writing material is required in the milking parlour.

### Methods

1. Data inspection for content, completeness and actuality,

2. Farm Inspection activities directed at risk factors in the environment that might influence udder health performance.

3. Clinical inspection activities.
   For this purpose a list of cows to be examined by the HH & PM practitioner is required. The composition of this list may be flexible, but usually contains the following categories:

– cows with clinical mastitis
– cows with a recent history of high SCC
– cows freshening with history of clinical mastitis and/or high SCC.

Sampling of abnormal quarters for bacteriological culture needs to be done on a regular basis. All cows with clinical mastitis events and cows with a history of high somatic cell counts should be sampled. Preferably, sampling is based on quarter milk CMT score to improve the probability of culture positive samples. Sampled cows need to be recorded in the farm diary.

4. Regular farm visits. Frequency of farm visits is usually determined by herd size and/or calving pattern. In herds of 80 to 100 cows a frequency of once in every 3 to 4 weeks seems optimal.

*Table 3. Further analytical options when primary udder health parameters are deviating*

**A. High Bulk milk Somatic Cell Count:**

$$\text{\% cows above SCC cut-off limit (e.g. 200,000)} \quad \frac{\text{\# cows with SCC} > 200}{\text{\# cows SCC tested}}$$

$$\text{Prevalence of high SCC per parity} \quad \frac{\text{\# cows positive in parity i}}{\text{\# cows tested in parity i}}$$

$$\text{Prevalence of high SCC per stage of lactation} \quad \frac{\text{\# cows positive in SOL j}}{\text{\# cows tested in SOL j}}$$

$$\text{Infection risk} \quad \frac{\text{\# cows} < 200 \text{ last sample } \textit{and} > 200 \text{ this sample}}{\text{\# cows} < 200 \text{ last sample}}$$

$$\text{Elimination ('cure') risk} \quad \frac{\text{\# cows} > 200 \text{ last sample } \textit{and} < 200 \text{ this sample}}{\text{\# cows} > 200 \text{ last sample}}$$

$$\text{Contribution of highest SCC cows} \quad \frac{\text{(SCC} * \text{Kg. milk) for highest SCC cows}}{\text{Sum of (SCC} * \text{Kg. Milk) for all cows}}$$

**B. High incidence of clinical mastitis:**

| | |
|---|---|
| Pathogen distribution<br>Parity distribution<br>Distribution of the cases over stages of lactation<br>Calving pattern in the herd<br>Incidence and prevalence of teat lesions | } Graphical or tabular display |

## Evaluation skills

1. Ability to interpret primary and secondary udder health indices as well as indications from mastitis detection aids, such as repeated somatic cell count measurements and electronic device (conductivity) readings. Further analysis should be done to describe the problem and to look for patterns in time, age, stage of lactation (When, Where, What). Some examples of further analytical options are shown in Table 3. Known risk factors such as failure to dip teats, or the presence of teat lesions should be evaluated based on indications from these analyses (see also part 4).

2. Familiarity with automated data processing and veterinary epidemiologic concepts. Familiarity with available software that analyses various sources of (electronic) data to help diagnose causes of decreased or improved udder health status (Thurmond, 1993).

3. Familiarity with interpreting udder health disorders and knowledge of effective treatments and/or herd udder health management strategies.

## EPILOGUE

The udder is in a central position on a dairy farm. It produces by far the greatest part of the farm income. Mastitis is the greatest cause of milk quality failures in the dairy industry. Somatic cell counts in milk can be used to measure subclinical mastitis statuses. Udder health should be seen as a part of a complete Herd Health and Production Management program. Path analysis studies have shown relationships between nutrition, fertility and udder health (Curtis et al., 1985; Erb et al., 1985). Genetic studies have shown genetic correlations between udder health and milk production potential (Emanuelsson et al., 1988). Hence udder health is central in herd performance and requires considerable attention from farm manager and herd health and production management advisors.

# 6.2 MONITORING UDDER HEALTH: EXECUTION

Ynte H. Schukken and Theo J.G.M. Lam

Department of Herd Health and Reproduction, School of Veterinary Medicine, University of Utrecht, Yalelaan 7, 3485 CL Utrecht, The Netherlands

## 6.2.1 INTRODUCTION

Execution of an udder health program within herd health and production management (HH & PM) services comprises three activities: 1) data inspection, 2) clinical inspection, and 3) farm inspection.

Data inspection is directed at assessing the accuracy and quality of data collected by the farmer and at getting insight in the current udder health performance. An important role of the practitioner is to continuously motivate the farmer in collection of relevant data. A useful mechanism for motivating the farmer to collect data is to provide regular feedback of information derived from farm and clinical inspection, and external collected data.

Clinical inspection of the herd is focused on udder health of cows and when necessary of young stock. Clinical inspection should not only be directed at clinically diseased cows, and cows with a history of udder health problems but also at health aspects that may be related to udder health such as metabolic diseases and lameness. On farms with specific problems clinical monitoring of teat-end conditions of all cows in the milking herd may be required. The clinician should be able to relate clinical findings with findings from other operational management functions such as: nutrition, milk production, and fixed assets and labor.

The farm inspection activity consists of a thorough inspection of management practices and of environmental conditions to detect risk factors that might influence the multifactorial background of udder health performance. The performance of the milking machine, and the execution of milking techniques and milking hygiene by the milkers are essential fields of attention with regard to udder health and milk quality.

Collection of cow and herd data by the farmer, and the clinical and farm inspection by the practitioner lead to three data sources. Data resulting from the farm and clinical inspection activities have to be recorded by the practitioner in the same way as the farmer is recording relevant data. Integration of the three data sources into the decision making process forms a key part of activities after the farm visit. In this part, the three inspection activities will be described and important elements emphasized.

## 6.2.2 INSPECTION OF HERD DATA

### Completeness and accuracy of data

Udder health events may be recorded in the farm diary, on individual cow cards, on a herd mastitis chart, or directly into a computer. The type of records kept and how those records are processed influence how data is monitored for completeness and accuracy. The veterinary practitioner should ensure that record keeping is adequate and correct. If needed the mastitis chart and/or the bulk milk somatic cell count chart and plate loop count chart should be updated with the latest data. The practitioner should convince the farmer of the importance of data collection.

### Data collection and data sources

Herd and farm data are very important in an udder health program. The farmer is the primary source for diagnosing clinical mastitis. The daily observation during milking is the most important way of obtaining data on clinical mastitis. As discussed before, the incidence of clinical mastitis is one of the four primary indices of udder health performance on a dairy farm. The collection of milk samples of abnormal secretum, before the treatment with antimicrobials, is the task of the milker. Data on the occurrence of clinical mastitis and the subsequent treatment can be recorded on a mastitis chart as shown below. To monitor the incidence of clinical mastitis, the number of clinical cases, and the number of cows at risk must be calculated (Erskine et al., 1988). In addition to the number of cases the number of cows affected should be known. Data on the number of cows at risk can be obtained from DHI records, fertility barn charts etc.

*Figure 1. Mastitis chart*

| | | | | |
|---|---|---|---|---|
| ** | ** | = | LF | RF |
| ** | ** | = | LH | RH |

| Cownr/Name | Par | Calving | DiM | Date-1 | | | Date-2 | | | Date 3 | | | Dry Cull |
|---|---|---|---|---|---|---|---|---|---|---|---|---|---|
| 45 LISA 12 | 6 | 6/7/95 | 292 | ** | ** | 1/2 | ** | ** | 2/5 | ** | ** | 23/5 | |
| | | | | Sau | ** | | Sau | ** | | Sau | ** | | 1/6/96 |
| 34 DIRKJE 106 | 1 | 4/4/96 | 2 | ** | ** | 6/4 | | | | | | | |
| | | | | Ec | ** | | | | | | | | |
| 13 JOZINA 36 | 3 | 9/12/96 | 34 | SU | ** | 12/1 | | | | | | | |
| | | | | SU | ** | | | | | | | | |
| 25 SNITSER 125 | 3 | 9/12/95 | 92 | Neg | ** | 15/3 | | | | | | | |
| | | | | ** | ** | | | | | | | | |
| 268 BRENDA 18 | 1 | 1/1/96 | 405 | ** | Neg | 10/2 | | | | | | | |
| | | | | ** | ** | | | | | | | | |

*Table 1. Herd clinical mastitis report/12 monthly list*

| | Months: | | | | | | | | | | | |
|---|---|---|---|---|---|---|---|---|---|---|---|---|
| | **1** | **2** | **3** | **4** | **5** | **6** | **7** | **8** | **9** | **10** | **11** | **12** |
| # Calvings | 3 | 4 | 3 | 5 | 2 | 2 | 3 | 2 | 4 | 5 | 5 | 3 |
| # clinical mastitis cases | 1 | 0 | 1 | 2 | 0 | 0 | 1 | 0 | 0 | 0 | 1 | 0 |
| # culls due to mastitis | 0 | 0 | 0 | 1 | 0 | 0 | 1 | 1 | 0 | 0 | 0 | 0 |

Next to recording of clinical mastitis, record keeping on culling and culling reasons is required. Culling data do often yield important additional information with regard to udder health performance (Fetrow, 1988). Udder health problems may remain unnoticed in disease prevalence when farmers tend to sell affected cows at a high rate. Hence, besides incidence of clinical mastitis, and prevalence of subclinical mastitis, cows culled for udder health problems have to be recorded.

Data from the clinical mastitis chart, relevant data from the fertility chart and other forms can be transferred to a herd clinical mastitis report 12 monthly list which provides information on udder health performance on a monthly basis. This report provides per month the number of cows that freshen, the number of clinical cases and the number of culls due to udder health problems. Seasonal trends in mastitis are easily detected, and the number of cows at risk is estimated by the number of cows that freshen.

Another source of farm data is the milk receipt from the milk processor. Milk is checked regularly to monitor quality of the raw product. These quality control measures are reported to the producer. Measures include: fat, protein and lactose content of bulk milk, bulk milk somatic cell count (BMSCC), plate loop count, freezing point, and the presence of inhibitory substance (Schukken et al., 1992).

*Table 2. List of cows in alphabetic and/ or numerical order with SCC counts or linear scores in the current lactation, parity and day of lactation. Dry period is indicated (D), as well as a fresh cow (F)*

| | | | | | | SCC | | |
|---|---|---|---|---|---|---|---|---|
| **cownr** | **parity** | **Calving date** | **12/5** | **8/4** | **9/3** | **14/2** | **11/1** | **12/12** |
| 23 | 3 | May 3 | 6650 | D | D | D | 230 | 125 |
| 25 | 3 | Dec 9 | 6140 | 2345 | 768 | 2357 | 1563 | F |
| 12 | 2 | Nov 12 | 124 | 34 | 12 | 54 | 8 | 98 |
| 6 | 3 | Oct 23 | 45 | 65 | 3219 | 96 | 88 | 23 |
| 56 | 5 | Jan 18 | 3869 | 6234 | 48 | 21 | D | D |
| 34 | 1 | April 4 | 4891 | F | - | - | - | - |
| 45 | 6 | July 6 | 3869 | 452 | 562 | 4378 | 934 | 2185 |

*Table 3. Mean SCC per test day and number of cows in the three SCC classes*

| Test day | N | mean SCC | Percent of herd: < 200,000 | 200,000-500,000 | > 500,000 |
|---|---|---|---|---|---|
| May 12 | 36 | 623 | 50 | 10 | 40 |
| April 8 | 32 | 357 | 43 | 14 | 43 |
| March 9 | 34 | 725 | 55 | 5 | 40 |
| Feb 14 | 37 | 854 | 47 | 16 | 37 |

*Table 4. Mean SCC per parity and number of cows in three SCC classes*

| Parity | N | mean SCC | Percent within each parity < 200,000 | | 200,000 - 500,000 | | > 500,000 | |
|---|---|---|---|---|---|---|---|---|
| 1 | 12 | 489 | 7 | 58% | 3 | 25% | 2 | 17% |
| 2 | 7 | 537 | 4 | 57% | 0 | 0 | 3 | 43% |
| 2 | 17 | 834 | 7 | 41% | 1 | 6% | 9 | 53% |

*Table 5. Mean SCC stage of lactation and number of cows in three SCC classes*

| Days in milk | N | mean SCC | Percent within stage of lactation < 200,000 | | 200,000 - 500,000 | | > 500,000 | |
|---|---|---|---|---|---|---|---|---|
| < 100 | 9 | 350 | 6 | 66% | 1 | 11% | 2 | 22% |
| 100 - 200 | 18 | 596 | 8 | 44% | 3 | 17% | 7 | 39% |
| > 200 | 9 | 978 | 4 | 44% | 0 | 0 | 5 | 56% |

The third source of herd data are the reports from Dairy Herd Improvement centers. These reports include milk production per cow, days in lactation, fat and protein content, and when requested individual SCC information. Several systems to report SCC data are currently used (Reneau, 1986; Dohoo and Leslie, 1991). Examples are presented in Tables 2 to 7. In Table 2 a list of all cows with their historical performance with regard to SCC is presented. Such a list allows the evaluation of patterns in SCC. Short term (acute) increases in SCC can be distinguished from long term (chronic) elevated counts.

Some DHI centers provide distribution of SCC (mean and 3 classes (< 200, 200 - 500, > 500) in the total herd, per test day (Table 3) parity (Table 4), and day of lactation (Table 5).

To be able to distinguish between bulk milk SCC increases that are caused by only a few cows, or bulk milk SCC increases caused by a large proportion of the herd, a list

*Table 6. List of cows over 200,000 somatic cells/ml, ranked in order of % contribution to the bulk milk SCC*

| Cownr | Parity | Calving date | Kg Milk | SCC | %Contribution | avg SCC |
|---|---|---|---|---|---|---|
| 23 | 3 | May 3 | 35.1 | 6650 | 18 | 6650 |
| 25 | 3 | Dec 9 | 32.4 | 6140 | 16 | 5084 |
| 56 | 5 | Jan 18 | 36.9 | 3869 | 10 | 2875 |
| 34 | 1 | April 4 | 18.6 | 4891 | 7 | 4891 |
| 45 | 6 | July 6 | 19.4 | 3869 | 7 | 2021 |

with the contribution of each cow to the bulk milk SCC is presented. When only a few cows are responsible for the high bulk milk SCC, the percentage contribution of these few cows will be high (i.e. three cows contribute > 40% of all somatic cells). This is shown in Table 6.

In Table 7 an estimate of the rate of new infection is presented for an example herd. This estimate is reported for the current sampling day and the previous sampling days. It refers directly to the formula presented by Natzke (1981): Prevalence = Incidence * Duration, and is therefore an important component in monitoring of subclincal infections. Since individual SCC measurements tend to be rather variable, it is advisable to observe SCC patterns within a cow and within a herd in time, and to make decisions based on these patterns rather than on single SCC measurements of cows.

Additional sources for farm data are farm computers and computerized devices in the milking parlor. Recent developments in on-line measurement of milk temperature and the Electrical Conductivity of milk (Nielen et al., 1992) may complement and eventually even replace clinical observations.

*Table 7. Estimate of the rate of new infections. (Number of cows that were < 200,000 in the previous sample and are now > 200,000 divided by the number of cows that were < 200,000 in the previous sample)*

| | Rate of new infections | | | | | | | |
|---|---|---|---|---|---|---|---|---|
| Test day | herd | | heifers | | parity 2 | | parity > 2 | |
| May 12 | 5/19 | 20% | 1/7 | 13% | 1/4 | 25% | 3/8 | 30% |
| April 8 | 4/18 | 23% | 1/7 | 13% | 1/4 | 25% | 2/7 | 28% |
| March 9 | 7/16 | 43% | 3/7 | 43% | 1/3 | 33% | 3/6 | 50% |

### 6.2.3 CLINICAL INSPECTION

A clinical inspection includes clinical examination and treatment practices on cows with clinical mastitis, and CMT testing or bacteriological evaluation of cows with a history of high SCC. In herds with mastitis problems observations on udder quality, teat shape (Agger et al., 1986) and teat lesions (Van der Geer et al., 1988) on all cows may be required. Other aspects that should be inspected are: identification of cows treated for mastitis, body condition of dry and lactating cows by scoring every individual cow in the herd, percent of blind quarters in the herd, percent of fresh cows with udder edema and broken udders, management of mastitic cows, cows that should be culled due to chronic mastitis and clinical and bacteriologic examination of cows purchased recently. Dry and lactating cows should be inspected for general cleanliness, milk leaking, presence of (many) flies on cows, and inspection whether hair is clipped from udders and surrounding.

When the udder health situation on a farm is suboptimal, it is important that the practitioner becomes involved in treatment regimes, sampling of treated quarters, scoring of udder and teat-end quality of all cows in the herd, observations on udder skin conditions and record keeping. Bacteriological analysis of bulk milk and quarter milk samples of individual cows in the herd is a prerequisite to detect major pathogens. Sampling of cows may involve the complete herd or may be guided by SCC, CMT or conductivity measurements. Bacteriological results often include sensitivity of pathogens towards antibiotics. This information may be used to evaluate antibiotic treatments, and to design a herd-specific treatment protocol.

High milk production, frequent milking (3 or 4 times daily) and a relatively high vacuum may cause a detoriation of teat-end shape in milking cows. Recent studies have shown that severe teat-end eversions may be a sign of dysfunctioning of the milking machine, and may have an important impact on the incidence of mastitis (reviewed by Hamann et al., 1994). Longitudinal follow-up of teat end shape may be required to monitor the performance of the milking machine by scoring keratinization of the teat opening (Figure 2) and by examining teat-end swelling, bleedings, and eversion of epithelium. Dry cows and heifers should be included since they form a natural reference category within each herd.

*Table 8. Teat end evaluation. See Figure 2 for scoring system*

| Score | Performance | Goal |
|---|---|---|
| 0 | % | > 60% |
| A | % | < 20% |
| B | % | <10% |
| C | % | < 5% |
| D | % | < 5% |
| Trauma | % | < 5% |

*Figure 2. Scoring system of teat-end keratinization. The top series refers to teat-ends with a smooth ring, whereas the lower series refers to teat-ends with an irregular ring (courtesy to Research station for Cattle, Sheep and Horses, Lelystad, the Netherlands)*

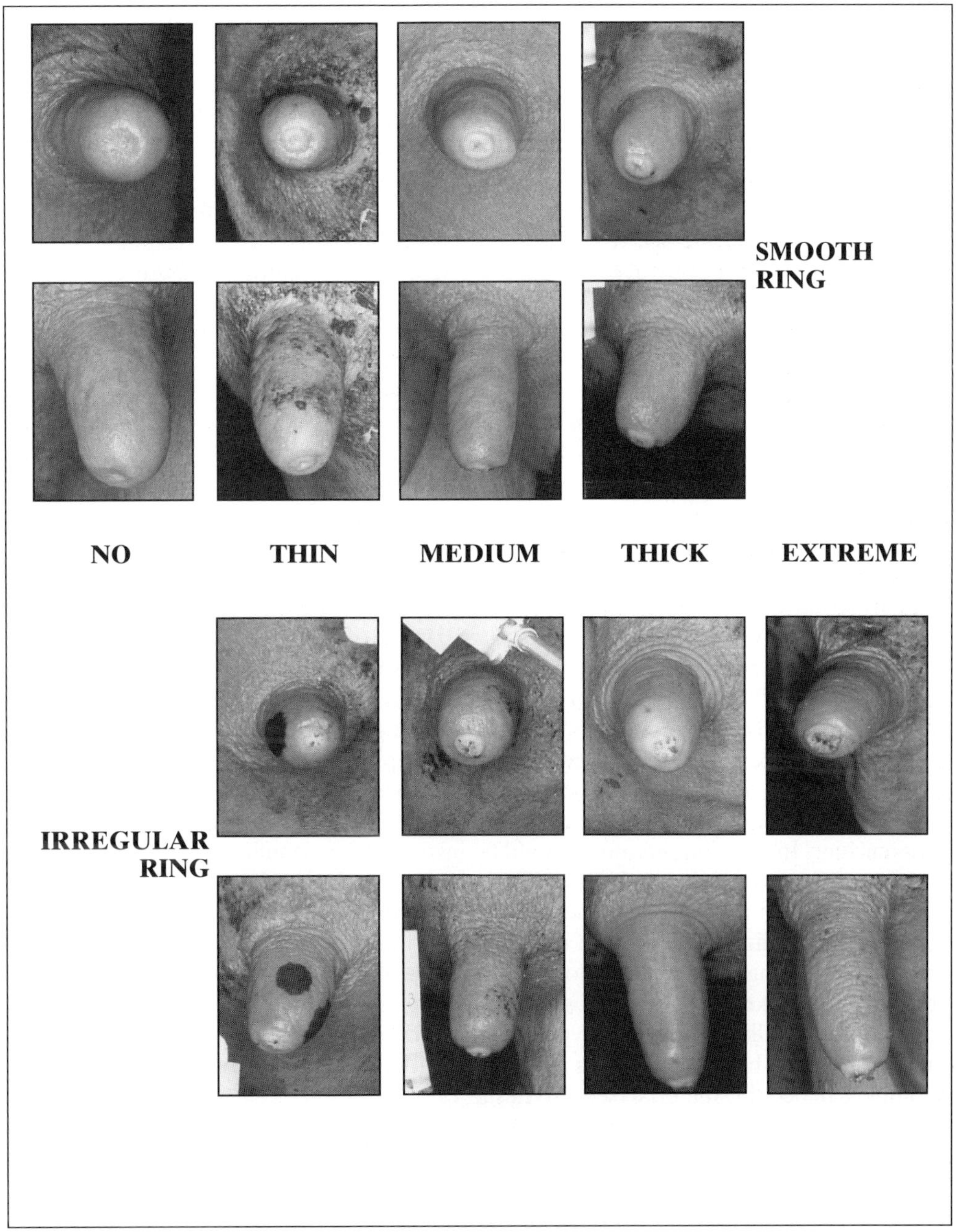

*Table 9. Teat condition*

| Score | Performance | Goal |
|---|---|---|
| Normal | % | > 80% |
| Dry cracks | % | < 5% |
| Warts | % | < 5% |
| Acute Lesion | % | < 5% |

Regular scoring of teat ends provides an estimate of % cows with teat injuries (goal: < 5%). In addition information can be gathered about the percent of blind quarters in the herd (goal: < 5%).

More in depth analysis of teat end swelling and lesions may be obtained with the use of ultrasonography of the teat (Spencer, 1995). Teat wall thickness before and after milking can be measured without distorsion of the teat due to this measuring device.

### 6.2.4 FARM INSPECTION

Farm inspection is an extremely important tool to obtain information on udder health. It should include surveys in various management categories. These categories can be divided into practices related to milking procedures, farm environment, milking system (checking functioning and maintenance) and management practices related to mastitis treatment and control procedures. A scoring system to identify factors in these fields that may contribute to a herd's udder health performance is discussed in part 4 of this Chapter. The quantitative scoring system is primarily usefull during the investigation process in a problem herd. Expansions or reductions of the system may be required depending on the type of problem or the specific skills of the investigator. Further investigations may be based on patho-physiologic knowledge of mastitis, or may be guided by epidemiologic investigation of risk factors (Bartlett et al., 1986; Thurmond, 1993). An example is given in part 5 of this Chapter.

A source of valuable information on the milk machine is the inspection sheet of the milking machine. In addition pulsators should be inspected for cleanliness, air, milk tubes and inflations for cracks and/or holes. The inspection also includes cleanliness of the milking parlor, milking equipment and of the milk filter. It is impossible to obtain a good overview of the milking technique without an actual observation of the milking process. An observation of the milking allows evaluation of the preparation of the udder, the technique of attachment, squaking of liners, blind milking, alignment of milking units with udders, amount of rest milk, post milking hygiene, and handling of the cows. Special attention also should be paid to hygienic practices in the maternity pens and dry cow facilities, including cleanliness of bedding material (see also Leslie, 1994).

Since economics are an important component of udder health, an economic analysis survey should be performed. An example is presented in Table 10. More complete evaluations on economics of mastitis are available (Dijkhuizen, 1977; Fetrow and Anderson, 1987).

*Table 10. Economic analysis survey*

**1. Bulk milk tank SCC**

(BMSCC - 150,000)/100,000 = ______ units
Total daily milk loss = ______ units * .015 * ______ kg shipped/day
= ______ kg

Total daily $ loss = ______ kg * ______ ct per kg = $______

**2. Individual cow SCC**

| SCC range | # cows | | % loss |
|---|---|---|---|
| 0 - 150 | ________ | x 0 | ________ |
| 151 - 250 | ________ | x 1.5 | ________ |
| 251 - 400 | ________ | x 3.5 | ________ |
| 401 - 1000 | ________ | x 7.5 | ________ |
| 1001 - 3000 | ________ | x 12.5 | ________ |
| > 3001 | ________ | x 17.5 | ________ |
| Sum | ________ (A) | | ________ (B) |

Average loss = ______ (B) / ______ (A)/100 = ______ (C)

Total daily milk loss = ______ (C) x ______ kg milk shipped/day

= ______ (D) ______

Total daily $ loss = ______ (D) x ______ ct per kg = $______

**3. Clinical cases**

\# clinical cases in last year ______ x $100,- = ______
\# involuntary culls due to mastitis in last year ______ x $750,- = ______
Total = $______

**4. Cost of mastitis control**

Dry cow therapy ______ cows x $ ______ = $ ______
Teat dip fluids $ ______
Paper towels $ ______
Cost of SCC measurements $ ______
Total = $______

## EPILOGUE

The importance of data collection and subsequent monitoring cannot be overestimated. Only with regular inspection and evaluation of performance indices, dairy farms can effectively assure udder health and excellent milk quality. Only high quality data will allow usefull monitoring. The maintenance of clinical records, milk production and SCC results, and other pieces of information is an essential part of farm management. Without data, effective herd health management is not possible. An essential component of dairy herd health is therefore assurance of sufficient data of high quality. These data are partly collected through milk recording systems, partly by the farmer and partly by the veterinary practitioner. Monitoring depends on the quality of these data. To be able to follow the udder health situation on a farm, a continuous flow of data is required. Only when this is guaranteed through a regular program, the quality of the product and the health status of the cows can be guaranteed.

*For references see part 5 of this Chapter.*

# 6.3 MONITORING UDDER HEALTH: DECISION MAKING, ANALYSIS, INTERVENTION AND FOLLOW-UP

Ynte H. Schukken and Theo J.G.M. Lam

Department of Herd Health and Reproduction, School of Veterinary Medicine, University of Utrecht, Yalelaan 7, 3485 CL Utrecht, The Netherlands

## 6.3.1 INTRODUCTION

Once a monitoring program is in place, evaluation of the data becomes the most important issue. The general process of the interpretation of data is shown in Figure 1. This process consists of several steps. The basic requirements are the preset targets for udder health of the farmer and the presence of sufficient data collected as herd data, clinical data, farm inspection data, or a combination thereof. The data will then be processed into the primary udder health performance indices, and compared to the preset targets. When the targets are met, data collection will continue, and, if necessary, the targets can be adjusted. When the targets are not met, further processing of the data to calculate secondary indices, or further data collection and analysis are necessary. In this part decision making, analysis, intervention and follow-up in udder health programs will be discussed.

*Figure 1. General process of the interpretation of Udder Health data*

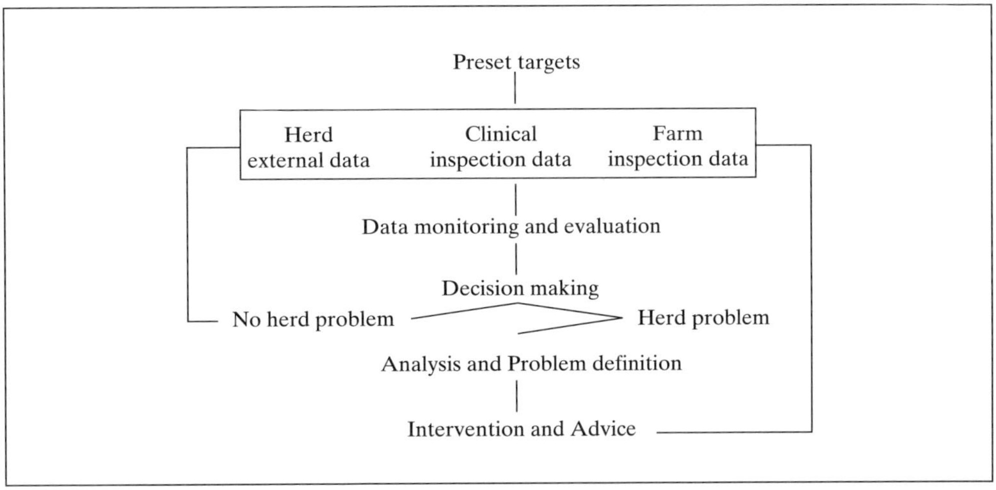

## 6.3.2 DECISION MAKING

After collection of data, primary udder health performance indices are calculated. Primary indices should be calculated from readily available data in farms participating in an udder health program. Any aberration of these performance indices should trigger further calculation and investigation of secondary more precise, but less general indices.

In part 2 of this Chapter, the BMSCC of a farm, the incidence of clinical mastitis, clinical cases per affected cow, and the number of culls due to udder health problems were defined as primary preset targets. To be able to evaluate short term effects and long term effects, these three primary performance indices should be calculated for three time periods; for example the last twelve weeks, the last 6 months and the last year. Indices calculated over the last 6 months and year provide trends towards a positive or negative development of udder health performance while calculations over a shorter period may indicate sudden drops or improvements. Also, when an index calculated over a short period deviates from preset targets, an acceptable annual rolling average may put the problem in perspective. Especially with bulk milk somatic cell count data, which tend to have a large variance, this is an important consideration.

Important secondary indices are the proportion of cows above a certain somatic cell count cut-off limit, the risk of "new infection", the risk of elimination, and the contribution of the highest SCC cows to the bulk milk SCC. These secondary performance indices are important, but can only be calculated in herds subscribing to cow-SCC service. More advanced tools like daily electrical conductivity measurements may yield other parameters (Nielen et al., 1992).

## 6.3.3 DECIDING ON THE EXISTENCE OF A HERD PROBLEM

The decision that a herd problem exists should be made by the farmer in conjunction with the HH & PM practitioner. This decision may be based on simple deviations from preset targets. Once the target is exceeded analysis will be started. Exceeding the penalty limits imposed on the industry by government regulations may be another reason to start further analysis. A third method to decide on the existence of a herd problem is based on the presence of a performance goal, and prior knowledge on the variability of the indices that are used. This latter method allows the farmer to define the amount of false-positive warnings. This method wil be explained in more detail below.

The variability of the indices that have been defined before is known from extensive field surveys. Bulk milk somatic cell count can be modelled by a log-normal distribution (Shook et al., 1982), while the incidence of clinical mastitis can be modelled using a Poisson distribution (Schukken et al., 1991) (see part 4, Chapter I). Most likely, the number of cull cows due to udder health problems can also be modelled using a Poisson distribution (Schukken et al., 1991). The application of this knowledge to a herd of approximately 50 cows is shown in Table 1. In this Table the preset targets have been defined by the farmer. For three time periods the expected annual performance

*Table 1. Evaluation of udder health indices to decide on the existence of a herd problem in a 50 - cow dairy herd. Action level refers to the level that, once exceeded, triggers further analysis. Actual refers to the actual data from a 50 - cow dairy farm*

| Index | Last 90 days | Last 6 months | Last 12 months | Preset target |
|---|---|---|---|---|
| BMSCC | | | | |
| Action level | 380 | 320 | 290 | |
| Actual | 210 | 205 | 190 | <240 |
| Clinical mastitis | | | | |
| Action level | 42% | 34% | 30% | |
| Actual | 48% | 40% | 32% | <18% |
| Culling due to mastitis | | | | |
| Action level | 24% | 15% | 11% | |
| Actual | 8% | 8% | 6% | <5% |

is calculated (e.g. the three months incidence is multiplied by 4) and compared to the preset target. Based on the variability of the index, an action level has been calculated.

In table 1 this process is illustrated for a 50 cow dairy. The preset target for clinical mastitis is this herd is 18% (or less), or 9 cases of clinical mastitis. Assuming a Poisson distribution, the standard deviation of this number equals 3 (square root of 9). The action level is defined as 2 standard deviations above the preset target. In the herd in table 1 this would mean 9 + (2*3) = 15 cases of clinical mastitis or 30%. The example farm in table 1 shows an incidence of 32%, and therefore further analysis is indicated.

The presence of some sort of formal decision making process allows the farmer and the advisor to think about the presence of false positive and false negative warnings. Neither of these are wanted, but it is likely that some of these errors will occur no matter what system is used. Once the decision making system is decided upon, it should be a very quick and easy process. Preferably this process is automated when the herd health data are already present in a computerized system.

When the evaluation process is finished, two options remain. It is either decided that there is currently no udder health problem, and the farmer will continue his activities as before. Or it is decided that an udder health problem is present on the farm. In the latter case, further analysis is indicated.

### 6.3.4 CONTINUOUS MONITORING

When the primary indices do not signal a problem, monitoring of the udder health situation continues. Monitoring consists of at least the following components:

BMSCC, based on monthly reports, number of cases of clinical mastitis, and number of culls due to udder health. A more complete monitoring system is advisable even when currently no udder health problems exist. Such a system adds to the afore mentioned components, regular evaluation of cow-SCC, sampling of clinical and subclinical affected cows, and evaluation of udder health management on a regular basis.

Individual cow SCC is usefull to detect cows with a prolonged high SCC. Prolonged high SCC may be defined as cow-SCC > 250.000 cells/ml. in two out of the last three samples. These cows should be evaluated by CMT and positive quarters should be sampled for bacteriological culture. Sampling of all clinical cases before treatment should be part of any treatment protocol. Udder health management may be evaluated using a checklist (Philpot and Nickerson 1991; Leslie 1994) or an evaluation tool as presented in part 4 of this Chapter.

This monitoring scheme services two goals, first it informs the farmer and the veterinary practitioner about the current udder health status and the level of management. Changes in management to optimise the situation, or the decrease the risk may be advised based on these data. Secondly, it provides historical data in the situation that an udder health problem does occur.

## 6.3.5 DATA ANALYSIS

When the primary indices signal a problem, more analysis of existing data may give information as to the source and the cause of the problem. Secondary indices as summarized in part 1 of this Chapter should be calculated and analysed. These secondary indices will yield additional information and can be used to define the problem more precisely. Investigations to describe the problem and to look for patterns in time, age, stage of lactation, place in the barn (When, Where, What) etc. should be undertaken (Thurmond, 1993).

Data derived from clinical and farm inspection activities also should be evaluated using the management evaluation tool that is described in part 4 of this Chapter. These data will yield information regarding proper or improper functioning of the milking machine, milking techniques such as failure to dip teats, or the presence of teat lesions, and the contribution of the environment to the mastitis problem. When leads are detected that point towards a certain causal mechanism for the mastitis problem, further data collection may be necessary. In a herd with a high incidence of clinical mastitis this may be the culturing of bedding samples or ventilation checks. The problem solving protocols for herds with either a high bulk milk SCC or a high incidence of clinical mastitis will be described in more detail.

## 6.3.6 PROBLEM SOLVING IN HERDS WITH HIGH BULK MILK SCC

The first step is to obtain a history. Historical bulk milk data may be used to define if a herd problem exists. For example, a long term high bulk milk SCC and a short term high bulk milk SCC may be differentiated. In the first situation likely a herd problem exists, while in the latter case some individual cows may have a large impact on the average SCC.

This can be defined more precisely by calculating the contribution of the highest SCC cows to the bulk milk SCC (see Table 7 in part 2). In the case that the highest three SCC cows (or 5% of all cows) contribute more than 30 - 40% of the bulk milk SCC, then these specific cows appear responsible for the problem, when this is not the case it is likely that a high prevalence of infection exists. The second step is to perform an inspection of relevant farm data, clinical data, and to perform a farm inspection. A high prevalence of subclinical mastitis is detected quite well by monitoring cow somatic cell counts (see Tables 3 - 8 in part 2). It is important to realize that the prevalence of any disease, but specifically of subclinical mastitis can be defined as:

Prevalence of disease = Incidence of disease * disease duration

This is an important relation for problem solving in high subclinical mastitis herds (Natzke, 1981). Prevalence may be estimated by calculating the proportion of cows with an individual SCC above a threshold. Often a threshold of 250,000 cells/ml. is used (Tables 3 - 6 in part 2). To impact this problem, both incidence and duration of the disease should be addressed. The important steps in subclinical mastitis control programs involve the reduction of the incidence, the shortening of the duration of infection or sometimes both. The most important components of the "seven point" program are:

1. Proper maintenance and use of the milking machine,
2. Proper milking procedures,
3. Employ post-milking teat disinfection,
4. Dry treatment of cows with quality antimicrobials,
5. Accurate treatment of clinical mastitis during lactation,
6. Culling of chronically infected cows,
7. Maintenance of a clean environment in barn and parlour.

Factors that affect the incidence of new infections are a proper functioning of the milking machine, proper milking procedures, post milking teat disinfection and the maintenance of a clean environment. In any program, the reduction of incidence should be the primary target. When the number of new infections does not decrease, a continuous process of treatment and culling will be the result. No obvious improvements will take place. From infectious disease epidemiology it is learned that the spread of any infection can only be reduced or eventually eliminated when the basic reproduction rate ($R_0$) of an infection is less than 1. The basic reproduction rate is defined as the number of new infections that results from one typical existing infection (Anderson, 1991). This parameter depends heavily (among other factors) on the probability of transmission and the density of susceptible and infectious hosts. Udder health programs try to increase the number of susceptible hosts (= uninfected cows), hence the major route to keep the $R_0$ value low is the prevention of transmission of infection. The infection risk as defined in Table 3 in part 1, and reported by DHI (Table 7 in part 2) is associated with $R_0$. When an average infection is assumed to have a duration of less than one lactation, the mean infection risk on a farm should be less than 10% (Dohoo and Morris, 1993).

Intramammary infections spread mainly during milking, consequently proper maintenance of the milking machine and milking techniques are essential. Known infected cows should be milked last, and clusters disinfected between cows. Despite these recommendations, the teat-end may still be infected after milking. Preventing the spread of teat-end infections into the mammary gland, post-milking teat disinfection has proven to be essential in these programs.

The elimination risk ("cure") may be estimated from individual cow SCC data. Factors that affect elimination of infection are dry treatment with antimicrobials, treatment of (sub) clinical mastitis during lactation, and last but not least culling of chronically infected cows. Although these measures are essential in reducing the prevalence, they merely support the measures taken to reduce incidence of new infections. Effective reduction of duration has a high impact on easily observable indices. Effective dry treatment, in combination with culling of high SCC cows may have a tremendous impact on the current bulk milk SCC. This may be an important aspect as to motivating producers to continue the program.

The third step is to define a differential list of causes based on the definition of the observed problem.

An example of a definition of the problem is: A 60 cow herd with a Bulk milk SCC of 560,000. The percentage of quarters above 250,000 cells is 60%, the majority is among the older cows in late lactation. The most important pathogen prevalences are: *S.aureus*: 20% of the cows, and *S.agalactiae* in 30% of the cows. The milking technique is not optimal and selective dry cow treatment is used. The estimated economic loss is $17,000 per year.

The fourth step is to perform additional laboratory examinations, additional measurement in milking machine function or other relevant parameters. In SCC problem herds it is advisable to sample all cows, or at least all cows with a high individual SCC during two or more sampling days. This may be done on a cross-sectional basis, but it is also advisable to continue to sample cows with repeated high SCC in a longitudinal follow-up program. Especially cows with two or more subsequent high cell counts should be sampled (see Table 3 in part 2). In this phase it may be useful to perform a teat-end inspection, to further analyse milking machine function during milking, and to observe the milking technique. The analytical method described in part 4 of this Chapter may be used for this purpose.

Finally, in the fifth step a list of causes of the problem will be reported. This list is explained to the farmer, and discussed in detail. The farmer should after this step be aware of the problem, and be aware of the causes of the problem. A list of recommendation is created and follow-up evaluations should be planned. Research has shown that the prevention and elimination of infection in high SCC herds is possible. A reduction of 100% of the *S.agalactiae* infections is feasible, and the prevalence of *S.aureus* can be reduced significantly. Bulk milk SCC can decrease to levels below

250,000 within one year of the program. The programs to be implemented in case of *S.agalactiae* and *S.aureus* will be discussed in more detail.

### S.agalactiae program

The goal of this program is to eradicate *S.agalactiae* from the herd. This is a feasible goal since it is a strictly intramammary pathogen. A benefit/cost ratio for such a program appears to be attractive (Erskine and Eberhart, 1990). The first step is to optimize management such that reintroduction and spreading of the microorganism will not occur. This includes the seven-point program as described above. In addition, no cows should be added to the herd unless proven to be negative for *S.agalactiae.* There is no sense in commencing with the next steps if the seven-point program is not executed according to standards.

The second step is to sample all lactating cows in the herd for bacteriological analysis. The sensitivity of bacteriological culturing for the detection of *S.agalactiae* is high, and all infected cows are likely detected. Thirdly, all infected cows should be treated with an appropriate antibiotic at the same point in time ("blitz" treatment). It is important to discuss this procedure with the milk processing plant. Approximately 10 days after treatment all infected cows should be sampled again for evaluation of treatment effect. Strict sampling of all cows that freshened for a period of 2 - 4 months is important to prevent reintroduction of the germ into the milking herd. Follow-up with individual cow milk SCC and sampling of all cows more than once over 200.000 cells/ml. is advised for early detection of new udder health problems.

### S.aureus program

In contrast to *S.agalactiae*, there is no simple eradication program for *S.aureus*. This microorganism also survives in the environment of cows or on the skin of cows. Chronically infected cows are extremely hard to cure. Both lactation therapy and dry cow therapy are not always successful (Sol et al., 1994). The central issues in the *S.aureus* program are prevention of new infections, and shortening of the duration of existing infections. Dynamics of *S.aureus* infections in a herd was described by Lam et al. (1996). It was shown that the number of new infections per unit of time could be modelled by:

# new infections = ß * # susceptible * # infectious,

where ß is a transmission "constant", that depends on the microorganism, management and herd specific circumstances. The # susceptible, and # infectious refer to the number of quarters that are respectively free of infection, or infected by *S. aureus*. Prevention of new infections may occur through reducing transmission by hygienic milking practices, optimal functioning of the milking machine, and most important, through practising of post-milking teat disinfection (Lam, 1996). Separation of infected cows from non-infected cows may have an impact on the number of new infections.

According to the above equation this should lead to a significant reduction in incidence (Wilson et al., 1996). In practice, detection of infected cows is difficult due to relative low sensitivity of bacteriological culture (Sears et al., 1990). Vaccination may play a role in future (Colditz and Watson, 1985). Recent studies have shown some effect of vaccination with a *S.aureus* vaccine in reduction of new infections under field conditions (Nordhaug et al., 1994).

Shortening of existing infections may occur through treatment of *S.aureus* infections during lactation (either clinical or subclinical), treatment of infections at dry off, or through culling of infected cows. Treatment success of *S.aureus* infected quarters depends on the height of SCC (higher SCC leads to lower treatment success), age of the animal (older cows have a lower treatment success), the number of infected quarters, and the germ count at the time of infection (Sol et al., 1994). Also, information on the susceptibility to antibiotics of *S.aureus* may be helpful in the selection of the proper treatment.

Eradication of *S.aureus* is not a realistic goal. Hence the goal of an udder health program is to reduce the reproduction ratio of *S.aureus* in the herd. A stable endemic situation with a low prevalence is then feasible. To obtain this a low incidence of new infections, and a relative short length of the average infectious period should be obtained (Lam et al., 1996).

## 6.3.7 PROBLEM SOLVING IN HERDS WITH A HIGH CLINICAL MASTITIS INCIDENCE

The first step is to obtain a history and to describe the complaint. Preferably, data should be present to quantify the clinical mastitis problem. Often there are no complete data available, and a prospective data collection system should be implemented.

The second step is to perform an inspection of relevant data, a clinical inspection and an inspection of the farm. With regard to the data, the incidence of clinical mastitis should be calculated, and specified with regard to microorganism, season, stage of lactation, parity, location of the affected quarters, and possibly other relevant factors. With regard to the clinical farm inspection, the epidemiological triangle of agent, environment and host should be kept in mind. A number of known risk factors for clinical mastitis will be discussed (see also Leslie, 1994; Philpot and Nickerson, 1991; Bramley et al., 1992; Sandholm et al., 1995).

### a. Agents

The mean incidence rate of clinical mastitis in herds with a low bulk milk SCC has been measured in only a few surveys. These are summarized in Table 2.

In all these surveys, *E. coli* was the most important pathogen together with the non-agalactia streptococci. These microorganisms are abundant in the environment of the dairy cow. It indicates that although the exposure may be reduced by management, it is not opportune to strive for elimination of the pathogen. Examples of high *E. coli*

*Table 2. Incidence rate and percentage distribution of mastitis pathogens in three surveys on clinical mastitis in herds with a low bulk milk SCC*

| Microorganism | Survey: I [1] | II [2] | III [3] |
|---|---|---|---|
| Incidence rate expressed as cases per 10,000 cow days at risk | 14.9 | 13.9 | 5.2 |
| Coliforms | 29.7 | 43.5 | 16.2 |
| Environmental streptococci | 25.4 | 12.3 | 12.8 |
| Staphylococcus aureus | 1.7 | 2.2 | 9.6 |
| Non-lactose fermenting rods | 6.5 | – | .4 |
| Other, incl. more than one pathogen | 1.7 | 5.4 | 14.2 |
| Staphylococcus spp. | 5.4 | 7.8 | 13.0 |
| Corynebacterium bovis | 1.7 | – | 2.4 |
| Contaminated | .6 | – | 8.5 |
| Negative | 27.2 | 28.6 | 22.9 |

Hogan et al., 1989 [1] – Erskine et al., 1988 [2] – Schukken et al., 1989 [3]

exposure leading to increased clinical mastitis have been documented. Philpot and Nickerson, (1991) describe a case where an udder ointment was heavily contaminated, leading to increased exposure and clinical mastitis. The data from Schukken et al. (1989) illustrate that in low bulk milk SCC herds, *S.aureus* may still play a role in the cause of clinical mastitis.

**b. Environment and Management**

Part 4 of this Chapter may be used to evaluate environment and management. Some components will be discussed here in more detail.

**Cubicles**

The cubicle and its bedding are an important part of the environment of the dairy cow. In several studies a relation between cubicle cleanliness, log cfu in the bedding and the rate of clinical mastitis was observed (Bramley and Neave, 1975; Dodd et al., 1984).

**Milking**

The milking machine may be an important cause of mastitis in herds with a high SCC (Natzke, 1981). However, the milking machine has also been identified as a cause of clinical mastitis in herds with a low SCC (Hoblet et al., 1988; Bramley et al., 1992). A similar argument holds for milking routine. Suboptimal milking procedures are especially prevalent in herds with a high SCC (Natzke, 1981). But in herds with a low SCC some milking procedures (wet udder preparation, check of first streams of milk, and machine maintenance) were also associated with an increase in clinical mastitis (Schukken et al., 1991).

**Dry cow management**

Management of the dry cow is an important factor in reducing the incidence of clinical mastitis in the subsequent lactation. The first seven days after cessation of milking and the days just before parturition are periods with a high rate of new infections (Eberhart, 1986). In general, management in the period of milk cessation, the dry period and the periparturient period should be focused on a low exposure of the udder to microorganisms and an optimalization of physical and immunological host defense mechanisms (Eberhart, 1986; Oliver and Sordillo, 1989).

It appears that dry cow antibiotics remain useful in herds with a low Bulk Milk SCC. Dry cow antibiotics not only remove most existing infections, but also decrease the number of new infections in the early dry period (Eberhart, 1986). Results from a field trial in an institutional herd, with a low prevalence of infection with major pathogens at drying off (< 10% of the quarters), revealed that the two quarters not treated with antibiotics at dry off showed a signifcantly higher incidence of clinical mastitis due to *S.uberis* than the two quarters in the same cows with an antibiotic dry cow treatment (Schukken et al., 1993). Similar results were reported by Robinson et al. (1988).

The method of antibiotic insertion is an important factor influencing the incidence of new infections. A study by Boddie and Nickerson, (1986) showed that a partial insertion of the dry cow syringe canula decreased the incidence of infections in the dry period. Destruction of the teat canal keratin plug and injection of microorganisms into the teat cistern may be the reason for this increase in infection rate.

**Nutrition**

Studies regarding nutrition and clinical mastitis have focused mainly on minerals and vitamins, especially vitamin E and selenium, and vitamin A and ß-carotene (Conrad and Smith, 1986). It has been shown that nutrition has an effect on the quality of the immune response (Boyne and Arthur, 1979). Several studies have related dietary components to the immune function or to the incidence of clinical inflammation (reviewed by Gershwin et al., 1985). Currently most evidence points towards selenium deficiency and negative energy balance (hypoglycemia and ketonemia) as the most likely nutritional components that influence udder health (Dohoo et al., 1984).

**c. Host**

Several host factors have been identified as risk factors in epidemiological studies on clinical mastitis. These factors will be reviewed with special attention to the biological explanation in the pathogenesis of clinical mastitis. Some of these factors may contribute to the infection opportunity of microorganisms (i.e. destruction or reduction of physical barriers), but most factors will be associated with non-specific host defenses. Important findings were the observations of Kremer et al., (1993); Lohuis et al.,

*Figure 2. The relation between pre-infection leukocyte function and killing of microorganisms (Kremer et al., 1993)*

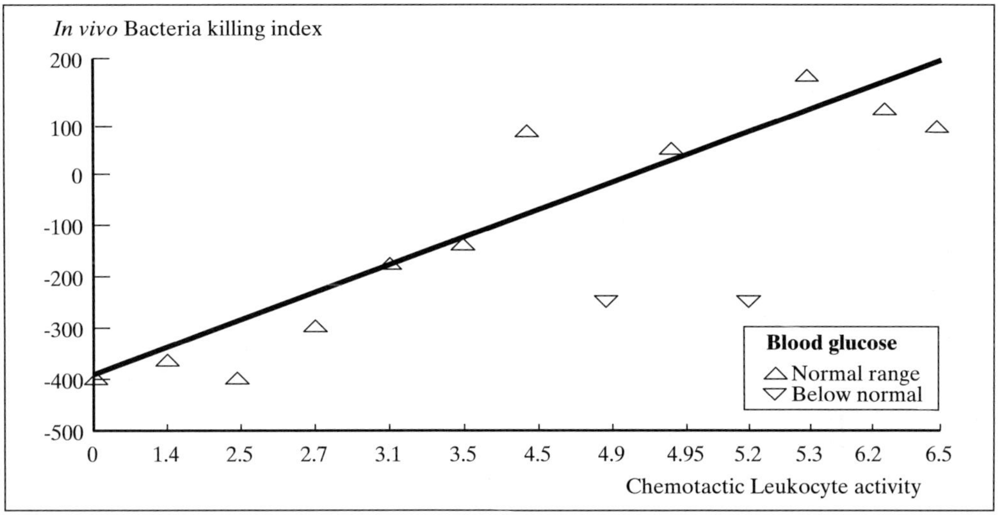


(1990); and Heyneman et al., (1988)) that respectively the preinfection chemotactic activity of PMNs, and the bactericidal potency of leukocytes were predictive of the clinical response after an experimental infection with *E.coli* in normoglycemic cows (Figure 2). In hypoglycemic (ketotic) cows this relationship disappeared and these cows showed a low bacterial killing capacity. Hence, it is likely that alterations in non-specific host defenses are relevant to clinical mastitis in well managed herds since mastitis in these herds is often caused by opportunistic infections.

**Parity**

Parity has been identified as a risk indicator in several observational studies. In most studies the incidence increased with increasing parity (e.g. Bendixen, 1988).

**Stage of lactation**

In all observational studies on clinical mastitis stage of lactation was an important determinant of clinical mastitis (Bendixen, 1988). The rate of mastitis during lactation follows a negative exponential distribution with the peak in the first days after calving. The first days after calving exhibit a decreased number of circulating neutrophils (Newbould, 1976). In addition a dramatic decrease in functionality and mammary influx of neutrophils and lymphocytes occurs shortly after calving (Kehrli et al., 1989).

**Level of milk production**

A high herd level of milk production was associated with an increased incidence rate of clinical mastitis (Schukken et al., 1991). Similarly, geneticists consistently find a genetic correlation between milk production and mastitis (Emanuelsson et al., 1988).

The genetic evidence is fairly consistent that selection for milk yield is accompanied by increased susceptibility to disease (Shook, 1989).

**Periparturient diseases**

Some periparturient diseases have been identified as risk indicators for subsequent occurrence of clinical mastitis. The most important of these diseases are: parturient paresis (Curtis et al., 1985), retentio secundinarum (Schukken et al., 1988; Gunnink, 1984), dystocia (Bendixen, 1988) and ketosis (Dohoo and Martin, 1984). This was also observed in a study by Dohoo et al. (1984), cows with a history of ketosis were at increased risk of mastitis. Negative energy (and protein) balances that exist during early lactation may contribute to impaired neutrophil function (Kehrli et al., 1989).

**Milk leaking and teat lesions**

Leaking of milk in between milkings has been associated with an increased risk of clinical mastitis (van de Geer et al., 1988). Obviously, teat lesions are an important risk factor for clinical mastitis (Agger and Willeberg, 1986; Grommers et al., 1971). The physical destruction of the first line of defence against infection contributes important to the incidence of clinical mastitis. Recently a scoring system to evaluate teat-end conditions was presented, and it may be used to evaluate teat condition in a herd (see part 2 of this Chapter).

**Colonization with minor pathogens**

In some recent studies the use of post milking teat disinfection has been hypothesized as an risk factor for clinical mastitis, especially the cases that are caused by opportunistic infections (Robinson et al., 1988). The experiments regarding the protective effect of colonization by minor pathogens (coagulase negative staphylococci, corynebacterium spp., other micrococci) on subsequent risk of clinical mastitis were not conclusive in their results: protective effects were observed by Linde (1982), while no effect was observed in a study by Doane et al. (1987). Recently, Lam (1996) reported a field study where in a within cow comparison, quarters that were disinfected after milking were compared with quarters that were not disinfected. In the not-disinfected quarters, an increase in the prevalence of minor pathogens was observed, and this was associated with a reduction of clinical coliform mastitis. At the same time increase in the prevalence of subclinical *S.aureus* infections occurred.

It is not possible to give a complete list of risk factors that are possibly associated with clinical mastitis. As mentioned before, in a problem solving approach, step one is to define the complaint, step to is to perform an inspection of clinical data, herd data and farm inspection data. The third step is to create a list of possible causes of the problem. Preferably the problem definition includes the major causal microorganisms. The definition should include the presence of seasonality, parity distribution, stages of lactation etc. when any of these factors are present in the herd. An economical definition of the problem is important to weigh the costs of a prevention program against the current amount of money lost.

Example of such problem definition is: A 50 cow herd with an incidence of clinical mastitis of 40%. The bulk milk SCC is 170,000. The distribution of pathogens shows a majority of *E. coli* (40%), and non agalactia-Streptococci (40%). The majority of cases occur in early lactation. The cow's environment is wet and dirty, the cows are soiled, an environmental problem exist. The estimate economic loss is $10,000 annually.

The fourth step is to perform additional investigations. This may include measurements of machine function, scoring teat-end condition, measuring the quality of management using the tools defined in part 4 of this Chapter, evaluating the existence of metabolic disorders and others.

In the fifth step a final list of causes is summarized. This list is explained to, and discussed with the farmer. Based on this list a series of recommendations is proposed. It is important to set reasonable goals for the intervention program. Reducing clinical mastitis is a challenging program. And to date no successful program with a guaranteed reduction in incidence has been described. Therefore, no high expectations should be allowed at the onset of the program.

Some recent experimental studies indicate that non specific stimulators of the immune function may decrease the number of clinical cases. Non specific immuno stimulation has been described with Levamisole (Flesh et al., 1982), Concanavalin A (Oliver and Sordillo, 1989), Colchicine (Oliver and Smith, 1982), and Interleukin-2 (Nickerson et al., 1989). Most non-specific immunostimulators have been tested under experimental conditions; field trials in herds with a low SCC have not been described yet. More field work has been published with regard to vaccination against coliform mastitis. A field trial using a mutant *E. coli* J5 antigen vaccine showed a decrease in incidence and severity of coliform mastitis (Hogan et al., 1992; Gonzalez et al., 1989). In these trials, the total mastitis incidence in the experimental and control group was not significantly affected, although a reduction in *E. coli* mastitis was observed. Also the severity of infection was significantly reduced in vaccinated animals compared to control animals.

### 6.3.8 FOLLOW-UP

To evaluate the intervention program, monitoring of progress is required. Therefore, at the beginning of such a program a system to monitor the identified problem should be implemented. Regular calculation of indices on incidence and prevalence of udder infections should take place. The indices defined in part 1 may be used for this purpose. When preventive udder health programs start, the main factor that will be influenced is the incidence of new infections. This means that the prevalence of infections will only drop slowly. Irrespective of the quality of the program. Analysis of the proper indices is therefore essential to evaluate the progress of the program. Follow-up sampling of either high SCC cows, or cows with clinical mastitis is an essential component of the follow-up program. For subclinical mastitis, regular evaluation of cow SCC is important, and for clinical mastitis a herd mastitis chart, or a similar monitoring tool should be implemented.

## EPILOGUE

In this chapter we have artificially divided the udder health problems into two main groups. Although this represents the majority of the problems that we have observed in our herds, there will be herds that show a combination of the two problems. Apart from these general categories there will always be outbreaks of some rare microorganisms. It was the intention in this chapter to emphasize a systematic herd health approach. Most likely, the problems due to rare events will eventually be solved through application of this general framework and creative thinking. The approach to herds with an udder health problem should be a team approach. Important members of such a team are the farmer, practitioner, milking machine technician, extension agent, and specific outside advisors such as bacteriologists, referral veterinarians or environmental specialists.

Udder health has great impact on the dairy farm. It influences farm economics, it influences animal welfare, and it also influences the quality of milk. These aspects combined indicate that udder health monitoring is important for both producer and consumer. Future developments in this field will be likely toward more automatic monitoring of cows in automated milking parlors or even in robotic milkers. Udder health should be closely watched in such systems. With regard to treatment, no major developments are currently expected. However with regard to prevention of infection, either through more precise management, or through vaccination or immune modulation further progress is to be expected. An integrated approach to udder health, combining nutrition, housing, hygiene, milking techniques, animal genetics and animal immunity will likely solve some of the major problems in todays dairy industry.

*For references see part 5 of this Chapter.*

# 6.4 MONITORING UDDER HEALTH: A SCORING SYSTEM TO IDENTIFY FACTORS CONTRIBUTING TO A HERD'S MASTITIS PROBLEM

William J. Goodger

Department of Medical Sciences, School of Veterinary Medicine, 2015 Linden Drive West
Madison, WI 53706, USA

## 6.4.1. INTRODUCTION

Two dairies with genetically similar herds of the same size in similar environments can have markedly different milk outputs. It is thought that this objective measurable difference in productivity may be due to a difference in management between two operations. This difference in management, however, is not easily measured. Clinicians should have a tool to assess the impact of management practices, because their importance as an input is similar to that of feed, labor, etc in harvesting milk. For instance, in the case of mastitis, veterinarians have not had an integrated quality control system to use in field investigations. Such a system would make use of a standardized reporting form to define the factors contributing to the herd's mastitis problem and would implement a plan providing management advice to control mastitis.

A standardized reporting form can be used on-farm, based on specific scoring criteria developed for the most important milking management practices associated with maintaining udder health. This form can be used to identify milking management factors associated with suboptimal udder health and monitor the effect of changing management practices over time. Because this standardized reporting form provides an objective and reproducible scale for measuring the adequacy of management practices, the form is referred to as an "instrument" as it functions in much the same way as other clinical instruments (stethoscope, thermometer, etc.). In other words, it measures deviations from normal or optimal practices that are associated with disease or the increased risk of it.

The approach to management taken here is to observe and score measures which are indicators of the quantity of management as opposed to assessing the quality of management in a simple yes/no checklist. Also, the dairy farm operator is interviewed and their verbal responses can be validated by scoring these readily observable indicators. For instance, the adequacy of post-milking teat dipping is an indicator in the postmilking procedures category. Its adequacy or quantity of management is determined by sampling 5 or more cows in the milk barn or exiting the parlor using the "coverage test". This is accomplished by observing the coverage of teat dip on a paper towel for each cow's teat end. This data will generate information on how much management is being applied as opposed to just knowing if the procedure is being utilized.

The purpose of this chapter is to describe an integrated quality control system which utilizes a scoring instrument to evaluate milking management practices.

*Scoring approach*

The scoring visit should occur during milking and would take the form of recording observations and making measurements for 46 questions in 12 management categories. The categories can be divided into practices related to milking procedures (category c6 to c9), practices related to the farm environment (c1, c4, c5), practices related to the milking system (c2, c3), practices related to mastitis treatment and control procedures, including the use of records (c10 to c12). Also, farm visits to dairies would include recording milking time vacuum tracings, reviewing milk processing plant test results, and collecting DHI data for scoring questions in the form. The format of the visit will be informal, with the veterinarian recording observations and measurements concerning each question. Following the farm visit the recordings/measurements will be reviewed, the scoring form will be filled out, and the dairy will be scored using criteria in the scoring manual. This scoring instrument has been validated for its content in that in its entire form it measures milking management. Its reliability between users has been tested and its ability to measure the result or output from management, in this case somatic cell count, has also been validated.

## 6.4.2. MILKING PRACTICES EVALUATION FORM (FOR SMALL DAIRIES)

The form for the "instrument" contains 3 - 4 questions in each category. Each of the 3 - 4 questions is assigned a scale from 0 - 20 points.

DAIRY: ______________________________

EVALUATOR: ______________________________

| **GENERAL SANITATION PRACTICES (C1)** | **COMMENTS** | **SCORE** |
|---|---|---|
| 1. Is there standing water, manure and mud in the alleyways, lanes, or corrals? | | |
| 2. What efforts does the manager take to keep the cow yard or freestall (loose housing system)/exercise yard clean and dry? | | |
| 3. What efforts does the manager take to keep the stall barn clean and dry or how frequently are the milking parlor floors and walls washed? | | |
| 4. Are the milking units (claw, teat cups, and liners) and equipment (system) rinsed, washed, and sanitized between shifts? | | |

**CATEGORY SCORE =**

## GENERAL SANITATION PRACTICES (C1)

**1. Is there standing water, manure and mud in the alleyways, lanes, or corrals?**

| Score: | | |
|---|---|---|
| | 20 | Clean |
| | 15 | 25% dirty |
| | 10 | 50% dirty |
| | 5 | 75% dirty |
| | 0 | All dirty |

Look at traffic lanes to barn, feed lanes and alleyways in corrals. Find out how often lanes or alleyways are scraped. When evaluating, consider time since last scraping.

**2. What efforts does the manager take to keep the cowyard or freestall (loose hou sing system)/exercise yard clean and dry?**

| Score | For freestall | | For cowyard |
|---|---|---|---|
| 20 | Adequate slope (exercise yard)<br>Alleys scraped 2x daily<br>Adequate bedding | 20 | Adequate slope (cowyard)<br>Scraped daily<br>clean yard |
| 15 | Adequate slope (exercise yard)<br>Alleys scraped daily<br>Bedding 75% | 15 | Adequate slope (cowyard)<br>Scraped every other day<br>25% dirty |
| 10 | Not adequate slope (exercise Yard)<br>Alleys scraped every other day<br>Bedding 50%<br>(1/2 length of bed scooped out) | 10 | Not adequate (cowyard) slope<br>Scraped weekly<br>50% dirty |
| 5 | Some slope (exercise yard)<br>Alleys scraped weekly<br>Bedding 25% (both ends scooped out) | 5 | Some slope (cowyard)<br>Scraped biweekly<br>75% dirty |
| 0 | No slope (exercise yard)<br>No schedule for scraping<br>No bedding | 0 | No slope (cowyard)<br>Scraped monthly<br>All dirty |

Look to see that cow yards or exercise yard associated with freestall are sloped in a proper manner, i.e. not toward drinking water troughs, but toward some drainage system. Ask how often the cow yard is scraped and verify by visual observation, taking into account the length of time since the last scraping. For freestalls, check for bedding used and maintained adequately (8 cm of bedding). Also, consider the cleanliness of the traffic lanes in the freestalls, score down if dirty. If observations are conducted during the summer, consider what the pens probably look like during the winter. Evaluate between score levels of adequate bedding by assessing the amount of manure in the bedding. Use common sense to score and combine the different situations.

**3. In case of a stanchion barn: what efforts does the manager take to keep the barn clean and dry?**

| | | |
|---|---|---|
| Score: | 0 - 4 | Gutter grates are present |
| | 0 - 4 | Soiled bedding scraped from rear of stall |
| | 0 - 4 | Lime (calcium carbonate) spread on alleyways |
| | 0 - 4 | Approximately 8 cm of bedding |
| | 0 - 4 | Cow trainers present and adjusted |
| | 0 - 20 | Total |

Question dairy operator as to when stalls and central alley are scraped and limed. Verify with visual observation as to whether there is a lot of manure in the gutters and in the stall especially toward the back end. Modify scores between ranges.

**In case of a milking parlor: how frequently are the milking parlor floors and walls washed?**

| | | |
|---|---|---|
| Score: | 20 | – Walls are washed between milkings and floors are washed during and between milking groups |
| | 15 | – Floors are washed during and between milking groups |
| | 10 | – Floors are washed only between groups |
| | 5 | – Floors are washed after each milking |
| | 0 | – Floors are not washed between every milking |

Bonus points to add: 4- walls washed once a week; 3- walls washed once every two weeks; 2- walls washed once a month; 1- wall washed once every two months. For example, score 10 because floors are washed only between strings and 2 because walls washed once a month for a final score of 12.

Question dairy operator as to when parlor floors and walls are hosed down. Verify with visual observation as to whether there is a lot of manure on the floors and walls while cows are being milked. Modify scores between ranges considering adequacy of wash-down procedure. Check to see if manager steam-cleans or otherwise sanitizes walls periodically.

**4. Are the milking units (claw, teat cups, and liners) and equipment (system) rinsed, washed and sanitized between milkings?**

Consider inside (CIP) and outside cleaning of individual machines. Check if milk lines are rinsed with a disinfectant solution (not just a detergent).

| | | |
|---|---|---|
| Score: | 0 - 5 | Runs sanitizer through machines before use |
| | 0 - 5 | Measures temperature of wash-up water periodically |
| | 0 - 5 | Immerses and flushes in wash and rinse between milkings |
| | 0 - 5 | Scrubs periodically |
| | 0 - 20 | Total |

## MILKING EQUIPMENT MAINTENANCE (C2)

| MILKING EQUIPMENT MAINTENANCE (C2) | COMMENTS | SCORE |
|---|---|---|
| 5. Are liners changed on a regular schedule that follows manufacturer's specifications for # milkings/liner? | | |
| 6. How frequently are pulsators cleaned or flushed? | | |
| 7. How frequently is the vacuum controller/regulator disassembled and cleaned? | | |
| 8. Is there a scheduled maintenance check by a qualified service technician? | | |
| | CATEGORY SCORE = | |

**5. Are liners changed on a regular schedule that follows manufacturer's specifications for number of milkings per liner?**

Get numbers for:
a. Cows milked
b. Milkings per day
c. Milking machines used
d. Frequency with which liners are changed

Calculate number of milkings per liner. Compare to values from manufacturers (average = 1000 uses between changes under USA conditions). Give 20 if under recommendations. If over, subtract recommendations from actual and divide by recommendations to obtain a % over recommendations. Multiply the % by 20 to get a product which is subtracted from 20 to get a score. (No negative points!)

*Calculations:*
Step 1—product = 20 x (Actual - recommendation)/recommendation
Step 2—20 minus product = final score

**6. How frequently are the pulsators inspected and/or cleaned/flushed?**

| | | |
|---|---|---|
| Score: | 20 | Monthly |
| | 15 | Quarterly |
| | 10 | Semi-annually |
| | 5 | Annually |
| | 0 | Never |

Find out how often pulsators are cleaned. Look at top of pulsator units to check if they are clean. Take into account the size of the dairy and environmental conditions. Note some pulsators have an air filter system. Units attached to a filtered-air system may not need to be cleaned as often. This is also the case with DeLaval sealed units (clean those every year).

**7. How frequently is the vacuum controller/regulator inspected and/or disassembled and cleaned?**

| | | |
|---|---|---|
| Score: | 20 | Monthly |
| | 15 | Quarterly |
| | 10 | Semi-annually |
| | 5 | Annually |
| | 0 | Never |

Procedure: Question dairy operator as to how often vacuum controller/regulator is disassembled and cleaned. Look to see that the vacuum controller is located in an area that is as free as possible from dust and water and see how clean filter is (modify score).

**8. Is there a scheduled maintenance check by qualified servicemen?**

Score: 5 – Regularly scheduled maintenance check
5 – Maintenance check by qualified personnel
5 – Maintenance check approximately once/month
5 – System checked in some manner

Ask how often and by whom is the equipment checked. Determine if the system is checked (pulsators, regulator, etc.) or if "supplies are dropped off." Find out what is included in the maintenance check i.e. filters, soaps, sanitizers, oil etc. Deduct if dairy operator does the maintenance him/herself exclusively.

## ADEQUATE MILKING SYSTEMS (C3)

| ADEQUATE MILKING SYSTEMS (C3) | COMMENTS | SCORE |
|---|---|---|
| 9. Are the number of cows milked & their production level within the specifications of the milking system? | | |
| 10. Does the milk flow as directly as possible from the udder to the milk line?<br>11. What is the cyclical vacuum fluctuation measured at the claw? | | |
| 12. Is there a constant release of air through the vacuum regulator even when milk flow is heaviest? | | |
| | **CATEGORY SCORE =** | |

**9. Are the number of cows milked and their production level within the specifications of the milking system?**

Identify milk line size and configuration of line. Use table to find number of milking units recommended:

### PARLOR CONFIGURATION

| Milk line size (internal diameter) | Dead-end | 1-row double slope 2-row double slope | 2-row double slope (close-loop) |
|---|---|---|---|
| 38 mm | 2 | 4 | 8 |
| 48.5 mm | 4 | 8 | 16 |
| 60 mm | 6 | 12 | 24 |
| 73 mm | 9 | 18 | – |
| 98 mm | 16 | – | – |

### STANCHION BARN CONFIGURATION

| Milk line size | Dead-end | 1 row double slope |
|---|---|---|
| 38 mm | not permitted | 4 |
| 48.5 mm | not permitted | 8 |
| 60 mm | not permitted | 12 |
| 73 mm | not permitted | 18 |

Give 20 for an adequate system. If more units than recommended are used, subtract recommendations from actual and divide by recommendation to obtain a % over recommendations. Then multiply % by 20 to get a product which is subtracted from 20 to get a score. If the situation doesn't fit above specifications, identify interim score from nearest configuration given. Also, a common fault is variable slope or flat spots. The milk line should have a uniform slope towards the receiver with a minimum fall of 2.5 cm and preferably up to 5 cm per 3 m of milk line. Calculate slope with a spirit level.

**10. Does the milk flow as directly as possible from the udder to the milk line?**

Make sure the milk does not have to go through loops and turns before reaching the milk line (assuming the long milk hose is the proper length). Look at the length of the milk hose, is it as short as possible without causing the unit to fall off during milking (when cow moves a little)? Also, the milk line should be mounted as low as is practical, never more than 1.2 m above the cow's standing level. Score how direct milk flows as follows:

| | | |
|---|---|---|
| Score: | 0 - 7 | No loops in the milk hose-direct path |
| | 0 - 7 | Long milk tube length between unit and milk pipeline (low or high line) =229 -279 cm and height of milk line < 1.2 m above the cow's standing level |
| | 0 - 6 | Support arm-hose present and used |
| | 0 - 20 | Total |

**11. What is the cyclical vacuum fluctuation measured at the claw?**

Measure at the unit or cow most distant from the receiver jar. Use either a "Detco" (Dairy Test Equipment Co., 14058 Euclid Ave., Chino, CA 91710) or "Dectrace" (Dairy Equipment Co., P.O.Box 8050, Madison, WI 53708) or similar recording device (digital readout). Identify two average producing cows in the herd. Then record during milking, pulsator tracings with pulsator line attached to a front teat cup and milking vacuum with milking vacuum line attached to the claw on the first cow. Next, record same on second cow with pulsator line on rear teat cup and milking vacuum line attached to the claw. Do not include fluctuations due to squawks on the claw where the measurements are being made.

| | | | |
|---|---|---|---|
| Score: | 20 | if | < 7 kPa |
| | 10 | if | 7-10 kPa |
| | 0 | if | >10 kPa |

**12. Is there a constant release of air through the vacuum regulator even when milk flow is heaviest?**

Listen to the sound of air entering the vacuum regulator while cows are milking. Down-grade for amount sound fluctuates from a constant hiss.

| | | |
|---|---|---|
| Score: | 20 | Constant hiss |
| | 15 | Few fluctuations per minute & still reserve air flow (When all units are on the cows the regulator should be admitting the reserve air or surplus vacuum pump capacity to stop the vacuum in the milking sys tem from exceeding a pre-set level). |
| | 10 | Lots of fluctuations (>10/min.) & still reserve air flow. |
| | 5 | Shuts down for a moment; beyond reserve air flow. |
| | 0 | No hiss at all, beyond reserve air flow constantly. |

**CONDITION OF COWS (C4)**

| CONDITION OF COWS (C4) | COMMENTS | SCORE |
|---|---|---|
| 13. Does the manager take note of the body condition of the dry cows? | | |
| 14. Does the manager monitor udder, quarter and teat condition? | | |
| 15. Are the stalls of adequate width and length to minimize teat injuries? | | |
| 16. How has the manager installed and use ventilation in the building housing the cows? | | |
| | CATEGORY SCORE = | |

## 6.4.3. MILKING TECHNIQUE AND MANAGEMENT

### 13. Does the operator take note of the body condition of the dry cows?

Find the average body condition score of the cows in the dry pen. Question the dairy operator as to what condition he/she considers the dry cows to be in terms of fleshing. Score body condition score as follows:

| Average Body Condition Score Ranges: | Operator's Response: |
|---|---|
| 3.76 - 4.00+ | Poor (too fat) |
| 3.51 - 3.75 | Good (a little fat) |
| 3.26 - 3.50 | Excellent |
| 3.01 - 3.25 | Good (a little thin) |
| 2.76 - 3.00 | Fair (thin) |
| 2.51 - 2.75 | Poor (skinny, bony) |

Find difference between ranges of BCS and operator's response. If they differ, subtract 5 points per row to obtain your numerical difference. Subtract numerical difference from 20 to get a score. If unable to obtain an operator's response with confidence then compare actual BCS with "Excellent body condition score = 3.26 - 3.5" to obtain numerical difference. Give 20 to the operator who views/condition scores the dry cows with a veterinarian or nutritionist at least once a month.

**14. Does the operator monitor udder, quarter and teat condition?**

Observe 20 teat ends in the stall barn or milking parlor following milking. The act of milking can aggravate all types of teat lesions. Subtract from 20 one point for each teat end exhibiting some inflammatory response. Look for signs of hyperkeratosis (teat canal erosion, or orifice erosion), petechial hemorrhages, eversions, bruising, and chapped teats or frozen teats (winter). Lesions on the upper barrel of the teat include warts, cuts and pox-like lesions. Palpate 5 udders for abscesses/scar tissue and collect data on the number of cows with blind quarters and/or light quarters. Adjust score obtained from observing 20 teat ends by down scoring one point for each udder with an abscess/scar tissue, each cow with a blind quarter, and each cow with a light quarter.

**15. Are the stalls of adequate width and length to minimize teat injuries?**

Use the following table to assess stall size, both width and length for different sizes of Holstein cows:

| Stall Type | Cows < 545 kg | 636 kg | > 727 kg |
|---|---|---|---|
| **Stanchion** | | | |
| width | 1.2 m | 1.35 m | not rec. |
| length | 1.65 m | 1.73 m | not rec. |
| **Tie-Stall** | | | |
| width | 1.2 m | 1.35 m | 1.5 m |
| length | 1.73 m | 1.8 m | 1.95 m |
| **Freestall** | | | |
| width | 1.13 m | 1.2 m | 1.2 m |
| length | 2.1 m | 2.4 m | 2.4 m |

Score: 6 points for adequate numbers of stalls = 1 per cow
6 points for adequate length
8 points for adequate width

**16. How has the operator installed and used ventilation in the building housing the cows?**

Score if building has mechanical ventilation:

20 – Building has continuing exhaust fans and intermittent exhaust fans which are thermostatically controlled with air inlets using summer modifications
15 – Building has continuing exhaust fans and intermittent exhaust fans which are thermostatically controlled with air inlets
10 – Building has intermittent exhaust fans which are thermostatically controlled with air inlets
5 – Building has exhaust fan with air inlet
0 – Building has no exhaust fan or air inlet.

Score if natural ventilation:

20 – Building has adequate size to side opening (2.5 cm/3 m of bldg. width) and rid ge cap (5 cm/3 m of bldg. width) with a 2.5 cm/3 m of barn width as the ope ning at the eave (between roof and side wall) which creates a chimney effect to air movement through the eave and out through the ridge cap of the buil ding
15 – Building has adequate size to ridge cap and the addition of curtains (which can be lowered or raised from the top or bottom of the side of the building) to open the side of the building depending on the season. A permanent opening in the side curtain will equal 2.5 cm/3 m of barn width
10 – Building has adequate size to ridge cap-opening 5 cm/3 m of building width
5 – Building has open ridge cap
0 – Closed building.

## EFFICIENT TRAFFIC FLOW (C5)

| EFFICIENT TRAFFIC FLOW (C5) | COMMENTS | SCORE |
|---|---|---|
| 17. Are the uninfected cows milked before the infected cows? | | |
| 18. Does the manager have a policy about handling cows and is it reflected in their behavior? | | |
| 19. How efficient is the traffic regulation system for getting cows into the barn or parlor for milking? | | |

**CATEGORY SCORE =**

**17. Are the uninfected cows milked before the infected cows?**

Optimum order: Fresh heifers
Fresh cows
High producers
Medium producers
Low producers/strippers
Staph cows (if identified and segregated)
Mastitic cows (cows being treated)

Some dairy operators will milk "uninfected cows" identified by their low somatic cell count (SCC) before higher SCC cows which may be potentially infected.

Score: 0 - 8 Mastitis cows under treatment milked last
0 - 8 Separate milking unit for infected/treated cows and/or unit is properly disinfected after use
0 - 4 Cows with low SCC milked before high SCC cows

0 - 20 Total score

**18. Does the manager have a policy about handling cows and is it reflected in their behavior?**

Score: 20 – Operator has a concern about how cows are handled and it is reflec ted in their behavior
15 – Operator has a concern about how cows are handled but it is not reflected in the behavior of the cows
10 – Operator does not care how cows are handled and the cows' behavior shows it
5 – Operator does not care how cows are handled, uses instruments such as sticks, prods, or canes; and the cows' behavior shows it

Ask dairy operator if he/she has a policy about how workers handle cows, e.g. how the milker brings them into the barn or parlor or how heifers are brought into the milking herd. Find out if use dogs, walking canes, electric prods or if tail cows (look if some cows have broken/short tails). Note if the cows are nervous or jumpy around people. Remember that cows will act more nervous around strangers than with milkers.

**19. How efficient is the traffic regulation system for getting cows into the barn or parlor for milking?**

**Stanchion Barn:**

Score: 7 – Stanchions or tie stalls numbers are adequate for milking herd
7 – Route from exercise yard is most direct to the barn given layout of dairy
6 – When milking herd is in the barn, cows are not loose in the barn

**Parlor:**

Score: 7 – Cows do not end up in the wrong corrals or freestall areas after milking
7 – Cows do not stand for long periods of time before and after milking
6 – Uses some type of gate and lane system

## MILKER PERFORMANCE (C6)

| MILKER PERFORMANCE(C6) | COMMENTS | SCORE |
|---|---|---|
| 20. How often does the milker keep his/her hands clean/dry during milking and exhibit personal cleanliness? | | |
| 21. How is the vacuum level monitored during milking? | | |
| 22. How frequently are the units (claw, teat cups, and liners), long milk hoses, CIP (cleaned in place) cups, and other machine operation/cleaning rubber goods checked for cracks and leaks? | | |
| 23. What is the ratio of the actual throughput (cows milked per hour) per unit compared to manufacturer's specifications? | | |

**CATEGORY SCORE =**

### 20. How well does the milker keep his/her hands clean/dry during milking and exhibit personal cleanliness?

0 - 5 – Milker(s) appear(s) clean and clothes not excessively wet/dirty
0 - 5 – Milker's hands are reasonably clean and not noticeably wet/dirty

**Dry preparation (Pre-dip)** **or**
0 - 10 Milker's hands remain dry

**Wet Preparation**
0 - 10 Milker's hands washed (immersed in solution) between each cow but remain dry

Total = 0 - 20 points

### 21. How is the vacuum level monitored during milking?

Score: 0 - 5 – Milker knows actual vacuum level
0 - 5 – Milker knows location of gauge(s)
0 - 5 – Gauges accurate and working
0 - 5 – Gauges are visible

0 - 20 Total

Farm gauges are often inaccurate. Sometimes the indicator needle sticks and it will not move above 50 kPa to indicate a high operating vacuum if the regulator malfunctions. Tap the face of the gauge to check for a sticking needle. See what the type of gauge is (deduct 2 points for a dial gauge, as it is less sensitive than a digital gauge), if it is working, and if it is accessible to be monitored.

**22. How frequently are the units (claw, teat cups, and liners) long milk hoses, CIP (cleaned in place) cups, and other machine operation/cleaning rubber goods checked for cracks and leaks?**

Visually inspect all milking units. Identify wear, cracks, tears, leaks, torn rubber, excessively soft rubber changing the cross-sectional area due to kinking, loose connections, and distortion or swelling due to fat absorption. Most common faults include reduction in cross-sectional area of milk hoses (due to kinking or bending near the milk line inlets) or of short milk tubes where these join the claw inlets (due to age or mismatching) or cracks or tears in short milk tubes and pulse tubes. Divide 20 by number of units and subtract points for each unit exhibiting any defects. Note the air vent in the claw should be clear and unblocked.

Example: 20 points/4 units = 5 points/unit
2 units with obvious cracks and worn rubber
= 20 - (2 x 5 points) = 10

**23. What is the ratio of the actual throughput (cows milked per hour) per unit compare to manufacturer's specifications?**

Need data from:
a. Number of cows milked
b. Milking time (excluding clean-up)
c. Number of milking units in use
d. Parlor or stanchion barn
e. Units per milker (if applicable)

Then to calculate the ratio:
Step 1: milking cows(a)/milking time(b) = cows/time
Step 2: cows/time x 60 = cows/hr
Step 3: cows/hr. divided by the # of milking units(c)

Assume specifications are optimal. Calculate throughput (number of cows milked per machine per hour) based on figures for number of cows milked, length of milking (excluding clean-up) and number of units milking reported by dairy operator. Specifications for parlor configuration are 4.5 cows/hr./unit and for a tie stall or stanchion barn are 7 - 10 cows/hr./unit (d).

$$\frac{\textit{actual throughput}}{\textit{manufacturers' spec}} \times 20 = \textit{score}$$

## PRE-MILKING PROCEDURES (C7)

| PRE-MILKING PROCEDURES (C7) | COMMENTS | SCORE |
|---|---|---|
| 24. What is the percent of udders that are grossly soiled before preparation for milking? | | |
| 25. Does the milker make sure teats are properly washed, sanitized, and dried (single service paper towel) prior to milking? | | |
| 26. Does the milker stimulate milk letdown before each teat cup is attached to the teats of each cow? | | |
| 27. Are the quarters and foremilk of each cow checked for abnormalities before every milking? | | |
| | CATEGORY SCORE = | |

**24. What is the % Fof udders that are grossly soiled before preparation for milking?**

Observe the udders in the milking barn or parlor before milking. Determine the approximate percentage of udders that are clean (numerator) by scoring 20 cows as either clean or dirty (denominator). Multiply the percentage clean by 20 to get a score. All mud and manure should not be present on the udders.

**25. Does the milker make sure teats are properly washed, sanitized and dried (single service paper towel) prior to milking?**

Score how dry and clean teats are following preparation for milking by: using white glove test or apply paper towel to the teats of 4 cows picked at random over milking time immediately following preparation for milking. Observe towel and score 3 for dryness and 2 for cleanliness/cow.

| | | |
|---|---|---|
| Score: | For dryness = | 0 - 3 |
| | For cleanliness = | 0 - 2 |
| | Each cow = | 0 - 5 |
| | Total = (0 - 5) x (4 cows) = | 0 - 20 |

**26. Does the milker stimulate milk letdown before each teat cup is attached to the teats of each cow?**

Does the milker have a consistent routine to prepare the teat end of each quarter? Observe the way the milker stimulates let down. Does the milker do it by stripping some milk from the quarter, wiping off dirt on the teat end with a towel, or applying pre-dip, etc. Also, to assess adequate letdown it is important when let down is done e.g. just before teat cups are placed on the teats of each cow's quarters or if he or she stimulates let down in a number of cows before putting milking units on a cow. Score milk letdown by observing 5 cows: consistent milking preparation routine = 12 points; adequate milk letdown procedure = 8 points.

**27. Are the quarters and foremilk of each cow checked for abnormalities before every milking?**

See if milker checks for abnormal milk (flakes, blood, gargot, etc.) by squirting first stream of milk onto floor (parlor) or strip cup (barn). Observe if milker looks for a swollen quarter or feels for a hard quarter to check for potential mastitis. Score based on approximate percentage of 20 quarters observed/checked or had milk observed from stripping multiplied by 20.

## MILKING PROCEDURES (C8)

| MILKING PROCEDURES (C8) | COMMENTS | SCORE |
|---|---|---|
| 28. Are teat cups applied gently and with a minimum of air admission within 1-2 minutes of milk letdown? | | |
| 29. Are teat cups kept aligned on the udder to prevent liner slips? | | |
| 30. Does the milker check for under milking of the cow before disconnecting the milking machine? | | |
| 31. Is the vacuum shut off before removal of teat cups? | | |

**CATEGORY SCORE =**

**28. Are teat cups applied gently and with a minimum of air admission within 1-2 minutes of milk letdown?**

Step 1: Watch for amount of air admission on 5 cows.The milker should cut off vacuum on other cups when attaching a teat cup (subtract 5 points) and should prevent air admission from the teat cup as much as possible when they are being aligned

Step 2: Then using a watch calculate the time from the stimulation of let down to the application of teat cups to the teat ends of the cow's quarter on 4 - 5 cows

Score teat cup application by:

20 – 1 - 1.59 minutes
15 – 2 - 2.59 minutes
10 – 3 - 3.59 minutes
5 – >4 minutes

**29. Are teat cups kept aligned on udder to prevent liner slips?**

Estimate the incidence of slipping or falling teat cups by listening and looking. See how quickly the milker realigns teat cups. Note the stage of milking when the slips occur. Slips are important toward the end of milking. As milk flow is reduced it is easier for liner slips to cause reverse jetting allowing milk laden with bacteria to penetrate the teat canal. Score slipping and realigning time. Score: amount of squawking (10 with 5 - 10 slips/100 cows milked); realigning time (10 if each slip is realigned immediately). Adjust scores appropriately.

**30. Does the milker check for under milking before disconnecting the milking machine?**

If cows are undermilking, subclinical infections may flare to a clinical stage. Check a representative sample of udders for completeness of milkout by hand stripping for a reasonable period of time or into a test bucket. Most cows should milk out in 6 minutes. A visual means to determine when milk flow stops should be available. If automatic take-offs are used, see if milker double-checks that all quarters are milked out.

| **Reasonable period of time:** | **or** | **Test Bucket:** |
|---|---|---|
| Score undermilking by: | | 20 - < .2 lbs/cow(96cc) |
| check 4 cows: 5 pts/cow = 20 | | 15 - < .5 lbs/cow(240cc) |
| hand strip quarters, | | 10 - .5 -.9 lbs./cow(240 - 432cc) |
| if 2 or more quarters can strip 5 | | 5 - > 1 lb./cow(480cc) |
| or more squirts (each) then -5 | | |

**31. Is the vacuum shut off before removal of teat cups?**

Watch for milker removing individual cups without shutting off vacuum. If automatic take-offs are used and placed on manual, the vacuum should be shut off before teat cups are removed. Score vacuum shut-off: observe 5 cows x 4 points/cow if vacuum is shut off properly. Deduct 5 points if machine stripping is practiced. Also, deduct 5 points if individual teat cups are removed individually without shutting off vacuum to milk cows with blind quarters or cows that don't milk completely from a quarter.

**POST MILKING PROCEDURES (C9)**

| POST MILKING PROCEDURES (C9) | COMMENTS | SCORE |
|---|---|---|
| 32. Are all teats dipped completely, immediately after milking with the proper strength of teat dip? | | |
| 33. What measures has management taken to keep cows from lying down immediately after milking? | | |
| 34. Are individual milking units kept clean between cows? | | |
| | CATEGORY SCORE = | |

**32. Are all teats dipped completely immediately after milking with the proper strength of teat dip?**

Determine approximate percentage of adequately dipped teats in a sample of cows (5 or more) in the milk barn or exiting the parlor. Do this by using the "coverage test." This is accomplished by covering the teat orifice with a paper towel following milking and a cow being post-dipped or sprayed. Observe the coverage on the paper towel for each teat end and record as adequate coverage or not. Multiply percentage of adequate coverage by 20 to get score. Be especially wary of a spray system. Note teats should be covered with dip for at least 2 inches above the teat orifice. This may be excessive but will ensure compliance. Check teat dip cups for residue.

**33. What measures has management taken to keep cows from lying down immediately after milking?**

See if cows are fed after milking (or feed is pushed up), are held in a clean lane or pen so that cows are kept standing up while teat sphincters are closing (about 1 hour).

Score: 20 – New feed after milking
15 – Pushed feed after milking
10 – Some feed leftover in manger
5 – Little feed leftover in manger
0 – No feed in manger

**34. Are individual milking units kept clean between cows?**

See if outside of milking units especially the teat cups and claw are kept clean by checking the units at the end of milking. Make sure that the teat cups are not dragged on the ground between cows or laid down in manure and/or bedding.
Score: % of milking units with clean teat cups and claws multiplied by 20.

**MASTITIS TREATMENT (C10)**

| MASTITIS TREATMENT (C10) | COMMENTS | SCORE |
|---|---|---|
| 35. Are antibiotics used on the farm in a proper manner? | | |
| 36. Are mastitis cows identified within the herd and the milk discarded? | | |
| 37. Are infected milking cows treated with a tested and FDA approved antibiotic? | | |
| 38. Are aseptic techniques used when treating cows? | | |

**CATEGORY SCORE =**

**35. Are antibiotics used on the farm in the proper manner?**

Score: 0 - 5 – Is milk from a treated cow tested before it goes in tank?
0 - 5 – Does the veterinarian or the drug directions decide the dosage rate?
0 - 5 – Are antibiotics discontinued based on label or veterinary instruc tions?
0 - 5 – Do labels or instructions have withdrawal times?

0 - 20 Total

**36. Are mastitic cows identified within the herd and the milk discarded?**

Score: 20 – Identified and milk discarded as soon as mastitis noticed.
15 – Identified and milk discarded after treatment at the next milking.
10 – Not identified and milk discarded after treatment.
5 – Not identified and milk discarded at the next milking.

**37. Are infected milking cows treated with a tested and FDA approved antibiotic?**

Watch out for "home brews" - even vet-compounded or mixed preparations. Look at drugs out of date and storage.

Score: 20 – Yes, FDA approved
15 – Extra label approved by vet
10 – Vet mixed prep
5 – Homebrew

**38. Are aseptic techniques used when treating cows?**

Person treating should wash hands between cows, wash teat end with alcohol-soaked cotton, used separate treatment tubes for each teat and dip teats after treatment.

Score: 0 - 5 – Wash teat end with alcohol soaked cotton
0 - 5 – Use separate treatment tubes for each teat
0 - 3 – Person washes hands between cows
0 - 5 – Dip teats after treatment
0 - 2 – Tubes in teat canal partially

0 - 20 Total

## MASTITUS CONTROL (C4)

| MASTITIS CONTROL (C11) | COMMENTS | SCORE |
|---|---|---|
| 39. What percent of mastitis treatment and control activities are carried out or are indirectly supervised by the veterinarian? | | |
| 40. Are all quarters of all cows dry-treated with a commercially prepared dry treatment? | | |
| 41. How is the maternity pen (close-up) managed? | | |
| 42. How are chronic (includes Staph cows) mastitis cows managed regarding the manager's policy on culling and segregation? | | |
| | CATEGORY SCORE = | |

**39. What % of mastitis treatment and control activities are carried out or are indirectly supervised by the veterinarian?**

Ask if a veterinarian is consulted in terms of maintaining mastitis control programs and if he/she is consulted for treatment/diagnosis of difficult clinical cases. Also ask if fresh and clinical cows are cultured or samples saved before treatment for later culturing. Score by taking % of activities as % of 20.

**40. Are all quarters of all cows dry-treated with a commercially prepared dry treatment?**

Score: 0 - 5 – Product approved for dry-cow use
0 - 5 – Single treatment at onset of dry period
0 - 5 – Use for all cows or selective based on culture
0 - 5 – All or none dry off versus gradual dryoff
——
0 - 20 Total

**41. How is the maternity pen (close-up) managed?**

Score: 0 - 5 – 1 maternity pen/25 cows
0 - 5 – Cleaned regularly between calvings
0 - 5 – Adequate bedding (8 cm)
0 - 5 – Strategically located and regularly observed
——
0 - 20 Total

Define maternity pen as where cows are last two weeks before calving. Note that calving on pasture may be cleanest. Verify with visual observation that maternity pen is clean, dry and uncrowded. Also may note if dry cows are monitored for mastitis. Modify score by looking at pen condition.

**42. How are chronic mastitis (includes Staph cows) cows managed regarding the manager's policy on culling and segregation:**

Score: 20 – Culled immediately when recognized as chronic mastitis (treated mul tiple times during a lactation, cultured as Staph aureus, and scc > 500,000 for 3 consecutive months

15 – Immediately segregated (milked with a separate unit or milked last) and culled when dry

10 – Segregated and no specific culling policy with regard to mastitis status

5 – No culling and no segregation

## RECORD USE (C12)

| RECORD USE (C12) | COMMENTS | SCORE |
|---|---|---|
| 43. Is SCC or CMT used monthly by the manager for management decisions such as culling or culturing cows with a high SCC or CMT 2/3? | | |
| 44. Are treatments of clinical cases recorded in some manner? | | |
| 45. Are milk processing plant (company) results on bulk tank samples monitored by the dairyman? | | |
| 46. Are there goal and alarm levels of udder health measures to monitor mastitis incidence? | | |
| | CATEGORY SCORE = | |

**43. Is SCC or CMT used monthly by the manager for management decisions such as culling or culturing cows with a high SCC or CMT 2/3?**

Score: 20 – Individual SCC or CMT are used to culture or cull and in addition the dairy operator uses further sub-population analyses such as using L2 scores to compare L1 vs 2, and L3 lactations, comparing to previous SCC, etc

15 – Operator receives SCC information & use individual data or CMT to culture or cull

10 – Operator receives SCC & uses herd average SCC

5 – Operator obtains SCC information & doesn't use

0 – Operator doesn't receive SCC & doesn't do CMT's

**44. Are treatments of clinical cases recorded in some manner?**

Score: 20 – Records are kept on an individual cow's permanent written record or on computer
15 – A transient piece of paper (e.g. list of mastitis cows)
10 – An erasable medium (e.g. blackboard) is used
5 – Some worker (e.g. herdsman, milker) remembers
0 – Not at all

Question dairy operator as to method of recording clinical case data. Add additional points for completeness of record, i.e. record includes condition, treatment used and time/date of treatment. Some operators record treated cows on a calendar.

**45. Are milk processing plant (company) results on bulk tank samples monitored by dairy operator?**

See if the dairy operator is aware of fluctuations. Ask him/her what is done about fluctuations. Find out which is looked at - Standard Plate Count, Bulk Tank Somatic Cell Count, and Post Incubation count and why. Creamery cards may not be posted or even saved. Score use of creamery results by:

0 - 7 – Manager posts current milk processing plant results in milk house
0 - 7 – Manager is aware and knows test results
0 - 6 – Manager understands and knows how to interpret results
------
0 - 20 Total

**46. Are there goal and/or alarm levels of udder health measures to monitor mastitis incidence?**

Score: 0 - 5 – There is a goal level for udder health
0 - 5 – Goal level is firm (Goal is realistic and not "soft")
0 - 5 – There is an alarm level for udder health
0 - 5 – Alarm level is firm
------
0 - 20 Total

Measures of udder health that can be monitored include % of herd being treated at any one time, incidence of mastitis in fresh cows, SCC levels, etc.

## EPILOGUE

The success of solving a multifactorial disease problem such as mastitis by identifying milking management practices is dependent on being able to elicit a change in management performance. The change that one would expect once a problem is identified does not occur expeditiously because there is a lag between when the problem was defined, the plan of action initiated, and when various stages of implementation have begun. This is not only time dependent but dependent on the type of bacteria causing the problem i.e., an environmental versus a contagious pathogen requires a much different scale of solution.

One of the challenges in clinical problem solving facing practitioners in mastitis investigations is the ability to integrate data from multiple sources with a disease with multiple causes. The challenge is to integrate the management factors responsible for the frequency of bacteria present either on the farm or cow environment with factors responsible for the pathogenesis of the disease. The pathogenesis depends on the bacterial numbers at the teat end, the method of bacterial penetration into the teat canal, and the cow's immune system (scc). The hope is that an instrument as described above can address the above challenge as a standardized recording form to measure actual management performance. To the extent that it does this, it becomes a clinical instrument measuring deviations from normal or optimal practices, that are associated with suboptimal udder health or the increased risk of it. This instrument can also be regarded as a qualitative precursor of the quantitative method of Hazard Analysis Critical Control Points, HACCP, operated at the farm level as described by Noordhuizen & Welpelo (1996). In this concept of HACCP, the critical control points may comply with some of the scoring items named here. But before such a method can be implemented at the farm, risk identification and quantification (see Chapter 1, part 4) has to be undertaken.

The compliance of the dairy farm operator in implementing a plan of action that has evolved from the output of the use of an instrument as has been described above is the most critical factor in the success of resolving a mastitis problem. Probably one important ingredient of compliance is having a motivated dairy farm operator. But being able to monitor progress in a "connected" manner i.e., connected to the dairy farm operator's management system is probably the most important ingredient. In a sense, the instrument as a standardized recording form functions to integrate data from multiple sources/causes over time and becomes a quality control system tracking success and failures as a surveillance system does in the case of an infectious disease. This function allows the further connection to financial measures by being able to measure the profit and return from the implemented management changes resulting from a plan of action.

Other scoring instruments can be developed for other health management areas (reproduction, replacements, etc.) as standardized recording forms or checklists by veterinary practitioners to enhance their problem solving abilities with diseases having multiple causes. One approach in developing a clinical instrument would be to develop a list of criteria which would measure deviations from optimal management practices via scoring by reviewing the literature and attempting to obtain a consensus from experts through interview. In addition, although not completely necessary, some analysis such as correlation analysis could be attempted to make sure that their criteria was not only associated with the management practices of the health management area in question but also with the output of those management practices. Reliability of the instrument becomes less of a concern because of being used by individuals in a practice where they can occasionally compare their scores as they already do in the use of other clinical instruments such as body condition scores (Goodger et al., 1988 a; Goodger et al., 1993).

## REFERENCES

*Goodger, W.J., R.Ruppaner, B.D.Slenning, and J.E.Kushman. 1984. An approach to scoring dairy management on large-scale dairies. J. Dairy Sci. 67:675-685.*

*Goodger, W.J., S.Repp, and J.C.Galland. 1988a. Toward developing an instrument for measuring milking management practices. Prev. Vet. Med., 6:109-126.*

*Goodger, W.J., T.Farver, J.Pelletier, P.Johnson, G.De Snayer and J.C.Galland. 1993. The association of milking management practices with bulk tank somatic cell counts. Prev. Vet. Med., 15:235-251.*

*Noordhuizen, J.P.T.M., and H.J.Welpelo. 1996. Sustainable improvement of animal health care by systematic quality risk management according to the HACCP concept. The Vet.Quarterly 18 (4) 121-126.*

# 6.5 MONITORING UDDER HEALTH: CASE STUDIES

Ynte H. Schukken and Theo J.G.M. Lam

Department of Herd Health and Reproduction, School of Veterinary Medicine,University of Utrecht, Yalelaan 7, 3584 CL Utrecht,The Netherlands

## 6.5.1 INTRODUCTION

In part 5 of this Chapter, two case studies will be presented. The first case study deals with a high bulk milk SCC farm, and the second with a farm showing a high incidence of clinical mastitis. In both cases the farmer is not participating in a HH & PM program.

## 6.5.2 CASE STUDY I

### Definition of the complaint

95 cow dairy herd is managed by two brothers. Apart from dairy cows they also have about 500 fattening hogs. The average milk production per cow is + 6200 kg milk, 4.3% fat and 3.5% protein. Cows are housed in a freestall barn. The cows are milked in a 2x6 milking parlor. The herd is in a regular herd health and production management program provided by the local practitioner. The herd obtains monthly DHI information, including individual SCC measurements. Udder health indices are shown in table 1.

The farmers expressed concern about the height of the Bulk Milk SCC. Based on these data, the problem in this herd can be decribed as a high bulk milk SCC.

### Disease history

After questioning the farmers, further information about the high bulk milk SCC problem was obtained. The problem of high bulk milk SCC has been present for a number of years. It has become more pressing due to the lower SCC limits that were

*Table 1. Udder health indices, Herd A*

| Indices | 1993 | 1994 | 1995 |
|---|---|---|---|
| Bulk Milk SCC | 497 | 426 | 350 |
| Incidence Clinical Mastitis | 8% | 14% | 8% |
| Culling due to udder health | 2 (2%) | 4 (4%) | 6 (6%) |

imposed on the industry by European regulations. Since approximately two years the farmers have been subscribing to the individual cow-SCC program. They have noted that a number of cows have been high in their SCC for a longer period of time. So far very few milk samples were collected for bacteriological analysis. There have always been relatively few cases of clinical mastitis.

Milking is done by both farmers. No post-milking teat disinfection is practiced. Dry cow antibiotic treatment is used selectively, most heifers are left untreated. Clinical mastitis is treated with antimicrobials when frequent stripping did not result in cure. Approved products are used for both clinical cases and treatment at dry-off. Milking is in a two times six herringbone parlor with automatic take-off. The milking machine is checked twice a year, and adjustments are made when required.

Record keeping is limited on the farm, monthly records on milk sampling are kept. However, some but certainly not all cases of clinical mastitis are reported in a farm diary. No records are kept on teat lesions, or other udder health disorders. Once in a while a new cow is added to the milking herd. These cows are not checked for udder health or any other disease before entry into the herd.

## INSPECTION

### Data inspection

Analysis of existing SCC data revealed a high prevalence of cows with an SCC above 200.000 cells/ml.: the prevalence ranged between 17% and 45%, and was on average 35%. Incidence of "new infections" ranged from 4% to 31% per milk recording, and was on average 17%. Elimination risk ("cure") ranged between 2% and 36% per milk recording, and was on average 10%. The cow with the highest SCC, contributed in general approximately 8% of all cells in the bulk milk. These data indicate that there was a herd problem. No individual cow caused the high bulk milk SCC by herself, and also the prevalence of cows with an increased cow milk SCC was always high. The incidence of new infections is approximately double of what is acceptable, the elimination risk is low and from the primary indices we learn that few cows are culled for udder health reasons.

### Farm inspection

Environmental assessment of the barn was done. The cows were reasonably clean (± 10% had dirty thighs), and the cubicles were dry and reasonably clean, bedded with rubber mats and some sawdust. Ventilation was sufficient in this barn at the time of the visit. The milking cows were housed in the same barn as the dry cows but separated by a gate. Calving occurred in a separate pen but within the same barn. The calving pen was also used for diseased cows. The milking parlor was dirty at the time of the visit, cleaning of the milking parlor was only done once a day. The milking machine itself was cleaned twice a day, using an automated washing program. Evaluation sheets of the milking machine were present in the milk house, and indicated no major problems.

The general hygiene level on the farm was substandard. Quality of the haysilage and cornsilage was acceptable, but not excellent.

### Clinical inspection

Inspection of the milking cows showed that they were reasonably clean, approximately 10% had dirty thighs. Body condition of the cows appeared to be somewhat below standard, some fresh cows went down to a score of 1.0. Clinical evaluation of the teats and the udder revealed that a number of cows had rather severe teat-end eversion. A number of cows also showed the presence of small flakes when the milk was checked. These quarters always showed a positive T-pol test (3+). Few cows showed teat lesions.

The dry cows were more dirty than the milking cows. The udders had dried-up nicely, and no teat-end eversions were seen in the dry cows. Body condition score of the dry cows was high (4 - 5). The general body condition of the milking cows appeared to be good.

### Differential cause list

Based on the analysis of data, and the evaluation of clinical, farm, and management data the cause of the problem is likely infection in a large proportion of the herd by a contagious microorganism. The microorganisms most probably involved are:

1. *S.aureus*
2. *S.agalactiae*

### Additional investigation

It was decided to culture all cows, observe the milking process, and evaluate milking machine performance during milking ("wet test"). All teats of all cows were scored with regard to teat-end eversions, and teat lesions. The formal scoring procedure presented in part 4 of this book will be performed.

The results from the bacteriological analysis showed that about 30% of the cows

*Table 2. Results of bacteriological analysis, Herd A (Sa = S.aureus)*

| | Days in Milk | | | | | | Parity | | | | | |
|---|---|---|---|---|---|---|---|---|---|---|---|---|
| SCC | 0 - 100 | | 100 - 200 | | > 200 | | 1 | | 2 | | > 2 | |
| | n | Sa | n | Sa | n | Sa | n | Sa | n | Sa | n | Sa |
| < 200 | 18 | 1 | 23 | 4 | 20 | 6 | 14 | 1 | 14 | 2 | 33 | 8 |
| 200 - 500 | 4 | 1 | 5 | 2 | 3 | 3 | 2 | 1 | 1 | 0 | 9 | 5 |
| > 500 | 2 | 2 | 5 | 4 | 3 | 2 | 0 | 0 | 3 | 2 | 7 | 6 |

*Table 3. Teat-end evaluation*

| Score | Performance | Goal |
|---|---|---|
| 0 | 30.6% | > 60% |
| A | 23.5 % | < 20% |
| B | 16.6 % | < 10% |
| C | 15.2 % | < 5% |
| D | 14.1 % | < 5% |
| Trauma | 5.2% | < 5% |

was infected in at least one quarter with *S. aureus*. There was no evidence of infection with *S. agalactiae* in the herd. The results of the bacteriological sampling are summarized in Table 2.

Observation of the milking process revealed that the cows were prepared for milking with a dry paper towel. About 6 cows were prepared with the same towel before units were attached. Units were attached according to standards, and in about 5% of cases some squaking was observed. The milking was rather unorganised, and the time between preparation of the udder, and attachment of the unit was considerably different between cows. Units were removed automatically. The cows were milked out rather well. The wet test revealed that milking vacuum was unstable, and showed large drops when one of the clusters dropped (this occurred 5 times during the milking). Vacuum below the teat was relatively high (46 Kpa) and dropped dramatically in high producing cows (to 30 Kpa).

*Table 4. Scoring udder health management on the farm*

| Category | Score | % of maximum |
|---|---|---|
| General sanitation practice | 17 | 21% |
| Milking equipment maintenance | 50 | 63% |
| Adequate milking system | 44 | 55% |
| Condition of cows | 40 | 50% |
| Efficient traffic flow | 17 | 28% |
| Milker performance | 46 | 58% |
| Pre-milking procedures | 43 | 54% |
| Milking procedures | 45 | 56% |
| Post-milking procedures | 10 | 17% |
| Mastitis treatment | 65 | 81% |
| Mastitis control | 31 | 39% |
| Records use | 25 | 31% |

Teat ends were in fairly poor condition with a large number of teat end eversions. The scoring of the teat-ends is presented in table 3.

The results of the scoring procedure of udder health management is presented in table 4.

This score indicates a general sub-optimal udder health management. Specific areas of concern are general sanitation practice, traffic flow, post-milking procedures and records use.

**Evaluation and synthesis of information**

The results in table 2 indicate that *S.aureus* is the main cause of intramammary infection in this herd. Infection prevalence is specifically high in older cows and cows later in lactation. This pattern is seen often when between cow infections are the main source of infection. The longer a cow is in the milking herd, the greater the probability of infection. Infection of quarters with *S.aureus* occurs specifically during milking and appears to follow the equation:

$$\text{Number of new infections} = \beta * N_{Susceptible} * N_{Infectious}$$

Where ß is a transmission parameter that depends on the microorganism involved and management procedures in the herd (Lam et al., 1996). Management procedures that have an effect on this transmission parameter are post-milk teat disinfection, efficient traffic flow of infected cows, vacuum stability, use of single towels etc. Another important component in the above equation is the number of infectious quarters in the herd($N_{Infectious}$). Culling of infected cows, treatment of infected cows during lactation or the dry-period, and finally complete separation of infected cows will lead to a reduction of the number of infectious cows, and thereby to a reduction in the number of new infections. The number of susceptible quarters ($N_{Susceptible}$) should be as high as possible. Without adequate reduction of the transmission parameter, a large number of susceptible quarters leads to a high number of new infections. This will occur when cows are culled, and replaced by clean cows without sufficient changes in management procedures.

The data inspection indicated a high proportion of new infections, indicating that either the transmission parameter or the number of infectious cows or both are too high. From the bacteriological sampling data we concluded that the number of infectious quarters is relatively high. The scoring system (Table 4) indicated that udder health management is weak on a number of points. The main issues appear to be general sanitation, traffic flow of infected animals, and post-milking procedures. These four factors are essential with regard to transmission of infection from one quarter to another, and the proportion of infected quarters in the herd.

Scoring of the teat-end revealed a relative high proportion of cows rather severe eversions (29.3% in category C and D). There are several possible causes for this problem. The vacuum level in the milking machine is high, and vacuum fluctuation is also high. This may lead to a high compressive load on the teat-end. A high compressive load increases the probability of teat-end eversion (Bramley et al., 1992). Another possibility is a relative late take-off of the clusters. In this farm the cows were milked out well, however, overmilking may lead to teat-end eversion.

### List of causes

The problem in this herd is a high BMSCC. The main cause of this is a high prevalence and infection risk of *S.aureus*. Additional causes are low general sanitation, absence of traffic flow with regard to infected cows, no post-milking teat disinfection, and little use of udder health records. Additionally, milking machine function apparently leads to teat canal eversion. Hence overmilking, vacuum height and liner design need careful review.

### Recommendations and intervention

Using this information, a preventive udder health program aimed at reduction of new infections, decrease of the number of infectious cows, and adequate monitoring was advised. this program consisted of the following components:

1. start post-milking teat dip with a registered (iodine) dip,
2. use individual paper towels,
3. have milking equipment checked and adjusted,
4. identify and milk *S.aureus* infected cows last,
5. diagnose and promptly treat clinical mastitis,
6. cull chronic infected *S.aureus* cows (list was made),
7. treat all cows at dry off (list provided for specific treatment of *S.aureus* infected cows),
8. monitor teat-end quality,
9. start an accurate record keeping program with regard to udder health.

### Follow-up

After about 8 months the results were evaluated. The BMSCC figures showed initially a slight drop, but this was followed by an increase later. When the data of the herd was split into two cohorts based on the *S.aureus* status at the time of sampling, it was observed that the mean SCC decreased rapidly in the infected group, but increased equally rapid in the initially uninfected group (Figure 1). Further investigation revealed that the recommendations regarding culling and early dry treatment were followed promptly (resulting in a drop in mean SCC in the initially infected cows). However, the recommendations regarding post milking teat dip, individual towels and separate milking were not implemented, resulting in a high infection rate in the initially clean cows.

This herd clearly illustrates the importance of the basic reproduction rate ($R_0$) principle. When the number of new infections per existing infection is not reduced below

*Figure 1. Mean SCC in cohorts that were initially infected, resp. uninfected with S.aureus*

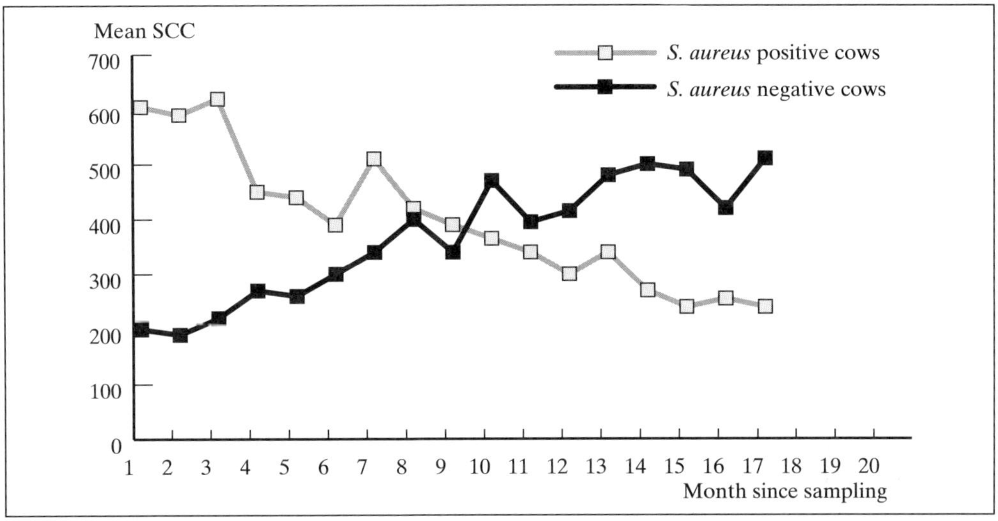


1.0, no effect may be expected from a prevention program. Culling and drying off of infected cows will only temporarily alleviate the problem. The key in reducing *S.aureus* prevalence is reducing transmission of *S.aureus* from an infected quarter to uninfected quarters.

### 6.5.3 CASE STUDY II

**Definition of complaint**

This is a 95 cow dairy farm, managed by the owner and a herdsman. In addition to dairy farming, they are also in the business of cash cropping. The farm is among the top producers in the area. The rolling herd average is 10,300 kg milk with 4.4% fat and 3.5% protein. The average Bulk milk somatic cell count averages approximately 150,000 and is always below 250,000. Culling in this herd is high mainly due to sales for breeding purposes. The incidence of clinical mastitis was 45% in the last 12 months. The farmer complains about a clinical mastitis problem, he also notes that sometimes germ counts are also high. The primary udder health indices during the last two years are shown in Table 5.

*Table 5. Udder health indices for herd B*

| Indices | 1993 | 1994 | 1995 |
|---|---|---|---|
| Bulk Milk SCC | 165 | 221 | 165 |
| Incidence Clinical Mastitis | 43% | 39% | 73% |
| Culling due to udder health | 6(6%) | 7(7%) | 4(4%) |

The problem on this farm can be defined as a clinical mastitis problem. No problem exists with regard to bulk milk SCC or culling due to udder health.

### Disease history

After questioning the farmer, further information about the clinical mastitis problem was obtained. The problem with the high incidence of clinical mastitis has been present for a number of years. The problem appears to increase as the average milk production per cow increases. Clinical mastitis cases tend to be rather severe. Clinical cases are promptly treated with antibiotics and anti-inflammatory agents. Frequent milking is practised in mastitic cows. Cases appear to occur throughout the year. Sampling for bacteriological analysis is standard.

Milking is three times a day in a 2 x 8 milking parlor. The cows are prepared with individual dry towels. Only when udders are dirty, water is used. The units are attached immediately after preparation. Clusters are removed by automatic take-off. All quarters are sprayed with chlorhexidine before and after milking. Milking is done by several milkers. All cows are dried-off abruptly, and treated with an approved antibiotic.

Approximately three years ago the milking machine was renewed, and partially replaced. No improvements have been observed after replacement of the milking machine. The milking machine is evaluated twice a year.

*Table 6. Herd B clinical mastitis report*

| | Months | | | | | | | | | | | |
|---|---|---|---|---|---|---|---|---|---|---|---|---|
| | **1** | **2** | **3** | **4** | **5** | **6** | **7** | **8** | **9** | **10** | **11** | **12** |
| # Calvings | 8 | 2 | 8 | 6 | 7 | 10 | 10 | 15 | 11 | 7 | 6 | 12 |
| # clinical mastitis cases | 1 | 2 | 1 | 6 | 8 | 8 | 8 | 9 | 7 | 6 | 6 | 3 |
| # culls due to mastitis | 0 | 0 | 1 | 0 | 1 | 0 | 1 | 1 | 0 | 0 | 0 | 0 |

*Table 7. Clinical mastitis per stage of lacation*

| Stage of lactation | # cases |
|---|---|
| 0 - 30 | 19 |
| 31 - 60 | 6 |
| 61 - 120 | 10 |
| 121 - 180 | 22 |
| 181 - 240 | 6 |
| 241 - 300 | 2 |
| > 300 | 0 |

*Figure 2. Microorganisms observed in samples from clinical cases in herd B*

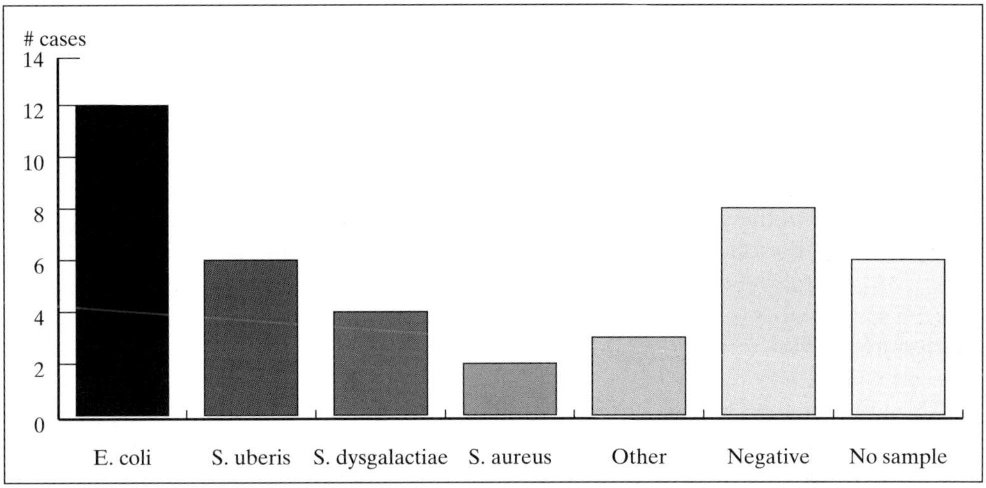


## INSPECTIONS

### Data inspection

Analysis of individual cow SCC showed that approximately 5% of the cows had a prevalence of SCC above 200.000 cells/ml., the incidence of "new infections" was always below 10%, and the elimination risk was always greater than 30%. Records on clinical mastitis are kept accurately. From almost all clinical cases, pretreatment samples are collected for bacteriological culture. The results of the cultures are shown in Figure 2. Clinical cases occur predominantly in cows in their second and higher lactation. There is a tendency towards a higher incidence in the summer months, as shown in the clinical mastitis report monthly list (Table 6). When the clinical cases are tabulated per stage of lactation, a first peak around calving, and a second peak at approximately 150 days in lactation is present (Table 7).

A relative high germ count is present, ranging from 5,000 to 45,000 with an average of 20,000 cfu/ml.

### Farm inspection

The herd is housed year round in a free stall. Grass is mowed daily, and fed inside the barn (zero-grazing). The barn is slightly overcrowded: 70 cubicles and 50 feeding places for 90 milking cows. Ventilation is natural. At the time of the visit the temperature in the barn was high (27°C) and ventilation was not sufficient. An environmental survey revealed that most cows were clean. The udders are clipped and generally clean at entrance in the milking parlor. The cubicles have a concrete floor and are bedded with chopped straw. Cubicles are not dry. The size of the cubicles is relatively small compared to the size of the cows. The farmer and herdsman are very conscious about general hygiene. Calving pens are cleaned after every calving. Diseased cows are housed in cubicles separate from the calving area.

The milking parlor is clean and well lighted. The parlor design is a two by eight herringbone with automatic take-off. Milk weights and milk temperature are measured on a daily basis. Recording of milk weights occurs in a weigh jar. When this jar was opened a large amount of black grease was present inside the jar. Automatic gates to lead the cows in and out of the parlor are used. These gates make use of the milking vacuum.

General sanitation on the farm is high. Quality of forage and concentrates is excellent.

### Clinical inspection

The milking cows in this herd are well fed. Frequent feed changes are practiced, and fresh cows are only offered fresh clean food. The cows are in good body condition relative to stage of lactation. Drop in body condition during early lactation is relatively small given the high production. Body condition score is measured every three weeks. At the time of the visit two cows with clinical mastitis were present. They were housed and milked seperately. Treatment was adequate, and these cows appeared to recover well. A number of cows was evaluated with regard to teat-end quality. A number of severe eversions were observed, also petechial hemorrhages and some chapped teats were present.

The dry cows were housed in a seperate barn, and have no contact with the milking cows. Body condition in dry cows averages at 3.5 to 4. The dry cows are clean, and teat-end quality in the dry cows was good.

*Table 8. Scoring udder health management on the farm*

| Category | Score | % of maximum |
|---|---|---|
| General sanitation practice | 55 | 69% |
| Milking equipment maintenance | 55 | 69% |
| Adequate milking system | 65 | 81% |
| Condition of cows | 32 | 40% |
| Efficient traffic flow | 51 | 85% |
| Milker performance | 65 | 81% |
| Pre-milking procedures | 74 | 93% |
| Milking procedures | 65 | 81% |
| Post-milking procedures | 55 | 92% |
| Mastitis treatment | 75 | 94% |
| Mastitis control | 72 | 90% |
| Records used | 70 | 88% |

*Table 9. Teat-end evaluation. See Figure 2 in part 2 for scoring system*

| Score | Performance | Goal |
|---|---|---|
| 0 | 15% | >60% |
| A | 25% | <20% |
| B | 35% | <10% |
| C | 15% | <5% |
| D | 10% | <5% |
| Trauma | 9% | <5% |

## Differential cause list

The results of the data, farms and clinical inspection reveals a high incidence of clinical mastitis, due to environmental microorganisms. Likely the environment of the cows contributes to this problem. Possible causes for the high incidence of clinical mastitis are a high incidence of teat lesions, sanitation of the cubicles, poor ventilation in the barn, shortage of cubicles, and possibly other aspects of housing and management.

*Figure 3. Teat-end keratinisation in a cow in herd B, photograph is taken shortly after milking (courtesy Research station for Cattle, Sheep and Horses, Lelystad, the Netherlands)*

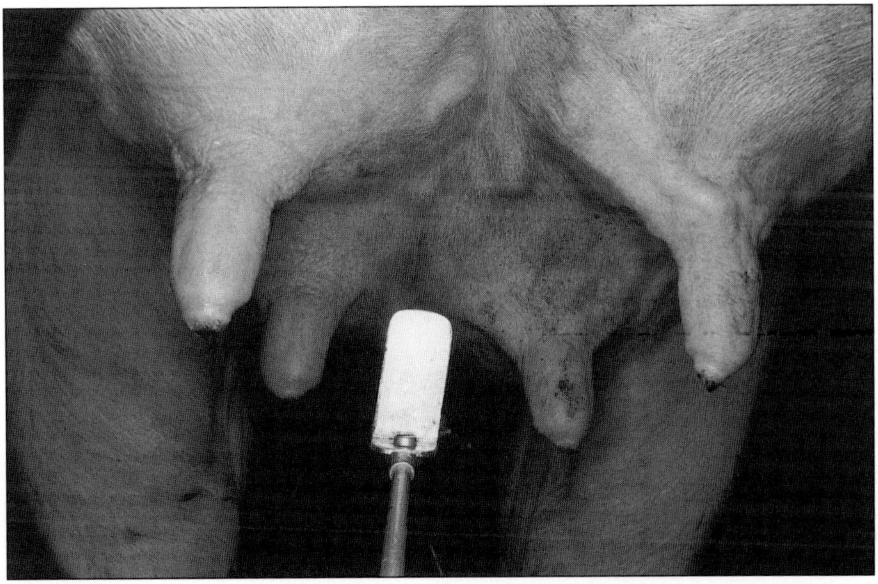

## Additional investigations

A formal evaluation of udder health management was performed. Teat-end condition was scored, and the milking machine was tested during milking ("wet test").

The results of the scoring procedure of udder health management is presented in Table 8.

Udder health management on this farm is relatively good. Most categories score high. The only exception is the category on condition of cows. Aspects of management that cause the low score in this category are the presence of teat lesions and teat-end eversions, the relative small stalls compared to the size of the cows, and the inadequate ventilation in the barn.

Teats are in rather bad condition, and more than 25% of teat-ends showed evidence of severe eversion (Table 9). Teat end quality was monitored longitudinally, and appeared to detoriate. Teat lesions due to trauma were present with a relative high prevalence (9%). No incidence data are present with regard to teat trauma.

The cows are not completely milked out, and teat ends are edemic and painfull after milking. Some of the teats are depicted in Figure 3.

The performance of the milking machine was evaluated during milking. Stray voltage was suspected and researched but was not observed. During the wet-testing it was observed that after milking during the washing procedure, some of the units were only sporadically washed. Sampling of the affected clusters revealed a high coliform count in the inflations at the start of every milking.

## Evaluation and synthesis of information

In this herd no single problem appears to be responsible for the high incidence of clinical mastitis caused by environmental microorganisms. Factors that are possibly contributing to the high incidence of clinical mastitis are: high level of milk production, the environment of the cow, failing of the washing system, and the teat-end eversion. These factors have been reported before as risk factors for clinical mastitis (see part 3).

In this herd there is a definite goal for maximum milk production per cow per year, consequently milk production level is not easily changed to prevent clinical cases of mastitis. Mechanisms behind higher risk for clinical mastitis in high producing cows are a negative genetic correlation between udder health and milk production, an increased risk for negative energy balance, possibly leading to a decrease in immune function, a higher risk of leaking milk, and thereby increasing the risk of infection. Factors in the environment certainly affect the incidence of clinical mastitis. Coliform count in the bedding will be higher in badly ventilated barns. Also small cubicles may increase the risk of trauma to the teat and/or udder. Teat-end eversions have been associated with a high compressive load on the teat end. Factors involved in a high compressive load are milking vacuum, design and flexibility of the liner, the number of cycles, the milking ratio, and a number of cow factors.

There is no evidence in this herd for contagious mastitis problems. Somatic cell counts are continuously low, and almost all cases of clinical mastitis are caused by either coliforms or environmental streptococci. Apparently, management on this farm is such that there is very little opportunity for microorganisms to spread between cows. This may even lead to a very low prevalence of minor pathogens, although no data were collected in this herd to substantiate that. A low prevalence of minor pathogens may lead to an increased susceptibility for infections with environmental pathogens.

### Final list of causes

Based on these further data, the clinical mastitis problem may be partly caused by the environmental problems in the herd, and relative bad teat-end condition. Also, the high coliform load in some of the clusters may increase the risk of coliform infection. The prevalence of teat trauma appeared to be high and is likely associated with a number of cases of clinical mastitis.

### Recommendations and interventions

It was advised to repair the washing problems of the milking machine. Liners and vacuum level should be adjusted such that teat-end condition improves. It may be advisable to work on the cubicle design to prevent teat lesions, and to increase ventilation in the barn. Washing and cleaning procedures of the milking machine should be adjusted to allow a better cleaning of all clusters. Finally, an advice with regard to housing of the cows was given. The present barn should be remodelled or replaced by a barn that is more suitable to house the larger number of cows. More suitable also refers to ventilation and cubicle size.

### Follow-up

Vacuum level was decreased, and a number of liners were tried, after some experimentation, the teat end condition improved. Several attempts were undertaken to increase hygiene in the cubicles. An outside exercise yard did not result in a drop of clinical mastitis. Mechanical ventilation was installed. After these changes, the incidence of clinical mastitis dropped somewhat. The incidence of clinical cases levelled off at about 30%. Searching continues to further decrease incidence of clinical cases. Adjustments to the cleaning process of the milking machine resulted in a rapid drop in germ count to an average of 5,000 cfu/ml.

This herd illustrates the lack of generality in problems that are present in these high incidence herds. No blanket advice can be given. Only a continuous effort to search for possible problems may eventually result in identifying the source.

## EPILOGUE

The two case studies presented here are two examples of farm-level udder health problems. Both cases are not easy to solve and require in-depth knowledge of the biology of mastitis and management of dairy herds. In the case of the high BMSCC problems a fairly standard protocol will often lead to an alleviation of the problem. However, as shown in the present study, the participation of the farmer is essential to obtain a long term solution. In contrast, high clinical mastitis problems require an in depth analysis and often non-standard solutions. Longitudinal follow-up of herds in a complete HH & PM program is a prerequisite to diagnose and solve these problems.

## REFERENCES

*Agger, J.F. and P. Willeberg. 1986. Epidemiology of teat lesions in a dairy herd, II. asso ciations with subclinical mastitis. Nord. Vet. Med. 38:220-231.*

*Anderson, R.M., 1991. Populations and infectious diseases: Ecology or Epidemiology. J.Animal Ecology. 60:1-50.*

*Bartlett, P.C., J.B. Kaneene, J.H. Kirk, M.A. Wilke, and J.V. Martenuik. 1986. Development of a computerized dairy herd health data base for epidemiologic research. Prev. Vet. Med. 4:3-14.*

*Bartlett, P.C, J. van Wijk, and D.J Wilson. 1991. Temporal patterns of lost milk production following clinical mastitis in a large Michigan Holstein herd. J.Dairy Sci. 74:1561-1568.*

*Becker, N.G. 1989. Analysis of infectious disease data. Chapman and Hall, London.*

*Bendixen, P.H. 1988. Risk indicators of disease occurrence in dairy cows in Sweden. PhD. thesis, Swedish university of Agricultural Sciences, Skara.*

*Boddie, R.L. and S.C. Nickerson. 1986. Dry cow therapy: effects of method of drug administration on occurrence of intramammary infection. J.Dairy Sci. 69:253-257.*

*Boyne, R. and J.R. Arthur. 1979. Alterations of neutrophil function in selenium deficient cattle. J.Comp. Path. 89:151-153.*

*Bramley, A.J. and F.K. Neave. 1975. Studies in the control of coliform mastitis in dairy cows. Br. Vet. J. 131:160-169.*

*Bramley, A.J., F.H. Dodd, G.A. Main, and J. A. Bramley. 1992. Machine milking and lac tation. Insight books, Vermont, USA.*

*Colditz, I.G. and D.L. Watson. 1985. The immunophysiological basis for vaccinating ruminants against mastitis. Aust. Vet. J. 62:145-165.*

*Conrad, H.R. and K.L. Smith. 1986. Selenium and Vitamin E in bovine mastitis. Page 43 in Proc. Symp. Mastitis Control Hyg. Production Milk. Espoo, Finland.*

*Curtis, C.R., H.N. Erb, C.J. Sniffen, R.D. Smith, and D.S. Kronfeld. 1985. Path analysis of dry period nutrition, postpartum metabolic and reproductive disorders, and mastitis in Holstein cows. J.Dairy Sci. 68:2347-2353.*

*Doane, R.M., S.P. Oliver, R.D. Walker, and E.P. Shull. 1987. Experimental infection of lactating bovine mammary glands with streptococcus uberis in quarters colonized by corynebacterium bovis. Am. J.Vet. Res. 48:749-751.*

*Dodd, F.H., T.M. Higgs, and A.J. Bramley. 1984. Cubicle management and coliform mastitis. Vet. Rec. 114:522-525.*

*Dohoo, I.R., S.W. Martin, and W.C.D. Sandals. 1983. Disease production and culling in Holstein-Frisian cows I. The data. Prev. Vet. Med. 1:321-334.*

*Dohoo, I.R. and S.W. Martin. 1984. Disease, production and culling in Holstein-Frisian cows, III. Disease and production as determinants of disease. Prev. Vet. Med. 2:671-681.*

*Dohoo, I.R., and K.E. Leslie. 1991. Evaluation of changes in somatic cell counts as indi cators of new intramammary infections. Prev. Vet. Med. 10:225-237.*

*Dohoo, I.R., and R.S. Morris. 1993. Somatic cell count patterns in Prince Edward Island dairy herds. Prev. Vet. Med. 15:53-65.*

*Dijkhuizen, A.A. 1977. Economic aspects of disease and disease eradication, with special regards to mastitis (in Dutch). Page 87 in Publication 2, Department of Agricultural Economics, College of Veterinary Medicine.*

*Eberhart, R.J. 1986. Management of the dry cow to reduce mastitis. J.Dairy Science 69:1721-1732.*

*Emanuelsson, U., B. Danell, and J. Philipsson, 1988. Genetic parameters for clinical mastitis, Somatic Cell Counts, and milk production estimated by multiple trait restricted maximum likelihood. J.Dairy Sci. 71:467-476.*

*Erb, H.N., R.D. Smith, P.A. Oltenacu, C.L. Guard, R.B. Hillman, P.A. Powers, M.C. Smith, and M.E. White. 1985. Path model of reproductive disorders and performance, milk fever, mastitis, milk yield and culling in Holstein cows. J.Dairy Sci. 68:3337-3347.*

*Erskine, R.J., R.J. Eberhart, L.J. Hutchinson, S.B. Spencer, and M.A. Campbell. 1988. Incidence and types of clinical mastitis in dairy herds with high and low somatic cell counts. J.A.V.M.A. 192:761-762.*

*Erskine, R.J., and R.J. Eberhart. 1990. Herd benefit to cost ratio and effects of bovine mastitis control program that include blitz treatment of S.agalactiae. J.A.V.M.A. 196:1230-1235.*

*Fetrow, J., and K. Anderson. 1987. The economics of mastitis control. Comp. Cont. Educ. Pract. Vet. 9:f103-f112.*

*Fetrow, J. 1988. Culling in Dairy Cows. Proc. Am. Assoc. Bov. Practitioner, 102-107.*

*Gershwin, M.E., R.S. Beach, and L.S. Hurley. 1985. Nutrition and disease. Academic press inc., New York, NY.*

*Gonzalez, R.N., J.S. Cullor, D.E. Jasper, T.B. Farver, R.B. Gushnell, and M.N. Oliver. 1989. Prevention of coliform mastitis in dairy cows by a mutant Escherichia coli vaccine. Can. J. Vet. Res. 53:301-306.*

*Goodger, W.J., S. Repp, and J.C. Galland. 1984. An approach to scoring dairy manage ment on large scale dairies. J.Dairy Sci 67:675-685.*

*Goodger, W.J., S. Repp, and J.C. Galland. 1988. Toward developing an instrument for measuring milking management practices. Prev. Vet. Med. 6:109-126.*

*Goodger, W.J., T. Farver, J. Pelletier, P. Johnson, G. DeSnayer, and J. Galland. 1993. The association of milking management practices with bulk tank somatic cell counts. Prev. Vet. Med. 15:235-251.*

*Grommers, F.J., E.A. vandeBraak, and H.W. Antonisse. 1971. Direct trauma of the mam mary glands in dairy cattle. Br. Vet. J. 127:271-281.*

*Gunnink, J.W. 1984. Retained placenta and leukocyte activity. Vet. Quart. 6:49-54.*

*Hamann, J., C. Burvenich, M. Mayntz, O. Osteras, and W. Halder. 1994. Macine induced changes in the status of the bovine teat with respect to the new infection risk. Bulletin of the IDF 297:13-22.*

*Heyneman, R., G. Vandeputte-Vanmessom, and C. Burvenich. 1988. Possible correlation between severity of experimentally induced E.coli mastitis and characteristics of peripheral leukocytes. Arch. Int. Pharmacodyn. Ther. 291:298-302.*

*Hoblet, K.H., J.S. Bailey, and D.E. Pritchard. 1988. Coagulase positive staphylococcal mastitis in a herd with low somatic cell counts. J.A.V.M.A. 192:777-778.*

*Hogan, J.S., K.L. Smith, K.H. Hoblet, P.S. Schoenberger, D.A. Todhunter, W.D. Hueston, D.E. Pritchard, G.L. Bowman, L.E. Heider, B.L. Brockett, and H.R. Conrad. 1989. Field survey of clinical mastitis in low somatic cell count herds. J.Dairy Sci. 72:1547-1559.*

*Hogan J.S., K.L. Smith, D.A. Todhunter, and P.S. Schoenberger, 1992. Field trial to deter mine efficacy of an E.coli J5 mastitis vaccin. J.Dairy Sci. 75:78-84.*

*Kehrli, M.E., B.J. Nonnecke, and J.A. Roth. 1989. Alterations in bovine neutrophil func tion during the periparturient period. Am J. Vet. Res. 50:207-211.*

*Kremer, W.D.J., Burvenich, C., Noordhuizen-Stassen, E.N., Grommers, F.J., Schukken, Y.H., Heeringa, R., and Brand, A. 1993. Severity of experimental E.coli mastitis in ketonemic and non-ketonemic dairy cows. J.Dairy Sci. 76:3428-3436.*

*Lam, T.J.G.M., 1996. Dynamics of bovine mastitis, a field study in low somatic cell count herds. Ph.D. thesis, Utrecht University.*

*Lam, T.J.G.M., DeJong, M.C.M., Schukken, Y.H., and A. Brand. 1996. Mathematical modeling to estimate efficacy of postmilking teat disinfection in split udder trials of dairy cows. J.Dairy Sci. 79:62-70.*

*Leslie, K.E., 1994. Mastitis control in dairy herds. In: Herd Health, 2nd edition, eds: Radostitis, O.M., Leslie, K.E., and Fetrow, J.,*

*Linde, C. 1982. The effect of coagulase-negative staphylococci in the cow's udder on experimental induction of mastitis and on milk production. PhD. thesis. University of Agricultural Sciences, Uppsala.*

*Lohuis, J.A.C.M., Y.H. Schukken, P.A.J. Henricks, R. Heyneman, C. Burvenich, J.H.M. Verheijden, A.S.J.P.A.M. van Miert, and A. Brand. 1990. Preinfection functions of blood polymorphonuclear leukocytes and the outcome of experimental Escherichia coli mastitis in the cow. J.Dairy Sci. 73:342-350.*

*Natzke, R.P. 1981. Elements of mastitis control. J.Dairy Sci. 64:1431-1438.*

*Newbould, F.H.S. 1976. Phagocytic activity of bovine leukocytes during pregnancy. Can. J. Comp. Med. 40:111-115.*

*Nickerson, S.C., P.A. Baker, and P. Trinidad. 1989. Local immunostimulation of the bovine mammary gland with interleukin-2. J.Dairy Sci. 72:1764-1769.*

*Nielen,M., H. DeLuyker, Y.H. Schukken and A. Brand. 1992. Electrical conductivity of milk: Measurement, Modifiers and Meta analysis of Mastitis detection performance. J.Dairy Sci 75:606-614.*

*Noordhuizen, J.P.T.M., and Welpelo. 1996. Sustainable improvement of animal health care by systematic quality risk management according to HACCP concept. The Vet. Quart 18(4) 121-126.*

*Nordhaug, M.L., L.L. Nesse, N.L. Norcross, and R. Gudding. 1994. A field trial with an experimental vaccine against Staphylococcus aureus mastitis in cattle. J.Dairy Sci. 77:1267-1284*

*Oliver, S.P. and K.L. Smith. 1982. Milk yield and secretion composition following intra mammary infusion of colchicine. J.Dairy Sci. 65:204-214.*

*Oliver, S.P. and L.M. Sordillo. 1989. Approaches to the manipulation of mammary invo lution. J.Dairy Sci. 72:1647-1657.*

*Paape, M.J., G. Ziv, and W.D. Schultze. 1988. Evaluation of polyethylene intramammary device in mastitis control. Isr. J.Vet. Med. 44:74-78.*

*Philpot, W.N., and S.C. Nickerson. 1991. Mastitis: Counter Attack. Babson Bros. Co. Naperville, Ill.*

*Reneau, J. 1986. Effective use of Dairy Herd Improvement Somatic Cell Count in Mastitis control. J. Dairy Sci. 69:1708-1720.*

*Robinson, T.C., E.R. Jackson, and A. Marr. 1988. Mastitis incidence in quarters with dif ferent infection status at drying off and calving in two,, treatment groups. Br. Vet. J.144:166-168.*

*Sandholm, M., Honkanen-buzalski, T., Kaartinen, L., and S. Pyorala. 1995. The bovine udder and mastitis. University of Helsinki, Helsinki.*

*Schukken, Y.H., H.N. Erb, and R.D. Smith. 1988. The relationship between mastitis and retained placenta in a commercial population of Holstein dairy cows. Prev. Vet. Med. 5:181-188.*

*Schukken, Y.H., F.J. Grommers, D. vandeGeer, and A. Brand. 1989. Incidence of clinical mastitis on farms with low somatic cell counts in bulk milk. Vet. Rec. 125:60-64.*

*Schukken, Y.H., G. Casella, and J. van den Broek, 1991. Overdispersion in clinical masti tis data from dairy herds: a negative binomial approach. Prev. Vet. Med. 10:239-245.*

*Schukken, Y.H., F.J. Grommers, D. vandeGeer, H.N. Erb, and A. Brand. 1991. Risk fac tors for clinical mastitis in herds with a low bulk milk somatic cell count, I. the data and risk factors for all cases. J.Dairy Sci. 74:1123-1129.*

*Schukken, Y.H. K.E. Leslie, A.J. Weersink, and S.W. Martin. 1992. Impact of reducing somatic cell count regulatory limits on milk quality and milk safety. Proc. 31st Nat. Mast. Counc. meeting, 63-72. Arlington, VA.*

*Schukken, Y.H., J. VanVliet, D. VandeGeer, and F.J. Grommers. 1993. A randomized blind trial on dry cow antibiotic infusion in a low somatic cell count herd. J.Dairy Sci. 76:2925-2931.*

*Sears, P.M., Smith, B.S., English, P.B., Herer, P.S., and R.N. Gonzalez. 1990. Shedding pattern of S.aureus from bovine intramammary infections. J. Dairy Sci. 73:2785-2789.*

*Shook, G.E., 1982. Approaches to summarizing somatic cell counts which improve interpretability. Page 150 in Proc. 21st Ann Meeting Nat. Mast Council. Arlington, VA.*

*Shook, G.E. 1989. Selection for disease resistance. J. Dairy Sci. 72:1349-1359.*

*Smith, K.L., D.A. Todhunter, and P.S. Schoenberger. 1985. Environmental mastitis: cau se, prevalence, prevention. J. Dairy Sci. 68:1531-1553.*

*Sol, J., O.C. Sampimon, J.J. Snoep, and Y.H. Schukken. 1994. Factors associated with bacteriological cure after dry cow treatment of subclinical mastitis with antibiotics. J. Dairy Sci 77:75-79.*

*Spencer, S. 1995. What happens inside and outside the teat. Page 41 in: Proc. NMC regional meeting, Harrisburg, PA.*

*Thurmond, M.C. 1993. Epidemiological methods in mastitis treatment and control. Vet. Clinics N. Am. 939-947.*

*Tyler, J.W., M.C Thurmond, and L. Lasslo. 1989. Relationship between test-day measure ments of somatic cell count and milk production in California dairy herds. Can. J. Vet. Res. 53:182-187.*

*VandeGeer, D., Y.H. Schukken, F.J. Grommers, and A. Brand. 1988. A matched case-control study on severe clinical mastitis. Page 60 in Proc. 6th Int. Conf. Animal Hygiene, Skara, Sweden.*

*Watson, D.L. 1988. Vaccination against experimental staphylococcal mastitis in ewes. Res. Vet. Sci. 45:16-27.*

*Wilesmith, J.W., P.G. Frances, and C.D. Wilson. 1986. Incidence of clinical mastitis in a cohort of British dairy herds. Vet. Rec. 118:199-204.*

*Wilson, D.J., Gonzalez, R.N., and P.M. Sears. 1995. Segregation or use of separate mil king units for cows infected with S.aureus: effects on prevalence of infection and bulk tank somatic cell count. J. Dairy Sci 78:2083-2085.*

# MONITORING FOOT HEALTH

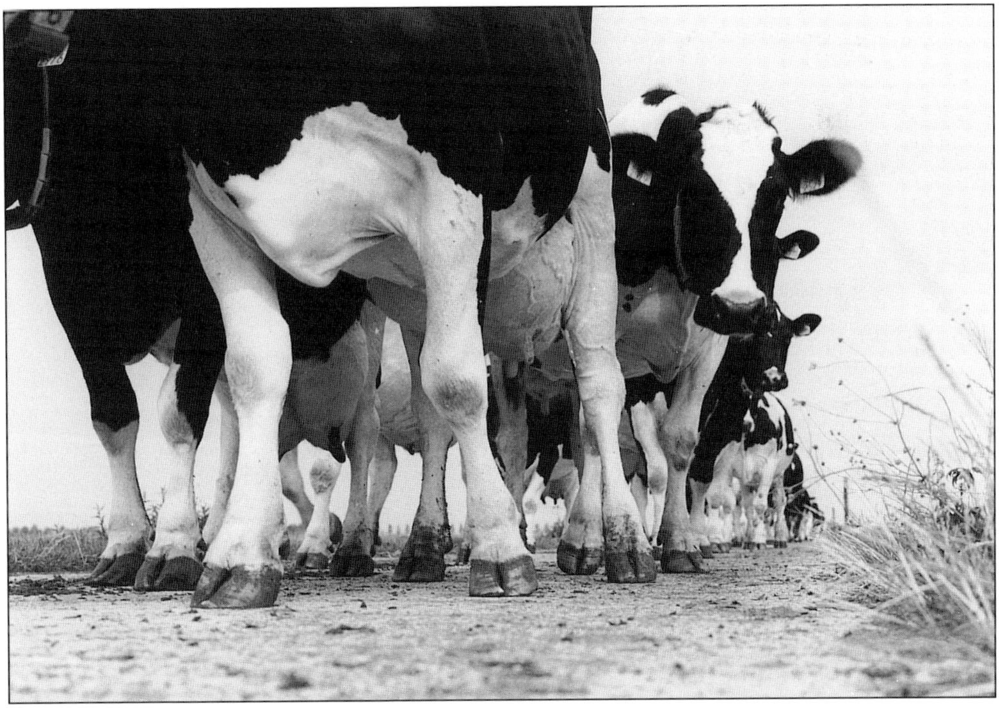

# 7.1 MONITORING FOOT HEALTH: OBJECTIVES, MATERIALS AND METHODS

Jos P.T.M. Noordhuizen[1], Elsbeth N. Noordhuizen-Stassen[2], Klaas Frankena[1], and Alberto Brizzi[3]

[1] Department of Animal Husbandry, Wageningen Institute of Animal Science, Wageningen Agricultural University, Marijkeweg 40, P.O. Box 338, 6700 AH Wageningen, The Netherlands
[2] Department of Herd Health and Reproduction, School of Veterinary Medicine, University of Utrecht, Yalelaan 7, 3584 CL Utrecht, The Netherlands
[3] Large Animal Practice, Via Gorizia, 16, 43100 Parma, Italy

## 7.1.1 INTRODUCTION

Sound feet and legs are of paramount importance to the cow for optimal productivity, and animal welfare, and for coping with day-to-day farming conditions and procedures. Regardless of the farming system, lameness can be a costly problem in a dairy herd (Greenough et al., 1981). The direct costs to the dairyman comprise costs for treatment and extra labor, reduced milk production, loss of body condition, a prolonged calving interval as a consequence of an estrous or suboptimal estrous expression, increased risk for teat lesions, and ultimately a higher culling risk together with reduced slaughter value. Lameness is the third economically most important disease category at the herd level in dairy cattle, after mastitis and subfertility (Dijkhuizen, 1987). For these reasons, a Herd Health and Production Management (HH & PM) program for lameness control should aim to minimize (sub)clinical lameness in order to optimize (re)production and animal welfare, thereby reducing forced culling and financial losses (Noordhuizen and Brand, 1983).

Lameness incidence and prevalence may show a wide variation between farms, as is shown in Figure 1 for dermatitis interdigitalis and dermatitis digitalis. This means that each farm has to be considered individually because of its specific situation.

Lameness is a multifactorial disease condition, caused by infectious and/or non-infectious factors which act together with environmental and host factors. It is a symptom of different processes and as such not a formal diagnosis (Espinasse et al., 1984). Based on an internationally agreed etiological and pathogenetic standard (Weaver, 1994; Mortensen, 1994), lameness can be split up in primary and secondary disorders. The following primary disorders (diagnoses) can be distinguished:

- Dermatitis interdigitalis (sometimes called footrot),
- Dermatitis digitalis (Mortellaro disease),
- Pododermatitis aseptica diffusa (laminitis),
- Phlegmona interdigitalis (sometimes called foul-in-the-foot)

Primary disorders can result in several secondary disorders or lesions, such as: pododermatitis circumscripta and septica (sole ulcer), solear contusion, white line zone

*Figure 1. Lameness prevalences of dermatitis interdigitalis (A) and dermatitis digitalis (B) in a group of dairy farms (after Smits et al., 1992)*

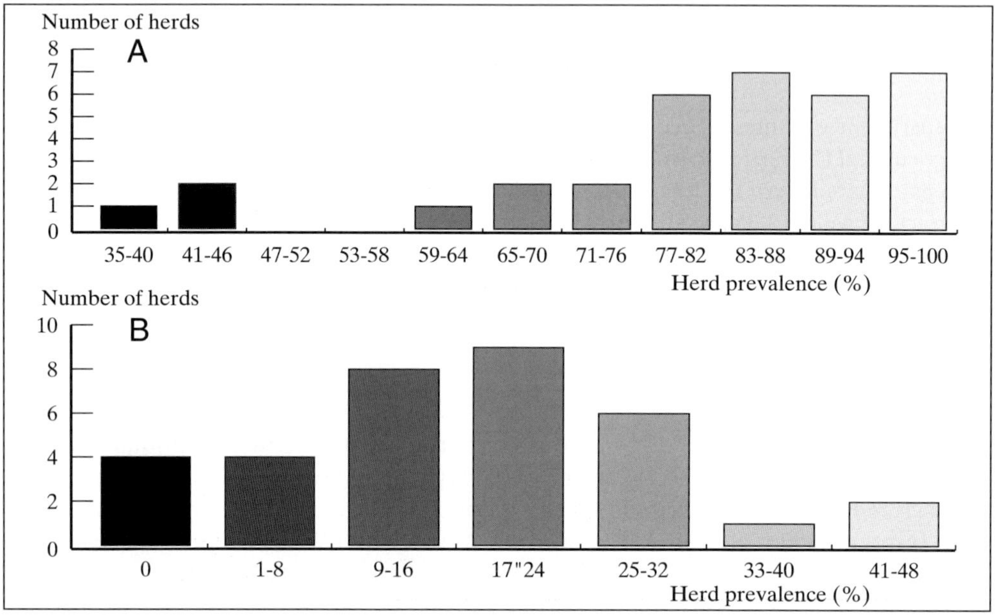


defects, heel erosion and interdigital hyperplasia. A secondary lesion may be caused by one or more primary disorders. For instance, sole ulcers might be derived from laminitis (pododermatitis aseptica diffusa) and/or foul-in-the -foot (dermatitis interdigitalis). The distinction between these underlying primary processes is very important if lameness problems have to be solved and whenever preventive intervention programs have to be implemented. Many factors at cow, management and environment level that contribute to the occurrence of lameness vary according to each lameness category. Furthermore, their effect can have a different direction (increasing or decreasing the risk).

In this part of the Chapter, the objectives or, more specifically, the preset targets, and the execution of the HH & PM protocol for monitoring claw health are outlined.

## 7.1.2 PROTOCOL

Health care of feet and legs is best conducted by following the basic herd health and production management (HH & PM) protocol outlined in Chapter 1, part 1, and presented in Figure 2.

*Figure 2. Herd health protocol for monitoring health of feet and legs*

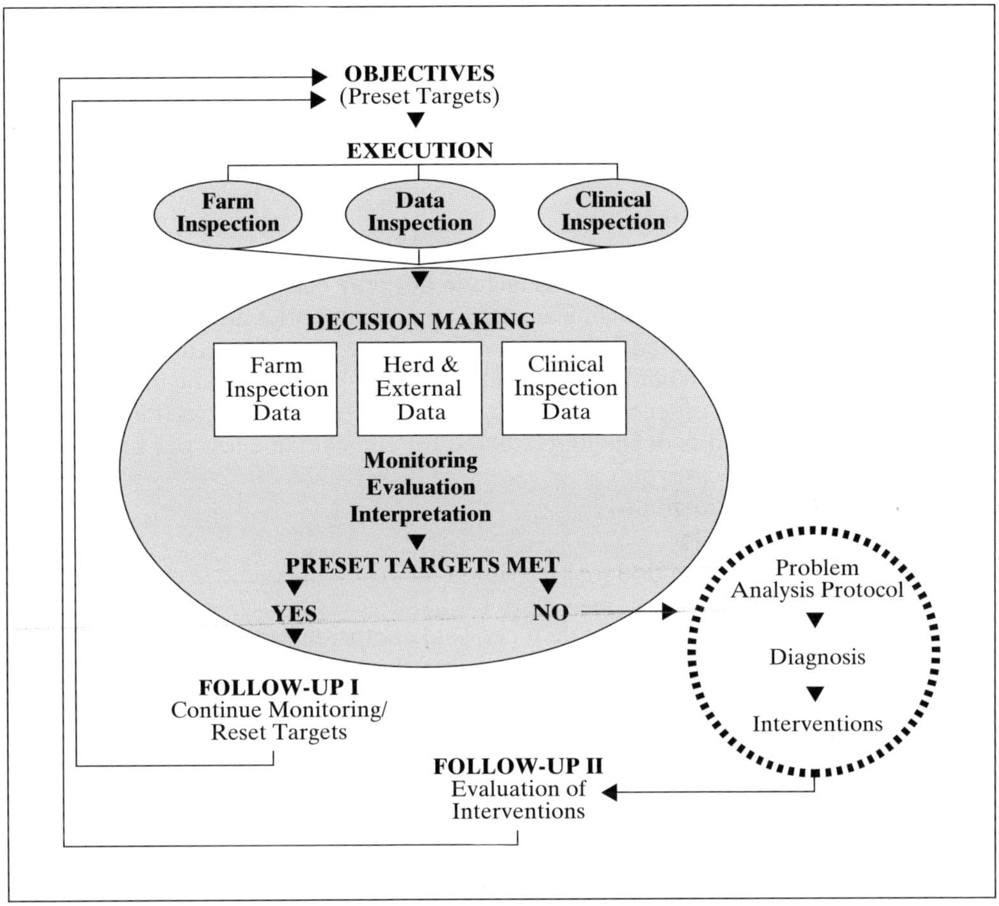


## 7.1.3 OBJECTIVES AND PRESET TARGETS

For each farm, primary and secondary preset targets are defined as performance indices. They comprise crude clinical observations, as well as primary and secondary digital disorders. The primary performance indices describe claw health care in broad lines. They enable us to monitor claw health during routine monthly herd visits. The primary performance indices, expressed as numbers or percentages comprise:

1. cows treated for clinical lameness either per 3, 6 or 12 months,
2. clinical cow cases either per 3, 6 or 12 months,
3. cows culled for lameness problems per 3, 6 or 12 months.

Minimal acceptable levels for these 3 primary performance indices should be defined for each individual farm, taking into account the general understanding of local conditions. For example, less than 20% for each index. However, the percentage level may vary between farms and over time as was stated before.

In addition to the primary performance indices secondary indices may be presented which are related to the primary lameness performance indices. They define, in more detail, the primary digital disorders, which may appear important to the farmer or practitioner. The following clinical performance indices, expressed as numbers or percentages per head (cows/young stock) present over a certain period of time include:
- clinical dermatitis interdigitalis (footrot) cases,
- clinical laminitis cases,
- clinical dermatitis digitalis cases.

A further extension can be made to include not only clinical performance indices in the preset targets, but also subclinical performance categories and secondary digital disorders. These can be derived from observations during routine farm visits or specific herd inspection visits. When both clinical and subclinical diagnostic information is made available, a full list of secondary performance indices may look as follows:
1. The percentage of cows of the herd treated for clinical lameness per time period, specified for clinical cases of:
   (a) phlegmona interdigitalis,
   (b) dermatitis digitalis,
   (c) dermatitis interdigitalis,
   (d) laminitis,
   (e) secundary lesions such as sole ulcer, sole contusion, white line process, white line separation, solear haemorrhages, interdigital hyperplasia.
2. The percentage of young stock treated for clinical lameness per time period, and specified for clinical cases of a, b, c, d, and e under (1),
3. The percentage of cows in the herd scored for subclinical disorders and lesions during routine claw inspection or routine herd claw trimmings, specified for cases of a, b, c, d and e,
4. The percentage of young stock scored for subclinical disorders and lesions during routine claw inspection or routine herd claw trimmings, and specified for cases of a, b, c, d and e,
5. The percentage of cows/young stock primarily culled for lameness reasons, and specified for cases of a, b, c, d and e.

It is very difficult to set out preset targets for an individual farm against average performance indices of a larger group of farms. Wide variations in incidence and prevalence of lameness occur among different farms and during time. It should be emphasized that for establishing performance targets, claw trimming conducted on a herd basis can be most beneficial to obtain data on clinical and subclinical disorders and lesions. Such data are supportive in determining preset targets more precisely.

In addition to these lameness monitoring indices, it is advisable to look at genetic aspects as well. The genetic make up of certain cow families and bulls appears to predispose for lameness if e.g. the heel height is too low, hocks are excessively straight or corkscrew deformity is present. Generally speaking, genetic improvement of conformation of feet and legs must be encouraged at any point of the evolvement of the HH & PM program.

## 7.1.4 EXECUTION: MATERIALS AND METHODS

### Records

Record keeping is the basis for any herd health protocol, as was already stated in Chapter 1, part 1. The following primary data recording systems can be distinguished:
*) the farm diary and herd fertility-health wall chart,
*) the examination list (clinical veterinary inspection),
*) the herd clinical lameness chart.

### The farm diary and the fertility-health wall chart

At the start of a HH & PM service, records are often not available and interviewing the dairyman about lameness cases during the past year usually does not yield any valid information about foot health. Therefore, both the dairyman and the professional claw trimmer must be convinced about the value of recording their own findings. In this way a historical database can be built up, which is essential in analysis and solving of lameness problems that might occur later in time.

The farmer should use the farm diary to record all cows which show clinical lameness specifying: date, foot, leg or claw involved, diagnosis if possible, treatment applied, date of clinical recovery and eventual relapse. Similar recording details should be kept of cows culled for lameness reasons. From time to time information from the farm diary, inclusive data originating from clinical inspections, is transferred to the herd fertility-health wall chart or herd clinical lameness chart or into a computerized database, in order to provide herd-time overviews of herd claw health. As pointed out earlier, a herd clinical lameness chart, together with a herd fertility-health wall chart serves the purpose of obtaining an overview of the whole herd performance with regard to the pattern of clinical lameness cases, and to the cows and feet/claws involved, together with the (re)production stage those cows are in. Trends can then be detected and problem areas or animal groups can more easily be identified.

### The examination list

The examination list largely meant for cows deserving a reproductive tract examination should be extended to those cows which should be examined for lameness. An example of such an examination list is given in Table 1. While the practitioner performes the examinations the farmer handles the list and records the findings reported by the practitioner.

Note that cow 4365 should be put on the list for the next visit to check her for recovery. In this way the examination list becomes more dynamic in nature.

*Table 1. Combined fertility lameness examination list*

| Cow ID | Calving date | Estrus/ AI dates | Fertility findings | Reason for examination | Findings of examination or treatment |
|---|---|---|---|---|---|
| **Date of Examination** | | | | | |
| 1267 | 1/5/95 | 20/6, 21/7 | PD- | estrus not observed | PGF treated |
| 4365 | 2/7/95 | 20/8, 11/9 | PD+ | lame left hind | sole ulcer |

**Herd clinical lameness chart**

For specific lameness problems, the practitioner can design a herd clinical lameness chart (Table 2) enlisting all those cows which experienced any clinical lameness, and all clinical cow cases in chronological order. This chart is very similar to the herd clinical mastitis chart (Chapter 6), and reports the cow's ID, the date of the lameness event, the foot/leg/claw affected, the diagnosis and the treatment, and preferably, the date of clinical recovery or culling. In this way a specific overview of the lameness problem is obtained and further analysis can be conducted into specific lameness diagnoses and on high risk cows. The list is updated with data from the farm diary and the examination list, by either the farmer or the HH & PM practitioner at the end of each farm visit. It is then used for specific discussion about decisions and actions to be taken.

*Table 2. Herd clinical lameness chart (general headings)*

| Cow ID | Data | Foot/Claw affected | Diagnosis | Treatment | Recovered or culled |
|---|---|---|---|---|---|
| 234 | 10/07 | left hind claw | sole ulcer | trimmed | |
| 321 | 12/07 | left hind claw | laminitis | trimmed | |
| 135 | 13/07 | right hind claw | phlegmona | tetracyclines | rec. 16/07 |

*Table 3. More specified herd clinical lameness chart*

| Cow ID | Date | Foot/Claw affected | Derm. interd. | Derm. Digit. | Lamin. | Phlegm. interd. | Second Lesion |
|---|---|---|---|---|---|---|---|
| 56 | 09/04 | left front | – | yes | – | – | – |
| 56 | 21/07 | right front | – | yes | – | – | sole ulcer |

For a better insight into the claw health situation and subsequent action it is, however, more indicated to use the more specific diagnoses mentioned in a previous paragraph. The herd clinical lameness chart may then have the following headings (Table 3).

This procedure allows for recording more than one diagnosis per animal at the same time, as usually occurs in the field. Meanwhile, the practitioner may record certain remarks which need specific attention during e.g. the next farm visit. For example: "concrete floors are slippery" or "foot prints point to heel erosion (erosio ungulae) among cows, need check next time".

After a given period of time it is easy to sum up the numbers of records in the respective columns, and detect which diagnostic category is most prevalent and which cows (parities) are most involved. Seasonal variations can also be detected. The advantage of this chart is that both at the start of a HH & PM service and at farms with lameness problems, an excellent overview of the current claw health situation is provided. The data originate from both the farm diary and veterinary inspection during farm visits. Additionally, this information can be used for further analysis of lameness conditions.

## Additional tools

On the farm, facilities for further claw inspection (e.g. a crush) should be available. It is advisable for larger herds to have their own facilities; the veterinary practice could provide a mobile facility as a service unit to farmers with smaller herds. The facility should provide for an easy examination of both hind and front feet. Furthermore, claw trimming tools should be available. Among these are: claw pincers, trimming knives of different design but always freshly sharpened, wooden or rubber claw blocks for treating severe lesions, surgical materials and bandages. The findings made during the inspection or trimming should be recorded.

A walk-through foot bath is also a very important tool. Its regular use (e.g. monthly) is very important in the prevention of dermatitis interdigitalis (Toussaint-Raven et al., 1985).

Other tools that can be used are the Risk Indicator Profile and Between Herd Comparisons. The Risk Indicator Profile (see Chapter 1, part 4) may represent a valuable tool in setting priorities in the health program for reducing lameness problems and preventing them from re-occurrence on a specific farm (see Part 2 and 3 of this Chapter). Greenough & Vermunt (1994) have presented a herd lameness checklist to evaluate potential stressors at the herd level. Between herd comparisons are useful tools in herd health psychology: they are best used to show a particular dairyman that results can be achieved and progress can be made, by showing him performances of other herds hence stimulating motivation. Such comparisons may also be used to rank herds participating in HH & PM services, according to their performance indices. As such they may help to keep up motivation among farmers. Between herd comparisons can also be used in the setting of study clubs of dairymen, to discuss mutual problems and alternative solutions and to show differences in husbandry systems.

It will be clear that the use of computer technology is largely time saving for analysis of lameness and inspection data, as for farm comparisons. At the same time one should be aware of the fact that the analysis features outlined above are hardly available in current veterinary computer software programs.

## Methods

While executing a foot health monitoring protocol the practitioner has to address three major areas:

1. data inspection before and during each farm visit. Data inspection is directed at (a) quality and accuracy of data recording, and (b) obtaining a proper insight into the claw health situation and trends. The latter will be discussed in parts 2 and 3 of this Chapter,
2. farm inspection related to managerial conditions and environmental factors, possibly associated with the occurrence of lameness, and
3. clinical inspection of cows and or young stock in order to detect different claw disorders and to make a herd inventory of subclinical conditions.

## Data inspection

HH & PM services are performed on the basis of information stemming from different data sources. Within a HH & PM service, time has to be made available to check for data quality. Data inspection should focus at actuality, accurateness and completeness of available data, recorded by the farmer and/or the herdsman and the HH & PM practitioner. Data quality may refer to the accuracy of diagnoses made by the farmer. For example for proper analysis and advice later on, it is most desirable that more than the complaint "lame" is noted in the diary. This is essential if reasons for lameness are to be investigated and potential risk factors are to be evaluated. Causes for lameness must be specified as diagnoses because risk factors for one disorder will be different or differently directed than those for another diagnosis. In some situations, the farmer may record his own diagnosis. If properly trained those diagnoses can be valid. If not, the practitioner has to check the reliability of those diagnoses before, or during the regular farm visits.

Records of disorders found in individual cows examined and treated for clinical lameness by the practitioner must be made available as additional data to those of the dairyman. They should be recorded on the farm diary and or the herd clinical lameness chart or in another database. The same procedure must be followed for clinical lameness diagnoses made during consultative visits. They may later be listed on a new examination list for further checking, e.g. for recovery, at the next farm visit.

The farm diary is also inspected for remarks by the farmer such as managerial events (changing rations or pasture plots; regrouping of cows; changing weather conditions) or notations about newly calved cows, complete with calving history and possibly metabolic diseases. This information is important to help the practitioner focus on underlying factors of lameness problems actually prevalent in the herd and on trends over time.

## The farm inspection

### General inspection

Since, in most cases, lameness is multifactorial in nature, adequate attention has to be paid by the HH & PM practitioner to farm conditions, the cow's environment and management strategies. Consequently, the practitioner should go around the farm together with the farmer to collect and discuss the information. The inspection will focus among others on: animal related factors, housing facilities and equipment, including level of maintenance and hygienic conditions, storage of bedding material, immediate cow environment, management, especially nutrition and pasturing related factors, feedstuff storage, and quality of forage. Each of these areas comprises more detailed, different environmental and management factors or conditions which may be related to the occurrence of lameness. Next to the qualitative role of the given factors, it appears highly relevant to have insight into their quantitative contribution to the lameness situation. Specific observations possibly related to lameness should be recorded on the clinical lameness list presented in Table 2, as remarks in order to facilitate problem analysis if needed.

Checking the environmental items by routinely making personal observations on the spot and by talking to the dairyman not only is a demonstration of interest, but is also useful in highlighting the negative aspects about deficiencies where attention should lead to improvement. This may regard a nutritional or an acute overt lameness problem. For example, an outbreak of phlegmona interdigitalis among heifers in a given pasture, could narrow down the attention to e.g. a high animal density per acre against too few drinking places in the plot; infection may build up.

### Specific inspection

If an overt severe lameness problem or situation appears not to be easily solved, it is strongly advisable to look into more detail to the potential conditions and risk factors on and around the farm that may affect the occurrence of both clinical and subclinical lameness situations. A more in-depth analysis, with regard to environmental aspects possibly involved in the occurrence of lameness, is part of a subsequent step: the environmental conditions or Risk Indicator Profile. Risk indicators are conditions in the cow's environment which may contribute to the occurrence of certain lameness diagnostic categories. In case of overt lameness problems it is indicated to study those factors which contribute most to the existence of a lameness problem in more detail (Wells et al., 1995). These issues will be further addressed in part 2 and 3 of this Chapter.

As a basis for this risk factor analysis, the practitioner may perform a field survey among the farms in his practice, investigating the effect of potential risk factors and then go back to the problem farm to check for the relevance of factors on that particular farm. To perform such studies, the practitioner should have the proper knowledge and skills. Additional training in applied quantitative veterinary epidemiology (see Chapter 1, part 4) is indicated. An example of a screening list with different conditions contributing to lameness is retrieved from literature and presented in part 3 of this Chapter.

Studying lameness and its respective causes requires excellent observational skills from the HH & PM practitioner. Lameness represents a multifactorial syndrome, which is hard to tackle. If needed, the practitioner can call for expert help from e.g. a cattle housing expert or a nutritionist. In all situations the information gathered should be properly used. That means that general inspection circumstances will yield advice of a more general nature, while detailed practice surveys, where more insight exists about potential risk factors, will result in more specific advice.

The findings coming from the general or specific farm inspection procedure are used for a further integral analysis of data, the subsequent discussion between farmer and practitioner and for decision-making by the farmer.

**The clinical inspection**

Before the farm visit physically starts, the practitioner should examine the updated farm diary and the herd clinical lameness chart in order to update him/herself on the pattern of clinical lameness cases over time and on the actual claw health status of the herd. This information may indicate whether some suspected cows should be added to the examination list, prepared by the farmer, and whether he/she needs to examine a sample of the herd for subclinical lameness evaluation. Subsequent actions often result from discussions with the farmer and are based on detected trends or needs expressed by the farmer or practitioner. The same applies for inspection of previously examined cows, in order to determine the level of recovery. As a result of this, a few cows may be added to the examination list.

Clinical inspection of lame cows on the examination list should be done after the reproductive examinations. The practitioner will look for subtle abnormalities in the walking and standing behaviour of cattle, and if present will add them to the examination list (Noordhuizen and Brand, 1983). There appears to be a wide variation in lame cow detection ability among farmers and practitioners, which indicates the need for specific training.

More important is to incorporate veterinary clinical inspection as a routine in the HH & PM services. During this routine, a cross-sectional examination of feet and legs of a certain sample of the herd, e.g. 5 or 10%, is checked for subclinical claw disorders, especially in case of suspect developments. For such purpose claw inspection and/or trimming equipment must be available at the farm. This procedure is comparable to the one followed in mastitis control (Chapter 6). All diagnoses or findings of clinical and subclinical diseased cows must be recorded by the farmer on an examination list, while the practitioner performs the examinations. The data from the examination list should be transferred to a specific herd clinical lameness list (see Table 2), which then becomes a subclinical disorder inspection chart.

Subclinical lesions inventory may disclose the early development of new problem areas, in need of prompt attention before becoming major clinical problems.

Results of cross-sectional examination or inventories may provide the practitioner

*Table 4. Example of a claw trimming scoring list for diagnosing clinical and subclinical lameness diagnoses and severity classes (Adapted after Noordhuizen et al., 1995)*

| | | |
|---|---|---|
| Date of: | Cow ID: | Parity: |
| herd claw trimming: | Pedigree nr.: | Breed: |
| Farm code: | Date of birth: | Sire: |
| Claw trimmer: | Date of calving: | Dry yes/no: |
| Observer: | | |

| **Diagnosis** | **Right rear** | | **Left rear** | | **Right front** | | **Left front** | |
|---|---|---|---|---|---|---|---|---|
| | **outer** | **inner** | **outer** | **inner** | **outer** | **inner** | **outer** | **inner** |
| | **1 2 3** | **1 2 3** | **1 2 3** | **1 2 3** | **1 2 3** | **1 2 3** | **1 2 3** | **1 2 3** |
| Footrot | ❑❑❑ | ❑❑❑ | ❑❑❑ | ❑❑❑ | ❑❑❑ | ❑❑❑ | ❑❑❑ | ❑❑❑ |
| Laminitis | ❑ | ❑ | ❑ | ❑ | ❑ | ❑ | ❑ | ❑ |
| Ital. footrot | ❑ | ❑ | ❑ | ❑ | ❑ | ❑ | ❑ | ❑ |
| Foul in foot | ❑ | ❑ | ❑ | ❑ | ❑ | ❑ | ❑ | ❑ |
| White line | ❑❑ | ❑❑ | ❑❑ | ❑❑ | ❑❑ | ❑❑ | ❑❑ | ❑❑ |
| Sole ulcer | ❑❑ | ❑❑ | ❑❑ | ❑❑ | ❑❑ | ❑❑ | ❑❑ | ❑❑ |
| Tyloma | ❑ | ❑ | ❑ | ❑ | ❑ | ❑ | ❑ | ❑ |

*Note: Figures 1, 2 and 3 point to severity classes, 1 being moderately affected and 3 severely affected. In cases where only option 1 is available this means "present".*

with indications of the current lameness status of the herd, especially when the pattern of development is evaluated over time. In this way certain areas needing attention may be identified and certain actions taken at early stages. Such a pattern is presented in Table 5. For evaluation purposes it usually is most appropriate to distinguish classes or categories per heading as is shown in Table 4. This short list originates from cross-sectional surveys into lameness prevalences in The Netherlands.

These surveys have been conducted among over 10.000 cows and 1200 replacement young stock. From the original 250 putative factors this short list was made, where factors are clustered per leading category (Frankena et al., 1991; 1992; 1993).

The herd (sub)clinical lameness list (Table 2 and 3) can also be handled during the regular claw trimming procedures on the farm twice a year. In such a way the herd prevalence of claw disorders can be determined and again areas in need for further attention can be distinguished. The advantage of this strategy is that impending problems can be detected at a rather early stage, that is before too many clinical cases arise.

At the end of the clinical inspection the number of cases are categorized and a possible problem is defined in more detail. This information is compared with the information about the pattern of clinical lameness over time determined before the farm visit and the actual situation at the start of the farm visit. Hence, the practitioner can better focus his attention on the real lameness problem on the farm.

*Table 5. Overview of findings with regard to subclinical digital disorders as established during veterinary clinical examination in a herd H*

| Farm visit: | 1 | 2 | 3 | 4 |
|---|---|---|---|---|
| **Digital disorder diagnosis:** | | | | |
| Interdigital phlegmona | 1 | 0 | 0 | 2 |
| Digital dermatitis | 0 | 0 | 0 | 3 |
| Laminitis | 6 | 3 | 2 | 1 |
| Interdigital dermatitis | 0 | 2 | 1 | 0 |
| Sole ulcer | 2 | 3 | 1 | 2 |
| White line defect | 0 | 0 | 1 | 1 |
| Tyloma | 1 | 2 | 0 | 1 |

*Herd N : 100 cows; sample: 10%*

**Regular, routine claw trimming**

The most important routine intervention for the maintenance of sound feet and legs is regular claw trimming. Environmental, managerial and etiological factors will dictate the required frequency of this management tool. Twice per year claw trimming for each animal over two years of age is the absolute minimum. In order to provide sufficient and reliable data it is strongly advisable, whenever possible, to involve a professional claw trimmer in the HH & PM service. He is the one that can perform routine claw inspection and make diagnosis on the majority of the cows during his routine trimming visits. The dairyman himself can also perform this kind of functional claw trimming for example at drying off. Skilled claw trimming rests on a solid and proper practical training which should on beforehand be followed in order to prevent claw health problems. It is then not important whether a professional claw trimmer or the dairyman performs this task. What is important is that the trimming be done in a skilled manner and on a regular basis.

Routine trimmings are also intended to facilitate a proper observation of the claws. The claw must be elevated, tied up, and cleaned with water and a brush for optimal observation and trimming conditions. In order to be able to evaluate the aspect of the bearing surface, excessive solear horn should be invariably cut away. Careful attention of the bearing surface (ground contact surface) of the claw is important, because the presence of haemorrhagic horn, horn defects and their localization is a useful indicator of problems. It is advisable to routinely trim a few millimeters of solear horn of each claw for better inspection and diagnosing. For those who are interested in functional trimming of claws the book by Toussaint-Raven et al. (1985) focusing on practical application is most worthwhile. It deals with all aspects of functional trimming and is completed by a section about trimming of diseased claws. Do it yourself trimming is the best way to understand the different types of lameness diagnoses and the behavior of affected cows.

After completion of the three inspections, a discussion has to be done with the farmer about the possible relationships between the recorded findings and the claw health status of the herd. This is followed by interpretation of the available datasets in order to come to a final herd diagnosis. Ultimately this should lead to providing the farmer with several alternative combat strategies, and to the discussion about what actions would be most appropriate, given the situation on the farm, the expected costs and benefits and the available managerial opportunities available (see part 2 of this Chapter).

## EPILOGUE

The herd health situation with regard to lameness is the ultimate result of biological, genetic, management, environmental and economic issues. This makes lameness, and its etiology a very complex problem area. The farmer cannot be expected to act as an expert on his own in this field. For this reason, and since cattle must always walk to function, the claw and leg health status should always be included in a comprehensive HH & PM service. A HH & PM service has to be implemented in such a way that it meets the mutually agreed preset targets of both the practitioner and the dairyman. These goals must be expressed in quantitative terms such as those outlined above, and adjusted depending on the conditions and changes that occur over time.

The evaluation of the herd's performance with regard to lameness problems requires more of the practitioner's time and effort than the occasional attention to a clinically lame cow or a stroll through the herd during herd health visits. The assistance that the practitioner has to provide, in order to solve a current problem, or preventing lameness from becoming a future cause of suboptimal feet and leg performance, also requires a thorough understanding of the pathogenesis of the disorders and of the factors involved at cow, herd, environment, human and economic level. Therefore, practitioners dealing with lameness, either at the clinical or the subclinical level, should be aware of the difficulties and seek proper additional training in diagnosing, treatment and prevention of these disorders. The aid of diagnostic labs and well trained experts in different fields should be encouraged. This is specifically true for training in applied veterinary epidemiology, meant for field surveys as pointed out above. Only with that training and skills the HH & PM practitioner is able to tackle the lameness problems adequately. Chapter 1, part 4 deals in more detail with those issues and provides more insight into principles and methods for application. This training is specially true when outbreaks occur and where detailed diagnosis and actions are needed, which goes beyond the regular and more general surveillance of a HH & PM service.

The practitioner must always find ways to improve the suitability of the information to the dairyman, to enhance his motivation in a positive sense and to provide him with advice that is soundly based on true arguments and is economically justified. If needed, the herd health practitioner should look for support from other experts in specific areas, such as genetics, housing design or nutrition.

A farmer may have saved direct expenses for veterinary interventions, such as herd claw trimming, on a short term, but at the same time his herd will become at higher risk for lameness problems in the long run. It is the task of the practitioner to show to the farmer what the benefits of a proper foot health status are in terms of production economics, estrus expression and behavior, and animal welfare.

*For references see part 3 of this Chapter.*

# 7.2 MONITORING FOOT HEALTH: DECISION-MAKING, PROBLEM ANALYSIS, FOLLOW UP

Jos P.T.M.Noordhuizen[1], Alberto Brizzi[2], Elsbeth N.Noordhuizen-Stassen[3], Klaas Frankena[1].

[1] Department of Animal Husbandry, Wageningen Institute of Animal Sciences, Wageningen Agricultural University, Marijkeweg 40, P.O.Box 338, 6700 AH Wageningen, The Netherlands

[2] Large Animal Practice, Via Gorizia 16, 43100 Parma, Italy

[3] Department of Herd Health and Reproduction, School of Veterinary Medicine, University of Utrecht, Yalelaan 7, 3584 CL Utrecht, The Netherlands

## 7.2.1 INTRODUCTION

In the preceding part 1 of this Chapter the outline of a herd health and production management (HH & PM) protocol for monitoring and control of lameness has been elaborated and the execution of this protocol addressed. In this part, the decision-making process, problem analysis and follow up are addressed.

Decision-making is based on monitoring raw data, evaluating processed data and analysing and interpreting performance indices. All preceding activities are aimed at one ultimate goal: decision support. Interpretation of the gathered information can be used to assess the actual claw health status or, in case of problems, to identify the most probable herd diagnosis. In this way it is possible to get a better insight into the potential causes of a problem. Through this knowledge the provision of alternatives for solution and or prevention of the problem can be facilitated. This is the point where the advice is substantiated and action prepared.

Therefore, this section of the protocol deserves specific attention of the practitioner, because different levels of availability of information may play a role in the process, and opportunities and limitations of decision-making, analysis and follow-up

The aforenamed steps are addressed through two example herds Z. These herds have the same background and set up. Different situations leading to different interpretations are highlighted by using the respective specification Z1 and or Z2 in the Tables, Figures and text.

## 7.2.2 DECISION MAKING

Decision-making is first based on the target performance indices set by the farmer together with his practitioner (see Chapter 7, part 1). These indices may be a reflection of average figures in the nearest population, e.g. in the region of the veterinary practice or a larger one. Information at farm level is needed for comparison with the target indices and for subsequent proper decision-making. This information originates from various sources in and around the farm.

**monitoring**

Monitoring is aimed at the collection and evaluation of raw data. Information can originate from different sources (see Chapter 7, part 1), subdivided into routine (a, b, c, d, e), lameness-specific (f, g) and additional records (h):

**(a) the farm diary.**
in which the farmer ideally records every clinical case of lameness occurring in his herd as well as certain farm events such as formalin foot bathing and routine herd claw trimming procedures. A farm diary at best will equally comprise information on other farming areas such as reproduction and feeding, which may be of importance to the solution of a lameness problem. A barn chart for herd fertility and health status is in service too.

**(b) the clinical examination list.**
Data on this list is meant for examining suspect cows and assessing the actual clinical claw health status during the farm visit. Data originate from the farm diary. This list comprises both new cases and a check for recovery of earlier cases in addition to cows due for reproductive examination. In more intensive HH & PM programs the practitioner may conduct more intensive examinations, such as a sample of the herd for checking the subclinical lameness status (see at g).

**(c) fertility health chart.**
which shows the herd performance in reproduction, health and dry off and culling in an overview. Problem cows in the different areas of dairy farming are easily identified.

**(d) herd and farm inspection survey.**
In case of overt lameness problems and in case of routine farm visits it is indicated that the practitioner makes an inventory of environmental conditions possibly related to a lameness problem. This comprises two levels: an extensive level meant for routine farm inspection; an intensive level (field survey) meant to contribute substantially to the solution of current lameness problems in the herd (see further paragraphs and Chapter 7, part 3).

**(e) the 12-monthly list.**
The 12-monthly list contains the primary and secondary performance indices which serve to assess the current situation with respect to lameness in the herd, to assess the evolution of the lameness prevalence/incidence over time and to cross-check the performance with performance indices in other areas such as reproduction.

**(f) herd clinical lameness list.**
This list is usually operational in case of manifest lameness problems. It serves to focus attention on the lame cows with respect to repeated cases and to recovery or culling. It is comparable to the herd clinical mastitis list (see Chapter 6).

**(g) subclinical lameness inventory.**
In case of overt clinical lameness problems in the herd or in situations where problems are expected or in situations where no information about claw health is available on the farm, this inventory may serve as a first overview of the current situation. At the same time the cows at high risk for clinical lameness are identified.

**(h) additional information sources.**
In the case of lameness it is indicated to check the herd performance in other areas such as milk production, reproduction, nutrition. For example: does the clinical lameness problem affect estrous detection efficiency on the farm? Comparison of farms, for example through study groups, with respect to their performance indices could be a subject for discussion and source of information as well, particularly because experiences can be exchanged among farmers.

## Data processing

In the most sophisticated situation, all information mentioned above is gathered by both the farmer and the practitioner and, at the same time, this information is stored in and processed by a computer program, specifically designed to support herd health and production management programs. Such computer programs should not only be designed to provide the farmer with action lists, or with herd performance reports (12 monthly list), but also for the analysis of data from herd level to group level, from group level to individual cow level, cross-checking information from various farming areas.
An example of a frequency distribution derived from such a computer program is given in Table 1. A histogram may provide individual cow numbers for proper analysis and interpretation.

*Table 1. Example of a frequency distribution produced by a computer program for supporting HH&PM programs. Numbers in the Table refer to individual cow numbers*

| | | | | |
|---|---|---|---|---|
| 136 | | | | |
| 195 | | | | |
| 210 | | | | |
| 189 | | | | |
| 173 | 156 | | | |
| 163 | 144 | 98 | | |
| 166 | 179 | 131 | | |
| 171 | 187 | 174 | 53 | |
| 176 | 186 | 86 | 99 | |
| 119 | 212 | 116 | 97 | |
| 215 | 312 | 321 | 211 | 191 |

**0 30 60 90 120 150 Interval calving-1st service (days)**

In non-ideal situations, the gathered information, shortly highlighted above from (a) to (h), may vary greatly. Many levels can be distinguished: from no information available at all (or "in the farmer's head") to gradual availability of parts of information (fertility health barn chart alone or in conjunction with farm diary or extended with other parts) up to the highly sophisticated situation where management information systems are coupled to computers in the veterinary practice and to agricultural computer networks in a region or state.

The most important issue of all information levels is that the practitioner is aware of the potentials and the limitations of these different levels, mainly with respect to analysis and interpretation of the findings, and, hence, decision-making and advice.

**Assessing the information**

The example herd Z is presented here in order to illustrate the different use of data in different situations. A differentiation between Z1 and Z2 has been made for specific conditions.

The basic situation of herds Z is as follows: Each herd comprises 60 dairy cows on a yearly basis and 30 head of young stock. The animals are of the Holstein-Friesian breed. The farm is family run and shows an average milk production of 8500 kg per cow per year. Animals are housed in a loose housing system and are milked in a 2 x 6 herringbone parlor. About 23 ha of grassland scattered around the farm house is exploited and 2 ha of corn are available. The farmer participates in a HH & PM program of his practitioner and applies a data recording system routinely (see Chapter 1, part 2). The farm is visited once every 4 weeks by the practitioner. As a routine procedure, the farmer applies formaline footbathing every month and calls the professional claw trimmer twice yearly for routine herd claw trimming. Together with his practitioner the farmer has set targets for performance of his herd with respect to claw health. These preset target indices are given in the respective Tables.

Given the fact that within a HH & PM program ample information is available on a farm diary, fertility health barn chart, 12 monthly list, examination lists and farm inspection records, the first task is to deduce the claw health situation from these datasets.
Therefore, the practitioner assesses the fertility health barn chart data over the past 6 and 12 months, together with the information from the 12-monthly list. The following "herd claw health overview" is derived for herd Z (Table 2).

Comparing the data in Table 2 with the preset target indices it can be concluded in situation Z1 that there exists a clinical lameness problem in the herd for quite some time somewhere in the year (see cows and cow cases of clinical lameness). Furthermore, it appears that several cows are affected by clinical lameness more than once in that year (see 139% cow cases). These chronic and or relapsing cases occurred inspite of routine claw trimming and frequent footbathing. Relatively many cows have been culled for lameness reasons. From the farm diary it can be seen since when this problem has increased substantially.

In situation Z2 the outcome is different. It may appear that a clinical lameness problem is pending given the fact that the cows and cow cases are at a high-normal level.

*Table 2. Herd claw health overview on clinical lameness in herd Z over the past year, given for the 2 situations Z1 and Z2, and the preset performance target indices for the herd*

| | Z1 | | Z2 | | target |
|---|---|---|---|---|---|
| Average number of cows present | 60 | | 60 | | – |
| Number of cows with clinical lameness recorded | 41 | (68%) | 12 | (20%) | <20% |
| Number of clinical cow cases | 84 | (139%) | 18 | (30%) | <25% |
| Number of clinical leg cases | 112 | | 21 | | |
| Number of foot cases without diagnosis | 2 | | 1 | | 0 |
| Number of missing diagnoses in total | 0 | | 0 | | 0 |
| Herd claw trimming frequency per year | 2 | | 2 | | 2 |
| Footbathing frequency per year | 12 | | 3 | | * |
| Number of cows culled in total | 22 | (37%) | 14 | (23%) | <25% |
| Number of cows culled for lameness reasons | 2 | (10%) | 3 | (21%) | <10% |

– *means: not applicable*
* *means: is depending on the situation (see text)*

It is equally possible that there is no real problem existing. Since formaline footbathing is rarely applied and the number of cullings for lameness relatively high, it seems appropriate that the practitioner conducts a further assessment in order to rule out a pending problem. This can be done by asking the farmer about his observations, by checking the farm diary (the practitioner will usually know whether or not the farmer is a "writer") and the 12-monthly list.

From the 12-monthly list where overall parameters are recorded (Table 3) additional information can be obtained in order to specify the need for further investigation and have better insight. In this example of situation Z1 only a part of this 12-monthly list is

*Table 3. Part of the 12-monthly list referring to the lameness situation Z1 in herd Z over the last 6 months*

| **Parameter** **date ->** | **6/7** | **3/8** | **5/9** | **10/10** | **5/11** | **7/12** | **8/1** |
|---|---|---|---|---|---|---|---|
| # milking cows | 47 | 48 | 48 | 49 | 47 | 51 | 51 |
| # dry cows | 14 | 10 | 13 | 11 | 8 | 6 | 8 |
| # cows calved | 1 | 4 | 0 | 2 | 5 | 4 | 2 |
| # clinical lameness | 5 | 1 | 0 | 1 | 1 | 4 | 7 |
| # culled for lameness | 0 | 0 | 0 | 0 | 0 | 1 | 1 |
| # culled in total | 1 | 0 | 0 | 1 | 2 | 2 | 1 |
| # cows treated for subestrus | 3 | 0 | 1 | 3 | 3 | 5 | 5 |

presented, mainly referring to the situation of lameness.

From Table 3 it can be read that there was a first peak in clinical lameness occurrence in the herd in July. These 5 cases appeared to be acute cases of footrot, as could be found in the farm diary. After treatment these cases disappeared. After July there was a steady but low level of clinical lameness up to November and December when suddenly the number of clinical cases increased substantially. The practitioner could have observed the 4 cases in November as indicator-cases (alarm phase 1) deserving extra attention at the following farm visit to determine either the alarm phase 0 of no longer a problem, or alarm phase 2, an increasing problem requiring action. Additionally it can be seen that there could be a concurrent problem of estrus detection. Because many disorders are strongly related to parity and lactation stage these factors should also be comprised in the analysis. Interrelations between health, reproduction and lameness should be accounted for too. Tools for executing this task are highlighted in part 3 of this Chapter.

### 7.2.3 PROBLEM ANALYSIS

**Problem specification**

– **herd diagnosis**

The potential problem detected in the preceding paragraph has to be defined in more detail in order to facilitate proper decision-making. It is not known sofar what the herd diagnosis is. Therefore, the practitioner decides to analyze the data one step further, that is drawing a frequency distribution of diagnoses set during this period. This is presented in Table 4.

**Situation in herd Z1:**
Digital dermatitis is the most frequently observed clinical diagnosis in this herd, followed by sole ulcers and laminitis cases. Since sole ulcers could originate from either dermatitis

*Table 4. Breakdown of clinical lameness cases into diagnosis categories in herd Z over 1 year; 2 situations Z1 and Z2*

| | Z1 | Z2 |
|---|---|---|
| Interdigital phlegmona | 6 | 6 |
| Interdigital dermatitis | 2 | 24 |
| Laminitis | 11 | 3 |
| Digital dermatitis | 45 | 2 |
| Sole ulcers | 32 | 32 |
| Arthritis/periarthritis | 6 | 2 |
| Miscellaneous | 10 | 4 |

interdigitalis or laminitis, the practitioner now knows where to focus his attention on. Although the number of interdigital dermatitis cases is low, the disorder still could be present at a subclinical level. For digital dermatitis a rapid diagnosis is warranted as well as a proper treatment. Subsequently, the practitioner has to focus on environmental aspects such as nutrition, housing, management (see at paragraph "farm inspection").

**Situation in herd Z2:**
In this situation the number of sole ulcers is highest, followed by interdigital dermatitis. It seems most probable that in this situation both diagnoses are related. On the other hand, the number of laminitis cases is relatively low. Attention should be focussed mainly on causes of interdigital dermatitis and sole ulcers.

If the practitioner is not too sure about his first conclusions, it can be indicated to examine a sample of the herd for either clinical or subclinical lameness diagnoses. The latter may also be valid in case the farmer's diagnosis has appeared not to be too reliable or in the case that no data are available at all. For that herd inspection, e.g. during farm visits or routine claw trimming procedures, a recording list is available (see Chapter 7, part 1). This action may provide information supportive to the final herd diagnosis setting.

- **identification of cows at risk**

Once a herd diagnosis has been set, the next action steps are determined by analysis of data. A further breakdown of the basic information from Tables 2, 3 and 4 (primary and secondary lameness indices) into frequency distributions about foot/legs involved, parities affected, lactation stages involved, seasons of occurrence will provide the practitioner with more insight into the problem. These frequency distributions are presented in Figure 5, 6, 7 and 8 for herd Z in different situations.

**Situation in herd Z1:**
From these Figures (left parts) it can be observed that hind legs are more affected than fore-

*Figure 5. Distribution of clinical lameness cases over legs in herd Z. Two different situations, Z1 and Z2 respectively, are given. RR= rear right, LR= rear left, RF= right front, LF= left front; X represents 3 cases of clinical lameness*

| | | | | | | | | |
|---|---|---|---|---|---|---|---|---|
| | | | | | | | | X |
| | X | | | | | | | X |
| X | X | | | | | | X | X |
| X | X | | | | | X | X | X |
| X | X | | | | X | X | X | X |
| X | X | X | X | | X | X | X | X |
| **RR** | **LR** | **RF** | **LF** | | **RR** | **LR** | **RF** | **LF** |

*Figure 6. Distribution of first clinical lameness cases over parity in herd Z. Two situations are given, Z1 and Z2. X represents 3 cases of clinical lameness*

| | | | | | | | | | | | |
|---|---|---|---|---|---|---|---|---|---|---|---|
| | | | | | | | | | | | X |
| | X | | | | | | | | | | X |
| | X | | | | | | | | X | | X |
| | X | | | | | | | | X | X | X |
| X | X | | | | | | | X | X | X | X |
| X | X | | | | | | | X | X | X | X |
| X | X | | X | | | | X | X | X | X | X |
| X | X | X | X | X | X | X | X | X | X | X | X |
| **1** | **2** | **3** | **4** | **5** | **6>** | **1** | **2** | **3** | **4** | **5** | **6> parity** |

*Figure 7. Distribution of clinical lameness cases over lactation stages in herd Z. Two different situations are given, Z1 and Z2. X represents 3 cases of clinical lameness*

| | | | | | | | | | |
|---|---|---|---|---|---|---|---|---|---|
| | X | X | | | | | X | X | X |
| | X | X | | | | | X | X | X |
| | X | X | | | | | X | X | X |
| | X | X | | | | X | X | X | X |
| **dry** | **0** | **100** | **200** | **300 days in milk** | **dry** | **0** | **100** | **200** | **300** |

*Figure 8. Distribution of clinical lameness cases over calendar months in herd Z. Two situations are given, Z1 (symbol X) and Z2 (symbol O). X represents 3 cases of clinical lameness*

| | | | | | | | | | | | |
|---|---|---|---|---|---|---|---|---|---|---|---|
| O | | | X | | | | | | | | |
| O | O | X | X | | | | | O | | | |
| O | O | X | X | | X | | | O | | | |
| O | O | XO | XO | | X | | | XO | O | | |
| O | XO | XO | XO | X | XO | XO | O | O | XO | O | |
| XO | XO | XO | XO | XO | XO | XO | XO | XO | XO | XO | XO |
| **1** | **2** | **3** | **4** | **5** | **6** | **7** | **8** | **9** | **10** | **11** | **12** |

**calendar months**

limbs, as would be expected from literature research (Russell et al., 1982; Smits et al., 1992). Parities 1 and 2 appear to be more involved than older parities. Younger cows with lameness problems could indicate a problem which possibly already exists and increases during the rearing period. Herd history or farmer's memory could answer this question.

Younger parities have been described in the literature as being more affected and more at risk for lameness (Frankena et al., 1992). Even in young calfhood, animals can already be heavily affected by lameness (Frankena et al., 1992). It should be noted, however, that these patterns of associations can be highly different between regions and definitely between farms. Therefore, within-herd analysis or so-called "site-specific analysis" is very important (Enevoldsen & Mortensen, 1995).

The early and mid-lactation stage cows were more frequently involved in the problem. The former possibly due to the periparturient stress and subsequent negative energy balance coupled to the increasing milk production of the cow. Mid-lactation stage clinical lameness may be the sequela of a preceding subclinical lameness.

The seasonal distribution of clinical cases points to spring and early summer as high incidence periods, which is according to literature reports.

The aforenamed findings of analysis in this herd Z indicate that the periparturient period of cows should be a period of extra attention and care. This attention and care refers to the housing and handling of cows, to nutrition around calving and in the dry period, claw condition. Action appears to be indicated among young stock as well. It is very possible that the origin of the problem of lameness is to be found there.

**Situation in herd Z2:**
In this situation, there is hardly any difference between rear and front legs affected. Front leg disorders often point to housing design failures, specifically of feedbunk height at the feed rack as compared to height of cow's standing floor. In principle, the floor surface behind the feedrack should be at the same height as the floor surface in front of the feedrack ("pasture level"). If not the case, then we may expect trauma in the front claws in cows reaching out for feed. One could say that this situation is a worsening of the situation in herd Z1.

Predominantly older parities are involved in this problem. This could mean that problems are at low level during the first parities and maybe even during the young stock rearing period. On the other hand, if disorders occur, maybe the follow-up and check on treatment effectivity is poor, leaving affected cows to become chronic problem cows with relapsing lameness cases.

The cases of clinical lameness are scattered over the different lactation stages which supports the previous finding of relapsed cases and possible poor treatment results. The problem mainly occurs during the winter or housing season, meaning that exposure to infectious agents is higher as well as to environmental stressors, which is in accordance with literature (Smits et al., 1992; Frankena et al., 1992, 1993; Vermunt & Smart, 1994).

Now that the high risk cows (groups) and periods have been identified, the next step in the decision-making process is to search for additional information at both the cow level and the environment level. This information is needed for determining the putative causes and synthesize conclusions for advice.

Additional information at the cow level refers to the subclinical lameness cases which may be prevalent among the herd. Since there is no correlation between the clinical incidence of lameness (diagnoses) and the prevalence of subclinical lameness (diagnoses), a certain clinical lameness problem may even be larger due to subclinical cases.

The practitioner can check this phenomenon by inspecting the claws in a sample of the herd, say 10% of the cows and record the findings on a herd inventory list (see Chapter 7, part 1). Suppose that in the example herd Z this inventory points to subclinical laminitis among 80% of the sampled cows. Then, the clinical herd diagnosis is extended with a subclinical herd diagnosis, which possibly broadens the scope of action for decision-making.

Furthermore, it is possible that the number of subestrus cows increasing over time, as is shown in Table 3, was a consequence of the lameness problem occurrence. Estrous detection could therefore be used as an indirect indicator for lameness problems. This could be estimated by using a 2 x 2 Table where cows with or without a certain lameness diagnoses are set against cows with low or high number of days open. The crude risk that lame cows are representing for delayed days open can be calculated. This is illustrated in Figure 9.

The aforegiven example of calculating risk is a very crude one. It is obvious that in the case of days open, different other factors may play a role which are left outside the calculation. Multivariate methods should be applied for such calculations but are outside the scope of this text. We refer to Chapter 7, part 3 and Chapter 1, part 4 for further details.

**Breakdown into causative factors: the environment (farm inspection)**

The search for potential causes in the environment has to be combined for both the clinical and the subclinical herd diagnosis.

The farm inspection follows the checklist of factors according to categories such as housing, pasturing, nutrition, microclimate, hygiene and manure handling, management strategies (sire selection, formaline footbathing, ration composition, feedbunk management, health care). An example of such a checklist is given in Appendix . The factors and conditions named in Appendix originate from field surveys among 10.000 cows and 1200 young stock (Frankena et al., 1992-92-93). Among the different surveys performed throughout the world many factors are identical, but sometimes differences occur due to variable husbandry conditions or geographical location (Greenough & Vermunt, 1994; Vermunt & Smart, 1994). Therefore, unambiguous and specific risk factors for all situations cannot be provided here.

*Figure. 9. Example of a 2 x 2 table for calculating crude relative risk in a herd. The relative risk of cows affected by clinical lameness for delayed conception (over 150 days) as compared to cows without a clinical lameness can be calculated as (19/23) / (11/12)= 1.9*

| | | **Cows with days open** | | |
|---|---|---|---|---|
| | | < 150 days | > 150 days | |
| **Cows without clinical lameness** | Yes | 19 | 12 | 31 |
| | No | 11 | 23 | 34 |
| | | 30 | 35 | 65 cows present |

The findings from this farm inspection, which best is done together with the farmer, provide often ample issues for discussion.

On farm Z, situation Z1, the nutrition should be scrutinized because of the laminitis problem. In this evaluation are comprised: ration composition for the different production stages, commodities used, proper mixing procedures, feedbunk management (is ad libitum truly ad libitum? are there feed remainders? are there feed refusals? which quality feed for which cow groups? how often are feeds changed? is it a rapid or gradual change?).

At the same time, the farmer has to decide about the actions to be taken for dermatitis digitalis. Among these are: hygiene improvement, proper manure handling, adjustment of slatters and slots, early diagnosis and treatment.

With respect to the sole ulcers related to either laminitis or interdigital dermatitis, a check has to be performed on proper claw trimming procedures for all those involved. The latter sometimes comprises the professional claw trimmer too!

In situation Z2, where the problem is mainly interdigital dermatitis and sole ulcers the attention has to be focussed on hygiene during the housing period and the provision of proper and functional claws during pasturing and before the housing period starts. Adequate claw trimming is a major element of this advice.

Usually the factors related to the occurrence of digital disorders are largely known. However, they are qualitative in nature, meaning that there is no ranking in relevance nor a priority setting possible on individual farms. For a more detailed elaboration of potential causes and quantification of disease risk contribution of factors we refer to the epidemiological survey mentioned in Chapter 1, part 4.

Such a survey on farms in a veterinary practice may be appropriate too in situations where no data at cow or environment level are available, e.g. on farms where no herd health and production management program is applied yet.

When the information from data inspection, general or specific farm inspection and clinical examination has become available, interpretation and decisions have to be made. This is the last step prior to advice and or action.

## 7.2.4 TREATMENT AND OTHER INTERVENTIONS (ADVICE), FOLLOW-UP

Once a herd lameness diagnosis has been set and potential contributory conditions from the environment identified, subsequent action for treatment or other intervention has to be defined and measures have to be taken for checking on recovery at next farm visits and consistently assessing the situation.

### Treatment and other interventions (advice)

For **digital dermatitis** early detection and rapid treatment is imperative. Local treatment with antibiotics is indicated, whereafter the cows should be brought into dry environment for at least 30 min. Close attention for detecting new cases is warrented. Hygiene standards should be screened on the farm, not in the last place among maiden heifers and pregnant heifers. Most of the outbreaks occur during the housing period. Irregular slatters causing at least microtrauma predispose for the disease; the same is valid for highly slippery concrete floors. Purchased animals may introduce the disease into a herd. Another factor is the manure handling. Cows standing in the slurry may experience a softening and weakening of the digital skin and adverse effects of ammonia on the skin. There seems to be a breed disposition for this disease with Holstein cattle being more affected than other breeds. Formaline foot bathing, if applied, should be withdrawn for at least 10 days in case of a dermatitis digitalis outbreak. The more chronic cases look like footrot. Therefore, proper diagnosing is paramount. Chronic cases often do not respond as desired, maybe because of induced resistance against the antibiotics applied. In cases of large outbreaks it can be indicated to treat the herd as a whole by applying antibiotic foot bathing for 3 days. Inspite of much research, the causative agent is not detected, spirochaetes being still the most likely causative organisms.

For **laminitis** the areas for attention are nutrition in general (feed composition; ration balancing) and rapid feed changes in particular (feed bunk management). Additionally, traumatic conditions in the pasture (metalled walking path) or the housing facilities (poor slatter conditions) may be involved. Especially around the calving period the cow is at highest risk for laminitis (Mortensen, 1994). Body condition during late lactation and in the dry period can be a signal for metabolic disturbances. The feed supply increase after calving should therefore be gradual. The feed of high quality, especially the roughage. Metabolic disorders should be avoided as much as possible (see Chapters 3 and 4 about nutrition and disorders). Functional trimming of all cows must be performed (Toussaint Raven et al., 1985).

For **interdigital dermatitis**, aspects of infection burden become more relevant. Hygiene standards in the cubicles and walking areas must be screened, as well as the manure handling on concrete floors. Infection burden is highest during the housing period due to infection build-up. Especially subclinical dermatitis interdigitalis is prevalent among cows during housing (sometimes upto 90% of the herd, Frankena et al. 1992). The higher the parity of cows, the higher the prevalence of the disorder. Screening should already be done during the rearing period of the calves (see Chapter 2). Formaline foot bathing is curative for the disorder; it should be applied every 3 weeks for 3 to 5 consecutive days at a concentration of 3 - 5%. At the same time the trimming technique of e.g. the farmer or professional claw trimmer should be evaluated.

The **phlegmona interdigitalis** is not a true claw disorder. It is the affected lamina propria which is causing the disorder involving Dichelobacter nodosus and Fusobacterium necrophorum. Claw horn production is not affected. Distinction should be made between this disorder and dermatitis (inter)digitalis for proper treatment and preventive action. Sometimes only one, other times several cows are affected. Clinical lameness is usually peracute. Treatment with antibiotics for 1 or 2 days makes the cow recover very rapidly without too much impact on milk yield. Claws are seldomly affected twice due to local immunity build-up (Peterse, 1992). Calves too may be affected severely. A relationship of this infection with the Dichelobacter nodosus infection in footrot points to poor hygienic conditions in the housing period.

## Follow up

After the advice has been given and measures taken, it is needed that the practitioner deals with a close follow up. This is necessary not only for checking on the effects of measures taken, but also for stimulating the farmer's motivation to keep on going. The latter is highly important because effects of measures against lameness are not to be expected on the short term. At the other hand, measures with regard to housing facilities and management are not expected to be taken all at once.

Therefore, the practitioner should pay attention to the evolution of the lameness problem and to the primary and secondary performance figures during subsequent farm visits. Essentially, he folllows the same routes of evaluation as pointed out in this chapter. During the farm visits he should also screen cows for recovery and check the farmer for having taken the measures advised earlier. It often is a matter of repeating the story and pressing the farmer to take action. This will work out easier if the farmer knows that his practitioner will turn back to the problem area each subsequent visit.

Evolution of the lameness problem can be evaluated by means of the *routinely available records* as presented in chapter 7, part 1 (farm diary, 12-monthly list, examination list, computer output). The practitioner has to stick to the problem, as long as parts of the problem remain. If the problem has been overcome it is equally important that the practitioner clearly discusses this with the farmer, praising him for the succesfull outcome of this efforts.

## EPILOGUE

Interpretation of analysis results requires skills, knowledge and experience of the practitioner or his consultants. When for example skills on applied epidemiology are not available, the practitioner should contact an epidemiological unit within a diagnostic lab or veterinary school. This, however, is only applicable if the farmer participates in a HH & PM program and, hence, data is available. This was shortly illustrated by using a 2x2 Table and estimating the crude relative risk of prolonged days open in case of clinical lameness as compared to cows without being affected by a clinical lameness.

If a farmer does not participate in a HH & PM program and confronts the practitioner with a lameness problem he wants to solve, the hampering of lack of information is substantial. Then first a herd inventory should be made for clinical and subclinical digital disorders, while at the same time the farm diary should be introduced to keep track of occurring lameness problems. Farm inspection is coupled to these activities next in order to obtain a herd diagnosis, broaden insight into animals at and farm areas of risk and provide the justified procedure for decision-making and follow up. The reliance on the memory of a farmer over the past 6 or 12 months with respect to lameness cases can be heavily biased (recall bias) and is therefore not advised here. If the basic information is collected and interpreted, the practitioner has to discuss with the farmer the target levels he wants to achieve. Sometimes this goal-oriented approach is not familiar to the farmer. In that case it is advisable to design a path where progression towards performance targets is set at low pace but gradually increasing depending on farmer's skills, motivation for cooperation and activity.

As can be noted from the preceding paragraphs, most analyses are retrospective in nature since they are based on historic data. Additional activities such as herd inventory of subclinical lameness cases, farm inspection or epidemiological survey are usually cross-sectional in nature. This means that the time component in the relationship between cause and disorder is missing, resulting sometimes in insufficiently conclusive or inconclusive findings. Often nothing better is available and therefore it provides a first practical tool to the practitioner to focus the farmer's attention on specific fields of dairy farming and on management topics, which often can easily be adapted to a better level. As such it contributes to an overall improvement of the health status of feet and legs.

Prevention of lameness problems on the other hand, starts at the point of potential risk factors on the farm (see Appendix and Chapter 7, part 3). An adequate preventive action leads to primary and secondary performance parameters which will be of good quality and according to preset target figures. This means that the practitioner has to monitor constantly what is going on at the different areas of farming, both cow and environment related. Farm inspection therefore has a major role in the prevention of lameness. Curative treatment of clinical lameness cases often comes too late and takes too much time to repair a problem. Especially when we know that lameness already occurs to a large extent among calves.

Risk factors for lameness diagnoses are many and are highly different between diagnoses, either in nature or in direction (risk increasing or decreasing). Therefore, one should address lameness not as a whole syndrome, but in a diagnosis-specific way. Large differences may exist between countries or states due to geographical or ecological differences or differing animal husbandry and management strategies. That is why an uniform checklist for all risk factors for all lameness diagnoses cannot be given.

Finally, it should be clear that a herd with a high incidence of clinical lameness is prone to problems in the area of estrus detection. Hence, it is warranted to check reproductive performance figures as well as a cross-check for (subclinical or clinical) lameness. The same is valid for body condition scores and, to a certain extent, for milk production. Therefore, an integrated approach to herd health and production management is in fact the only way to deal with a lameness problem adequately.

*For references see part 3 of this Chapter.*

# APPENDIX

## GENERAL OVERVIEW OF CONDITIONS RELATED TO LAMENESS

* **Animal related conditions:**

| | |
|---|---|
| Parity: | 1 |
| | 2 |
| | 3 and higher |
| Lactation stage: | < 30 days |
| | 31 - 60 days |
| | > 60 days |
| Production stage: | lactating |
| | dry |
| Breed: | > 50% Holstein Frisian |
| | > 50% Dutch Frisian |
| | > 50% MeuseRhineYssel |

* **Environment related conditions:**

| | |
|---|---|
| Herd size: | 41 - 50 cows |
| | 51 - 60 cows |
| | 61 cows and more |
| Stocking density: | > 2 cows/ha |
| | < 2 cows/ha |
| Milk yield: | < 8000 kg/cow |
| | > 8000 kg/cow |
| Calving interval: | < 391 days |
| | > 391 days |
| Disinfection tub used for claws: | 3 days |
| | > 3 days |
| | < 3 days |
| Average concentrates supply: | < 5 kg/cow/day |
| | > 5 kg/cow/day |
| Concentrates supply at 30 kg milk: | < 7.7 kg/cow/day |
| | > 7.7 kg/cow/day |

| | |
|---|---|
| Barn floor condition: | smooth |
| | rough |
| Loose slatters: | yes |
| | no |
| Cubicle bedding: | straw |
| | woodshaves |

Cubicle floor: Enkamat/concrete/rubber/soil.
Cubicle width and length in cm.
Use of chalk in the boxes: yes or no.
Feed bunk level higher/equal to/lower than exercise area.
Grassland soil type is: sand, clay, sandy clay, or peat.
Land heigth is high or low.
Liver fluke history present on farm: yes or no.

| | |
|---|---|
| Cubicle cleaning performed: | once daily |
| | twice daily |
| Slatter cleaning performed: | once daily |
| | twice daily |
| Walking distance to pasture: | < 200 m |
| | 200 - 400 m |
| | > 400 m |

*Note: commonly one class per item is chosen as reference class*

# 7.3 MONITORING FOOT HEALTH: CASE STUDY ON LAMENESS

Jos P.T.M. Noordhuizen[1], Klaas Frankena[1], Elsbeth N. Noordhuizen-Stassen[2], and Carsten Enevoldsen[3]

[1] Department of Animal Husbandry, Wageningen Agricultural University, Marijkeweg 40, P.O. Box 338, 6700 AH Wageningen, The Netherlands
[2] Department of Herd Health and Reproduction, School of Veterinary Medicine, University of Utrecht, Yalelaan 7, 3584 CL Utrecht, The Netherlands
[3] Danish Institute of Animal Science, Department of Animal Health and Welfare, Research Centre Foulum, P.O.Box 39, DK-8830 Tjele, Denmark

## 7.3.1 INTRODUCTION

Lameness is a complex disease syndrome, with different problem areas (Greenough et al., 1981). The HH & PM practitioner may be asked regularly to analyse and to solve specific lameness problems. Lameness problems should be analysed following a protocol consisting of description of the complaint, history taking, clinical and farm inspection, probabilistic herd diagnosis, inventorying contributing factors, and intervention. Recommendations to the farmer should be based on the outcomes of the whole process of analysis. They may be aimed at intervention or preventive actions. The lameness problem described in part 3 of this Chapter is based on a herd lameness problem that is fictitious but based on field data.

## 7.3.2 COMPLAINT OF THE FARMER

The farm comprises 59 Holstein-Friesian dairy cows, 15 maiden heifers between 1 and 2 years of age, and 20 dairy calves less than 1 year old. The average milk production per cow per year is 8300 kg, with 4.92% butterfat and 3.57% milk protein.
Lactating cows and heifers and dry cows are housed in a loose housing system with slatted floor. All lactating cows and heifers are kept in one production group, and dry cows in a separate group. Pregnant heifers are housed in a separate barn. During the winter housing period the cows are fed grass and corn silage, while concentrates are fed through two automatic concentrates supply units in the barn. During the summer season the cows are pastured day and night.
The farmer is managing the milking process, grassland utilization and grassland care, and animal nutrition, while the farmer's wife assists in feeding the calves and in other incidental tasks on the farm.

During a visit to farm H, the farmer confronts the practitioner with a recent outbreak of clinical lameness. The number of cows seen in estrus has declined also.

The practitioner has been consulted with some frequency lately for lameness cases in individual cows. The current outbreak occurred despite regular formaline footbathing, and a twice-yearly, whole-herd claw trimming strategy. During a discussion between farmer and practitioner it was agreed that the problem should be analyzed and solved.

### 7.3.3 HISTORY TAKING AND PROBLEM DEFINITION

The following primary parameters were derived or calculated from the recorded data (see Tables 1, 2, 3):

a. The average number of cows present over the preceding year: 43
b. The number of cows with one or more clinical lameness events: 12 (or 28% over cows present)
c. The total number of clinical cow cases: 23 (or 53% over cows present)
d. The number of individual legs with lameness (including repeated cases): 31
e. The number of cows culled for reasons of lameness: zero.

The farm's annual target indices for clinical lameness were 20%, 25% and 10% for categories (b), (c) and (e) respectively. Actual lameness occurrences exceeded two out of these three indices, substantiating the existence of a clinical lameness problem on farm H.

Secondary performance indices were as follows:

f. 21 cases of sole ulcer
g. 3 cases of dermatitis interdigitalis
h. 1 case of laminitis
i. 1 case of Mortellaro disease (dermatitis digitalis).

Other diagnoses were not recorded. Most clinical lameness cases occurred in older cows and in hind claws. About the same number of cases was observed during the housing period (November - April) as during the pasture period (May - November). Clinical lameness cases were not evenly distributed over the entire lactation period; no cases were seen during the dry period.

The next step in the investigation procedure is to check whether certain cow groups experienced more lameness than others. Therefore, the herd is split into a group with, and a group without clinical lameness cases. The results are shown in Table 3. It appeared that 5 cows from the lameness group have been kept open by the farmer versus 1 cow from the no-lameness group, all for different reasons.

Other disease, such as mastitis (9 cows) and cystic ovarian disease (12 cows) occurred twice and three times more often among lame than among no-lame cows, respectively. Total number of services and number of services per conception were higher in the lame group, while 1-st service pregnancy rates were comparable. There were 4 cases of milk fever in the herd over the preceding year, all in the lame group. Twice as many cows in the lameness group have been culled than from the no-lame group; although the reason for culling was never given as lameness.

*Table 1. Analysis of clinical claw disorders over 1 year (lactation stage; legs; diagnoses)*

| **Distribution of first lameness cases over stage of lactation** | | **Distribution over legs** | |
|---|---|---|---|
| 0 - 30 days: | 4 cows | Right front: | 6 cases |
| 31 - 60 days: | 3 cows | Right rear: | 8 cases |
| 61 - 90 days: | 1 cow | Left rear: | 10 cases |
| 91 - 120 days: | 1 cow | Left front: | 7 cases |
| 121 - 210 days: | 1 cow | | |
| 211 - 300 days: | 1 cow | | |
| > 300 days: | 1 cow | | |
| dry period: | 0 cows | | |
| Total: | 12 cows | | |

| **Distribution over diagnoses** | | **Symptoms** | |
|---|---|---|---|
| Interdigital: | 0 | Sole ulcer: | 21 |
| Phlegmona: | 5 | Laminitis: | 1 |
| Interdig derm: | 3 | Digital dermatitis: | 1 |
| Periarthritis: | 0 | Other: | 0 |

First conclusion is that a clinical lameness problem exists on this farm. The lameness problem also seems to be associated with the performance in fertility, health, and milk production. More information is needed to arrive at a proper diagnosis and to identify potential contributory factors. Therefore, further clinical and possibly subclinical inspection is warranted.

## 7.3.4. INSPECTIONS

### Data inspection

In order to establish the presence and extent of a lameness problem, the available data including primary and secondary herd performance parameters (see Chapter 7, part 1) need to be screened. The usefulness of data inspection depends on the quantity and quality of data available on the farm. Relevant information can be obtained from computerized records if available, or taken from a fertility-health wall chart if one is kept. A more laborious method is to collect the data from a farm diary, if one exists. Data covering one full year period is necessary to evaluate seasonal effects and to obtain a general overview of the herd's performance indices. Data should be grouped according to diagnoses, cow groups affected, legs or claws affected, season of occurrence, parity and stage of lactation, and cullings for lameness reason, such as elaborated in

*Table 2. Analysis of clinical claw disorders over 1 year in herd H (parities; seasons)*

**Distribution over Parities**

| Parity | no. Cows | Lameness (lactation) | Lameness (dry-period) |
|---|---|---|---|
| 1 | 18 | 1 | – |
| 2 | 12 | 2 | – |
| 3 | 4 | 2 | – |
| 4 | 6 | 4 | – |
| 5 | 6 | 1 | – |
| 6 | 2 | 2 | – |
| ≥7 | 0 | – | – |

**Distribution over Seasons**

| | Jan | Feb | Mar | Apr | May | Jun | Jul | Aug | Sep | Oct | Nov | Dec |
|---|---|---|---|---|---|---|---|---|---|---|---|---|
| Cows/month | 41 | 39 | 37 | 38 | 39 | 38 | 40 | 42 | 48 | 50 | 52 | 55 |
| Cows calved | 2 | 4 | 1 | 2 | 6 | 3 | 3 | 3 | 7 | 5 | 0 | 4 |
| Heifers calved | 1 | 0 | 0 | 1 | 1 | 0 | 0 | 6 | 3 | 0 | 4 | 1 |
| Cases | 0 | 5 | 3 | 1 | 3 | 1 | 1 | 4 | 2 | 1 | 1 | 1 |

Chapter 7 part 2. With the aid of computer programs (management information systems) categorisation of the information is simplified.

If records have not been kept, the intensity of the investigation will be diminished and, accordingly, the recommendations will be more tentative. Improved record keeping should be recommended in order to support evaluation and refinement of the diagnosis, and recommendations in the future, while concurrently addressing the original complaint. This is called parallel tracking of immediate and midlong term objectives.

In this problem herd, data collected during regular herd health and production management services will be used. The approach to be followed when good records are not available has been addressed in part 2 of Chapter 7.

### Clinical and subclinical inspection

The most prevailing clinical diagnosis was sole ulcer. Sole ulcers originate from either dermatitis interdigitalis or laminitis. These latter could be diagnosed subclinically by further clinical inspection of a sample of the herd during the farm visit. Since there is no correlation between typical clinical and subclinical digital disorders, investigation of the predominance of clinical or subclinical claw disorders is indicated.

An inventory of all subclinical diagnoses during the twice-yearly routine herd claw trimming by the professional trimmer can be made for that purpose. An example of

*Table 3. Cows with clinical lameness (Lame) and cows without lameness (L-No). "Farm" includes all cows, C = cows, H = heifers*

| Period is 1 year<br>Calving Data | | Farm | Lame | L-No |
|---|---|---|---|---|
| (1) | # C/H calved | 40/17 | 16/7 | 24/10 |
| (2) | calving-calving interval | 374 | 370 | 378 |
| (3) | kept open | 6/1 | 5/1 | 1/0 |
| (4) | cystic ovarian disease | 12 | 9 | 3 |
| **Insemination Data** | | | | |
| (1) | no. C/H inseminated | 33/16 | 11/5 | 22/10 |
| (2) | efficiency figure | 1.57 | 1.46 | 1.68 |
| **Udder Health** | | | | |
| (1) | C/H clinical mastitis (%) | 7(12) | 4(17) | 3(9) |
| (2) | cow cases mastitis | 9 | 6 | 3 |
| **Claw / Leg Disorders** | | | | |
| (1) | C/H lameness | 15 | 15 | – |
| (2) | cow cases | 23 | 23 | – |
| (3) | leg cases | 31 | 31 | – |
| **Metabolic Diseases** | | | | |
| (1) | hypocalcemia | 4 | 4 | – |
| **Culling Data** | | | | |
| (1) | avg. no. of cows present | 43 | 21 | 22 |
| (2) | death | 1 | – | 1 |
| (3) | udder health | 3 | 3 | – |
| (4) | reproduction | 2 | 1 | 1 |
| (5) | age | 1 | 1 | – |
| (6) | other disorders | 1 | 1 | – |
| (7) | low production | 5 | 3 | 2 |

such an inventory list was given earlier (see in part 1 of this Chapter).

The hind claws of 40 cows were inspected during routine herd claw trimming on farm H. The results of this procedure were:

- dermatis digitalis: 1 clinical and 3 subclinical cases
- dermatitis interdigitalis: 1 clinical and 35 subclinical cases
- laminitis: 18 subclinical cases and 1 clinical case
- sole ulcer: 4 clinical cases
- other non-specific disorders: 6 cases in combination with dermatitis interdigitalis.

Subclinical dermatitis interdigitalis was the predominant diagnosis, followed by subclinical laminitis. Both of these conditions may lead to sole ulcers. The results also show that predominant clinical diagnoses and subclinical diagnoses are not necessarily the same. Furthermore, the lameness problem is larger at the subclinical level than at the clinical level. This is of great importance to both the practitioner and the farmer. The results direct the practitioner's attention to dermatitis interdigitalis and demonstrate to the farmer that a well-defined problem exists in his herd. Since causality of most digital disorders is multifactorial in nature, addressing the factors contributing to the occurrence of the specific lameness problem is indicated. In this case this refers to factors contributing to the occurrence of dermatitis interdigitalis and of laminitis.

### Farm inspection

The next step in the procedure is to perform a farm inspection together with the farmer, examining farm conditions, environmental and management factors known to be potentially related to the occurrence of dermatitis interdigitalis and laminitis. In Appendix of part 2 of this Chapter a putative list of factors was presented. Factors fall into categories such as housing and equipment, nutrition, management. The farm inspection might yield other, relevant information for proper decision-making and advice.

**Housing:** Cows and young stock are housed together in a freestall barn, with the dry cows housed separately in the same barn. Pregnant heifers are housed in a separate barn. Calves up to 10 weeks of age are kept in individual boxes with straw bedding. Older young stock are kept in pens with slatted floors. For the 49 lactating cows there are 50 places available at the feed rack and 48 cubicles. The barn is equipped with 2 concentrate supply stations and 3 drinking water troughs. Cubicles are of the Super Comfort type, measuring 110 x 225 cm (wxl) and a shoulder rail height of 110 cm. Cubicle floor is concrete; sawdust bedding material is added by the dairyman twice daily. The exercise area behind the feed rack is 285 cm wide and equipped with a slatted floor, without a manure shovel. Slats are 13 cm wide, slots are 4 cm wide. Many slats appeared to be irregular, sometimes loose and in many cases worn out. The pregnant heifer barn was more or less in the same situation.
**Nutrition:** The basic ration for lactating animals comprised 10 kg corn silage,

*ad libitum* grass silage and 0.6 kg soya during the housing period. Dry cows and pregnant heifers received grass silage of lower quality. Dry cows are introduced into the lactating herd about 1 week prior to expected calving, and pregnant heifers about 1 week after calving. During the pasture season cows are grazed day and night. The distance between pasture plots and milking parlor is 600 m in average. The path is of stones mixed with grass. Pasture soil type is clay.

Concentrates are supplied individually using the 2 supply stations in the barn. Cows receive between 0.5 and 14 kg of concentrates. Dry cows do not receive concentrates. At the day of calving the cows receive 2 kg of concentrates; this supply is increased 1 kg per day thereafter until a level determined by production is reached.

**Hygiene:** There is a stationary walk-through type footbath (110 x 72 x 15 cm, lxwxd) at the exit of the milking parlor. The footbath content is replenished every 3 - 4 weeks with 3 - 5% formaline. The formaline content of the solution lasts about 2 days. Twice yearly, the hind claws of all cows in the herd are trimmed. Footbathing is resumed two weeks after this routine trimming. Walking areas and cubicles are manually cleaned each day, while the whole barn is fully cleaned once a year using high pressure hot water cleaning.

### 7.3.5 EVALUATION OF INFORMATION

Summing up the information gained this far in the investigation process leads to the following preliminary conclusions as to link factors to both dermatitis interdigitalis and to laminitis:

- clinical lameness was observed in 28% of the cows during one year. In the lame group of cows more animals were culled; albeit for stated reasons other than lameness. More animals in the group with lameness were affected by mastitis, milk fever and cystic ovarian disease, which could have contributed to the culling. During routine claw trimming, subclinical lameness diagnosis was established in 90% of the cows.
- cubicles are 10 cm narrower than the recommended width. Condition of the exercise area was poor. The footbath was smaller than the recommended size of 100 cm width, 300 - 500 cm length and 15 cm deep. The fluid level and concentration of the fluid was not adjusted from day to day.
- the maximum concentrate supply was achieved in 14 days after calving, meaning that daily increase was more than the recommended 0.5 kg increase. Heifers were brought into the lactating herd rather late, resulting in possible stress situations at the beginning of their lactation.

Following this, more general inspection of the different farming areas it is up to the practitioner, in discussion with the farmer, to either initiate a more in-depth survey of risk factors or proceed with recommendations on the basis of the information already gathered. For a more in-depth survey we refer to the respective paragraph later in this Chapter.

Basis for further activity is that the probable herd diagnosis is that clinical cases of sole ulcer are caused primarily by dermatitis interdigitalis and secondarily by laminitis.

### 7.3.6 DIFFERENTIAL LIST OF CAUSES

Laminitis is primarily a metabolic disorder of the deeper layers under the sole horn. Hind claws are predominantly affected. Local edema is a first sign of disturbance in the peracute stage, which usually begins around calving. The subacute stage is seen most often. Haemorrhages in the sole can be found during claw inspection. Overt lameness is seldom seen, but this type may lead to deviating standing posture and hence disturbed weight bearing, deviating horn shoe and careful walking ("walking on eggs"). Due to edema and disturbed horn growth, mainly in the outer rear claws, lesions such as sole ulcers and double sole may develop. These lesions may lead to overt lameness.

Laminitis is a multifactorial disorder (Mortensen, 1994). Main contributing factors include stress due to calving, udder edema, infections (e.g. elsewhere in the body), digestive and metabolic disorders (ketosis), suboptimal nutrition, claw trauma. Recent publications have reported an estimated laminitis prevalence of 37% among calves between 2 and 12 month of age (Frankena et al., 1992), while cows on pasture had an estimated prevalence of 15% versus 77% during the housing period (Frankena et al., 1991).

Dermatitis interdigitalis is caused by an infection of the interdigital skin and tissues at the rear of the claw with Dichelobacter (Bacteroides) nodosus. Horn growth is affected by the initial inflammation. Excess and abnormal horn growth in the rear of the claw leads to deviating standing posture and to loss of horn function. Lameness is often seen in the development of dermatitis interdigitalis, but also when sole ulcers gradually develop. The main contributing factors are: high animal density leading to a build-up of the infectious agent, poor floor conditions, suboptimal hygienic standards, and breed. Recent studies have indicated that 66% of calves between 2 and 12 month were subclinically affected by the disorder (Frankena et al., 1993), while over 90% of the cows were affected (Frankena et al., 1991). The foregoing conditions largely apply to the farm under investigation.

### 7.3.7 FINAL CAUSE LIST

Based on the analysis of available information and the farm and clinical inspection findings it is concluded that the lameness problem at farm H is caused by dermatitis interdigitalis and laminitis.

### 7.3.8 INTERVENTION AND PROGNOSIS

To combat the dermatitis interdigitalis several measures have to be taken. The path between the milking parlor and pasture should be restored. The footbath is too small to be effective and the formaline should be replenished according to recommendations.

It seems worthwhile to trim the claws of pregnant heifers before introduction into the lactating herd. Introduction of heifers into the herd should be done no later than 3 - 4 weeks before calving to allow the rumen to adapt and avoid metabolic stress. Routine herd claw trimming should be done twice yearly with regular intervals in between. Manure handling in the barn should be carried out properly. Floor conditions in the exercise area and cubicle floors should be adjusted when and where possible, because e.g. irregular slats may lead to trauma and lesions.

To prevent laminitis it is most important that the herd health status is kept at the highest level. Prevention of milk fever, bacteriological infections (retained afterbirth, endometritis, mastitis), and ketosis should be given high priority since laminitis is also a secondary complication.

Nutrition should be discussed with an expert nutritionist. Feeding management deserves attention too because the maximum concentrate supply appears too high for the farm's production level and the increase to full feed after calving is too rapid.

In addition to the predominant (subclinical) lameness problem, the practitioner must address the current clinical problem which originally was the basis for the farmer's complaint. Proper treatment of the sole ulcers by the practitioner and or a professional claw trimmer is the first intervention for these cows. Subsequent follow-up of recovery of these cows the next step. It should be made clear to the farmer that clinically lame cows need more time to recover than the time it takes to prevent subclinical cases from becoming clinical.

Furthermore, it is obvious that in this case the attention of the practitioner goes beyond the lameness problem itself. Therefore, the integrated farm approach as proposed through Herd Health and Production Management programs is important for a high succes rate.

When these issues are addressed properly and advice is translated into action, a reduction in the number of clinical and subclinical lameness cases in this herd can be expected.

### 7.3.9 FOLLOW-UP OF THE LAMENESS PROBLEM

During regular herd health visits to the farm, the herd performance with regard to the occurrence of lameness should be checked by means of the primary and secondary performance indices. At the same time the performance indices in the area of reproduction, milk production and health can be monitored to indirectly assess the occurrence of events that increase the risk of dermatitis interdigitalis and laminitis. If performance indices remain at an unsatisfactory level, the recommendations have to be revisited. Effects of recommended measures should be evaluated; proper implementation of recommended measures should be evaluated. These recommendations should be written again on the farm visit reports and/or examination list to properly follow through and to serve as a reminder for the farmer. This is an important motivation to carry on for the farmer. At the same time it helps convince him, by means of repetition, that action is mainly focused on the newly calved cows and far less on the existing clinical cases. The former are indicators for the success rate of recommendations and preventive measures taken, while the latter should be checked as a measure of recovery and to evaluate the effectiveness of the recommended corrective measures. Usually it will take some time before effects are observed; the farmer should be made aware of this fact in order to avoid unrealistic short-term expectations (Vermunt and Smart, 1994).

### 7.3.10 IN-DEPTH SURVEY FOR RISK FACTORS

A further investigation of risk factors potentially related to digital disorders could be indicated if more farms in the veterinary practice suffer from severe lameness, if the lameness problem situation in a herd is especially severe, or if the general inspection and clinical inspection followed by advice and measures appear not to yield the desired improvement in the performance indices. In such an instant, an epidemiological survey is indicated. Examples are given by Greenough and Vermunt (1994) and Wells et al. (1995). Such a survey is an observational study (see Chapter 1, part 4) with 2 major elements: (1) an inventory of clinical/subclinical cases of a given disorder, (2) a questionnaire comprising more detailed questions directly related to risk factors. Such questions may be interview based or based on the practitioner's own observation or on-farm measurement.

The objectives of such a survey are to:

(a) obtain a better description of the lameness problem,
(b) define high risk cow groups more specifically,
(c) get more insight in those factors that contribute to disease occurrence and to quantify that contribution. The latter can be used to rank the factors according to their impact and hence set priorities in the program of combat/prevention of the disorder.

The inventory list used for recording disorders at the routine herd claw trimming can be used for recording the claw health state of animals upon examination, either having or not having a lameness diagnosis (see part 1 of this Chapter). Then, the practitioner has to develop the questionnaire. Categories of questions can be derived from a general list of putative factors such as presented earlier (Appendix in part 2 of this Chapter). However, in this case the categories have to be more refined and the questions detailed. The practitioner has to select the most relevant items from this list and convert these into questions. The questionnaire is administered by the practitioner or one of his (trained!) technicians on the farms in the survey. The data from the questionnaire are entered into a computer, e.g. using a spreadsheet program, and analyzed according to valid methods. If needed, support for such analyses can be obtained

*Table 4. An example of results from a survey on risk factors potentially contributing to the occurrence of dermatitis interdigitalis in dairy herds*

| | | **ß** | **OR=e$^{ß}$** | **AF%** |
|---|---|---|---|---|
| Parity | 1 | 0.92* | 2.5 | 60 |
| | 2 | 0.72* | 2.1 | 52 |
| Lactational stage | < 60 dim | 0.47$^{o}$ | 1.6 | 38 |
| | 60 - 120 dim | 0.19 | 1.2 | |
| Breed | > 50%HF | 0.21 | 1.2 | |
| | > 50%FH | -0.28 | 0.7 | |
| | > 50%MRIJ | -1.04* | 0.5 | |
| | other | -2.08* | 0.1 | |
| | 50%HF x 50%FH | 0 | 1 | |
| Herd size < 50 | | -0.06 | 0.9 | |
| > 70 | | -0.94* | 0.4 | |
| Ave. milk yield (continuous) | | -0.0 * | < 1 | |
| Footrot present | | 0.72* | 2.1 | 52 |
| Sole ulcer present | | -0.56$^{o}$ | 0.5 | |
| Interdigital hyperplasia present | | 1.82* | 6.2 | 84 |
| Selection for better leg conformation | | -0.01 | 0.99 | |
| Selection on claw pigment | | -0.61$^{o}$ | 0.5 | |
| Cubicle cleaning | > twice/day | 0.16 | 1.2 | |
| Cows sleeping on slatters | | 0.87* | 2.4 | |
| Use of chalk | | 0.28 | 1.3 | |
| Formalin foothbath present | | -0.24 | 0.7 | |
| Slat width | < 126 mm | -0.22(*) | 0.8 | |
| Slat width | < 40 mm | 0 ($^{o}$) | 1 | |
| Slat surface rough | | 0.30 | 0.30$^{o}$ | 1.3 |
| Irregular slatters present | | -0.21 | 0.8 | |
| Cubicle width | < 110 cm | -0.46 | 0.8 | |
| | > 110 cm | -0.30 | 0.7 | |
| Cubicle length | < 220 cm | 0.11 | 1.1 | |
| | > 220 cm | 0.55* | 1.7 | |
| Shoulderrail height (continuous) | | -0.05* | 0.9 | |
| Cubicle partition type: R-type | | 0.47* | 1.6 | 38 |
| other: | | 0.50* | 1.6 | 38 |
| Access to pasture limited | | 0.78$^{o}$ | 2.2 | 55 |
| Soil type grassland: peat | | 0.08 | 1.1 | |
| Walking distance on stony path | | 0.0 | 1 | |
| Hours outside in pasture (continuous) | | 0.08* | 1.1 | 9 |

*Remarks:*

** = significance level $P < 0.05$*

*$^{o}$ = significance level $P < 0.10$*

*OR > 1 means the risk is increased in the exposed animals (risk factor)*

*OR < 1 means the risk is decreased in the exposed animals (preventive factor)*

*OR = 1 means: no association between exposure to the factor and the disease*

*AF is the percentage of the disease occurrence which can be attributed to the exposure to the specific factor.*

through diagnostic labs or veterinary schools with an epidemiology unit.

Basic measures of epidemiological effect are the relative risk (RR) and the Odds Ratio (OR), an approximation of the RR. Also logistic regression coefficients, Beta, which can be converted into OR, and confidence intervals are obtained or statistical significance (p-value) tested. Attributable fraction (AF) can also be estimated. These parameters have been addressed in part 4 of Chapter 1 and have been further elaborated by Martin et al. (1987).

For this particular situation we retain OR as the outcome parameter for reasons of clarity and simplicity. The OR expresses the likelihood that the presence of a factor increases (OR > 1) or decreases (OR < 1) the likelihood of occurrence of a disorder as compared to the likelihood when that factor is absent. It is always a matter of comparison. In the example dermatitis digitalis is the outcome parameter (the disorder), while the answers to the questions are the various (classes of) factors involved. An example of the results of analysis of potential risk factors for dermatitis interdigitalis is given in Table 4. Complex interrelations among different health disorders and claw health and development in claw health over time in a herd can also be described effectively through such a within and between herds approach (Enevoldsen and Mortensen, 1995).

Factors increasing the risk for dermatitis digitalis in this survey population (Table 4) of herds appear to be, among others:

- parity 1 and 2 (as compared to older parities),
- the first half of the lactation period (as compared to the second half),
- Holstein breed (as compared to other breeds),
- concurrent dermatitis interdigitalis (as compared to the absence of it),
- presence of interdigital hyperplasia or tyloma (as compared to the absence),
- the phenomenon that cows sleep on slats (as compared to cows not sleeping onslats),
- the use of chalk in the cubicle bedding (as compared to the non-use),
- rough slat surface (as compared to good slat condition),
- cubiciles too long or too short (as compared to a proper size), and
- limited access to pasture (as compared to free access).

As stated before, there can be large differences in risk factors between regions as can be learned from literature (Frankena et al., 1992/1993, Wells et al., 1995). These are the factors that could be suitable for corrective or preventive action. Complex interrelations in herds between different health disorders and both claw health and change in claw health over time can also be described effectively through within and between herds approaches (Enevoldsen and Mortensen, 1995). Next step is to go back to the farm of concern and evaluate which factors from the survey apply specifically to that particular farm. Discussions between farmer and practitioner can be strongly supported by presenting cow lameness records together with other health related events in a graphical format (Thysen and Enevoldsen, 1996). A further discussion with the farmer about the risk factors which are prevailing on a particular farm may lead to a plan of action, that is tailor-made to that farm.

## EPILOGUE

Practically spoken, the exposure factor with the highest OR will also show the highest AF. Those factors could be the focus of the first step in the problem solving approach. Eliminating or manipulating those factors may substantially contribute to resolution of the dermatitis digitalis problems. Yet, this approach is not a panacea. Causality cannot always be established in a justified way. For example, the presence of sole ulcer does not indicate the cause or the consequences. Was sole ulcer prevalent before the occurrence of dermatitis digitalis? Or, was it vice versa? In the case of interdigital hyperplasia it can be different. Since this is a chronic condition that spreads the digits of the foot, both mechanical problems and increased susceptibility may occur. When interpreting this type of survey data, one should always bear in mind the most important of Evans' postulates regarding the aspects of causality (see Chapter 1, part 4 on applied epidemiology):

- are the results of the study repeatable and consistent when the survey is performed at another location but under identical conditions?
- does exposure to the factor preceed the disease occurrence (time component)?
- is the strength of the association between factor and disease great (narrow confidence interval)?
- is there a dose-effect relationship (more exposure = more disease)?
- is the outcome of the analysis biologically plausible?

Only with a sound logical and biological reasoning is it feasible for the practitioner to design a solution for the problems encountered during his herd health and production management program. There are always management factors or housing conditions that can be altered. At the same time there are always factors that cannot be changed, such as breed or housing system. Finally, there are factors that can only be changed slowly, such as genetic resistance (McDaniel, 1994).
When proposing changes to the farmer, the decision must be justifiable and based on cost-effectiveness. This can be done by presenting the proposed changes together with their estimated costs and potential benefits. Techniques of partial budgetting, cost-benefit analysis or simulation can be used to estimate returns on investments in proposed changes (Dijkhuizen et al., 1992; see also Chapter 1, part 5). Items on the list should be considered from the standpoint of greatest return on investment and also considered with regard to the willingness of the farmer to adopt the suggested changes (Enevoldsen & Mortensen, 1995; see also Chapter 1, part 5). However, it is important to note that such economic analyses are only valid and trustworthy to the farmer if they are based on a thorough analysis of his specific situation. For that purpose, the clinical diagnoses and observations made during farm visits are invaluable and indispensable (Enevoldsen & Mortensen, 1995).

Additionally, we always have to bear in mind that the results from cross-sectional inventories for subclinical lameness and related risk factors do not necessarily represent causal relation;, even when the impact of certain conditions has been quantified and they show an association with the prevalence of lameness. The effect of subclinical lameness on e.g. reproductive performance and milk production, for example, is very hard to establish. Nevertheless, such results can be useful in determining priorities for intervention, as part of a HH & PM program. Often obvious examples of cows with severe lameness producing much less milk can be identified during herd visits. Such examples are useful for discussing the relations between claw health and milk production with the farmer.

## REFERENCES

*Dijkhuizen, A.A., Huirne, R.H.M., Hardaker, J.B. (1992) Scope of management and management decisions. In: Prospects for automatic milking. Proc.of the internatl symposium on prospects for automatic milking. Wageningen, Netherlands. Ipema, Lippus, Metz & Rossing (Eds). EAAP Publ.65. Pudoc Sci. Publ. Wageningen, 299-309*

*Dijkhuizen, A.A. 1987. Bedrijfseconomische schade van klauwgebreken is aanzienlijk. Veehouderij 72:14-15.*

*Enevoldsen, C., Mortensen, K. (1995) Epidemiologic analyses of digital disorders in cattle. Relevance for research and herd health management. In: Orthopaedie bei Huf- und Klauentieren. P.F.Knezevic, ed. Schattenauer Stuttgart, 186-198*

*Enevoldsen, C., Mortensen, K. (1995) Epidemiologic analyses of digital disorders in cattle. Relevance for research and herd health management. In: Orthopaedie bei Huf- und Klauentieren. P.F.Knezevic, ed. Schattauer, Stuttgart, 186-198*

*Espinasse, J. 1984. Colour atlas on disorders of cattle and sheep digits. Intern. Terminology. Soc. Francaise de Buiatrie, 31 pages.*

*Frankena, K., Van Keulen, K.A.S., Noordhuizen, J.P.T.M., Stassen, E.N., Gundelach, J., De Jong, D.J., Saedt, I. (1992). A cross-sectional study into prevalence and risk indicators of digital hemorrhages in female dairy calves. Prev. Vet. Med. 14:1-12.*

*Frankena, K., Van Keulen K.A.S,, Noordhuizen, J.P.T.M., Stassen, E.N., Gundelach, J., De Jong, D.J., Saedt, I. (1993). A cross-sectional study of prevalence and risk factors of dermatitis interdigitalis in female dairy calves in the Netherlands. Prev. Vet. Med. 17:137-144.*

*Frankena, K.. E.N. Stassen, J.P. Noordhuizen, J.O. Goelema, J. Schipper, H. Smelt and H. Romkema (1991). Prevalence of lameness and risk indicators for dermatitis digitalis (Mortellaro disease) during pasturing and housing of dairy cattle. In: Proceedings of the annual meeting of the Society of Veterinary Epidemiology and Preventive Medicine, held at the Royal Veterinary College, University of London, April 17-19, 1991: 107-118*

*Frankena, K., E.N. Stassen, J.P.T.M. Noordhuizen, J.O. Goelema, J. Schipper, and H. Smelt. 1991. Prevalence of lameness and risk indicators for dermatitis digitalis (Mortellaro disease) during pasturing and housing of dairy cattle. In: Proc. Soc. Vet. Epid. & Prev. Med., London, pp. 107-118.*

*Greenough, P.R., Vermunt, J.J. (1994) In search of an epidemiologic approach to inves tigating bovine lameness problems. In: Proc. VIII-th Intern. Sympos. on Disorders of the Ruminant Digit, P.R.Greenough (Ed.) Banff, Canada, pp 186-196*

*Greenough, P.R., MacCallum, F.J., Weaver, A.D. (1981) Lameness in cattle. 2-nd edition, Wright-Scientechnica, Bristol*

*Martin, S.W., A.H.Meek, and P.Willeberg. 1987. Veterinary Epidemiology. Iowa State University Press, Ames. Iowa, USA.*

*McDaniel, B.T. (1994) Feet and leg traits of dairy cattle. In: Proc. VIII-th Intern. Symposium Disorders of the Ruminant Digit, P.R.Greenough (Ed.) Banff, Canada, pp 102-109*

*Mortensen, K. (1994) Bovine laminitis (diffuse aseptic pododermatitis): clinical and pathological findings. In: Proc.VIII-th Intern.Sympos. on Disorders of the Ruminant Digit, P.R.Greenough (Ed.) Banff, Canada, pp 210-226.*

*Mortensen, K. (1994) Bovine laminitis (diffuse aseptic pododermatitis): clinical and pathological findings. In: Proc. VIII-th Intern. Sympos. on Disorders of the Ruminant Digit, P.R.Greenough (Ed.) Banff, Canada, pp 210-226*

*Noordhuizen, J.P.T.M., and A. Brand. 1983. Veterinary herd health and production control on dairy farms. III: Index list on reproduction and lameness. Prev. Vet. Med. I:215-223.*

*Noordhuizen, J.P.T.M., K.D.C. Staerk, and M.V. Thrusfield. 1995. Applied epidemiology for the veterinary practice. Diergeneeskd. Memorandum. (42) 2:1-60. Amsterdam (in Dutch).*

*Peterse, D.J. (1982). Formaline footbath in the prevention of interdigital dermatitis in cattle. Neth.J.Vet.Sci. 107: 835-840.*

*Russell, A.M., Rowlands, G.J., Shaw, S.R., Weaver, A.D. (1982) Survey of lameness in British dairy cattle. The Vet.Record 111: 155-160*

*Smits, M.C.J., K. Frankena, J.H.M. Metz and J.P.T.M. Noordhuizen. 1992. Prevalence of digital disorders in zero-grazing dairy cows. Livestock Production Science 32:231-244.*

*Thysen, I., Enevoldsen, C. (1996) HERDVIEW: a PC program for interactive analysis of reproduction and health in dairy herds. At the INTERNET http://www.foulum.min.dk/~iver/herdview. Research Centre Foulum, Denmark*

*Toussaint-Raven. E., R.T. Haalstra and D. Peterse (1985). Cattle foot care and claw trimming. Farming Press, Ipswitch UK*

*Vermunt, J.J., Smart, M.E. (1994) The impact of a lameness management programme. In: Proc. VIII-th Intern. Sympos. on Disorders of the Ruminant Digit, P.R.Greenough (Ed.) Banff, Canada, pp 275-298*

*Weaver, A.D. (1994) International terminology of digital disease. In: Proc. VIII-th Intern.Sympos. on Disorders of the Ruminant Digit, P.R.Greenough (Ed.) Banff, Canada, pp 25-28*

*Wells, S.J., Trent, A.M., Marsh, W.E., Williamson, N.B., Robinson, R.A. (1995) Some riskfactors associated with clinical lameness in dairy herds in Minnesota and Wisconsin. The Vet.Rec. 136: 537-540*

# APPROACH FOR CONTROL OF INFECTIOUS DISEASES IN CATTLE HERDS

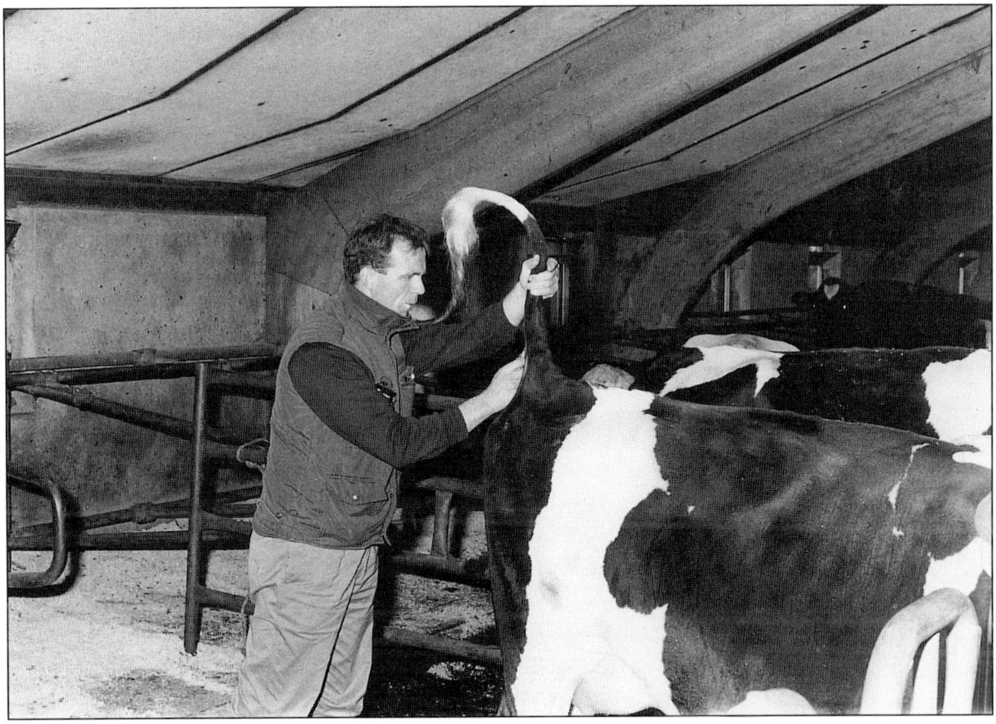

# 8 APPROACH FOR CONTROL OF INFECTIOUS DISEASES IN CATTLE HERDS

Wim H.M. van der Poel[1] and Daniel T. Scholl[2]

[1] Department of Herd Health and Reproduction, School of Veterinary Medicine, University of Utrecht, Yalelaan 7, 3485 CL Utrecht, The Netherlands

[2] School of Veterinary Medicine, Louisiana State University, Department of Epidemiology and Community Health, United States of America

## 8.1 GENERAL INTRODUCTION

Performance indices that are routinely monitored in HH & PM programs, such as abortions, reproductive failure, diseased animals, mortality, early culling or retarded growth may point to impending problems with regard to specific diseases. In addition to managerial deficiencies, it appears to be highly indicative of the specific disease state of the herd under HH & PM service. A variety of diseases have been selected to discuss differences in etiology, impact and diagnosis, and opportunities and limitations for control. The approach to the control of the diseases, in general, follows a basic outline:

1. herd screening (diagnosis)
2. removal of test positives
3. preventive measures (management, vaccination), and
4. monitoring.

Most of the selected diseases interfere dramatically with routine HH & PM procedures for adult and young dairy cattle performance improvement. Therefore, the practitioner must properly address these diseases for optimal control and the farmer must be made aware the application and the limitations of control measures. Many issues related to agent transmission should be assessed through farm inspection as a component of disease risk management.

The next paragraphs focus specifically on infections in dairy cattle herds. It should be noted that differences in the approach of such infections in beef cattle herds could occur.

The following infections are addressed: Bovine Virus Diarrhea virus (BVDV), leptospirosis, Johne's disease (*Mycobacterium paratuberculosis*), Bovine Herpes Virus-1 (Infectious Bovine Rhinotracheitis, IBR), Bovine Respiratory Syncytial Virus (BRSV), and bovine salmonellosis.

## 8.2 BOVINE VIRUS DIARRHEA VIRUS (BVDV)

Bovine virus diarrhea virus (BVDV) causes a complex disease syndrome with a worldwide distribution in cattle. It is very important to know the BVDV status of a herd. An unknown positive BVDV status interferes dramatically with a routine HH & PM program. Performance indices which are routinely measured in a HH & PM program such as number of abortions (Chapter 5), diseased animals, and poor growth (Chapter 2) may indicate impending problems with regard to BVDV. Within HH & PM services each herd should be monitored continuously for the presence of BVDV and measures should be taken to eradicate existing infections and to prevent new infections.

### 8.2.1 EPIDEMIOLOGY

BVDV is distributed worldwide. Prevalence of BVDV in cattle herds is over 80% in a number of states in Europe and North America (Niskanen et al., 1993). Some countries (Iceland) are free of BVDV. Over 2% of newborn calves may be persistently infected in regions with a high BVDV prevalence (Bolin et al., 1985). Persistently infected carriers continuously shed large amounts of virus in their environment and therefore play a major role in the spread of BVDV (Houe et al., 1993).

In BVDV positive herds it is possible to reach a situation of endemic stability. After a natural BVDV infection, cows normally develop a persistent, lifelong immunity and offspring of seropositive cows normally will not be persistently infected. Although in these BVDV seropositive cows, transplacental infection has not been observed, it cannot be excluded after infection with a heterologous strain. After accurate detection and culling of persistently infected cattle, transmission of BVDV in the herd can be continued by transient infections. During an outbreak in a dairy herd of about 200 cows in the Netherlands for example, the basic reproduction ratio ($R_0$) was estimated to be 3.9, meaning that on average 3.9 secondary cases were caused by one infectious animal. In this outbreak the spread of BVDV ceased after about 400 days (Moerman et al., 1993). Virus spread through transient infections might be reduced by vaccination, but this has not been documented to date.

### 8.2.2 ECONOMIC IMPORTANCE

Important economic losses due to BVDV infections have been described (Wentink and Dijkhuizen, 1990; Moerman et al., 1994). Acute disease, abortion, mummification and early embryonic death or congenital defects result in considerable reproduction losses (Dubovi et al., 1994). A significant number of infected lactating cows may develop a serious decrease in milk yield (Moerman et al., 1994). Even in herds where acute infections run an inapparent course, some cattle will have to be culled because of mucosal disease or detected persistent BVDV infections.

## 8.2.3 ETIOLOGY

Bovine virus diarrhea virus (BVDV), genus pestivirus, family Flaviviridae, is a single stranded RNA virus with a positive sense (Horzinek et al., 1991). Two biotypes of BVDV exist which can only be differentiated in cell cultures (Lee and Gillespie, 1957). Differentiation between cytopathogenic and non-cytopathogenic strains is very important to the pathogenesis and epidemiology of BVDV (McClurkin et al., 1984). This classification only refers to the behavior of specific isolates in cell culture, not to the behavior in the host animal (Jewett et al., 1990). The predominant circulating biotype is non-cytopathogenic. The cytopathogenicity of BVDV strains is always correlated with the appearance of the non-structural BVDV p80 protein (Ridpath et al., 1994). Differences between field isolates have been determined serologically. Isolates normally do not show major differences in virulence, but an extra virulent strain has been recently described (Pellerin et al., 1994).

## 8.2.4 CLINICAL SIGNS

Clinical signs of BVDV infections strongly vary in occurrence and severity. Clinical signs can be absent or non specific like inappetence and pyrexia. Gastrointestinal signs can consist of diarrhoea, mucosal erosions, ulcers and blunting of oral papillae. Respiratory signs such as ocular discharge, dyspnoea, and tachypnoea can be observed. Thrombocytopenia can cause persistent bleeding. Hemorrhages which mainly occur in calves can lead to deaths. Embryonic death, abortion, and/or calves born with neurologic disorders are usually the most costly disease symptoms. Mucosal disease develops in persistently infected cattle. It is characterized by severe leucopenia and thrombocytopenia. Persistently infected carriers can develop the same clinical signs, and in these animals there is also a strong variation in occurrence and severity of these signs. Mucosal lesions can be found in the entire gastrointestinal tract and the Peyer's patches become necrotic (Liebler et al., 1995). The animals usually die within 3 to 10 days.

When a seronegative pregnant animal gets infected, the outcome for the conceptus depends on the stage of gestation (before or after 120 days) and the biotype of the virus. Mucosal disease occurs in persistently infected immunotolerant animals (non-cytopathogenic BVDV) through development of cytopathogenic BVDV, which arises by RNA recombination in these animals (Tautz et al., 1994). Insertion of cellular RNA, in the BVDV genome results in the processing of p125 to p54 and expression of the nonstructural p80 protein by cytopathogenic BVDV strains (Tautz et al., 1993, Qi et al., 1992). Development of mucosal disease has been described after superinfection with a cytopathogenic homologous BVDV strain (Brownlie et al.,1984). It has not been investigated whether RNA recombination occurred after these superinfections.

### 8.2.5 DIAGNOSIS

For definitive diagnosis of BVDV outbreaks, antigen detection and serological examinations are the best approaches. Definitive diagnosis of a BVDV infection is made by isolation of the virus in cell culture in the acute phase of infection and by antibody detection. Animals which are detected BVDV positive twice in a one month interval are persistently infected carriers. These carriers often show serologically negative test results, but they can develop antibodies after infection with a heterologous BVDV strain (Westenbrink et al., 1989). Non-cytopathogenic strains can be identified by staining after culturing the virus (Bezek, 1992). Screening of large numbers of cattle for BVDV in serum, can be performed using recently developed antigen ELISAs (Bezek et al., 1992). Antibody development is measured by serum neutralisation tests or Enzyme Linked Immunosorbent Assay (ELISA). Immunoperoxidase staining and fluorescent antibody test (FAT) can be used for detection of the antigen (Vickers et al., 1990). These staining techniques can also be used on tissues during necropsy. Polymerase chain reaction (PCR) assay has been described (Hooft van Iddekinge et al., 1992), but is not (yet) used for routine diagnosis.

### 8.2.6 BVDV CONTROL OUTLINE

A herd becomes suspected of BVDV infection in the case that fertility problems or abortions and congenital defects occur in the herd. Hemorrhagic disease or respiratory disease in calves may also indicate an outbreak of BVDV infections. Development of mucosal disease in a persistently infected carrier in the herd, indicates a former congenital infection with a non cytopathogenic BVDV strain.

When a herd is suspected of BVDV, infections should be confirmed by virus isolation or testing of acute and convalescent serum samples at 4 week intervals. A fourfold rise in antibody titer indicates a recent infection. If infections are confirmed, the herd must be screened for persistently infected carriers by repeated virus isolation or antigen detection technique (see screening and diagnosis). Persistently infected carriers must be culled and as soon as new infections are no longer observed a monitoring program must be started (see below).

#### Screening

In dairy cattle BVDV can be screened by bulk milk testing using an antigen ELISA. In non-lactating cattle, BVDV can be screened by blood testing for BVDV antibodies. Positive detection of BVDV in bulk milk or antibodies in young stock older than 8 months of age, indicate excretion of BVDV in the herd and the presence of persistently infected cattle or acute infections. To identify all persistently infected cattle, individual blood samples of all cattle in the herd older than 6 months of age, must be tested for BVDV. Calves must be tested before receiving colostrum, or as soon as they are 6 months old. Calves can be tested for BVDV at a younger age, but in that case a negative result should be regarded with caution because maternally derived antibodies can interfere with virus detection techniques. After a one-month interval a second blood sample must be obtained from all cattle in which tests detected BVDV in the first blood sample. Calves can also be tested for precolostral antibodies. Precolostral antibodies indicate intrauterine infections after about 120 days in gestation (McClurkin et al., 1984).

### Eradication

Standard procedures for sampling of cattle within a herd (Chapter 1, part 4) are not applicable to eradication of BVDV. This is because seropositivity of individual cattle does not equate to viral infection, necessitating the use of more costly viral or antigen detection tests. Use of antigen detection methods to find the rarely occurring persistently infected carriers would require very large sample sizes, approximately as large as the herd. In addition, too much time would elapse before all sequential sampling would yield satisfactory results and the infection might have spread within the herd by the time results are available. On a regional basis, sampling of herds within a region to determine the herd prevalence is another issue. Nevertheless, eradication of the pathogen must be focused on identification and subsequent culling of persistently infected carriers.

### Prevention

#### – management

Confirmed persistently infected carriers should be culled immediately or at least kept strictly separated from pregnant dams until they are culled. Housing of persistently infected carriers with seronegative young stock is sometimes done to achieve natural herd-immunity, but spread of this virus is a threat for seronegative pregnant dams. After culling of carriers, reintroduction of BVDV must be aggressively prevented. Maintaining a closed herd is best. Purchased animals must be tested for BVDV before introduction in the herd. BVDV can be introduced in herds with contaminated needles, semen or embryos. Therefore, semen and/or embryos from BVDV negative cattle only should be used and the utmost hygienic technique must be employed. This latter point must be strictly observed by practitioners as well. Young stock must be housed separately from older cattle to make sure that new persistently infected virus carriers among calves and replacement heifers cannot transmit BVDV to pregnant dams. Measures must be taken to avoid contact with animals from potentially BVDV infected herds. Appropriate hygienic measures must also be taken to prevent introduction of the virus by visitors. Since sheep and perhaps other species can act as reservoirs for BVDV, cattle should not be kept in contact with other animal species.

– **vaccination**

A vaccination program can be used to induce immunity in seronegative animals. Vaccination of young stock can be useful to prevent the immunosuppressive effects of the virus after infection has occurred. In adult cattle the main goal of vaccination is to protect unborn calves from congenital infection in order to prevent abortion, development of congenital defects or persistent infection. Because of the large antigenic variety of BVDV strains most vaccines are probably not completely protective (Roeder et al., 1986). Vaccines which have demonstrated complete protection against BVDV transmission to the fetus have not been described and are most likely not available. The vaccine of choice for a vaccination program must be safe and must not induce mucosal disease.

### 8.2.7 MONITORING

In the beginning, monitoring by bulk milk testing or blood testing (see screening) can be done at six month intervals. In a later stage of the program, the intervals can be prolonged. Sampling of newborn calves should be continued until BVDV has not been detected on the farm for at least 1 year, since BVDV can circulate in a herd for more than a year even when persistently infected animals are absent (Moerman et al., 1993). During a vaccination program the screening for BVDV antibodies is not useful and monitoring therefore must be focussed on detection of BVDV antigen. Moreover, vaccine derived antibodies may interfere with virus detection tests.

## REFERENCES


*Bezek, D.M. 1992. Induction of thrombocytopenia in calves acutely and persistently infected with bovine viral diarrhea virus. PhD dissertation, Cornell University, Ithaca, NY,*

*Bezek, D.M. and G.D. Mechor. 1992. Identification and eradication of bovine viral diar rhea virus in a persistently infected dairy herd. JAVMA 201(4):580-586.*

*Bolin, S.R., A.W. McClurkin, E.T. Littledike, and M.F. Coria 1985. Frequency of persis tent bovine viral diarrhea virus infections in selected cattle herds. Am. J. Vet. Res. 11:2385-2387.*

*Brownlie. J., M.C. Clarke, and C.J. Howard. 1984. Experimental production of fatal mucosal disease in cattle. Vet. Rec. 114:535-536.*

*Dubovi, E.J. 1994. Impact of bovine viral diarrhea virus on reproductive performance in cattle. Vet. Clin. North Am. Food Anim. Pract. 10:503-514.*

*Hooft van Iddekinge, B.J.L., J.B.L. Wamel, H.G.P. Van Gennip, and R.J.M. Moormann. 1992. Application of the polymerase chain reaction to the detection of bovine viral diarrhea virus infections in cattle. Vet. Microbiol. 30:21-34.*

*Horzinek, M.C. 1991. Pestiviruses- Taxonomic perspectives. Arch. Virol. Suppl. 3:1-5.*

*Houue, H. and V.T.I. Palfi. 1993. Attempts at preventing further spread of bovine virus diarrhoea virus (BVDV) infection in 5 Danish dairy herds in which BVDV had been isolated. Acta Vet. Scand. 34:139-144.*

*Jewett, C.J., C.L. Kelling, M.L. Frey, and A.R. Doster, 1990. Comparative pathogenicity of selected bovine viral diarrhea virus isolates in gnotobiotic lambs. Am. J. Vet. Res. 51 (10):1640-1644.*

*Lee, K.M., and J.H. Gillespie. 1957. Propagation of virus diarrhea virus in tissue culture. AM J Vet Res 18: 952-953.*

*Liebler, E.M., C.Kusters, and J.F. Pohlenz. 1995. Experimental mucosal disease in cattle changes of lymphocyte subpopulations in Peyer's patches and in lymphoid nodules of large intestine. Vet Immunol. Immunopath. 48:233-248.*

*McClurkin, A.W., E.T. Littledike, R.C. Cutlip, R.C. Frank, G.H. Coria, and S.R. Bolin. 1984. Production of immunotolerant carriers to bovine viral diarrhea virus. Can. J. Comp. Med. 48:156-161.*

*Moerman, A., P.J. Straver, M.C.M. De Jong, J. Quak, T. Baanvinger , and J.T. Van Oirschot. 1993. A long-term epidemiological study of bovine virus diarrhea virus infections in a large herd of dairy cattle. Vet. Rec. 132:622-626.*

*Moerman, A., P.J. Straver, M.C. de Jong, J. Quak, T. Baanvinger, and J.T. van Oirschot. 1994. Clinical consequences of a bovine virus diarrhoea virus infection in a dairy herd: a longitudinal study. Vet Quart. 16:115-119.*

*Niskanen R. 1993. The relationship between the levels of antibodies to bovine virus diar rhoea virus (BVDV) in bulk milk and the prevalence of cows exposed to the virus. Vet Rec 133: 431-344.*

*Pellerin, C., J. Van den Hurk, J. Lecomte, and P. Tijssen. 1994. Identification and charac terisation of a new group of BVDV associated with high mortalities in calves. Proceedings of the 3rd congress of the European society for veterinary virology, Interlaken, 4-7 September 1994 pp 272-275.*

*Qi, F., J.F. Ridpath, T. Lewis, S.R.Bolin, and E.S. Berry. 1992. Analysis of bovine viral diarrhea virus genome for possible cellular insertions. Virol. 189:285-292.*

*Ridpath. J.F., F. Qi, F, S.R. Bolin, and E.S. Berry. 1994. Natural recombination in bovine viral diarrhea viruses. Arch. Virol. Suppl. 9:239-244.*

*Roeder, P.L. and J.W. Harkness. 1986. BVD virus infection: prospects for control. Vet. Rec. 118:143-147.*

*Tautz, N., H.J. Thiel, E.J. Dubovi, and G.P. Meyers. 1994. Pathogenesis of mucosal disea se: a cytopathogenic pestivirus generated by an internal deletion. J. Virol. 68:3289-3297.*

*Tautz, N., G. Meyers, and H.J. Thiel. 1993. Processing of poly-ubiquitin in the polypro tein of an RNA virus. Virol. 197:74-85.*

*Vickers, M.L. and H.C. Minocha. 1990. Diagnosis of bovine viral diarrhea virus infec tion using monoclonal antibodies. J. Clin. Diagn. Invest. 2:300-302.*

*Wentink, G.H. and A.A. Dijkhuizen. 1990. Economic consequences of infection with bovi- ne diarrhoea virus in 14 dairy herds (in Dutch). Tijdschr. Diergeneesk. 115:1031-1040.*

*Westenbrink F, Straver PJ, Kimman TG, de Leeuw PW (1989) Development of a neutra lising antibody response to an inoculated cytopathic strain of bovine virus diarrhoea virus. Vet Rec 125: 262-265.*

## 8.3 BOVINE HERPESVIRUS 1 INFECTION, BHV-1 (INFECTIOUS BOVINE RHINOTRACHEITIS, IBR)

BHV1 is widely distributed among cattle on all continents (Straub, 1990). Since its epidemic appearance in the seventies, the disease has currently changed into an endemic type of disease.

### 8.3.1 EPIDEMIOLOGY

Infected animals can shed virus for 1 to 14 days (Kaashoek, 1995). Like all Alphaherpesviridae, BHV1 establishes latency. After respiratory infection in cattle, the DNA of the virus is detectable in the trigeminal ganglia (Van Engelenburg, 1994). Latent virus can be reactivated and shed into the environment (Gibbs et al., 1977). BHV1 survival in the environment is optimal at 90% relative humidity (RH) and low temperature. Reactivation can be induced by stress such as parturition and corticosteroid treatment (Kaashoek, 1995; Thiry et al., 1987). Infected animals therefore are lifelong potential shedders of the virus, and can be regarded as carriers. Direct contact with shedding cattle is the most effective mode of transmission, but transmission by aerosols may also play a role (Wentink et al., 1993). Transport and introduction of animals into a new herd can be considered important triggers for reactivation of latent virus (Pastoret et al., 1984).

### 8.3.2 ECONOMIC IMPORTANCE

Clinical outbreaks of IBR can cause considerable losses mainly because of abortions, decreased milk production and costs of treatments. Wiseman et al. (1979) estimated the losses caused by 15 incidents of IBR. The number of cattle at risk was 2207 and the cost per animal was £ 27 in the UK (100 US$). In the Netherlands losses during outbreaks of IBR were estimated at 300 Dutch Guilders (200 US$) per milking cow (Dijkhuizen, personal communication, 1995). Besides economic losses due to clinical disease, exporting countries can expect increasing economic losses due to trade regulations and bans.

### 8.3.3 ETIOLOGY

Bovine herpesvirus 1 (BHV1) is a member of the family of the Herpesviridae and the subfamily of Alphaherpesviridae (Roizman et al., 1992). BHV1 has a linear double stranded DNA genome that codes for approximately 75 proteins, including at least 9 transmembrane glycoproteins. These transmembrane proteins are embedded in the viral envelope and form projecting spikes. Glycoproteins play a role in virus cell interactions (Spear, 1993), and interactions with the immune system, like binding immunoglobulin (Dubin et al., 1991). So far these glycoproteins are only distinguishable by their different endonuclease fragment patterns. Two major subtypes of BHV1 have been described: subtype BHV1.1 and subtype BHV1.2 (Misra et al., 1983). It has been demonstrated that 0.5% NaOH, 0.01% HgCl2, 1% CaOCl2 (chlorinated lime), 1% phenol derivatives and 1% quaternary ammonium base inactivate BHV1 within seconds and that 5% formalin does so within 1 minute (Straub, 1965).

## 8.3.4 CLINICAL SIGNS

Bovine herpesvirus 1 infections cause an acute inflammation of the mucous membrane of the respiratory tract or the genital tract resulting in infectious bovine rhinotracheitis (IBR), infectious pustular vulvovaginitis (IPV) or infectious pustular balanoposthitis (IPB). Acute infections are characterized by fever, depression, decreased appetite, hyperaemic mucosae, mucosal lesions, and nasal discharge (Wiseman et al., 1978). Obstruction of the upper respiratory tract can lead to seriously hampered breathing. Signs like decreased production, conjunctivitis, multisystemic disease in young calves, enteritis, abortions and mastitis have also been reported (Gibbs et al., 1977). BHV1.1 strains are associated with the respiratory infections and BHV1.2 strains with the milder genital infections, but both subtypes can be isolated from both tracts (Edwards et al., 1991).

## 8.3.5 DIAGNOSIS

The virus can readily be isolated from nasal or vaginal swabs. Samples should be collected from animals in the acute stage of the disease, showing respiratory signs and fever. The material should be kept at approximately 4°C and be prevented from drying during transport to the laboratory. Diagnostic laboratories can provide a virus diagnosis 24 - 48 h after samples have arrived. Viral antigen can also be identified from swabs and is even more rapid. Methods of choice include the immunofluorescence (IF) technique (Silim et al., 1983), PCR (Van Engelenburg et al., 1993), or immunoperoxidase staining (Collins et al., 1985). For detection of viral antigen PCR is the most sensitive technique available (Van Engelenburg, 1994). For antibody detection in blood serum or milk all laboratory diagnostic methods have been employed. The serum neutralisation (SN) test is commonly used and reliable, but ELISAs have been developed which have proven to be more sensitive than the SN test (Kramps et al., 1994).

## 8.3.6 BHV-1 CONTROL OUTLINE

### Screening and eradication

There is still a number of countries where IBR has not been diagnosed.

Some countries in Europe like Denmark, Switzerland and Austria have eradicated BHV1 by detecting and subsidized culling of infected cattle. Most of these countries have enacted trade and other regulations to protect their BHV1 free status. To get around export restrictions and to improve the health status of cattle, other countries, like The Netherlands, have recently initiated eradication programs. In countries with a high prevalence, culling of seropositive cattle is hardly economically feasible. Moreover, cattle are often vaccinated to prevent outbreaks of IBR and to reduce spread of the virus. To allow differentiation between infected and vaccinated cattle so called marker vaccines (see vaccination) have been developed. When marker vaccines are used, eradication campaigns can be instituted parallel to vaccination programs (Kaashoek et al., 1995). Specific eradication protocols differ between countries and are not further elaborated here (Kaashoek, 1995; Van Engelenburg 1994; Straub et al., 1982).

## Prevention

### – management

Purchase of infected cattle or the use of infected semen are probably the most important means for introducing BHV1 in a cattle herd. Therefore, herds should be closed, and purchased cattle should not be introduced into the herd without a quarantine period and not before they have been serologically examined for antibodies against BHV1. On infected farms in particular, young stock should be housed separately from adult cows. Herds should be closed and non milk producing cattle must be housed separately from adult cattle. Hygienic measures must be taken to prevent introduction of the virus by visitors. It is advisable to force visitors to change boots and to put on clean overalls at the entrance of the cattle barn.

### – vaccination

Since the beginning of the sixties, several attenuated vaccines have been developed for intramuscular and for intranasal use. Although some live virus vaccines have shown abortifacient effects, all currently available IBR vaccines have been proven safe in this regard. In most countries application of attenuated vaccines have proved satisfactory as a prophylactic measure. Protection has been reported to occur within 72 hours after intranasal or intramuscular vaccination with modified live virus vaccines (Sutton, 1980; Todd et al., 1972). When only a few animals of a herd show IBR disease, emergency vaccination is recommended to protect the rest of the herd from infection and disease. Intranasal administration leads to rapid production of interferon and may induce stronger immunity directly after vaccination. There also are numerous inactivated vaccines in many countries. Most modern inactivated vaccines available have proven to be safe and efficacious (Hjerpe, 1990; Kaashoek, 1995). Inactivated vaccines are preferred when spread of attenuated vaccines is regarded a disadvantage. In regions that are free of BHV1, introduction of live vaccine strains will be unwanted. Moreover, animals vaccinated with a live vaccine become latent carriers and potential shedders of the vaccine strain. Therefore inactivated vaccines are often preferred in cattle for export.

### Monitoring

Antibodies induced by conventional vaccines cannot be distinguished from antibodies induced by field virus. Therefore, all cattle vaccinated with conventional vaccines must be regarded as infected. Moreover, live vaccines can be reactivated and transmitted, and keep up the level of infection (Thiry et al., 1987; Van der Poel et al., 1995). In dairy herds screening of BHV1-infections can be performed by bulk milk testing for antibodies using ELISA. In non milk producing cattle, ELISA screening for serum antibodies can be performed by testing a sample of the herd (Chapter 1, part 4). At least 3 head of cattle per cow-house must be sampled. For monitoring of BHV1-free herds ELISA screening should be performed every month for bulk milk and every 2 months for serum samples.

## REFERENCES

*Collins, J.K., A.C. Butcher, and C.A. Riegel. 1985. Immune response to bovine herpesvirus type 1 infections: virus specific antibodies in sera from infected animals. J. Clin. Microbiol. 21:546-552.*

*Dubin, G., E. Socolof, I. Frank, and H.M. Friedman. 1991. Herpes simplex virus type 1 Fc receptor protects infected cells from antibody-dependent cellular cytotoxicity. J. Virol. 68:7046-7050.*

*Edwards, S., R.H. Newman, and H. White 1991. The virulence of British isolates of bovine herpesvirus 1 in relationship to viral genotype. Brit. Vet. J. 147:216-231.*

*Gibbs, E.P.J., and M.M. Rweyemamu. 1979. Bovine herpesviruses. Part I. Bovine herpes virus 1. Vet. Bull. 47:317-343.*

*Hjerpe, C.A. 1990. Bovine vaccines and vaccination programs. Vet. Clin. N. Am. Food. Anim. Pract. 6:188-194.*

*Kaashoek, M.J.K. 1995. Marker vaccines against bovine herpesvirus 1 infections. PhD thesis, Utrecht 1995.*

*Kramps, J.A., A. Magdalena, J. Quak, K. Weerdmeester, M.J. Kaashoek, M.A. Maris-Veldhuis, F.A.M. Rijsewijk, G. Keil, and J.T. van Oirschot. 1994. A simple, specific and highly sensitive blocking enzyme-linked immunosorbent assay for the detection of antibodies to bovine herpesvirus 1. J. Clin. Microbiol. 32:2175-2181.*

*Misra, V., L.A. Babiuk, Q. Le, and C. Darcel. 1983. Analysis of bovine herpesvirus type 1 isolates by restriction endonuclease fingerprinting. Arch. Virol. 76:341-354.*

*Pastoret, P.P., E. Thiry, B. Brochier, G. Derboven, and H. Vindevogel. 1984. The role of latency in the epizootiology of infectious bovine rhinotracheitis. In: Latent herpesvirus infections in veterinary medicine. G. Wittmann, R.M. Gaskell, H.J. Rziha (Eds.) Martinus Nijhoff Publishers, Dordrecht, pp. 211-227.*

*Roizman, B., R.C. Desroziers, B. Fleckenstein, C. Lopez, A.C. Minson, and M.J. Studdert. 1992. The family of Herpesviridae: an update. Arch Virol 123: 425-449.*

*Silim, A, and M.A.S.Y. Elazhary. 1983. Detection of infectious bovine rhinotracheitis and bovine viral diarrhea viruses in the nasal epithelial cells by direct immunofluorescence technique. Can. J. Comp. Med. 47: 18-22.*

*Spear, P.G. 1993. Entry of alphaherpesviruses into cells. Seminars in Virology 4: 167-180.*

*Straub, O.C. 1990. Infectious bovine rhinotracheitis virus. In: Virus infections of vertebrates. Z. Dinter and B. Morein (Eds.) pp. 71-108.*

*Straub, O.C. 1965. In vitro untersuchungen über die Wirkung einiger Desinfectionsmittel auf ein zur Herpesgruppe gehörende Virus der IBR-IPV-virusgruppe (Rhinotracheitis- und Bläschen-ausschlagviren der Rinder). Tierärtzliche Umschau 20: 568-573.*

*Straub, O.C., B. Schmidt, and H. Liebke 1982. Ein Beispiel zur sanierung IBR-IPV-virusverseuchter Bestände. Tierärtzliche Umschau 37: 319-324.*

*Sutton, M.L. 1980. Rapid onset of immunity in cattle after intranasal injection with a modified live virus IBR vaccine. Vet. Med. 75: 1447-1456.*

*Thiry, E, J. Saliki, M. Bublot, and P.P. Pastoret 1987. Reactivation of infectious bovine rhinotracheitis virus by transport. Comp. Immunol. Microbiol. Inf. Dis. 10:59-63.*

*Todd, J.D., F.J. Volenec, and I.M. Paton 1972. Interferon in nasal secretions and sera of calves after intranasal administration of a virulent infective bovine rhinotracheitis virus : association of interferon in nasal secretions with early resistance to challenge with virulent virus. Infec. and Immun. 5: 699-706.*

*Van der Poel, W.H.M., J.A. Kramps, J. Quak, A. Brand, and J.T. Van Oirschot 1995. Persistence of bovine herpesvirus 1 specific antibodies in cattle after intranasal vaccination with a live virus vaccine. Vet. Rec. 137: 347-348.*

*Van Engelenburg, F.A.C. 1994. Pathogenesis of bovine herpesvirus 1 infections, prospects for a gE-negative marker vaccine and molecular diagnosis, PhD Thesis, Utrecht 1994.*

*Van Engelenburg, F.A.C., R.K. Maes, J.T. van Oirschot, and F.A.M. Rijsewijk. 1993. Development of a rapid and sensitive polymerase chain reaction assay for detection of bovine herpesvirus 1 in bovine semen. J. Clin. Microbiol. 31: 3129-3135.*

*Wentink, G.H., J.T. van Oirschot, and J. Verhoeff. 1993. Risk of infection with bovine her pesvirus 1 (BHV1): A review. Vet. Quart. 15: 30-33.*

*Wiseman, A., P.M. Msolla, I.E. Selman, E.M. Allan, H.J.C. Cornwell, H.M. Pirie, and W.S. Imsay. 1978. An acute severe outbreak of infectious bovine rhinotracheitis: clinical, epidemiological, microbiological and pathological aspects. Vet. Rec. 103: 391-397.*

*Wiseman A., I.E. Selman, P.M. Msolla, H.M. Pirie, and E. Allan. 1979. The financial burden of infectious bovine rhinotracheitis. Vet. Rec. 105: 469*

## 8.4 BOVINE RESPIRATORY SYNCYTIAL VIRUS (BRSV)

Bovine respiratory syncytial virus causes yearly epidemics of respiratory disease in cattle all over the world. Most severe bovine respiratory syncytial virus (BRSV) associated disease is observed in calves under 6 months of age (Kimman et al., 1988). Seasonal periodicity of BRSV infection normally occurs with highest incidences in autumn and winter (Van der Poel et al., 1993). Stress factors like shipping, crowding and temperature changes are considered to play a role in outbreaks.

### 8.4.1 EPIDEMIOLOGY

Primarily infected calves are the most important source of BRSV during epidemics. The role of other species in the epidemiology of BRSV is most likely of minor importance (Van der Poel et al., 1995).

The protective efficacy of maternally derived antibodies is considered to be incomplete and these maternal antibodies do not reduce virus shedding after BRSV infection (Kimman et al., 1988). BRSV is often transmitted by contact with nasal secretions, but can also be transmitted by aerosols. Seroprevalence of BRSV in adult cattle is over 70% and is always higher than in younger individuals. Reinfections regularly occur in cattle of all ages (Van der Poel et al., 1993) and probably play an important role in the persistence of BRSV specific antibodies in cattle. During BRSV reinfection in adult cattle, respiratory signs and virus shedding have not been observed. Even in a completely seropositive herd the basic reproduction ratio ($R_0$) is estimated to be greater than 1, (meaning that one infectious animal causes more than one secondary infection) and the infection may not become extinct (De Jong et al., 1996).

### 8.4.2 ECONOMIC IMPORTANCE

Bovine respiratory syncytial virus is one of the most frequently observed respiratory infections in cattle (Stott et al., 1980; Caldow et al., 1993). Especially in young stock, respiratory disease is a costly disease problem (Kaneene et al., 1990; Verhoeff et al., 1989). The total costs due to BRSV infection in replacement calves are mainly caused by growth retardation, extra labor required for care and veterinary costs (Verhoeff et al., 1989).

### 8.4.3 ETIOLOGY

Bovine respiratory syncytial virus (BRSV) is an RNA virus classified in the genus Pneumovirus of the sub-family Pneumovirinae of the family Paramyxoviridae (Collins, 1991). The BRSV genome codes for ten virus proteins, of which eight are structural proteins. Of the structural proteins, the attachment protein G and the fusion protein F, both associated with the virus envelope, play a major role in the infectivity and immunogenicity of BRSV. The function of the 2 nonstructural proteins is unknown (Collins et al., 1991). The virus is sensitive to low pH, ether and chloroform, and is inactivated by heating at 56 °C (Paccaud and Jacquier, 1970).

### 8.4.4 CLINICAL SIGNS

Bovine respiratory syncytial virus is a major cause of clinical respiratory disease in cattle throughout the world (Stott and Taylor, 1985). BRSV can induce an acute interstitial pneumonia with alveolitis and bronchiolitis, especially in calves and yearlings (Van den Ingh et al., 1982). Elevated body temperatures and increased respiratory rates are the most frequently observed clinical signs during BRSV associated respiratory disease (Bryson et al., 1978). Outbreaks of BRSV infections can be inapparent but coughing or even respiratory distress can also be found (Van Bekkum et al., 1977). Calves can show inappetence, abdominal breathing, nasal discharge, and develop red mucosae. During auscultation increased respiratory sounds and rales can be observed, especially in the cranioventral parts of the lungs (Holzhauer and Van Nieuwstadt, 1976).

### 8.4.5 DIAGNOSIS

Laboratory investigations are needed for diagnosis of BRSV associated disease because clinical signs are often non-specific. In the acute phase of the disease BRSV can be isolated from nasal swabs and lung lavage fluid (Kimman et al., 1988). Lung lavage fluids are preferred for virologic examinations because the highest concentration of the virus is found in the lungs. BRSV shows a wide range of susceptible host cells; in cultures of bovine fetal trachea cells maximum titres of 105 plaque forming units per ml can be reached. The culture time needed for BRSV to develop cytopathologic effect (cpe) in cell culture can be more than 2 weeks. For serological examinations, blood samples of diseased animals should be collected. Acute phase and convalescent sera should be obtained from at least 5 animals per pen. Specific BRSV antibodies can also be determined in nasal fluids. To prevent drying, nasal swabs should be kept in test fluid (type of fluid depends on the test) during transport to the laboratory. Immunofluorescence assays or polymerase chain reaction (PCR) assays can be used to detect the antigen in nasal fluids, lung lavage fluids and lung tissue (Kimman et al., 1986; Van der Poel et al., 1994).

## 8.4.6 BRSV CONTROL OUTLINE

### Screening

In some cattle herds, outbreaks of BRSV infections run an inapparent course, whereas in others, serious BRSV associated disease is observed (Bohlender et al., 1982). Frequently occurring respiratory tract disease, in calves and young stock, especially in late autumn and winter, makes a herd suspect of regular outbreaks of BRSV infections. In a running HH & PM program this season is an important observation period for this disease. For accurate diagnosis of BRSV infections, acute phase and convalescent serum samples should be obtained. For virus isolation lung lavage fluids can best be obtained according to the method described by Fogarty et al. (in: Kimman et al., 1986).

### Eradication

In many countries in Europe and North America BRSV is endemic. The virus can be transmitted through aerosols (Sauber, 1986) and in regions where farms are situated close to each other airborne transmission may play a role (Van der Poel et al., 1993). Since even seropositive and vaccinated cattle are regularly reinfected, a steady incidence rate of reinfections cannot be halted; especially in large herds. Moreover, since the virus is easily transmitted among cattle (De Jong et al., 1996), it will be extremely difficult to eradicate the virus in areas with dense cattle populations.

### Prevention

#### – management

Housing and management are considered to play a role in the outcome of BRSV associated respiratory disease (Bryson et al., 1978). Because adult cattle are considered to be an important virus reservoir (Van der Poel, 1995), young stock should be housed separately from adult cattle. Considering susceptibility for respiratory infections, young stock should be housed in at least 3 separated age groups: 0 - 2 months of age, 2 - 6 months, and 6 months and older. To prevent shedding of large amounts of virus, it is preferable to keep no more than 10 calves in one pen. Ventilation is important but airflow must not exceed 0.5 m/sec. Humidity should be under 75% (Dodd, 1992). See also Chapter 2, part 2.

#### – vaccination

Both live and inactivated virus vaccines are available for vaccination against BRSV. Vaccines can reduce clinical BRSV associated respiratory disease (Stott et al., 1984; Zygraich et al., 1982) but are unable to protect against infections or reinfections. Vaccination should be performed at a minimum age of 3 months because immunologic response after vaccination (or field virus infection) is incomplete or absent in maternally immune calves (Kimman et al., 1988). Since BRSV infections mainly occur in autumn and winter (Van der Poel et al., 1993), vaccination is most effectively performed in the beginning of autumn or end of summer. Year-round vaccination of calves as soon as they reach the age of three months can also effectively reduce BRSV associated disease in herds. This can be easily integrated into a HH & PM program. During acute BRSV outbreaks, vaccination must be postponed, because enhancement of respiratory disease by BRSV vaccination has been observed (Kimman et al., 1989). In infected regions, vaccination of cattle older than 2 years of age will not enhance immunity, because all adult cattle will be seropositive, and regular reinfections will continuously stimulate BRSV immunity in the herds.

### Monitoring

Apart from diagnosis of BRSV infections during acute outbreaks of respiratory disease, monitoring and screening of BRSV is not very useful. In a herd, that once experienced an outbreak, BRSV infections can regularly return with or without causing overt disease. Hence the farm history is important to estimate disease risks when starting a HH & PM program. Reinfections run an asymptomatic course in adult cattle (Van der Poel, 1995).

## REFERENCES

*Bryson, D.G., J.B. McFerran, H.J. Ball, and S.D. Neill. 1978. Observations on outbreaks of respiratory disease in housed calves. Epidemiological and clinical findings. Vet. Rec. 103: 485-489.*

*Bohlender, R. E., M. W. McCune, and M.L. Frey. 1982. Bovine respiratory syncytial virus infections. Mod. Vet. Pract. 63: 613-618.*

*Caldow, G.L., S. Edwards, A.R. Peters, P. Nixon, G. Ibata, and R. Sayers. 1993. Association between viral infections and respiratory disease in artificially reared calves Vet. Rec. 133: 85-89.*

*Collins, P.L. The Paramyxoviruses (D. Kingsbury Ed.) New York: Plenum, 1991.*

*De Jong, M.C.M., W.H.M. Van der Poel, J.A. Kramps, A. Brand, and J.T. Van Oirschot. 1996. A quantitative investigation of population persistence and recurrent outbreaks of respiratory syncytial virus on dairy farms. Am. J. Vet. Res. (in press).*

*Dodd, V.A. 1992. Calf housing principles. Irish Vet. J. 45: 91-104.*

*Holzhauer, C., and A.P.K.M.I. Van Nieuwstadt. 1976. The etiological role of bovine respiratory syncytial virus in "Pinkengriep" (in Dutch). Tijdschr. Diergeneesk. 101: 1023-1031.*

*Kaneene, J.B., and H.S. Hurd. 1990. The national animal health monitoring system in Michigan. III. Cost estimates of selected dairy cattle diseases. Prev. Vet. Med. 8: 127-140.*

*Kimman, T.G., J. Sol, F. Westenbrink, and P.J. Straver. 1989. A severe outbreak of respiratory tract disease associated with BRSV probably enhanced by vaccination with modified live vaccine. Vet. Quart. 11:250-253.*

*Kimman, T.G., G.M. Zimmer, P.J. Straver, and P.W. de Leeuw. 1986. Diagnosis of bovine respiratory syncytial virus infections improved by virus detection in lung lavage samples. Am. J. Vet. Res. 47:143-147.*

*Kimman, T.G., G.M. Zimmer, F. Westenbrink, J. Mars, and E. van Leeuwen. 1988. Epidemiological study of bovine respiratory syncytial virus infections in calves; influence of maternal antibodies on the outcome of disease. Vet. Rec. 123:104-109.*

*Paccaud, M. F., and C.L. Jacquier. 1970. A respiratory syncytial virus of bovine origin. Arch. Ges. Virusforschung 30:427-442.*

*Sauber, C.E. 1986. A closer look at bovine respiratory syncytial virus Vet. Med. 81:947-956.*

*Stott, E.J., and G. Taylor. Respiratory syncytial virus. Brief review. Arch. Virol. 1985; 84: 1-52.*

*Stott, E.J., L.H. Thomas, A.P. Collins, S. Crough, J. Jebbett, G.S. Smith, P.D. Luther, and R. Caswell. 1980. A survey of virus infections of the respiratory tract of cattle and their association with disease. J. Hyg. Camb. 85:257-270.*

*Stott, E.J., L.H. Thomas, G. Taylor, A.P. Collins, J. Jebbett, and S. Crough. 1984. A comparison of three vaccines against respiratory syncytial virus in calves. J. Hyg. 93:251-261.*

*Van Bekkum, J.C., C. Holzhauer, P.J. Straver, and A.P.K.M.I. Van Nieuwstadt. 1977. Viral infections of the respiratory tract of cattle in the Netherlands. Bull. Off. Int. Epizoot. 88:69-79.*

*Van den Ingh, T.S.G.A.M., J. Verhoeff, and A.P.K.M.I. Van Nieuwstadt. Clinical and pathological observations on spontaneous bovine respiratory syncytial virus infections in calves. Res. Vet. Sci. 1982; 33:152-158.*

*Van der Poel, W.H.M., J.P.M. Langedijk, J.A. Kramps, and J.T. Van Oirschot. A sensitive reverse transcription polymerase chain reaction assay for detection of bovine respiratory syncytial virus in cattle. Proceedings IIIrd International congress of the European Society of Veterinary Virologists, Interlaken 1994.*

*Van der Poel, W.H.M., J.P.M. Langedijk, J.A. Kramps, W.G.J. Middel, and J.T. Van Oirschot JT. 1995. Bovine respiratory syncytial virus antibodies in sera of non-bovine species. Arch. Virol. 140:1549-1555.*

*Van der Poel, W.H.M., J.A. Kramps, W.G.J. Middel, J.T. Van Oirschot, and A. Brand. 1993. Dynamics of bovine respiratory syncytial virus: a longitudinal epidemiological study in dairy herds. Arch. Virol. 133:309-321.*

*Van der Poel, W.H.M, Epidemiology of bovine respiratory syncytial virus infections. PhD thesis, Utrecht 1995.*

*Verhoeff, J., M. Dijk, and A.A. Dijkhuizen. 1989. Short and long term aspects of bovine respiratory syncytial virus infections in dairy cattle. Proc. Soc. Vet. Epid. & Econ. Utrecht 1989: pp 43-51.*

*Zygraich, N. 1982. Vaccination against RS virus: A five year experience with Rispoval. Proceedings of the 12th World Congress on Diseases of Cattle, Amsterdam, The Netherlands.*

## 8.5 LEPTOSPIROSIS

*Leptospira hardjo* infections in cattle are common throughout the world and are only found in sheep and cattle (Gerritsen et al., 1994b). *Leptospira* serovar *hardjobovis* is pandemic in cattle, whereas the predominant serotype in Europe is *L. hardjo* type bovis. *L. hardjo* infections in cattle are mainly observed in temperate climate zones (Miller et al., 1991). Introduction of or contact with infected cattle is probably the most important means for introducing leptospires in cattle herds. *Leptospira* might also be introduced by the use of infected semen and interfacing with infected wildlife and rodents.

### 8.5.1 EPIDEMIOLOGY

Bovine leptospirosis is a zoonosis. *Leptospira* strains can penetrate intact mucosal membranes of the conjunctivae and nasal cavity, or abraded skin (Sullivan, 1974). *Leptospira* can persist in the kidneys and genitals without causing clinical signs. Carrier cows are an important source of infection, not only for other cows but also for dairy farm workers. Chronically infected carriers can shed leptospires for more than 150 days (Gerritsen, 1994; Leonard et al., 1992). Clinical epidemics of bovine leptospirosis only develop in naive herds and have most commonly been described in Europe and Australia (Ellis et al., 1985). In endemically infected herds an increase in prevalence of agalactiae and abortions due to leptospirosis may occur in association with humid environmental conditions (Heath et al., 1994).

### 8.5.2 ECONOMIC IMPORTANCE

Mastitis, agalactia, weak calves, abortions and fertility disorders are the most costly signs of leptospirosis in cattle. However, economic losses due to outbreaks of leptospirosis are hard to assess, because most infections are asymptomatic (Bennett et al., 1993). *Leptospira hardjo* can cause influenza-like symptoms in man. Because *L. hardjo* infections are often reported in man (Terpstra et al., 1991), reduction of the prevalence of bovine leptospirosis has become an important issue in countries with a high prevalence of leptospirosis.

### 8.5.3 ETIOLOGY

*Leptospira* are Gram-negative, motile, obligately aerobic, long (6 - 10 fm), helicoidal rods. The genus *Leptospira* is divided into 7 pathogenic and 4 non-pathogenic species. On the basis of antigenic differences, about 200 serotypes can be discriminated. At low temperatures *Leptospira* can survive for months in a humid environment. The bacterium is readily inactivated by desiccation, UV-light, acids, 1% NaOH and detergents (Faine, 1994).

### 8.5.4 CLINICAL SIGNS

*Leptospira hardjo* infections in cattle may cause abortion, stillbirth, retained placenta and other fertility problems (Ellis et al., 1976). Mastitis and epidemics of agalactiae have also been reported (Higgins et al., 1980) but most infections are asymptomatic (Ellis et al., 1985). Abortions are usually observed 6 - 12 weeks after the initial infection. Acute clinical leptospirosis in cattle is only observed in calves. Calves can become icteric and develop haemoglobinuria and fever (Ellis et al., 1985).

### 8.5.5 DIAGNOSIS

The small diameter of 0.1 fm of *Leptospira* does not allow observation with a normal light microscope. The bacteria can be observed with a dark-field microscope, using the 'Tindall-effect' (Birch-Anderson et al.,1973). Conventional diagnosis of leptospirosis relies on the detection of serum antibodies. The microscopic agglutination technique (MAT) is the basic diagnostic procedure of choice (Schuffner et al., 1927). In recent years, Enzyme Linked ImmunoSorbent Assays (ELISA) have been developed for serological diagnosis of leptospirosis in cattle (Bercovich et al., 1990, Thiermann et al,. 1983, Trueba et al., 1990). Because IgM and IgG response can be detected separately, immune responses caused by an acute or chronic infection can be differentiated (Cousins et al., 1985). Because serologic methods do not provide reliable information on the carrier or shedding state of an infected animal, direct demonstration of pathogenic *Leptospira* in urine can be required (Gerritsen, 1994). Isolation of *Leptospir*a organisms by culturing from urine samples has been described but is too laborious for routine diagnosis (Wagenaar, 1994). Recently Polymerase chain reaction assays (PCR) have been developed to detect *Leptospira* in urine samples of cattle. These PCR assays provide a rapid diagnostic method with a sensitivity and specificity comparable to bacteriological culture (Van Eys et al., 1989; Wagenaar, 1994).

### 8.5.6 LEPTOSPIROSIS CONTROL OUTLINE

**Screening**

Once a herd becomes suspected of leptospirosis on the basis of observed clinical signs, acute infections in individual cattle can be identified by detection of high IgM titers using an ELISA. For herd screening, reliable results can be obtained by serological testing using MAT or ELISA (Trueba et al., 1990). ELISAs can also be used on bulk milk samples. The presence of antibodies in fetal serum samples demonstrates an infection; however, absence of antibodies in fetal serum does not exclude infection (Ellis et al., 1982). As *Leptospira* infections are confirmed in a herd the seroprevalence should be estimated by serologic investigation of a sample of a herd (see Chapter 1, part 4). During outbreaks serological investigation of affected cows and newborn calves is the best approach in cattle herds. Definite detection of the carrier state in individual cattle is difficult because both seronegative carriers and seropositive non-excreting animals occur (Gerritsen et al., 1994 a). Therefore in general it is not feasible to focus the control of the spread of leptospirosis on culling or treatment of individual carriers.

**Eradication**

In herds with an estimated prevalence below 15%, serological screening of individual cattle is indicated. When there are only a few seropositive animals, they can be culled within a short period. These seropositive cattle can be treated with antibiotics (and vaccinated) to prevent shedding to seronegative herdmates (see above). To investigate whether the eradication program has been successful, serological follow up will have to be done. In vaccinated herds serological follow up is not useful within at least one year after the last vaccination because serological tests are unable to differentiate titers due to infection and titers due to vaccination, which can persist for up to 12 months. In herds with a low prevalence, repeated individual screening is needed to decide whether the herd is free of leptospires. In herds with repeated negative bulk milk screening results, outbreaks almost certainly have not occurred during the investigation period.

**Prevention**

– **management**

An increased prevalence of bovine leptospirosis can be observed during humid environmental conditions. The likelihood of infection with *Leptospira* organisms increases during periods of high rainfall, in environments where there is poor drainage, high water holding capacity of the soil, or flooding. Stagnant waters can be contaminated with leptospires (Bennett, 1993). Therefore humidity in housing systems must be prevented and drainage of pastures must be optimized. Introduction of infected cattle is probably the most important means for introduction of leptospires in a cattle herd. Therefore herds should be closed, and purchased cattle should not be introduced into the herd without a quarantine period and not before they have been serologically examined for antibodies against leptospires. Young stock should be housed separately from adult cows, especially on infected farms. Hygienic measures must be taken to reduce the contact of cattle with urine of herdmates as much as possible in order to prevent contamination with leptospires. Dairy farm workers must avoid contact of skin and especially mucosae with urine. In infected herds farmers can be advised to wear glasses in the milking parlour to prevent contamination by urine splashes or droplets.

The emphasis of the control of infection should be to reduce transmission of leptospires from infected to naive cattle. In endemically infected herds antibiotic treatment can reduce shedding of leptospirosis in urine of cattle (Gerritsen et al., 1994 a).

Shedding of leptospires is stopped by a single treatment with 25 mg/kg dihydrostreptomycin (Gerritsen et al., 1994 a). Antibiotic treatment of the whole herd is the quickest way to control *L. hardjobovis* infection in cattle (Gerritsen et al., 1994 a). In herds with an estimated prevalence over 50%, the whole herd must be treated with dihydrostreptomycin and a vaccination program is indicated (see vaccination).

– **vaccination**

A vaccination program can increase herd immunity and reduce the number of new infections in a herd (Little et al., 1992). Many vaccines for bovine leptospirosis have been developed and evaluated (Ellis et al., 1986, Flint et al., 1980, Bolin et al., 1989 ab). Although vaccination does not always protect against infection (Prescott, 1991) and although there are reports that vaccinated cows can continue shedding after experimental infection (Bolin et al., 1991), results of vaccination in field experiments are promising (Hancock et al., 1984, Marshall et al., 1979, Little et al., 1992). However, in the Netherlands good results have been achieved in leptospirosis control without vaccination (see monitoring). To prevent calves from infection and becoming chronically infected carriers, these animals should be vaccinated at 4 to 5 months age. Economic losses caused by abortion and decreases of milk production attributable to leptospirosis may be minimized by strategically timed vaccination of cows at the beginning of the dry period and at calving.

### Monitoring

The leptospirosis status of a herd can be determined by the detection of antibodies in bulk milk (Dom et al., 1991). In the Netherlands, a program organised by the animal health service to control *L. hardjo* infections in cattle is based on detection of anti-hardjo antibodies in bulk milk 3 times per year. Antibody negative herds receive a certificate. This program, which was started in 1993, has helped to reduce the prevalence of bovine leptospirosis in The Netherlands from 30% in 1993 to 5% in 1995.

## REFERENCES

*Bennett, R.M. 1993. Decision support models of leptospirosis in dairy herds. Vet Rec 132:59-61.*

*Bercovich, A, R. Taaijke,and B.A. Bokhout. 1990. Evaluation of an Elisa for the diagnosis of experimentally induced and naturally occurring Leptospirosis hardjo infections in cattle. Vet. Microbiol. 21:255-262.*

*Birch-Anderson, A, K. Hovind Hougen, and C. Borg-Peterson. 1973. Electron microscopy of Leptospira. 1. strain pomona. Acta Pathol. Microbiol. Scand. 81:665-676.*

*Bolin, C.A., A.B. Thiermann, A.L. Handsaker, and J.W. Foley. 1989[a]. Effect of vaccina tion with a pentavalent leptospiral vaccine on Leptospira interrogans type hardjobovisinfection in pregnant cattle. Am. J. Vet. Res. 50:161-165.*

*Bolin, C.A., R.L. Zuerner, and G. Trueba. 1989[b]. Effect of vaccination with a pentavalent leptospiral vaccine containing Leptospira interrogans serovar hardjo on type hardjo-bovis infection of cattle. Am. J. Vet. Res. 50: 2004-2008.*

*Bolin, C.A., J.A. Cassells, R.L. Zuerner, and G. Trueba. 1991. Effect of vaccination with monovalent Leptospira interrogans serovar hardjo type hardjo-bovis vaccine on type hardjo-bovis infection of cattle. Am. J. Vet. Res. 52: 1639-1643.*

*Cousins, D.V., G.M. Robertson, and L. Hustas. 1985. The use of the enzyme-linked (ELISA) to detect the IgM and IgG responseto Leptospria interrogans serovas hardjo, pomona, and tarrassovi in cattle. Vet. Microbiol. 10: 439-450.*

*Dom, P.P., R. Haesebroeck, R. Vandermeersch, J. Descamps, and K. Van Ommeslaeghe. 1991. Prevalence of Leptospira interrogans serovar hardjo antibodies in milk in Belgian dairy herds. Vet. Quart. 13: 118-120.*

*Ellis, W.A., and S.W. Michna. 1976. Bovine Leptospirosis: infection by the Hebdomadis serogroup and abortion - a herd study. Vet. Rec. 99: 409-412.*

*Ellis, W.A., S.D. Neill, J.J. O'Brien, J.A. Cassells, and J. Hanna. 1982. Bovine leptospiro sis: microbiological and serological findings in normal fetuses removed from uteri after slaughter. Vet. Rec. 110: 192-194*

*Ellis, W.A., J.J. O'Brien, and D.P. Mackie. 1985. Bovine Leptosirosis: some clinical features of serovar Hardjo infection. Vet. Rec. 117: 101-104.*

*Ellis, WA, and N. Zygraich. 1986. Experimental studies with Leptospira interrogans serovar hardjo vaccine. Proc. World Congress on disease of cattle, Dublin: 971-974.*

*Faine, S. 1994. Leptospira and leptospirosis. CRC Press, Boca Raton, USA.*

*Flint, S.H., and D.M. Liardet. 1980. A trivalent leptospiral vaccine with emphasis on a Leptospira interrogans serovar hardjo component to prevent leptospiruria. New Zealand Vet. J. 28: 263-266.*

*Gerritsen, M.J. 1994. Bovine Leptospirosis, Aspects of shedding, antimicrobial Therapy, and genomic characterisation. PhD thesis, Utrecht 1994.*

*Gerritsen, M.J., M.J. Koopmans, T.C.E.M. Dekker, M.C.M. De Jong, A. Moerman, and T. Olyhoek. 1994[a]. Effective treatment with dihydrosteptomycin of naturally infected cows shedding Leptospira borgpeterenii serovar hardjo type hardjobovis. Am. J. Vet. Res. 55: 339-343.*

*Gerritsen, M.J., M.J. Koopmans, D.J. Peterse, and T. Olyhoek. 1994[b]. Sheep as maintenan ce hosts for Leptospira borgpetersenii servar hardjo type hardjobovis. Am. J. Vet. Res. 55: 339-343.*

*Hancock, G.A., C.R. Wilks, M. Kotiw, and J.D. Allen. 1984. The long term efficacy of hardjo-pomona vaccine in preventing leptospiruria in cattle exposed to natural challenge with Leptospira interrogans serovar hardjo. Aust. Vet. J. 61: 54-56.*

*Heath, E.S., and R. Johnson. 1994. Leptospirosis, clinical update. J. Am. Vet. Med. Ass. 205: 1518-1523.*

*Higgins, R.J., J.F. Harbourne, T.W.A. Little, and A.E. Stevens. 1980. Mastitis and abor tion in dairy cattle associated with leptospira of the serotype Hardjo. Vet. Rec. 107: 307-310.*

*Leonard, F.C., P.J. Quinn, W.A. Ellis, and K. O'Farrell. 1992. Duration of urinary excre tion of Leptospira interrogans serovar hardjo. Vet. Rec. 131: 435-439.*

*Little, T.W.A., S.C. Hathaway, E.S. Broughton, D. Seawright. 1992. Control of Leptospira hardjo infection by beef cattle by whole herd vaccination. Vet. Rec. 131: 435-439.*

*Marshall, R.B., E.S. Broughton, and J.S. Hellstrom. 1979. Protection of cattle against natural challenge with Leptospira interrogans serovar hardjo using a hardjo pomona vaccine. New Zealand Vet. J. 27: 114-116.*

*Miller, D.A., M.A. Wilson, and G.W. Beran. 1991. Relationships between prevalence of Leptospira interrogans in cattle, and regional climatic and seasonal factors. Am. J. Vet. Res. 52: 1766- 1768.*

*Prescott, J.F. 1991. Treatment of leptospirosis. Cornell Vet. 81: 7-12.*

*Schuffner, W. 1927. Zur mikroskopischen Fruhdiagnose von Leptospirose. Munch. Med. Wschr. 74: 857.*

*Sullivan, N.D. 1974. Leptospirosis in animals and man. Aust Vet J 50: 216-223.*

*Terpstra, W.J., C. Gravekamp, and M. Brok-van Merriënboer. 1991. Leptospirose. Bull. Infectieziekten 2: 2-12.*

*Thiermann, A.B., and L.A. Garret. 1983. Enzyme-linked immunosorbent assay for the detection of antibodies to Leptospira interrogans serovar hardjo and pomona in cattle. Am. J. Vet. Res. 44: 884-887.*

*Trueba, G.A., C.A. Bolin, and C.O. Thoen. 1990. Evalution of an enzyme immunoassay for diagnosis of bovine leptospirosis caused by Leptospirosis interrogans serovar hardjo type hardjo-bovis. J. Vet. Diagn. Invest. 2: 323-329.*

*Van Eys, G.J.J.M., Gravekamp C., M.J. Gerritsen, W. Quint, J. Cornelissen, J. Ter Schegget, and W.J. Terpstra. 1989. Detection of leptospires in urine by polymerase chain reaction. J. Clin. Microbiol. 27: 2258-2262.*

*Wagenaar, J.A. 1994. Leptospirosis-diagnosis and pathogenesis. PhD thesis, Utrecht 1994.*

## 8.6 JOHNE'S DISEASE (MYCOBACTERIUM PARATUBERCULOSIS; PARATUBERCULOSIS)

Johne's disease, shortly called paratuberculosis, is distributed worldwide and is most prevalent in temperate climate zones. Reported prevalence figures range from 1.6% to 18.7% in the US (Whitlock et al., 1985; Braun et al., 1990), and prevalence estimates from 0.1 to 4.9% have been reported in The Netherlands on the basis of the number of vaccinated herds (Meulenberg, 1991).

### 8.6.1 EPIDEMIOLOGY

Ingestion of bacteria after contact with contaminated feces is suggested to be the most important mode of transmission, but transmission via milk or colostrum may also be important. Infected cattle can shed large numbers of bacteria for more than a year; clinically affected cows may especially shed large numbers of bacteria. Resistance to infection increases with age: calves less than 30 days old are most susceptible and only animals infected in calfhood develop clinical disease (Julian, 1975). Congenital infections have been induced experimentally but the role of congenital infections in the spread of paratuberculosis in cattle is of very limited importance compared to oral infection (Benedictus, 1985; Merkal et al., 1983; Reinders, 1963). A particular point of interest is the possible relationship between *M. paratuberculosis* and Crohne's disease in humans. However this needs more investigation of the possible role of *M. paratuberculosis*, and research is still on-going (Thompson 1994).

### 8.6.2 ECONOMIC IMPORTANCE

Paratuberculosis causes considerable economic losses in cattle production (Reinders, 1963). These losses are due to decreased milk production, decreased feed efficiency, reduced slaughter value, increased culling rate and costs of treatments (Whitlock et al., 1985; Benedictus et al., 1987). Reported estimates of losses due to paratuberculosis vary considerably (Whipple, 1991). In the US losses due to paratuberculosis have been estimated at 1 billion dollars annually (Merkal, 1983; Chiodini et al., 1984). In The Netherlands Benedictus et al. (1987) estimated losses due to paratuberculosis at 650 (US$ 400) per average cow with clinical symptoms.

### 8.6.3 ETIOLOGY

*Mycobacterium* is the only genus listed in the family Mycobacteriaceae. Mycobacteria are aerobic, Gram-positive acid-fast non-motile rods (0.2 - 0.6 x 1.0 - 10 fm) (Goodfellow and Cross, 1984). The lipid-richness of the cell wall makes stained bacteria resistant to the decolorization, even under strong decolorizing conditions (hydrochloric acid-alcohol). This acid-fastness has been considered a feature of mycobacteria, and can be used for rapid identification, for instance by Ziehl-Neelsen staining (Barkdale and Kim, 1977). *Mycobacterium paratuberculosis* grows extremely slow, taking 6 weeks to 6 months to grow, and it requires the growth factor mycobactin (Goodfellow and Wayne, 1982). To culture *M. paratuberculosis* from feces, decontamination procedures are needed, otherwise the mycobacteria will be overgrown (Whipple and Merkal, 1983). *M. paratuberculosis* is extremely resistant to many disinfectants: only phenol (1:40), creosol (1:32), and formalin (5%) can be used to kill *M. paratuberculosis*. The bacteria can survive for several months in the environment (Benedictus, 1985).

### 8.6.4 CLINICAL SIGNS

Paratuberculosis spreads very slowly, and a herd can be infected for years before clinical signs are manifested. Paratuberculosis disease occurs only in 3 to 10% of infected animals (Julian, 1975; Chiodini et al., 1984) and the incubation time varies from 6 months to 15 years. The terminal stage of the disease occurs in most cattle between 3 and 5 years of age (Benedictus, 1985). The disease can be precipitated by stress factors like parturition or other infections. A decrease in milk production is normally the first sign, and indicates the start of bacterial shedding (Benedictus et al., 1987). A chronic intermittent diarrhea develops (Gilmour, 1965) and affected cattle loose weight despite a good appetite. The clinical stage of the disease can last for 3 to 6 months (Chiodini et al., 1984). During the terminal stage of the disease, milk production decreases tremendously (Reinders, 1963) and diarrhea becomes watery. Cattle start to show edema and emaciation and eventually die (Chiodini et al., 1984).

### 8.6.5 DIAGNOSIS

Microscopic examination of Ziehl-Neelsen stained fecal smears is one of the oldest tests and is still routinely used. This method however has a limited sensitivity compared to culturing of the pathogen, especially in subclinically infected animals. Culturing the pathogen is still considered the most reliable diagnostic method and many culture methods have been described (Van der Giessen, 1993). A culture time of 6 - 8 weeks is needed for the development of *M. paratuberculosis* colonies and culture time of at least 6 months is needed for a reliable definite negative result. Enzyme-Linked Immunosorbent Assays (ELISAs) for detection of antibodies against paratuberculosis, have been developed but most of these ELISAs lack sensitivity and specificity in subclinically infected animals (Collins et al., 1991; Bech-Nielsen et al., 1992). A modified ELISA, based on detection of bovine gamma-interferon (IF- gamma) released by Johnin-PPD stimulated lymphocytes, showed a sensitivity of 72 - 93% and a specificity of more than 90% in infected animals (Wood et al., 1991). The measurement of the cellular immune response by a delayed type hypersensitivity (DTH) test, intradermal johnin, has limited value, because the reaction is distinctly positive only early in infection. Moreover, false-positives frequently occur due to cross-reactions (Benedictus, 1985). Since 1987 DNA probes have been developed for diagnosing paratuberculosis (Van der Giessen, 1993).

### 8.6.6 PARATUBERCULOSIS CONTROL OUTLINE

#### Screening

Control of paratuberculosis must be focused on early culling of shedders and on strict hygienic measures to prevent infection of susceptible young animals. Because most infected animals are subclinically infected, shedders have to be identified by the use of diagnostic tests. Because of the lack of reliable and rapid techniques for detection of subclinically infected animals, control of paratuberculosis in cattle herds is very difficult (Chiodini et al., 1984; Benedictus, 1985). For this reason, test and culling programs have not been very successful. Research is underway to improve diagnostic methods; in the meantime control of paratuberculosis relies on utmost hygienic measures on cattle farms.

#### Eradication

Eradication of paratuberculosis in the cattle population of a region will only be feasible when a reliable and inexpensive diagnostic test has been developed. Since the majority of infected animals shed bacteria without developing clinical disease, detection techniques are needed which can identify infected animals in an early stage of infection or at least as soon as they shed bacteria. As long as diagnosis of the infection in an early stage of the disease is not possible, eradication of the pathogen will be extremely difficult.

#### Prevention

**– management**

To prevent contact of newborn calves with feces of adult cattle, dams must be housed in a separated clean calving pen. To prevent transmission of paratuberculosis, newborn calves must be separated from their mother immediately after birth. Transmission to calves may be reduced by pasteurisation of colostrum (Benedictus, 1985) and calves should always be fed from clean buckets. Herds should be closed and cattle under 1 year of age must be housed separately from adult cattle and must not be pastured in fields which have recently been manured with manure of adult cattle. Hygienic measures must be taken to prevent introduction of bacteria by farm visitors such as practitioners, AI technicians, and salesmen.

– **vaccination**

The incidence of clinical cases can be reduced significantly by vaccination (Larsen et al., 1978; Wentink et al., 1991), but vaccinated animals are not protected against infection and may still shed bacteria. Another disadvantage is that vaccinated animals respond to immunologically based diagnostic tests, and therefore carriers can only be recognized in vaccinated herds by fecal culture or antigen detection tests. In some countries vaccination against paratuberculosis is prohibited because vaccinated animals cross-react in the intradermal tuberculin test.

### Monitoring

Research workers have developed sensitive assays for detection of antibodies against *M. paratuberculosis* in milk (Sweeney et al., 1994). Unfortunately these tests are not yet suitable for bulk milk screening. Therefore monitoring and screening must be performed with methods that have limited sensitivities and that can only be performed on blood and feces. Annual testing of pools of five fecal smear samples from all cattle over two years old in a herd is the most feasible monitoring and screening program at the moment. Sensitivity of three of these screenings in a herd at one year intervals is estimated to be 95 percent (Schukken, personal communication).

## REFERENCES

*Barkdale, L., K.S. Kim. 1977. Mycobacterium. Bacteriological Reviews 41:217-372.*

*Bech-Nielsen, S., J.B. Jorgensen, P. Ahrens, and N.C. Feld. 1992. Diagnostic accuracy of a Mycobacterium-phlei absorbed serum enzyme-linked immunosorbent assay for diagnosis of bovine paratuberculosis in dairy cows. J. Clin. Microbiol. 30:613-618.*

*Benedictus, G. 1985. Some aspects of bovine paratuberculosis. PhD Thesis, Utrecht.*

*Benedictus, G., A.A. Dijkhuizen, and J. Stelwagen. 1987. Economic losses due to paratuberculosis in dairy cattle. Vet. Rec. 121:142-146.*

*Braun, R.K., C.D. Buergelt, R.C. Littel, S.C. Linda, and J.R. Simpson. 1990. Use of an enzyme-linked immunosorbent assay to estimate prevalence of paratuberculosis in cattle in Florida. J. Am. Vet. Med. Ass. 196:1251-1254.*

*Chiodini, R.J., H.J. Van Kruiningen, and R.S. Merkal. 1984. Ruminant paratuberculosis (Johne's disease): the current state and future prospects. Cornell Vet. 74:218-262.*

*Collins, M.T., D.C. Sockett, S. Ridge, and J.C. Cox. 1991. Evaluation of a commercial enzyme-linked immunosorbent assay for Johne's disease. J. Clin. Microbiol. 29:272-276.*

*Giessen, van der J.W.G. 1993. A molecular approach to the diagnosis and control of bovine paratuberculosis. PhD thesis, Utrecht.*

*Gilmour, N.J.L., D.I. Nisbet, and J.G. Brotherston 1965. Experimental oral infection of calves with Mycobacterium Johnei J. Comp. Path. 75:281-286.*

*Goodfellow, M., and Cross T. 1984. The biology of actinomycetes. In: M. Goodfellow, M. Mordaski, and S.T. Williams (Eds.) Classification. pp:8-164. Academic press, London*

*Goodfellow, M., and L.G. Wayne. 1982. Taxonomy and nomenclature. In: C. Ratledge, and J. Stanford (eds.) The biology of mycobacteria. Physiology, identification and classification. pp: 471-521. Academic press, London.*

*Julian, R.J. 1975. A short review and some observations on Johne's disease with recom mendations for control. Can. Vet. J. 16: 33-43.*

*Larsen, A.B., A.I. Moyle, and E.M. Himes. 1978. Experimental vaccination of cattle against paratuberculosis (Johne's disease) with killed bacterial vaccines: a controlled field study. Am. J. Vet. Res. 39: 65-69.*

*Merkal, R.S. 1983. Paratuberculosis, Proc. Intern. Coll. Paratuberculosis, Ames, IA.*

*Meulenberg, J. 1991. Paratuberculose bij rundvee, hardnekkig en springlevend. Referaat, Vakgroep Infectieziekten en Immunologie, Faculteit Diergeneeskunde, Universiteit Utrecht.*

*Reinders, J.S. 1963. Control of clinical Johne's disease in cattle. PhD thesis, Utrecht.*

*Sweeney, R.W., R.H. Whitlock, C.L. Buckley, P. Spencer, A.E. Rosenberger, and L.J. Hutchinson. 1994. Diagnosis of paratuberculosis in dairy cattle, using enzyme-linked immunosorbent assay for detection of antibodies against Mycobacterium paratuberculosis in milk. Am. J. Vet. Res. 55: 905-909.*

*Thompson, D.E. 1994. The role of mycobacteria in Crohn's disease. J. Med. Microbiol. 41: 74-94.*

*Whipple, D.L., and R.S. Merkal. 1983. Modifications in the techniques for cultivation of Mycobacterium paratuberculosis. Proc. Intl. Colloq. Res. Paratb., Ames IA. pp: 82-92.*

*Whipple, D.L. 1991. Prevalence and economic impact of paratuberculosis. In: RG Chiodini and JM Kreeger (eds.), Proceedings of the third International Colloquium on Paratuberculosis, Orlando USA, pp: 381-388.*

*Whitlock, R.H,, L.T. Hutchenson, R. Merkal, L.T. Glickman, R.C. Rossiter, S. Harmon P. Spencer, J. Fetrow, J. Bruce, C.E. Benson, and J. Dick .1985. Prevalence and economic considerations of Johne's disease in the northeast US. Proc. 89th An. Mtg. US Animal Health Assoc. Milwauki Wi. pp 848-490.*

*Wood, P.R., H. Billman-Jacobe, A.R. Milnerr, and M. Carrigan. 1991. Serological and cellular assays for the diagnosis mycobacterial infections in cattle. In: R.G. Chiodini and J.M. Kreeger (eds.), Proceedings of the third International Colloquium on Paratuberculosis, Orlando USA, pp: 12-21.*

## 8.7 SALMONELLOSIS

Salmonellosis is an important disease in cattle, and infections caused by *Salmonella dublin* in particular, are common the world over (WHO, 1988). *S. dublin* is more or less adapted to cattle and outbreaks of infections most likely originate, either directly or indirectly, from cattle. *S. dublin* seems to establish itself in endemic areas where extensive, rough grazing is common, where cattle drink from streams, or where liver fluke parasitosis occurs.

### 8.7.1 EPIDEMIOLOGY

Peak incidences of salmonellosis in dairy cattle are observed in autumn or winter (Visser 1994b). Adult cows which recover from clinical disease caused by *S. dublin* may become permanently infected and excrete salmonellae. Such latent infections may be activated during periods of stress, for example, at parturition, and infected cows can be intermittent shedders for life (Wray et al., 1977). Contamination of buildings, pasture and streams may lead to further dissemination and infection of livestock (Noordhuizen and Frankena, 1994). Salmonellae can be excreted in milk for three to four weeks and transmitted to calves by feeding milk. Salmonellae have been isolated from mummified fetuses and still-born calves and it has been suggested by several authors that latent carriers might produce congenitally infected calves (Richardson et al., 1973; Counter et al., 1980). However, an important role of congenital infection in the epidemiology of *S. dublin* has not been reported.

### 8.7.2 ECONOMIC IMPORTANCE

*Salmonella dublin* belongs to the group of zoonotic salmonella species which are associated with human food poisoning (Werner et al., 1979). Poultry, pork and cattle and their products are the most important source of salmonella infections in humans (D'Aoust, 1989). Human beings can be infected by drinking unpasteurised milk but fecal contamination of milk probably presents the greater risk for infections in humans. Outbreaks of milk-borne *S. dublin* infections in humans have been observed. Veterinarians can develop pustular dermatitis caused by *S. dublin* after forced delivery of dead or emphysematous calves (Visser, 1991). In a number of countries, therefore, programs have been started to reduce prevalence of salmonellosis in cattle.

### 8.7.3 ETIOLOGY

Salmonellae are facultative anaerobic rods. The genus *Salmonella* is a member of the family Enterobacteriaceae and is divided into 2 species, *S. enterica* and *S. bongori* with *S. enterica* subdivided into 6 subspecies. Most salmonellae belong to *S. enterica* subspecies *enterica*. It is common practice to identify the organisms by the genus followed by the serovar (*S. typhimurium*). Approximately 2300 serovars have been described on the basis of somatic (O), flagellar (H), and capsular (Vi) antigens (Leminor et al., 1983). *Salmonella dublin* belongs to the serogroup D1 with the O:9,12 antigenic factors (Popoff et al., 1992). *Salmonellae* are ubiquitous organisms that cause infections in various animal species and in humans.

*S. dublin* is the predominant serotype in dairy cattle. S. dublin may survive for several months in faeces and slurry. The bacterium can be inactivated at 60 °C in 20 minutes. Inactivation can also be achieved with standard disinfectants such as formalin (5%) and chloride (0.2%) but the efficacy of disinfectants is strongly reduced in the presence of organic substances such as feces.

### 8.7.4 CLINICAL SIGNS

Acute outbreaks of *Salmonella dublin* enteritidis in dairy herds are characterised by septicaemia and gastroenteritis. Acute watery diarrhoea, fever, and abortions may be observed (Visser et al., 1993). Young cattle may develop arthritis or meningitis and nasal or ocular discharge. In calves, *S. dublin* is a common cause of pneumonia, often seen in combination with gastro-enteritis resulting in diarrhoea (Visser et al., 1992). Arthritis and osteomyelitis and occasionally peripheral necrosis of limbs or tail may be observed.

### 8.7.5 DIAGNOSIS

*Salmonella* is readily cultured from feces or rectal swabs in cases of clinical salmonellosis before antibiotic treatment is started. Culture from fetuses is important for diagnosis of salmonella abortions. Direct culture can be performed on brilliant green agar. Selective enrichment media (e.g. selenite broth or tetrathionate broth) can be used for accumulation of *salmonellae*. To identify carriers, individual fecal samples are needed and direct culture should be performed from these samples. By the use of serological assays, antibodies against lipopolysaccharides (LPS) of *S. dublin* can be determined. Cattle normally respond promptly to LPS antigen of *Salmonella* (Segall et al., 1991; Roden et al., 1992) and *Salmonella* LPS (O-antigen) is thought to be of major importance in the host defence against salmonella (Roantree et al., 1971). There are several reports on application of serological methods, such as ELISA, to detect antibodies to *S. dublin* LPS in cattle. Most of these ELISAs are designed to identify individual carriers in cattle herds (House et al., 1993), but some ELISAs are also suitable for serological screening in large series of cattle herds (Hoorfar et al., 1993).

## 8.7.6 SALMONELLOSIS CONTROL OUTLINE

### Screening

During an outbreak of *S. dublin* infections in a herd, diseased animals can be effectively treated with antibiotics (Wray et al., 1993). After an outbreak a herd can be infected for years, even when the herd is closed, because some cows may become permanent carriers (Wray et al., 1989). In this stage, control of the infection must be focused on hygienic measures (see management) and detection of carriers. Recently, sensitive ELISAs have been developed which can be a useful method to trace previous Salmonella infections in cattle herds (Hoorfar et al., 1993) and to identify *S. dublin* carrier cattle (House et al., 1993; Konrad et al., 1994). However, the bacteria are often shed intermittently, making it difficult to isolate *Salmonella* from fecal samples. Therefore, only active shedders can be identified by culturing *Salmonella* from fecal samples, and shedding carriers can be discriminated from transiently infected cattle only by repeated positive detections of *S. dublin* in feces.

### Eradication

To eradicate *S. dublin* from a herd, utmost hygienic measures must be taken and farm management must be altered to prevent dissemination of the pathogen (see management) over the farm. To stop shedding of *salmonellae* into the environment, acutely infected animals must be isolated and treated with antibiotics. Shedding carrier cows must be culled. Shedding carriers are identified by a repeated positive culture from their faeces. Cultures of feces of all animals in the herd must be performed and positive cows must be sampled again. Carrier cows can also be detected by monthly serological investigations but most of these carriers shed bacteria for limited periods or do not shed bacteria at all (House et al., 1993). Removal of shedders is fundamental to control and elimination of *S. dublin* and removal of carriers in conjunction with hygienic management and good nutrition has been successfully applied for elimination of *S. dublin* from infected herds (Nielsen et al., 1992)

### Prevention

#### – management

To prevent introduction of *Salmonella*, herds should be closed and if stock are purchased they must be quarantined for at least 7 days and their health monitored daily. Fecal and serological examination for *S. dublin* are worthwhile for purchased cattle. Surface water can be contaminated with salmonella and therefore cattle should be provided with ground water from clean drinking troughs or buckets. After application of slurry or manure, pastures should be rested for at least six weeks. In regions where liver flukes are prevalent, a fluke control program should be instituted (Wray, 1993). Visitors who have been to other farms should be provided with protective clothing and clean disinfected boots. Footbaths with active disinfectants should be provided at the entries of the livestock houses. Calves and young stock should be housed strictly separated from adult cows to prevent transmission between adult cows and calves and young stock.

– **vaccination**

Vaccination of calves has been shown to be helpful during an outbreak and also to provide passive protection. Parenterally as well as orally administered vaccines are available (Bauerfeind et al., 1995). Live attenuated, orally administered Salmonella vaccines provide the best protection against infection, especially when large doses are used. This superior protection is due to the ability of live vaccines to stimulate a more effective cell-mediated immune response when compared with killed preparations. The oral route allows the attenuated vaccine strain to utilize natural routes of invasion, thereby presenting antigen to lymphocytes in the gut-associated lymphoid tissue, and inducing production of secretory IgA on mucosal surfaces throughout the body (Clarke and Gyles, 1993). Vaccination of calves with live attenuated Salmonella vaccines have been shown to induce a mucosal immune response and to successfully reduce clinical signs of *S. dublin* infections (Jones et al., 1991; Segall et al., 1994; Segall et al., 1993). During the last decade a number of strategies have been used to construct live vaccines and to design mutations for vaccine constructs (Chatfield et al., 1992; Carrier et al., 1992). This has resulted in development of efficacious oral vaccines with minimal undesirable effects (Clarke and Gyles, 1993). In herds with a high salmonella prevalence, all cattle, including pregnant cows and calves, should be vaccinated at the end of the summer (Visser, 1994ab). In a salmonella control program it is preferable to vaccinate all herds in high prevalence regions. However protection against infection and excretion of salmonella by vaccination is incomplete and therefore a vaccination program should always be accompanied by hygienic measures.

## Monitoring

In naive herds salmonellosis can be monitored by ELISA screening (Hoorfar et al., 1993). Effective milk screening has been reported (House et al., 1993). In vaccinated or infected herds accurate serologic diagnosis requires a test that can differentiate chronic infections, convalescence, and vaccination responses. Differentiation of these groups can be made by serial testing: antibody responses to vaccination and infection often differ from antibody levels of carriers (House et al., 1993). Monitoring for shedding of bacteria by repeated culture of faeces of individual cattle can also be done but will be costly.

## REFERENCES

*Bauerfeind, R., and H.G. Baljer. 1995. Salmonellose beim rind - Gegenwärtige erreger resistenzsituation und kritische bewertung der impfmöglichkeiten. Coll. Vet. XXV: 11-17.*

*Carrier, M.J., S.N. Chatfield, G. Dougan, U.T. Nowicka, D. O'Callaghan, J.E. Beesly, S. Milano, E. Cillari, and F.Y. Liew. 1992. Expression of human IL-1 beta in Salmonella typhimurium. A model system for the delivery of recombinant proteins in vivo. J. Immunol. 148:1176-1181.*

*Chatfield, S., J.L. Li, M. Sydenham, G. Douce, and G. Dougan. 1992. Salmonella genetics and vaccine development. In: Molecular biology of Bacterial Infection: Current Status and Future Perspectives. Eds. C.E. Hoermache, C.W. Penn and C.J. Smyth, pp. 299-312. Cambridge: Cambridge University Press.*

*Clarke, R.C., and C.L. Gyles. 1993. Salmonella in: Pathogenesis of bacterial infections in animals. Eds. C.L. Gyles and C.O. Thoen, Iowa state university press, Ames.*

*Counter, D.E., and E.A. Gibson. 1980. Salmonella dublin infection in self contained dai ry herds in East Anglia: excretion at calving. Vet. Rec. 107:191.*

*D'Aoust, J.Y. 1989. Salmonella. In: Foodborne bacterial Pathogens. Ed. M.P. Doyle, pp327-445. New York: Marcel Dekker.*

*Hoorfar, J., N.C. Feld, A.L. Schirmer, V. Bitsch, and P. Lind. 1993. Serodiagnosis of Salmonella dublin infection in danish dairy herds using O-antigen based enzyme-linked immunosorbent assay. Can. J. Vet. Res. 57:268-274.*

*House, J.K., B.P. Smith, G.W. Dilling, and L.A. Roden. 1993. Enzyme-linked immuno sorbent assay for serologic detection of Salmonella dublin carriers on a large dairy. Am. J. Vet. Res. 54:1391-1399.*

*Jones, P.W., G. Dougan, C. Hayward, N. Mackensie, P. Collins, and S. Chatfield. 1991. Oral vaccination of calves against experimental salmonellosis using a double aro-mutant of Salmonella typhimurium. Vaccine 9:29-34.*

*Konrad, H., B.P. Smith, G. W. Dilling, and J.K. House. 1994. Production of Salmonella sero group D (09)- specific enzyme-linked immunosorbent assay antigen. Am. J. Vet. Res. 55:1647-1651.*

*Leminor, L., and M.Y. Popoff. 1987. Designation of Salmonella enterica sp. nov. as the type and only species of the genus Salmonella. Int. J. Syst. Bacteriol. 37:465-468.*

*Nielsen, B.B., and E.M. Vestergaard. 1992. Use of ELISA in the eradication of Salmonella dublin infection, in Proceedings Symp. Salmonella and salmonellosis. Plouragan-France, pp 220-224.*

*Noordhuizen, J.P.T.M. and K.Frankena. 1994. Salmonella enteritidis: clinical epidemio logical approaches for prevention and control of S. enteritidis in poultry production. International J. of Food Microbiology 21:131-143.*

*Popoff, M.Y., and L. Leminor. 1992. Antigenic Formulas of the Salmonella Serovars, 6th Revision. Paris: Pasteur Institute.*

*Richardson, A. 1973. The transmission of Salmonella dublin to calves from adult carrier cows. Vet. Rec. 92:112-115.*

*Roantree, R.J. 1971. The relationship of lipopolysaccharide structure to bacterial virulence. In: G. Weinsbaum, S. Kalis, Eds. Bacterial Endotoxins. New York: Academic Press, pp. 1-37.*

*Roden, L., B.P. Smith, S.J. Spier, and G.W. Dilling. 1992. Effects of calf age and salmonella bactericin type on ability to produce immunoglobulins directed against salmonella whole cells or lipopolysaccharide. Am. J. Vet. Res. 53: 1895-1899.*

*Segall, T., S.O. Jacobsson, K. Karlsson, and A.A. Lindberg. 1994. Mucosal immune responses in calves orally vaccinated with a live auxotrophic aroA Salmonella dublin strain. Zentralbl. Veterinarmed. B 41: 305-312.*

*Segall, T, and A.A. Lindberg. 1991. Experimental oral Salmonella dublin infection in cal ves: A bacteriological and pathological study. J. Vet. Med. B. 38: 169-185.*

*Segall, T, and A.A. Lindberg. 1993. Oral vaccination of calves with an aromatic-dependent Salmonella dublin (O9,12) hybrid expressing O4,12 protects against S. dublin (O9,12) but not against Salmonella typhimurium (O4,4,12).*

*Visser, I.J.R. 1994a. An outbreak of Salmonella dublin (in Dutch) Tijdschr. Diergeneesk. 119: 101.*

*Visser, I.J.R. 1991. Cutaneous salmonellosis in veterinarians. Vet. Rec. 129: 364.*

*Visser, I.J.R. 1994b. Salmonellosis in dairy cattle and small ruminants (in Dutch) Dier en Arts 9: 313.*

*Visser, I.J.R., M. Veen, and J.W.B. Van der Giessen. 1992. Salmonella dublin infections in dairy cattle, a review (in Dutch) Tijdschr. Diergeneesk. 117: 730-735.*

*Visser, I.J.R., M. Veen, J.W.B. Van der Giessen, D.J. Peterse, and W. Wouda. 1993. Salmonella dublin in dairy farms in the north of the Netherlands (in Dutch) Tijdschr. Diergeneesk. 118: 84-87.*

*World Health Organisation, Salmonellosis control: The role of animal product hygiene. Technical Report Series 774, Geneva, Switzerland, 1988.*

*Werner, S.B., G.L. Humprey, and I. Kamei. 1979. Association between raw milk and human Salmonella dublin infections. Br. Med. J. 2:238-241.*

*Wray, C. 1993. Bovine salmonellosis: an update. Ir. Vet. J. 46: 137-140.*

*Wray, C., and W.J. Sojka. 1977. Research of the progress of dairy science: bovine salmonellosis. J. Dairy Res. 44: 383-425.*

*Wray, C., Q.C. Wadsworth, D.W. Richards, and J.H. Morgan. 1989. A three year study of Salmonella dublin infection in a closed dairy herd Vet. Rec. 124: 532-535.*

# ANIMAL HEALTH AND DAIRY PRODUCTION IN DEVELOPING COUNTRIES

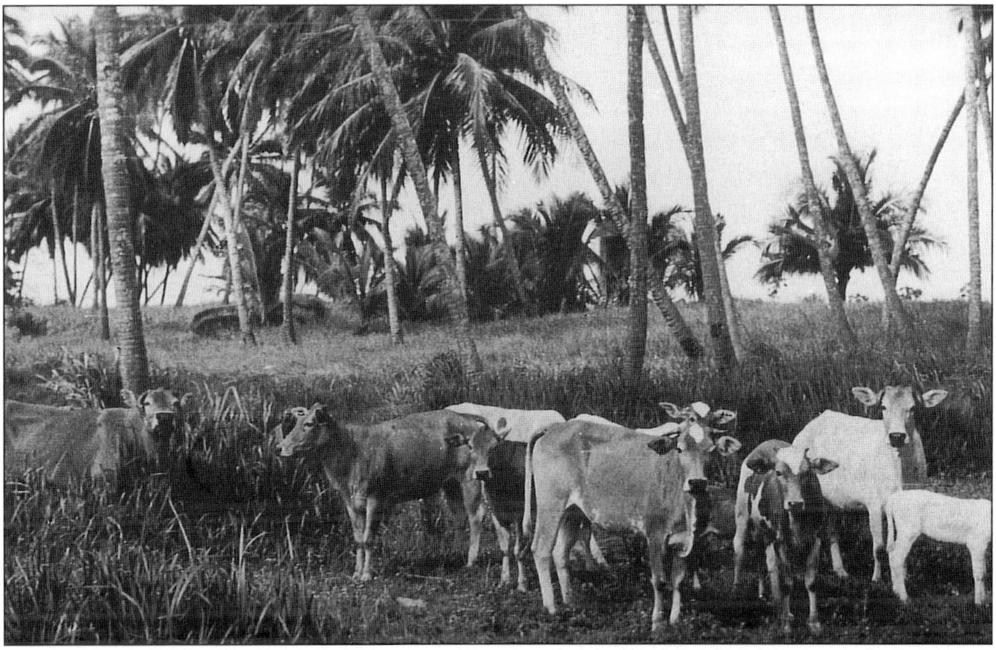

# 9 ANIMAL HEALTH AND DAIRY PRODUCTION IN DEVELOPING COUNTRIES

Dick Zwart and Rijk de Jong

Department of Animal Husbandry, Section of Animal Production Systems, Tropical Animal Husbandry division, Wageningen Institute of Animal Sciences, Agricultural University, P.O.Box 338, 6700 AH Wageningen, The Netherlands

## 9.1 INTRODUCTION

Herd health and production management (HH & PM) programs such as those being implemented in intensive dairy husbandry systems, cannot be strictly transferred to developing countries (Kaasschieter et al., 1992; Jong, 1996). This is based on several reasons. Among these are macro-economic and socio-economic aspects, the complexity of dairy development and the multifunctional roles of cattle. Moreover, dairy production takes place in different ecological zones and under quite different production conditions. This in contrast to developed countries, whereby in a continously improving infrastructure, much attention was paid to health care. In addition, HH & PM programs were developed, with the aim to support the daily management to the farmers.

In this chapter we address animal health and dairy production in developing countries from the point of view where the current situation differs from developed countries. From there we will discuss how dairy production fits into a farming system approach. Such an approach requires a surveillance system with different technical parameters. These will be placed in the context of possibilities in developing countries.

## 9.2 CURRENT SITUATION OF DAIRY PRODUCTION

Dairy production in developing countries differs in many respects from that in developed countries.

### (a) Macro-economic aspects

It is expected that developing countries will consume 37 kg milk equivalents (including non food use) per caput in the year 2000. In addition to an increase of local milk production from 143 million tons in 1988 to 187 million tons in 2000, a net import in these countries of 23 million tons of milk equivalents is expected in the year 2000 (Phelan, 1994).

The total trade in dairy products on the world market (outer inter-European

Union transactions) accounts, however, for less than 6% of the total production. Food aid amounts to 20% of the imports of developing countries, but varies greatly depending on domestic surpluses in North America, Europe and New Zealand. The small proportion of milk products on the world market and the increasing demand has led in many developing countries to political pressure for self-sufficiency, whereby a livestock policy was developed, with the aim to increase the supply of dairy products by expansion of the number of dairy cows and/or an increased production per animal.

The increase in demand will partly come from higher consumption per caput, but mainly from a larger, more or less affluent population in urban centres. This higher income of the urban dwellers will create a bigger demand for livestock products and this market is expected to increase even more rapidly than the urban population. The temptation is then great to supply the local urban elite with cheap imported dairy products, at the detriment of the local farms. The long term negative aspects for the local dairy industry of relying on reconstituted milk from the heavily subsidized imported or donated dairy products is now widely recognized (Walshe, 1994).

In many developing countries dairy development offers a real opportunity to increase economic growth and reduce poverty in rural areas. Aimed at small farmers, where milk production is labor-intensive, it contributes to both income and employment generation. Devendra (1993) estimates that approximately 76 - 95% of the animal population in South-East Asia is owned by small farmers with an average farm size of 1 - 2 ha and similar figures apply for Africa south of the Sahara (Grijseels, 1988).

### (b) Ecological zones

Dairy production in developing countries takes place in different ecological zones. Winrock (1992) distinguishes five zones, i.e. arid, semi-arid, sub-humid, humid and highlands. These ecological zones influence the plant growth and hence the availability of protein. They also have an influence on disease vectors and thereby the distribution of tick-borne diseases, trypanosomiasis and internal parasites (Table 1).

*Table 1. Animal health constraints in different ecological zones*

| Constraints | Arid | Semi-arid | Sub-humid | Humid | Highlands |
|---|---|---|---|---|---|
| Epidemic infectious diseases | + | + | + | + | + |
| Vector borne diseases | + | + | +++ | +++ | +++ |
| Parasitic diseases | - | + | +++ | +++ | +++ |
| Production/ Management diseases | - | ++ | +++ | + | +++ |

*+ = some importance; ++ = moderate importance; +++ = very important*

### (c) Dairy development projects

Dairy development projects require much more time, are more complex in nature than in developed countries and require an intensive and keen interest in monitoring data of progress in technical and economic productivity (Jong, 1996). Efforts to get true information on land size, livestock and details on income take time due to smallholders' fear that such information will be used for taxation. Data on performance of calf rearing require a long term monitoring from birth to age at first calving, and preferably longer to include lactation details and overall inputs during the whole period to make a sensible comparison between common and improved practices.

Temperature and humidity also determine whether purebred European cattle can be kept, e.g. in the highlands. Purebred Bos indicus or their crosses are kept in zones with high temperature and/or humidity.

### (d) Multifunctionality of cattle

Cattle have many functions, especially amongst smallholders. One of them is to supply draught power even by female crossbred dairy animals. However, a combination of poor nutrition and hard work has a detrimental effect on the ovarian activity and milk production (Zerbini et al., 1993 a,b). Manure production is another purpose of keeping cattle and farmers do appreciate its value for their crops (Ifar, 1996). In Kenya for example, cow manure is widely used for coffee plants, whereby the soil fertility for the fodder grasses is often neglected.

### (e) Production systems

Dairy production takes place in different production systems. Milk production and consumption by (agro) pastoralists in Africa and Asia is from large herds with seasonal surplus of milk products sold to towns or exchanged for grain with agriculturalists. In Latin America large dual purpose Zebu/Criollo ranch herds are seasonally milked mainly for supply to milk (powder) plants. Landless labor (mainly in Asia) and smallholders produce milk from a few cattle as a supplementary business to off-farm and arable cropping activities. Small and medium-scale commercial dairies are found in towns and peri-urban areas. In addition, large-scale farms, mainly private ones in Latin America or (para)statal farms in Africa and Asia are found around urban centres (Winrock, 1992; Jong, 1996). In one country different livestock production systems may exist side by side and it is mainly the government policy that will decide which system will survive at the end.

### (f) Governmental attitude to smallholders

The intensive commercial farms were established in the colonial period to meet the demand of the army, cities and even to provide a surplus for export. The institutions and services that were established closely copied western institutions. Parastatals, cooperatives and dairy boards were designed to serve the large colonial farms, but did not foster and serve the needs of the smallholders (Walshe, 1994). In some instances smallholder farmers could, however, make use of the veterinary services through vaccination and dipping facilities, and sometimes these services were even compulsory, e.g. dipping for tick control, foot and mouth disease vaccination.

After the colonial period the negative attitude to smallholder development was exacerbated in most countries by two unjustified policy decisions. First, a decision was made that the colonial dairy farmers (e.g. in Zambia) would be replaced by parastatal dairy farms. Where colonial farms did not exist (e.g. in Tanzania, Tunisia and Ethiopia) dairy development would be based primarily on parastatal or state farms. It was argued that the skills and management capabilities needed for successful dairying could be replaced or developed under a parastatal structure, but it is now clear that this approach was mistaken. The problems experienced by dairy parastatals are similar to those experienced by all parastatals: political interference (e.g. concerning milk prices), inadequate management, low productivity and poor economic performance. Second, governments were encouraged to rely on reconstituting cheap imports (donated or purchased at low world market prices and distorted exchange rates) to meet the growing urban demand. Thus sophisticated milk processing plants, often funded by donor agencies, were established in many major cities. The familiarity of the industrialized countries giving technical assistance based upon an intensive dairy model and the ready supply of equipment from the commercial sector, reinforced the newly independent countries' tendencies to build large-scale facilities under government control (Development Cooperation, 1992; Walshe, 1994).

Although the colonial legacy was negative in terms of its influence on the policies that governments followed (even after the colonial era) and on the culture and outlook of the dairy institutions that were established, it had many positive aspects. For example, specialized dairy breeds were introduced, and research was undertaken on dairy production and management (e.g. grass and forage production, animal nutrition, crossbreeding and animal health). Input supply services, artificial insemination, extension and milk collection services were also organized in a number of countries. Colonial farmers showed what could be achieved with improved dairy stock and good management under tropical conditions. It is regrettable that few countries have been successful in switching their emphasis to smallholder dairy development and combining the relevant parts of the pre-independence experience into strategies aimed at smallholders (Walshe, 1994). Most developing countries have now realized that these large parastatals are not the best solution for the dairy industry, and have made a switch to the smallholder farmers. India and Kenya are countries where this has been more or less successful (Banerjee, 1994; Walshe, 1994; Mc Dermott et al., 1993).

In conclusion, it can be said that, given all these differences, a western style of intensive commercial dairy production cannot always simply be transfered to tropical countries and that there are different solutions possible for dairy development in developing countries.

## 9.3 FARMING SYSTEMS APPROACH AND SURVEILLANCE SYSTEMS

The introduction of new technologies in smallholder dairy systems did not always bring the desired results. Similar experiences were found in the crop sciences, and it was first in this field that the term farming systems analysis or approach (FSA) was used. The FSA concept was later followed by animal scientists (Grijseels, 1988; Schiere, 1995). A systems approach implies that the farm household is studied as an entity which is made up of different interacting components (Rheenen, 1995). Livestock improvements cannot be considered separately from the effects it may have on other components. For example, zero grazing may be excellent for the control of ticks and other parasites, but the increased labor requirements may conflict with existing cropping patterns and household activities.

After an identification of the farming system and the identification of constraints, the next step is the introduction of management strategies and technical innovations into the system. Schiere (1995) distinguishes three systems. Open systems can import resources to satisfy their demands, the so-called high external input agriculture (HEIA). In closed systems, the demand has to be adjusted to the resources, the so-called low external input agriculture (LEIA). In general terms it can be stated that the western oriented dairy enterprise is based on HEIA, whereas the small farm is based on LEIA. A third intermediate system consists of a relative access to labor and capital. Examples for this system are the fodder banks in Nigeria, aimed at increasing milk production in the dry season or straw treatment with ureum in India. Trypanotolerant or tick resistant cattle, whereby the need for drugs is reduced, can also be considered as an intermediate system.

FSA has faced criticism that it is mainly crop-oriented and has rarely been applied to livestock processes, despite the similarities between the two (Schiere, 1995). FSA has also been accused of being too qualitative in its approach, and the problem of collecting reliable data and more specifically which data should not be underestimated (Udo & Brouwer, 1993). FSA is also mainly farmer oriented, but there are other actors in the field. Animal feed supply and animal health for example are certainly considered important by the farmer, but he has many more elements to deal with, as can be seen in Figure 1, adapted from Grijseels (1988). This is at least partly related to the fact that extensive operations are commonly multifunctional (for producing crops, milk, meat) comprising major socio-economic and cultural or religious constraints. Figure 1 is a simplification of the major elements characterizing the intensive systems in the developed countries and those in developing countries.

Another major difference is that more elements are beyond managerial control in extensive operations in developing countries than in intensive operations in developed countries. This relatively low level of control is related to the sociological, economic, cultural, religious and political structures prevailing in a certain region which are impacting livestock production more heavily in developing than in developed countries (Grijseels, 1988). In Figure 1 this is illustrated by component C.

*Figure 1. A simplified representation of the elementary differences between intensive, monofunctional farming systems in developed countries (parts A and B) and more extensive, multifunctional farming systems in developing countries (part C added to parts A and B). (Adapted by Noordhuizen after Grijseels, 1988). Part C largely comprises constraints*

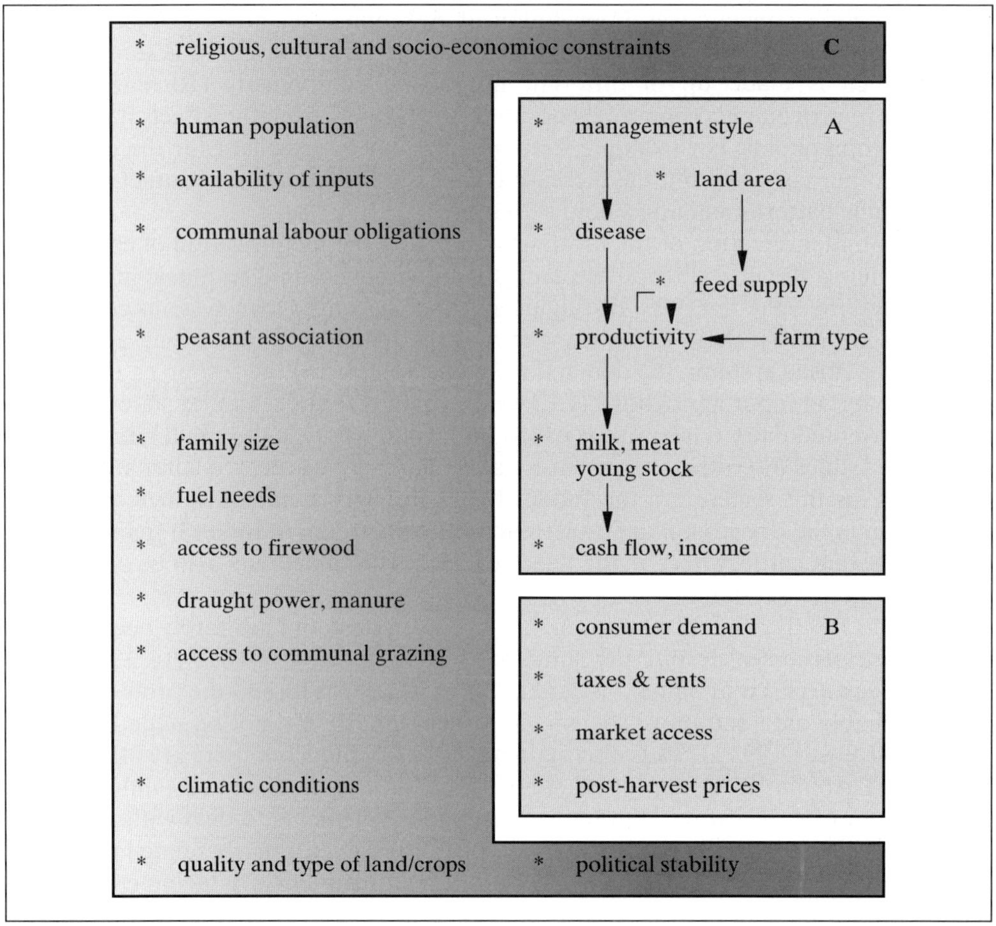


Zwart (1994) considers the farmgate price of the milk as an important factor which can determine failure or success of a dairy enterprise. There are also the policy makers in the region to reckon with. They can have certain objectives, e.g. development of rural dairy production, an activity which may formerly be unknown to the farmers. Typical examples in this respect can be found in areas of Indonesia, Kenya, Sri Lanka and Tanzania, where dairy farming was unknown and only introduced in the last decennia (Jong, 1996).

Moreover, a farmer is not a scientist, and what he considers "normal", like a low milk production, a low fertility etc. can in a common dialogue with him be identified as a "problem" (Zwart, 1994). Important in this respect is also his knowledge about diseases. Ethnoveterinary surveys (i.e. surveys based on local knowledge systems) can provide useful information on local perceptions of livestock diseases and their control. The main value of these studies for delivery of veterinary interventions may lie in tabulating and elucidating the ways in which disease are perceived locally and in identifying the discontinuities with veterinary concepts promoted in the region by outsiders (Curry et al., 1993).

Disease and animal surveillance must have clear objectives and as such can be mentioned:

1. it must help to understand the role of animals in farming systems and offer options for improvement.
2. it must furnish sufficiently reliable figures on disease prevalence which can be used by farmers and public organisations to control diseases.
3. it must offer a good analysis of the cost and benefit ratio for disease control.

*Figure. 2. Generalistic outline of a Farming Systems Approach in Herd Health and Production Management*

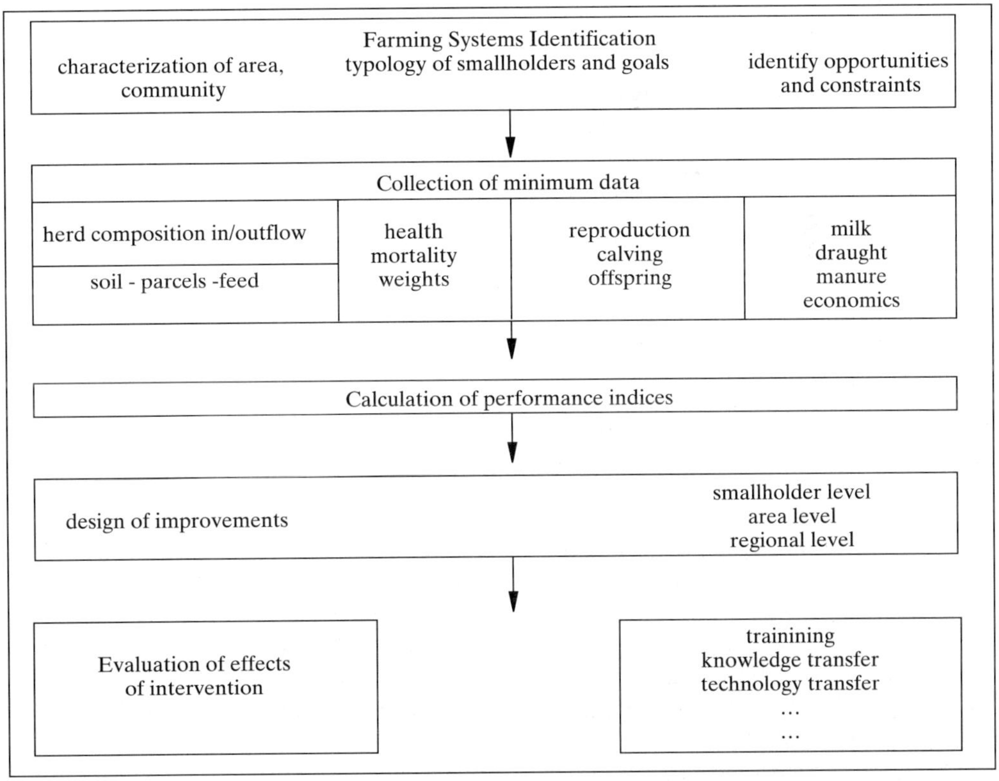

Any herd health and production management protocol meant for implementation on smallholder farms in developing countries should specifically be designed and tailor-made for local conditions. Among others this means that not only veterinary-technical issues must be addressed (as usual is in western situations) but also socio-economic, cultural and religious ones. The aforenamend means that specific protocols cannot be presented here. We have tried to design a more generalistic approach, adapted from Udo and Brouwer (1993) and outlined in Figure 2. You might make a comparison with the protocol in Chapter 1.

From Figure 2 it can be read, that the farming systems identification comprises both characterization of the area and community, and the typology of the smallholders. Involving objectives, opportunities and constraints means that the background for and the socio-economic conditions of a particular farming system in a particular area can be depicted. Against this background, a more specific protocol can be designed, hence being more tailor-made. The component of training of smallholders, and the transfer of technology is an essential element in the HH & PM service in the (sub-)tropics. It assists in improving skills and provides a better basis for future cooperation and development.

As can be seen from Table 2, the level of detailing in herd performance indices for pastoral systems or mixed farming systems is much lower than in specialized systems presented in the preceding Chapters. It is rather difficult to collect sufficient data which is reliable or representative for a regional population. Nevertheless it has been proven that the generalistic approach as given above can be adequate (Desai, 1986; Klink, 1994; Jong, 1996).

Udo and Brouwer (1993) stressed the fact, that the use of a database system might help to define a clear and feasible aim in analysing farming systems, whereby databases and simulation models interact. Reproduction and mortality are in this respect important parameters. Without further analysing the cause of mortality Hermans et al. (1989) and Udo et al. (1990, 1992) could calculate for Bangladesh that in some villages where grazing lands are present, the available feed would be sufficient to allow milk production, draught, weight gain and reproduction. In other villages the herds would not be able to replace themselves. This combined approach of information gathering for health and (milk)production has been used in many countries (Wilson and Clarke, 1976; Pullan, 1980) and is an important tool to set priorities in controlling diseases.

The next step then is to investigate the causes of mortality and poor reproduction. Veterinary services have always concentrated on aspects of mortality caused by infectious or notifiable diseases. They relied and should still rely on the activity of well trained animal health assistants in the field. This approach works reasonably well for the control of major epizootics like rinderpest, foot and mouth disease and contagious bovine pleuropneumonia through vaccination and quarantine measures.

It should be realised, however, that on a worldwide scale, none of the major animal diseases has been eradicated, but that on the contrary more diseases have emerged and new regions have become infected (Scott, 1988). Especially after the re-occurrence of rinderpest in large areas of Africa in the '80s, it was realised that the control and/or eradication of infectious diseases involves more than making a good vaccine or development of a

*Table 2. Relative relevance of herd/flock parameters for different production systems*

| Major objectives | Pastoral system<br>capital asset, meat, milk | Mixed system<br>intermediate pr, capital asset, milk | Specialized farms<br>milk; meat |
|---|---|---|---|
| **Herd parameters** | | | |
| **Reproduction** | | | |
| calving interval | – | – | ++ |
| calving rate | ++ | ++ | ++ |
| offspring weaned | ++ | + | ++ |
| age first calving | + | + | ++ |
| **Offtake** | | | |
| sales | – | – | ++ |
| all outflow | ++ | ++ | – |
| **Mortality** | **++** | **++** | **++** |
| **Body weights** | **+** | **+** | **++** |
| **Growth rate** | **–** | **–** | **++** |
| **Milk** | | | |
| yield | – | – | ++ |
| offtake | ++ | ++ | – |
| % in milk | + | + | ++ |
| **Indices** | **++** | **+** | **–** |
| **Feed consumption** | **–** | **++** | **++** |
| **Draught** | **+** | **++** | **–** |
| **Manure** | **+** | **++** | **–** |
| **Economics** | | | |
| cost-benefits | ++ | ++ | ++ |
| finance/insurance | ++ | ++ | – |

*– : not relevant  + : relevant  ++ : highly relevant*

good drug to control them. More emphasis is now placed on reorganisation of veterinary services, e.g. through privatization and full cost recovery (Haan, 1993). Moreover, non-infectious diseases and diseases related with management begin to play a more important role with the intensification of livestock production. This goes hand in hand with the development of diagnostic tests to support the diagnosis based on chemical and post-mortem examination. A central better equipped laboratory could carry out more complicated tests and confirm field diagnosis (Ozawa, 1991). Great distances and a poor distribution network limited in some countries their function and to overcome this the number of decentralized diagnostic centra were greatly enlarged. This policy brought the diagnostic centres closer to the farmers. This stressed the fact that this decentralisation will enhance the service delivery between farmer and service provider and as such it will improve the quality of service by ensuring what the clients wants i.e. providing them with a choice and dealing with the diversity of production-and ecosystems. Based on computerized Herd Health and Production Programs they have developed a so called "Animal Health and Production Improvement Model" (AHPIM) to strengthen this procces of decentralised decision making and service delivery. It does not prescribe a uniform procedure or data-set, neither is it accompanied by a computer software, but rather an approach with a set of guidelines for reorientating the delivery of health and production services.

Reports from Kenya (McDermott et al., 1993), Colombia (Otte and Lobo, 1984), Thailand (Morris and Leidl, 1993), Costa-Rica (Perez, 1994), all strongly suggest that the farmer is only interested in disease surveys when the link with production is clear to him. Over recent years complex multifactorial disease problems have grown rapidly in importance. Management assessment is in this respect an important factor. McDermott et al. (1993) report that on the initial visit farmers would answer questions about their management procedures by describing what they thought was the correct procedure, not what they did. The actual management practice was uncovered on subsequent visits. Perez (1994) in Costa-Rica has overcome this problem through a regular, planned herd health advisory program

When production data are linked with economic data, farmers are very often reluctant to participate, because they fear financial influences from outsiders. Farmers are only willing to cooperate when these two are separated.

Analysis of data from smallholder farmers for calculating indices is difficult because of the small number of animals (sometimes less than four) per farm. Thus, one animal's performance is extremely influential. For predicting mean responses the problem can be overcome by collecting data from more farms (Jong, 1996). An assessment of an individual farm's result, as is done in herd health and production management programs for larger farms, may be relatively unhelpful. Nevertheless data from small farms can be used to find correlations with identifiable groupings like extension areas, dairy societies, artificial insemination and inputs of veterinary services (McDermott et al., 1993; Klink, 1994; Schreuder et al., 1996). Nasir Hussain Shah (1990) working with smallholder milk buffalo farmers in Pakistan, could by a combination of progesterone determinations, good clinical examination, higher attention to the individual animal, hormonal treatment and extension, greatly improve the reproduction capacity of these animals.

Mukhebi (1992) combined epidemiological and economic data and came to an assessment of the impact of theileriosis and its control. The multipurpose use of cattle, the lack of reliable data, the estimation of the value of manure and draught power, make such a cost/benefit analysis often difficult.

In summary, it can be said that data collection is required for a good insight in the measures which should be taken to prevent losses and implement improvement in the system. This can be done at village level by non-academic staff (Haan and Bekure, 1990) or by private farmers' organisations (Desai, 1986). It is only based on this grassroot level data collection that intelligent measures can be taken in the form of disease control, cost-benefit analysis, extension, etc. (Otte and Lobo, 1984).

## 9.4 CLASSIFICATION OF DISEASES AND THEIR CONTROL

In view of the developments in livestock production and animal health care described above, there was a need for another classification of animal diseases than is usually done in textbooks. In its constraint analysis of animal agriculture in Sub-Sahara Africa, Winrock (1992) used a classification system whereby ecosystems and the multifactorial influences come more on the foreground. In the next section we have followed in great lines Winrock's ideas as they were summarized by Doyle (1992).

**Group 1**

Diseases like rinderpest, contagious bovine pleuropneumonia, and foot and mouth disease, which are independent of ecozones or production systems and cause high mortalities and severe economic loss. The technical solutions are largely known, and control depends mainly on socio-economic circumstances. There is a need, however, for (multivalent) thermostable vaccines. Promising results are, e.g. a thermoresistant Rinderpest vaccine, whereby the genome of the Rinderpest virus is incorporated into the Cowpox (vaccinia) virus (Pritchard, 1988).

**Group 2**

Diseases which are mainly vector transmitted. Their presence and severity is often ecozone dependent due to the environmental requirements of their insect vectors, e.g. tick-borne diseases. Control requirements are multifactorial, and changes in land use can greatly influence parasitic diseases. They are partly independent of the production system and partly dependent, e.g. in intensive dairy production with exotic animals. The tick-borne diseases are in this respect very important (Uilenberg et al., 1993). Farmers with valuable exotic dairy cattle generally prefer intensive spraying or dipping, although indigenous herds also benefit from working dip tanks (Table 3).

Intensive tick control through acaricides can now be supplemented by attenuated schizont vaccine against *T. annulata*, while immunization against East Coast Fever is

*Table 3. Technical parameters in 496 indigenous herds comparing villages with working and non-working dips in Kagera region of Tanzania in 1990 and 1991 (Jong, 1996)*

| Parameter | Dips working 1991 | Dips not working 1991 |
|---|---|---|
| Calf mortality % | 23.3 | 34.7 |
| Adult mortality % | 3.1 | 5.7 |
| Overall mortality % | 7.0 | 11.5 |
| Calving rate % | 41.2 | 40.7 |
| Off take % | 9.6 | 7.8 |
| Migration out % | 27.3 | 20.7 |
| Migration in % | 24.9 | 18.9 |

carried out on a limited scale using virulent sporozoite infection and treatment. Prevention of Heartwater, caused by the rickettsia *Cowdria ruminantium*, also still relies mainly on acaricidal tick control; an infection and treatment method is only used on a limited scale. Antigenic diversity is a complication for immunisation procedures in Heartwater and Theileriosis, although research on recombinant vaccines using a common antigen, is promising (Uilenberg et al., 1993; Jongejan and Uilenberg, 1994; Vliet, 1995).

Losses due to trypanosomiasis can be reduced by the use of trypanotolerant cattle (Paling and Dwinger, 1993), trypanocidal drugs and tsetse control (Brandl, 1988). The potential for milk production from trypanotolerant cattle is low and their role in commercial scale production is limited (Walshe et al., 1991). The use of trypanocides is practised in areas with a low tsetse challenge and can result in an acquired immunity in Sahiwal crossbred cattle (Paling et al., 1987). Currently, there are four methods available for the control of the tsetse fly:

1) the sterile male technique,
2) odour and insecticide impregnated traps and sheets,
3) application of insecticide/acaracide on the animal,
4) aerial spraying of insecticides (Brandl, 1988).

The odour-impregnated traps have the big advantage that they will allow participation of the cattle farmer in the control of the tsetse fly. Non cattle owners show far less interest in traps and traps tend to be stolen in some areas. Leak (1996) therefore prefers the "pour on" of acaricides under supervision, because cattle owners can see for themselves the effect on tsetse flies, ticks and other biting insects.

Parasitic diseases can be dramatic through the acute losses they cause, but their most important impact is on the productive performance of the animal without killing it (Klink, 1994). The importance of nutrition may in this respect be more important to counteract the consequences of the parasitic infection than to counteract the establishment of that same infection. The lower feed intake in parasitized animals is the major factor limiting the availability of energy. Added to this are the lower efficiencies with which apparently digestible and metabolisable nutrients are used for fat and protein deposition (Preston and Leng, 1987).

**Group 3**

Other diseases which are largely independent of the ecozone, and their importance increases as production systems are intensified. They cause low mortality except under neo-nates. They are multifactorial in nature and solutions are based on the application of known technical solutions. A few of these production/management diseases will shortly be discussed in more detail.

## 9.4.1. FOOT CARE

Exotic blood in dairy cattle goes along with foot and legs problems. Causes vary from infective agents in wet environments and after wounds from insects and small

*Table 4. The relation between claw problems (and other conditions), fertility and calculated losses of Friesian cattle imported in Sri Lanka (Nell, 1986)*

| Condition | No. of animals | Days between calving/conception | Calving interval | Extra loss in DFl at Dfl 2.50/day |
|---|---|---|---|---|
| Claw problems | 50 | 274 | 559 | 485 |
| Poor condition | 30 | 301 | 586 | 558 |
| Endometritis /Pyometra | 18 | 268 | 553 | 470 |
| Healthy animals | 52 | 91 | 376 | 28 |

stones, to overgrown claws from lack of wear and foot pad erosion associated with feeding (McDowell, 1989). Provision of a dry surface or dry bedding helps as well as regular trimming and walking the animals through a formalin bath. The latter has to be refreshed regularly to remain effective and should have an adjacent clean area for the animals to let the formalin do its weak disinfectant work.

Management practises related to prevent claw disorders and to carry out claw care are economically beneficial. Poor feet will reduce milk yield, longevity at the farm and rate of re-breeding (McDowell, 1989). An example from Sri Lanka illustrates the effects of claw problems, poor condition, pyometra in cows on calving interval and economic loss against the parameters of healthy cows in Table 4.

### 9.4.2 MASTITIS

Mastitis is often mentioned by smallholders as a problem in their cows, especially when calves are hand reared. They refer to clinical mastitis as the visible form, but it is estimated, like in the temperate areas, that sub-clinical mastitis has, however, a much higher prevalence causing higher losses per affected cow. For Indonesia, Ibrahim et al. (1992) cite a study indicating 10% and 14% of cows being affected by clinical and sub-clinical mastitis, respectively. In general this relatively low evidence may also be related with poor diagnostic facilities, but despite the low milk yields in developing countries, farmers cite mastitis as one of their major problems. In practising restricted suckling of calves during the lactation, mastitis can be reduced (Preston, 1989), but also mistakes of farmers resulting in poor and irregular milking can easily be corrected by the calf. Poor milkers, milking techniques and hygiene, which are no exception at smallholder level, cause damage to the teat leading to withholding of the milk by the cow, lower milk yields, mastitis and dirty milk. Cleanliness of the cow, the utensils, the milking area, the milker, and timely milk transport are essential for clean milk production, reasonable keeping quality and safety of the milk for the consumer.

### 9.4.3 DYSTOCIA, CALVING EASE AND REPRODUCTION

Many dairy farmers in the tropics experience with their improved cattle dystocia or difficult calving. Many cases are caused by steaming-up (especially with concentrates) of too small animals or animals in poor condition. It is also common in animals in an overfat condition after a very long dry period. The incidence is high in the case of well-to-do farmers and/or (para)statal farms that tend to follow the theory of steaming-up too much. Smallholders can often not afford the extra feeding at the time, since the cow is not producing cash revenue. According to personal experience at the Egerton College farm in Kenya during the early seventies, it was better to avoid steaming-up, especially in heifers, and let them produce a small calf at the early age of 2 years. Despite the fact that the heifers were not fully grown, dystocia was not a problem. After delivery, calved heifers should be fed properly, but preferably extra to produce a reasonable lactation and to get them in calf again at three months after calving. In order to allow them to reach mature weight an extra month of dry period before the second calving was more effective than late steaming up.

### 9.4.4 NUTRITIONAL DISEASES

Of the nutritional diseases, the metabolic diseases are the most important. Chase (1989) and Monfore (1989) in their epidemiological studies of dairy cows in Java, mention in this respect a few diseases. Inadequate energy and protein intake will produce (secondary) ketosis; inadequate calcium and phosphorus intake predisposes for milk fever. High grain levels, lack of long fibrous material and abrupt changes in the diet are important factors for rumen acidosis and displaced abomasum. Laminitis (pododermatitis aseptica diffusa) is often seen in *Bos taurus* animals after a sudden change in the diet with concentrates.

Deficiency diseases resulting from a lack of sodium, potassium, cobalt, copper (Sutmüller, 1961) have a regional distribution, although phosphorus (Carillo, 1993) and iodine (Zwart, 1959) are perhaps the most important ones on a worldwide scale. There is in this respect an urgent need for field or cow-side tests of metabolic markers in order to identify the consequences of sub-optimal mineral intake before productivity declines (Carillo, 1993). Prevention of these nutritional disorders depends greatly on improvement of the management and farming conditions.

## 9.5 HOUSING AND RELATED EFFECTS

Housing or confinement of livestock has many and important effects in livestock production. In the tropics, various types of housing and confinement exist, which vary according to type of animal, climate, production purposes and the socioeconomic environment. Most of these carry a considerable cost to the farmer in investment and/or labor. The effects of confinement on production can be distinguished in physical aspects of climate, feeding, breeding, disease control, type of housing, investments and labor.

In practical farm management, much depends on traditional knowledge and customs, individual attention and affinity, type of manager, the complex relationships between the "decision maker" and the "decision implementer", etc.

### 9.5.1 PHYSICAL ASPECTS OF CLIMATE

Warm climates (0 - 350 latitude) exhibit direct effects on animals, but these climates also have an indirect effect on cow performance through lower quality forages and

*Table 5A. Effect of environmental conditions on the ratio between dam's weight at 30 days postpartum and birthweight of female calves, and rate of development to 15 months of age (Holstein Frisian breed; weight in kg)*

| Country/state | breed | age of dam | weight of dam | birth weight calf | birthweight to dam weight ratio (%) | weight at 3 mths./birth weight (%) | weight at 15 mths./mature weight (%) |
|---|---|---|---|---|---|---|---|
| New York | Holstein | all | 680 | 42.1 | 6.2 | 234 | 54 |
| N.Carolina | Holstein | 1-st | 522 | 32.5 | 6.1 | | |
| Puerto Rico | Holstein | all | 620 | 38.4 | 6.1 | | |
| Venezuela | Holstein | all | 524 | 30.3 | 5.8 | 254 | 49 |
| Jamaica | Holstein | all | 511 | 28.4 | 5.6 | 235 | 56 |

*Table 5B. Effect of latitude on milk production and reproductive performance of Holstein cattle (all herds are commercial dairies except for Venezuela; all sires originate from USA and Canada AI stations)*

| country/state | latitude ('N) | climate type | milk yield (kg) | age at 1-st calving | days open | calving interval (days) | days dry | survival rate (%) (1) |
|---|---|---|---|---|---|---|---|---|
| New York | 40-42 | cool | 7718 | 28.8 mths. | 116 | 396 | 63 | 53.3 |
| N.Carolina | 35 | warm, humid | 7528 | 29.1 | 122 | 401 | 60 | 51.6 |
| Mexico | 18-28 | hot, dry | 7156 | 28.2 | 162 | 442 | 81 | 45.8 |
| Puerto Rico | 18 | hot, humid | 5464 | 31.2 | 157 | 437 | 108 | 46.1 |
| Colombia | 3-7 | warm, humid | 4771 | 36.1 | 179 | 459 | 87 | 42.2 |
| Venezuela | 8 | hot, humid | 3656 | 28.7 | 206 | 486 | 181 | 38.3 |

*(1) calculated as the proportion of those calving which survive to 54 months of age*

higher incidence of parasites and health problems (McDowell, 1989).
Some examples of different productivity and reproduction parameter outcomes under different environmental conditions are presented in Tables 5.A and 5.B (after McDowell, 1989). It would be too easy to attribute all differences to these environmental conditions; managerial qualities will undoubtedly play a substantial role as well, but the overall illustration is clear.

### 9.5.2 EFFECTS OF HOUSING ON FEEDING

In confining ruminants, generally the quantity and quality of the diet is affected by reduced feeding times (restricted grazing and at the stall) and reduced opportunities to the animals to select a more balanced diet. Stall feeding in the warm humid tropics can save on trampling losses during grazing. Also if ruminants are not contained properly they may damage the environment by destroying crops and through overgrazing, with risks of erosion, compaction of clay soils, etc. (Durning and Brough, 1991). On the other hand, stall feeding normally leads to less feed and water offered, with less variability and possible selection, leading to lower intake and, consequently, production. Production systems, like feedlots for beef cattle and intensive dairy production systems in developed countries relying on mechanically harvested feed (green chop, chopped maize, silage and hay) and concentrated feeds like agro-industrial by-products from processed grains and oilseeds, and ad libitum water, prove that under certain conditions stall feeding is not necessarily detrimental to productivity and has also been applied in (sub-) tropical climates.

### 9.5.3 EFFECTS ON BREEDING

Animals tied in a stall can hardly express the easily recognisable estrus signs like mounting and being mounted. Much more knowledge on recognizing other estrus signs like bellowing, drop in production, mucus discharge, etc and on correct timing of service or insemination is required by the farmer. Estrus is easier detected in animals in free stalls, and can be easier timed for service during the latter part of standing heat. In loose stalls the assistance of a teaser or young bull to spot cattle in estrus is less labor intensive and dangerous than it is to pass with the breeding bull twice or thrice a day along the cows in a stanchion barn.

### 9.5.4 EFFECTS ON DISEASE CONTROL

Exercise of cattle in loose barns is considered valuable for more appropriate wear of the growing hooves, access to sun light (if part of the loose barn is uncovered), exercise before calving, etc.

Housing can protect the animals from direct harmful effects of the environment like too much heat, moisture, wind, but especially from vector diseases transmitted by ticks and tsetse flies (only relevant for large parts of Africa). It creates, however, animals without acquired immunity. If by circumstances they are let out to graze,acute diseases may occure. Worm and liver fluke burdens can be reduced by housing as well, if farmers avoid to cut and carry fodder contaminated with manure. On the other hand, most smallholder stables or kraals experience an increased incidence of diseases (lung, intestinal, udder, claws and reproduction disorders) through closer animal contact, poor ventilation, dust, muddiness, lack of proper bedding and cleanliness, and poor hygiene. Especially poor hygiene around milking and calving in housed cattle causes many problems like mastitis and uterine infections.

### 9.5.5 OTHER ASPECTS OF HOUSING

Housing further assists in keeping out predators and thieves, can reduce the burden of day to day herding (enabling children to follow formal education), and helps in the protection of growing crops.

Increased pressure from population and cropping is leading to a reduced or nil fallow period. Farmyard manure is getting more important to maintain soil fertility in the absence of fallow crops and due to low availability and/or expensive artificial fertilizers. Scarcity of firewood also leads to more emphasis on manure for energy in the form of dried cakes or biogas. However, the application of manure or biogas slurry to crops requires a lot of work, hence farmers apply the organic fertilizer mainly for increased yields of quickly responding vegetables and other cash crops (bananas, coffee, fruit trees) and hardly to fodders or slow responding crops.

### 9.5.6 TYPES OF HOUSING

In many farmyards in the tropics trees, preferably a little elevated on a mount, are a cheap and comfortable form of housing. The slope provides easy drainage of urine and water wastage, and manure dries out faster. Ruminants can go there for shade, water troughs, for a breeze, or for protection against heavy rain to feel comfortable. This reduces the effect of direct radiation heat, improves heat exchange through cooling, and protects against too strong under-cooling, respectively.

For more confinement of a few animals for handling (breeding, milking, slaughtering) farmers go for ropes and/or simple crushes. When more animals are kept, a poled shade building is used with feeding provisions in the centre against the sun and rain or along the outside with(out) shade of the "corral", "kraal", "dry lot" or grassless paddock.

In dairy production at smallholder farms four main types are in use;

a. cattle are tethered with ropes and sticks, and moved once or more during the day;
b. cattle are tied under trees and hand fed;
c. cattle are housed in stanchion type barns with facilities of a gutter to collect manure (Sri Lanka model); and

d. cattle are housed in a shed with cubicles for resting and an area for walking and feeding (Kenya model).

Open sheds are preferred for cattle and buffaloes to facilitate heat exchange and fresh air, although in (peri) urban centres, farmers prefer closed housing to prevent intrusions from outside, and to protect themselves against complaints from neighbours. Some farmers also prefer closed housing to hide their animal possession for outsiders (e.g. devil eye in Sri Lanka) and/or to cut down on flies to create an environment for easy milking and less feed wastage.

If real protection against the hot climate is necessary, farmers put their animals underground like the Dagons in Mali for fattening of oxen on crop residues. For calf housing in the tropics, thick walled clay huts and grass/straw/stover thatches (e.g. with the Pokot in Kenya, and the farmers in the hills of Iringa, Tanzania) are very comfortable against the heat and the cold. The tendency to go for more durable roofs of corrugated iron should be discouraged. This roofing is less comfortable due to more heat accumulation during the day, and in the highlands due to very low temperatures at night. Most important is however that this system encourages draughts detrimental to good calf health. Individual housing for young calves on a wooden slatted floor or on sufficient deep litter is recommended to reduce the incidence of navel suckling, omphalitis as well as calf diarrhea.

Another point that requires attention regards feed troughs for roughage feeding:

a. a sloping feed platform towards the cattle assists in reducing the wastage of feed as may elevated feed troughs and feed gates.

b. feed gates that can separate animals avoid stiff competition for feed related to animal size, sex and behaviour (social order).

### 9.5.7 COSTS OF HOUSING

Although farmers, due to pressure from agriculture and increased population, are forced more and more towards a form of zero-grazing, the adoption is slow because of the extra labour and costs involved. The tendency towards stall feeding for manure collection to facilitate crop land fertilization, production of manure cakes and or biogas energy, is not strong either for the same reasons. Roughly, zero-grazing sheds cost between US$ 100 - 500 per cow, and minimum size biogas plants of 6 - 12 $m^3$ amount to US$ 150 - 500. These investments require cash while returns are long-term, mainly not in cash (at least not in the short run) but in kind (biogas, slurry) or in reduction of future expenditure (firewood, fertilizer).

For smallholders, investments in additional buildings range from 12 - 100% of the price of a dairy animal (Dairy India, 1987). An additional biogas plant to benefit more from zero-grazing, costed the value of about 1,000 litres of milk.

## 9.6 DAIRY DEVELOPMENT AND MANAGEMENT

Practical farm management is basically the organisation of inputs like resources of land, labor, capital and livestock, the choice of technology such as low input-low output, high input-high output, mechanisation, all within the limits of the physical, economic, social, and legislative environment.

In Indonesia, the main constraints in dairy development identified in Bandung area and East Java by a FAO mission in 1986 were the following managerial issues:

a. a low land availability; so expansion in dairying is dependent on off-farm carrying capacity for fodder such as weeds and regrowth in rice and other crops, forest fod der and fodder intercropping in plantations;
b. wasteful feeding practises by not chopping the fodder;
c. unbalanced cattle rations;
d. partly utilization of crop residues and little or no use of upgrading techniques;
e. poor calf rearing practices such as underfeeding, resulting in slow growth rates and poor quality heifers;
f. poor hygiene and inadequate preparation for milking, leading to contamination of milk and mastitis;
g. inadequate breeding practices leading to low conception rates of 40% or lower and long calving intervals of 15 - 18 months or longer;
h. lack of bull selection for size, type and ease of calving, and general lack of keeping records; and
i. farmers training with little analyses of farmers needs, not very practical program mes, little follow-up and inadequate supply of hand-outs.

In 1991, Ibrahim et al. (1992) reviewed 10 years of dairy development in East Java, and concluded that increase of dairy production has been mainly through imported dairy cattle, but that productivity was low, at only one third of their genetic potential. Main reasons are lack of sufficient high quality feed, poor adaptability of imported stock to local conditions, poor housing and management, more attention of cooperatives to marketing and little extension effort to cow problems, failure to repay dairy cattle credit in view of low productivity and milk price.

### 9.6.1 OVERALL MANAGEMENT

Improved dairy production depends on a wide range of environmental conditions. Berman and Wolfenson (1988) describe the phases of development of the dairy industry in Israel from 1930 - 1990. Initially, improvement of local breeds adapted to the Mediterranean environment (dry and hot) was tried with improved housing, feeding and cattle selection. However, results were little impressive with productions going slowly from 300 towards 1,000 kg of milk/cow/year. Secondly, the introduction of productive breeds from temperate zones resulted in high mortalities mainly due to tick-borne diseases. Thirdly, the improvement of veterinary services combined with

*Table 6. Comparison of farm performance of three different projects in Iraq (2 years after import of 800 in-calf Friesian heifers each)*

| | Project 1 | Project 2 | Project 3 |
|---|---|---|---|
| Percentage of cows in milk | 84 | 67 | 71 |
| Average dry period in days | 73 | 201 | 156 |
| Calves under 1 year | 616 | 484 | 506 |
| Milk production/cow/day in kg | 16.0 | 9.0 | 9.0 |
| Annual production per cow in kg | 4,906 | 2,201 | 2,592 |
| Annual milk production in "000 kg | 3,500 | 1,765 | 1,750 |
| Expected calving percentage | 85 | 60 | 68 |
| Expected calving interval in days | 429 | 608 | 538 |

crossbreeding of exotic blood into local cows showed more perspective up till 2,000 - 2,500 kg/cow. Only during the fourth phase, a real breakthrough was achieved from 3,200 kg/cow (irrigated fodder) to 8,000 kg/cow (including concentrate feeds). During the last phase, the stanchion barn was changed for the loose stall which reduced heat stress. Parallel development took place of better roughage, more adapted to soil and climate conditions, and availability of concentrate feeds. In the grade cattle population (mainly of Holstein Friesian blood), over time, no differences could be traced any more in heat regulation capacity and the percentage of exotic blood. Better adaption to heat meant in practice a lower milk production, and little improvement in milk yield when environmental conditions improved. To improve the housing climate of these highly productive cows, forced ventilation over the lying area of the cows is used. In addition, sprinklers are used to wet the cows at regular intervals.

It is well known that large differences exist in productivity and income between farms. Not many of the different on-farm practices have been investigated by research, because of difficulties with on-farm research. Particularly, on small farms the numbers are limited, and research facilities in transport and money are in short supply. Farmers, when they see some effects from treatments tested (like deworming, mineral supplementation), prefer the control animals to join the treatment too, and experiments end half way.

Technical and economic parameters in the tropics are scarce due to limited numbers of records kept and analysed, and the absence of systematic recording of economic performance through lack of book keeping bureaus. Information kept by projects is usually only available in the grey literature. A few examples indicating large differences in management are given in Tables 6 (Velzen, 1988) and 7 (Valk, 1987).

The main difference in management between the projects in Iraq (Table 6) was the feeding of hay and silage from stocks in Project 1. Projects 2 and 3 relied for roughage mainly on freshly cut green forage every day, which proved difficult to organize properly at that scale.

*Table 7. Performance comparison between good and poor management at recording smallholder farms of the Kenya Dairy Development Project*

| **Technical and economic parameters** | **Poor management** 1985/86 | 1986/87 | **Good management** 1985/86 | 1986/87 |
|---|---|---|---|---|
| Number of recording farms | 40 | 31 | 48 | 39 |
| Average number of cows | 2.40 | 2.38 | 2.55 | 2.57 |
| Milk production per cow (L) | 1,975 | 2,207 | 2,857 | 3,130 |
| Milk per cow sold (L) | 1,250 | 1,366 | 1,891 | 2,043 |
| Milk per cow for calf (L) | 181 | 215 | 219 | 249 |
| Milk per cow for home use (L) | 544 | 626 | 746 | 837 |
| Milk price per litre milk sold | 4.15 | 3.88 | 3.67 | 3.75 |
| Total sale of milk in Ksh* | 5,181 | 5,302 | 6,942 | 7,671 |
| Cattle sales-purchases in Ksh | 634 | 941 | 877 | 1,547 |
| *Total receipts in Ksh* | *5,815* | *6,242* | *7,819* | *9,218* |
| Supplements fed in Ksh | 701 | 1,102 | 1,539 | 1,723 |
| Other current expenditures in Ksh | 1,268 | 1,180 | 1,496 | 1,513 |
| *Total expenditure in Ksh* | *1,969* | *2,282* | *3,035* | *3,236* |
| Receipts - expenses in Ksh | 3,846 | 3,960 | 4,784 | 5,982 |
| Non current expenditure in Ksh | 235 | 110 | 339 | 282 |
| *Net cash flow per cow in Ksh* | *3,611* | *3,850* | *4,445* | *5,700* |
| Net cash flow per acre roughage | 3,109 | 3,476 | 3,976 | 6,035 |
| Cash flow dairy/total farm in % | 69 | 67 | 56 | 52 |

** 1 Ksh is about 0.10 US $*

### 9.6.2 BIRTH WEIGHT AND RATE OF DEVELOPMENT

McDowell (1989) indicates that the birth weight of female calves in temperate areas should preferably be 6 - 6.5% of the dam's weight at 30 days postpartum. At 3 months of age calves should weigh 225 - 250% of birth weight to arrive at 50 - 55% of mature weight at 15 months. With evidence from (sub)tropical areas in the USA and from countries like Jamaica, Puerto Rico, Colombia and Venezuela birth weights in the warm humid tropics are much lower than in temperate areas. This is considered due to maximum day temperatures over 27°C which during late pregnancy may reduce nutrient allocation to the calf.

For an illustration of calf weight and calf growth, Figure 1 provides the difference

*Figure. 2. Live weight development (kg) of Friesian cattle at "De Marke" in the Netherlands (including 3 calvings), offspring of imported Dutch Friesians at New Zealand farm in Sri Lanka, and of crossbred calves ("Kerala" and "MIDCOMUL" schemes) at smallholder farms in Sri Lanka (Source: Jong and Ariyaratne, 1996)*

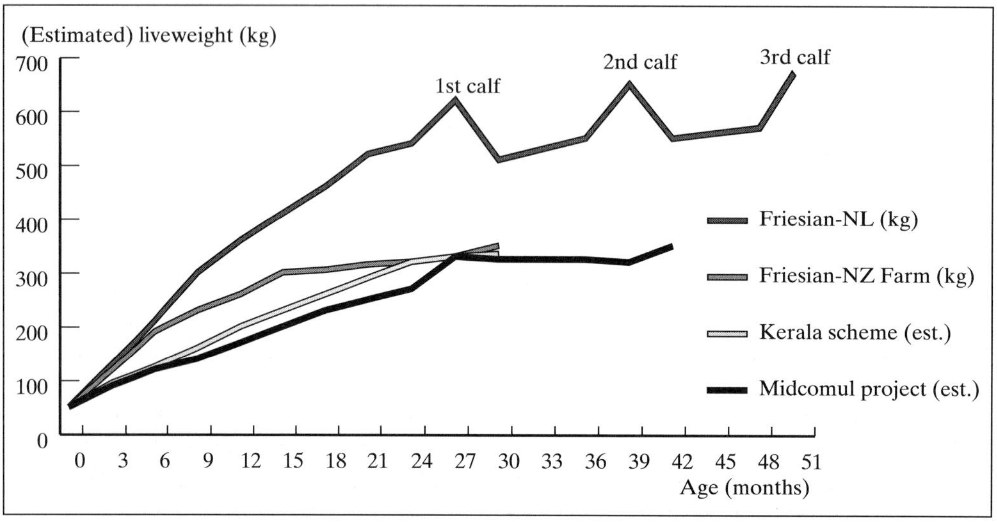


in growth between Friesian calves at the regional research centre "De Marke" in the Netherlands, calves from imported Friesians into Sri Lanka (at New Zealand farm) and crossbred calves of the "Kerala" scheme with subsidized feeds and the "MIDCOMUL" scheme based on three monthly target chest birth measurements at smallholder farms in Sri Lanka.

Large differences exist in birth weight between the temperate and tropical zones. This implies that calves in the tropics require much more time to reach weaning weights than in the temperate zone. Other factors are also more challenging in the tropics, like poorer feeding and higher risks of worm infestation, and ticks and tick-borne diseases.

Ibrahim (1988) gave the following hints for proper calf rearing and weaning:

1. Feed colostrum as soon, often and much as possible during the first 4 days;
2. When suckling is practised on one quarter to provide the milk, rotate the teat during the first month to avoid a pendulous teat/quarter;
3. When bucket feeding is applied, feed milk at the rate of 10% of body weight (5 - 30 days);
4. Introduce daily good quality, leafy roughage and palatable concentrate for early and ample development of the rumen, and to reduce calf diarrhea;
5. After 30 days reduce milk feeding gradually to 5% of body weight or reduce suc kling gradually to only before and after milking;
6. Provide daily fresh, clean drinking water and minerals next to the concentrates;

*Table 8. Age at different stages in reproductive life of dairy cattle in Latin America*

| Reproductive parameters | Months ± Sd |
|---|---|
| Age at puberty | 17 ± 4.4 |
| Age at first service | 24 ± 3.5 |
| Age at first conception | 25.5 ± 4.4 |
| Age at first calving | 34.7 ± 4.4 |
| Productive life (number of calvings) | 3.4 ± 1.1 |

7. Wean calves at:
   - 8 months (when suckling, and cow is to be dried off)
   - 6 months (when quantity and quality of roughage/concentrate is poor)
   - 4 months (when quantity and quality of roughage/concentrate is medium)
   - 2 months (when quantity and quality of roughage/concentrate is very good)

Adequate colostrum feeding is very important to reduce calf mortality. Age of puberty, first service, first conception and at first calving for dairy stock in Latin America (Russell et al., 1990), indicated in Table 8, is about 8 to 10 months higher than for temperate dairy stock, although a wide variation may exist (Perez, 1994).

### 9.6.3 HERD REPRODUCTION MANAGEMENT

Observation of estrus is more difficult in the tropics due to anestrus in case of poor nutrition and/or intensive suckling; the estrus period is shorter (average duration 12-14 hours), signs are less pronounced or mainly shown at night (buffaloes and indigenous cattle), and farmers are less keen on, or active in, heat detection. The frequency of estrus observation is important and when combined with a small bonus to farmlaborers can result in high pregnancy rates (pers. comm. Roest and Pieterse).

Experience from Tanzania indicates that in parastatal farms with employed labor, an incentive scheme for heat detection or better for conception assist very much in arriving at higher reproduction rates. Organisation of actual breeding at smallholder farms is more difficult due to low availability of the desired dairy type of bulls, poor communication with and functioning of the AI organisation. The best results are obtained in cool periods (of the day, season). Conditions of heat stress (standing in the sun or warm shed, walking to and from the bull) should be minimized. The activity of bullying should be reduced to avoid heat stress and low feed intake. The fertility of the bull and the quality of semen is reduced too during hot periods and seasons. Zebu and buffalo bulls are known to be in-active breeders during the hotter parts of the day, while they become very active at night, or when brought out of a dark and cool bull house.

Management of herd reproduction is very difficult in the absence of records kept or utilized. Cow calenders, if kept up to date, are good instruments for medium to large

*Table 9. Comparison of basic and improved (re)production performance indices*

| (Re)production parameters | Basic | Improved |
|---|---|---|
| Age at first calving (months) | 36 | 24 |
| Calving interval (months) | 18 | 14 |
| Lactation yield (kg) | 2500 | 2500 |
| Culling age (years) | 9 | 9 |
| Number of lactations | 4 | 6 |
| Total milk yield (litres) | 10000 | 15000 |
| Average number of female replacement stock per cow | 2 | 3 |

scale dairy farms to know the status of the herd, and to facilitate management. For smallholders, often with little formal education, herd reproduction management is more difficult and requires a lot of extension effort. A sociological study in Tanga area also indicated that although women did the cattle work, still the man had to arrange for breeding of the cow.

In Kenya and Tanzania intensive use is made of fertility cards to follow up the reproduction status monthly (observed in heat, served, outcome pregnancy diagnosis, etc). Experience from Kenya (Valk, 1987) indicates that calving intervals at smallholder farms are long (about 450 days), that it is difficult to improve on the situation over years, and that small farmers are reluctant to cull their infertile cows. Supply of phosphorus, especially of high biological quality, is often a simple but effective method to improve the reproductive status of the herd.

The effect of improved reproduction on milk production and the amount of replacement female stock required, can be considerable as is illustrated in Table 9 for smallholders in Sub-Sahara Africa (Walshe et al., 1991).

## 9.7 NUTRITION

Nutrition is the most important constraint in improving milk production and reproduction. Demand for feed is constant throughout the year, but supply of roughage fluctuates with the seasons. Planning a year round feed supply is one of the major objectives in dairy cattle nutrition. Providing the animals with a sufficient quantity of feed as well as with feed of sufficient quality are both important. Feed rations recommended to farmers based on western standards often assume maximum intake levels and feed of a certain good quality, while in practice most animals receive insufficient feed of lower quality.

What is required is a balance between amino acids, carbohydrates, minerals and long-chain fatty acids in the feed. Nutrient requirements for a particular productivity purpose must take into account the interaction among these critical nutrients (Preston and Leng, 1987). As such, feeding standards based on assigned nutritive values can be misleading when unconventional feed resources are used.

### 9.7.1 FEED RESOURCES

Walshe et al. (1991) gives the following division of feed resources:

- poor quality roughage (crop residues, natural grazing),
- good quality roughage (fodder crops, leys, fodder legumes, fodder trees),
- agro-industrial byproducts (sugarcane tops, sisal waste, canning waste, bran, oil cakes, molasses),
- concentrates (balanced mixtures of agro-industrial byproducts and grains),
- supplements (not-protein-nitrogen compounds, vitamin and mineral mixtures).

In many areas there is a surplus, either seasonal or permanent, of poor quality roughage. Its quality is often insufficient to meet maintenance requirements. Economics will decide the feasibility of supplementation or treatment of the poor quality roughage (Schiere, 1995). It is therefore necessary to have an insight in the seasonal availability of feed resources. Illustrative is the study by Ibrahim et al. (1992) in East Java. They considered the deficiency of high quality roughage as a major problem for the Javanese dairy farmers. There simply is not enough roughage available in the area to meet the needs for high milk production. Farmers feed a large amount of concentrates to compensate for the roughage nutrient deficiencies, and it is estimated that 25% of these concentrates is used for maintenance. On the other hand, grains are often exported in order to earn foreign exchange (Walshe et al., 1991).

### 9.7.2 ON-FARM FEED PRODUCTION

Walshe et al. (1991), Preston and Leng (1987), Orskov (1993), Preston (1991) and Leng (1991) all favour on-farm feed production in order to promote biomass production, whereby legumes are also important as a source of protein.

Fodder trees and shrubs produce good quality feed, remain green during the dry season and can be used in alley farming systems. Moreover fodder trees like Leucaena and Gliricidia can be used for boundary fences, firewood and wind breaks. Sugarcane remains in the field and its by-products can be used for feeding in the dry season.

Small farmers in Africa and Asia plant grasses for cutting to feed their dairy cows, although production is very seasonal and maintenance of fertility remains a problem.

Crop rotation should include fodder crops or food crops, whereby a crop residue is left over which is suitable for feeding cattle, like soybean or groundnut straw.

Pasture improvement for grazing is not easy, although Ibrahim (1994) claimed success in the Atlantic zone of Costa Rica with the introduction of grass-legume mixtures.

### 9.7.3 IMPROVEMENT OF FEED QUALITY

Several techniques exist to improve the quality of poor quality roughage. Preston and Leng (1987), Leng (1991), Orskov (1993) and Singh and Schiere (1993) give some biological, technical and socioeconomic considerations which should be taken into account when improvements of feed quality are introduced at a farmer's land.

For the synthesis of microbial protein from different nitrogen sources (ureum, peptides, proteins) a good carbohydrate energy source, e.g. molasses, is required. This microbial protein is later digested in the small intestines and absorbed as amino acids. A proportion of the dietary protein passes from the rumen into the small intestines without alternations, the so-called by-pass protein. This is also digested by enzyme hydrolysis and absorbed as amino acids. The amount of protein available for enzyme hydrolysis therefore depends on the efficiency of microbial growth in the rumen, and there is a need to determine the ratio of rumen degradable and undegradable protein of conventional and non-conventional feed, e.g. rubber seed meal, shrubs and tree fodders, for different production aims (Preston and Leng, 1987; Perera et al., 1992).

Where the diet contains a high proportion of fibre and therefore is only slowly fermented, the volume of the rumen (a physical factor) and the composition of the diet (chemical factor) set limits to the amount that can be consumed daily. A good overview of all factors influencing feed intake is given by Ketelaars and Tolkamp (1991). It will be clear, however, that when low grade fibrous forages are the main component of the diet, current feed evaluation systems are inappropriate since the potential intake is not measured.

The final criteria for the farmer to adopt a feeding system is not based on only biological parameters, but on economics, risk avoidance and common sense. It is therefore not surprising that in the world different feeding strategies exist or are tried at the farmer's level.

Chopping is practised in many countries and has the additional advantage that it is more difficult for the animal to select from the feed.

Steam treatment has proved feasible for sugarcane bagasse, but the quantity available is only 10% of total bagasse production and its use is limited to the immediate surroundings of the sugar factory.

Low level supplementation of sole crop residue rations with the specific objective of stimulating rumen function improves the ration to approximately maintenance level; medium or high levels of production cannot be achieved. In case of supplementation at higher levels the effects become additive and no special effect of improved rumen function is to be expected.

Treatment of crop residues with ammonia or urea has proved to be useful and shown good possibilities at smallholder level (Schiere, 1995; Singh and Schiere, 1993). Economics of feeding treated straw, the need to select grains with better quality and higher quantity of straw, its place in the production system and price relations between milk, concentrates and straw are all factors which require further investigation (Singh and Schiere, 1993).

### 9.7.4 FEED CONSERVATION

In temperate areas, hay and silage making are common practices for feed conservation. Hay making in the tropics is difficult, as the surplus grass is only available during the rainy season. Silage making is more suitable for large scale mechanized operations. Some experience exists at smallholder dairy operations in Malawi with fodder maize, and in Kenya with Napier grass. The system in Kenya is based on the use of molasses and on the cooperation between farmers in filling the pit in a short time. Other possibilities are storing of crop residues followed by treatment, cultivation of special dry season fodder, e.g. oats or pearl millet for silage. Establishment of fodder banks is promoted in West Africa (Preston and Leng, 1987). At large scale operations in South America and the Philippines sugarcane is successfully grown for feeding dairy cattle (Preston and Leng, 1987).

### 9.7.5 FEEDING SYSTEMS

Roughage is in most cases the cheapest feed available and it is sufficient to meet maintenance requirement up to maximum 5 litres of milk depending on the quality. Roughage rations can be supplemented with a range of agro-industrial byproducts (brans, oil cakes, brewery waste, molasses, etc.). In the (peri-)urban production systems where supplements are cheap or roughage expensive, it could be economical to reduce roughage to a minimum and increase the supplements to a maximum. Fluctuations in roughage production can be balanced by increasing supplements. Economic levels of supplementation depend on quality, the prices of supplements and the milk price (Walshe et al., 1991; Singh and Schiere, 1993). Increased feeding of supplements will reduce intake of roughage, although the rate of substitution is not clear. Production levels are often disappointing as compared to the theoretically expected production. The explanation for this is that the animals receive or eat less roughage than the recommended levels. Animals receive or eat insufficient roughage because it is not available, requires too much labor to cut, is not palatable and dirty, or because the animals are given insufficient time for grazing. Providing clean feed from a well designed feeding trough to avoid spoilage is necessary to reach maximum intake levels.

Molasses-urea-mineral blocks are a good feed supplement, and are carriers of non-protein nitrogen and minerals. The blocks are solid, fairly easy to manufacture, transport and store. Molasses intake should not exceed 20% of total intake, at higher levels it will depress digestibility (Preston and Leng, 1987).

In a peri-urban dairy project in Senegal a complete feed for dairy cattle has been developed based on groundnut shells as the source of crude fibre, mixed with groundnut cake, wheat bran and molasses. Regular manufacturing and distribution were the main bottlenecks (Walshe et al., 1991).

Problems often exist in distribution of feed (concentrates) to the individual dairy farmer. Quantities required are small and transportation costs are high. Distribution should be implemented as far as possible through the milk market channel and combined with the provision of credit by private traders or farmers' organizations and with deductions for repayments from milk sales. In the peri-urban areas with direct marketing of milk, farmers' organizations can still play a role in providing feed, e.g. by making contracts with food processors, e.g. vegetable oil extraction plants, breweries etc. Drying of brewery waste will help to reduce transportation cost and make handling easier as well as improve keeping quality.

Rations for dairy cattle based on average to good quality grass as the main source of roughage and supplemented with small quantities of concentrates, resulting in yields of 5 to 10 litres, are more often deficient in energy than in protein.

## EPILOGUE

The demand for milk and milk products is increasing in developing countries, but mainly in urban centres. This demand is covered either by import of milk products (often subsidised in the country of origin), by local production or a combination of the two. A good milk price for the farmer is an important stimulating factor and will largely determine the sustainability of technical inputs, as shown in countries like India, China, Kenya and Cuba (Kaasschieter et al., 1992; Jong, 1996). Moreover, milk production has benefits to the producer because a regular income can be maintained, which has advantages over irregular cashflows of meat and crop production, and also because cattle improves soil fertility.

Dairy production in developing countries takes place in different ecological zones. This means that there is not a single extension message as far as nutrition, health care and management are concerned. Crop residues and fodder trees play a much more important role than in Western countries. Ecological zones also determine the existence of tick-borne diseases, trypanosomiasis and other vector-borne diseases; these zones may equally be associated with certain management styles. It is likely that vaccines against all tick-borne diseases will be available in the next 10 - 20 years, but this is unrealistic for trypanosomiasis, neither can we do without acaricide for the next 20 years.

The type of housing also varies with the ecological zones. Housing indirectly influences the prevalence of diseases. Vector-borne diseases and helminthiasis will be reduced with confinement in stables, but others, like pneumonia, diarrhea and claw problems will increase with confinement.

For infectious diseases like rinderpest, foot and mouth disease, technical solutions for their control are available and their persistence in some regions is largely due to socioeconomic constraints and neglect of cost-benefits analysis (Haan and Bekure, 1990). With intensification, the emphasis will shift to disease-causing risk factors, such as under-nutrition, poor hygiene and management, that affect the productivity of the herd.

Data collection, linked with analysis and simulation models, are essential to gain an insight in the role of animals in farming systems. They are also necessary for disease control purposes and the costs involved in disease control and other inputs. Quite a number of surveys, however, lack well defined aims to meet these objectives (Udo and

Brouwer, 1993).

The more intensive the dairy system becomes and the greater the herds, the higher will be the need for more sophisticated herd health and production management programs as, e.g. is demonstrated by the work of Perez (1994) in Costa Rica.

Specialized commercial dairy systems can only be sustainable if there is adequate marketing, a good price policy, infrastructure, continuous supply of quality feed and concentrates, adequate veterinary services (vaccines, medicines, cost recovery), availability of breeding stock and control of pollution (Kaasschieter et al., 1992; Jong, 1996). If the hidden costs of these infrastructural requirements are all reflected in the milk price, it will make it possible for the small-scale farmers, which form the majority in developing countries, to compete on the market. A sustainable dairy production, without detrimental effects on the environment, is certainly within reach of the smallholder dairy farmer (Kaasschieter et al., 1992).

The challenge of the intensification of livestock production on smallholder mixed farms is to improve the efficiency of the production system. Anderson (1992) expects the greatest economic returns if money would be invested in development of feed resources and animal health-feed efficiency interactions.

The increased interdependence within farming systems requires a systems approach. In this respect animal health aspects have to be regarded as increasingly important. They are strongly interlinked with feeding, breeding, management, housing and the type of farmer. These interactions need more recognition and modification in institutional set-up, curricula development, research and extension efforts (Kaasschieter et al., 1992). Copies of Western-styled solutions are rarely suitable without major modifications. It is clear that for (sub-)tropical conditions the basic HH & PM protocol could be used, as long as the farm is approached in an integrated manner as is illustrated by the farming systems approach, FSA. In that way it is close to the ecosystem health concept as presented by Nielsen (1992).

## REFERENCES

*Anderson, J.R. 1992. Difficulties in African agricultural systems enhancement? Ten hypotheses. Agric. Syst. 38: 387-409.*

*Banerjee, A. 1994. Dairying systems in India. p.307. In: Dairy development and implementation. Sharing of experiences between Africa and Asia. E. Mann and B. Brooks (Eds.), FAO, Rome.*

*Berman, A. and Wolfenson, D. 1988. Climate influences in Tropical Animal Production. World Rev. Anim. Prod.: 24: 27-32.*

*Brandl, F.E. 1988. Economics of Trypanosomiasis control in cattle. In: Farming Systems and Resource Economics in the tropics. Vol. 1., W. Doppler (Ed.), Wissenschaftsverlag Vauk, Kiel, pp 220.*

*Carillo, B.J. 1993. Food losses due to mineral deficiencies and programme for their reduction. p.104. In; "Food losses due to non-infectious and production diseases in developing countries". FAO Animal Production and Health Paper, 114, Rome.*

*Chase, L.E. 1989. Metabolic disorders in dairy cattle nutrition. International Seminar on Holstein Friesians "Dairying in Tropical Environment". p.4. Seminar Pajajaran University. 22-25 May 1989, Bandung.*

*Curry, J.J.; Perry, B.D., Delehanty, J.M. and Mining, S. 1993. Improving animal health care delivery through the use of etnoveterinary knowledge in coastal and highland Kenya. p.220. In: Livestock services for smallholders: A certain evaluation. Editors: Daniels et al. Proceedings of a seminar held in Yogyakarta, Indonesia.*

*Dairy India, 1987. National Dairy Development Board, Anand, India.*

*Devendra, C. 1993. Sustainable animal production form small farm systems in South East Asia. FAO Animal Production and Health Paper, 106, Rome.*

*Desai, M. 1986. Livestock production and disease in the tropics. p.164 In: H. Kuil, R.W.Paling & J.E. Huhn (Eds.), Livestock production and diseases in the tropics. Faculty of Veterinary Medicine, Utrecht, pp. 157-161.*

*Development Cooperation, Ministry of Foreign Affairs. 1992. Livestock Production in developing countries. Policy Document nr.1, The Hague.*

*Doyle, J.J. 1992. What kind of animal health strategies for different agricultural production systems? A discussion paper. Page 391. In: Livestock production and diseases in the tropics. Editor CIRAD/EMVT. 7th International Conference of institutions of tropical veterinary medicine. Yamoussoukro.*

*Durning, A.B. and Brough, H.B. 1991. Tacking Stock: Animal Farming and the Environment. Worldwatch Paper 103, July 1991.*

*Gryseels, G. 1988. Role of livestock on mixed smallholder farms in the Ethiopian highlands. Ph.D. Thesis, Wageningen, pp.249.*

*Haan, C. de. 1993. The delivery of livestock services to smallholders. p.33. In: Livestock services for smallholders: A certain evaluation. Daniels et al. (Eds). Proceedings of a seminar held in Yogyakarta, Indonesia.*

*Haan, C. de and Bekure, S. 1990. Animal health services in Sub-Saharan Africa. World Bank Technical Paper 134, Washington D.C.*

*Hermans, C., Udo, H.M.Y. and Dawood, F. 1989. Cattle dynamics and their implications in Pabna district, Bangladesh. Agr. Syst. 29: 371-384.*

*Ibrahim, M.A. 1994. Compatibility, persistence and productivity of grass-legume mixtures for sustainable animal production in the Atlantic zone of Costa Rica. Ph.D. Thesis, Wageningen, pp. 129.*

*Ibrahim, M.N.M. 1988. Feeding tables "a practical guide". Editors: E.T.I. Division Animal Production and Health. Kandy, Sri Lanka, pp. 71.*

*Ibrahim, M.N.M.; Wassing, G.J.; Widodo, M.W. and De Jong, R. 1992. Dairy cattle development in East Java: A decade of progress and future prospectives. p.23. In; Livestock and feed development in the tropics. M.N.M. Ibrahim, R. de Jong, J. van Bruchem and H. Purnomo (Eds.), Malang.*

*Ifar, S. 1996. Relevance of ruminants in upland mixed farming systems in East Java, Indonesia. Ph.D. Thesis, Wageningen. pp. 139.*

*Jong, R. de and Ariyaratne, M.G. 1996. Performance and progress of dairy stock development in Sri Lanka. PGIA Occasional Series.*

*Jong, R. de. 1996. Dairy stock development and milk production with smallholders. Ph.D. Thesis, Wageningen. pp. 308.*

*Jongejan, F. and Uilenberg, G. 1994. Ticks and control methods. Rev. Sci. Tech. Off. int. Epiz. 13: 1201-1226.*

*Kaasschieter, G.A.; De Jong, R; Schiere, J.B. and Zwart, D. 1992. Towards a sustainable livestock production in developing countries and the importance of animal health strategy therein. Vet. Quart. 14: 66-75.*

*Ketelaars J. and Tolkamp, B. 1991. Toward a new theory of feed intake regulation in ruminants. Ph.D. Thesis, Wageningen. pp. 253.*

*Klink, E. van. 1994. Aspects of productivity traditionally managed Barotse cattle in the Wester Province of Zambia. Ph.D. Thesis, Wageningen, pp. 227.*

*Leng, R.A. 1991. Feeding strategies for improving milk production of dairy animals by small-farmers in the tropics. p.82. In: "Feeding dairy cows in the tropics". A. Speedy and R. Sancourcy (Eds.). FAO publication no. 86, Rome.*

*Mc Dermott, J.J.; Gitau, G.K.; O'Callaghan, C.Y; Omore, A.O.; P.A. Odima; Kyule, M.N. and Kilungo, J.K. 1993. Field research project to assess health and production indices on Kenyan smallholder dairy farms. p.77. In: Livestock services for smallholders: A certain evaluation. Daniels et al. (Eds.). Proceedings of a seminar held in Yogyakarta, Indonesia.*

*Mc Dowell, R.E., 1989. Environmental and genetic influencing performance in Holstein in warm climates. In: Proceedings of the International Seminar on Holstein Friesian "Dairying in Tropical Environments". Seminar Pajajaran University. 22-25 May 1989, Bandung, Indonesia.*

*Monfore, G.R. 1989. Diseases of U.S. cattle in the highlands of Cental Java, Indonesia. p. 1. In: Proceedings of the International Seminar on Holstein Friesian "Dairying in Tropical Environments". Seminar Pajajaran University. 22-25 May 1989, Bandung, Indonesia.*

*Morris, A.S. and Leidl, K. 1993. Structured data collection for animal health production in smallholder livestock production. p.69. In: Livestock services for smallholders: A certain evaluation. Daniels et al. (Eds.). Proceedings of a seminar held in Yogyakarta, Indonesia.*

*Mukhebi, A. 1992. Economic impact of Theileriosis and its control in Africa. p. 380. In; "The epidemiology of theileriosis in Africa". R.A.I. Norval, B.D. Perry and A.S. Young (Eds.). Academic Press. London.*

*Nasir Hussain Shah, S. 1990. Prolonged calving interval in the Nili Ravi Buffalo. Ph.D. Thesis, Utrecht. pp. 162.*

*Nell, A.J. 1986. Final report of the Netherlands Dairy Development Project 1978-1986 of the National Livestock Development Board and the Sri Lanka-Netherlands Livestock Development Programme.*

*Nielsen, N.O. 1992. Ecosystem health and veterinary medicine. Can. Vet. Journal 33:23- 26.*

*Orskov, E.R. 1993. Reality in rural development aid with emphasis on livestock. Rowett Research Ltd. Aberdeen. pp. 88.*

*Otte, E. and Lobo, C.A. 1984. Research needs of Colombia in the light of the activities of the Colombo/German project for the intensification of animal disease control. Prev. Vet. Med. 3: 109-121.*

*Ozawa, Y. 1991. A new concept in developing diagnostic services in tropical countries. p. 383. In; Livestock production and diseases in the tropics. H. Kuil, R.W.Paling and J.E. Huhn (Eds.). Faculty of Veterinary Medicine, Utrecht. pp. 385.*

*Paling, R.W. and Dwinger, R.H. 1993. Potential of trypanotolerance as a contribution to sustainable livestock production in tsetse affected Africa. Vet.Quart. 15: 60-67.*

*Paling, R.W.; Leak, S.G.A.; Katende, J. and Moloo, S.K. 1987. Epidemiology of animal trypanosomiasis on a cattle ranch in Kilifi, Kenya. Act.Trop. 44: 67-82.*

*Perera, A.N.F.; V.M.K.Y. Aparatne and Van Bruchem, J. 1992. Characterization of protein in some Sri Lanka tree fodders and agro-industrial by-products by nylon bag degradation. p.17. In: Livestock and feed development in the tropics. M.N.M. Ibrahim, R. de Jong, J. van Bruchem and H. Purnomo (Eds.), Malang.*

*Perez, E. 1994. Epidemiological aspects of morbidity, mortality and growth of calves in Costa Rica. Ph.D. Thesis, Utrecht. pp. 166.*

*Phelan, J.A. 1994. Milk supply networks for urban centres. p. 235. In: Dairy development policy and implementation. Sharing of experiences between Africa and Asia. Mann, E.J. and B. Brooks (Eds.), FAO, Rome.*

*Preston, T.R. 1989. The Development of Milk Production Systems in the Tropics. Technical Centre for Agriculture and Rural Cooperation.*

*Preston, T.R. 1991. Matching livestock systems with available resources. p. 56. In: "Feeding dairy cows in the tropics". A. Speedy and R. Sancourcy (Eds.). FAO publi cation no. 86, Rome.*

*Preston, T.R. and Leng, R.A. 1987. Matching ruminant production systems with available resources in the tropics and sub-tropics. Penambul Books, Armidale. pp. 245.*

*Pritchard, W.R. 1988. Ways that veterinary medicine can help alleviate hunger in Africa. J. Am. Vet. Med. Ass. 192: 1701-1705.*

*Pullan, N.B. 1980. Productivity of white Fulan; cattle on the Jos Plateau, Nigeria. III. Disease and management factors. Trop. Anim. Hlth. Prod. 12: 77-84.*

*Rheenen, T. van. 1995. Farm household level optimal resource allocation. An explorative study in the limestone area of East Java. Ph.D. Thesis, Wageningen. pp. 145.*

*Russel, J.M.; Galina, C.S.; Anta, E.; Porras, A. and Zarco, L. 1990. Parameters in Cattle under tropical conditions. In: Livestock reproduction in Latin America. Proceedings of the final research co-ordination meeting, Bogota, September 19-23, 1988. Joint FAO-IAEA, Vienna.*

*Schiere, J.B. 1995. Cattle, straw and system control. A study of straw feeding systems. Ph.D. Thesis, Wageningen. pp. 216.*

*Schreuder, B.E.C., Moll, H.A.J.; Noorman, N. Halimi, M. Kroese, A.H. and Wassing, G. 1996. A benefit-cost analysis of veterinary interventions in Afghanistan based on a livestock mortality study. Prev. Vet. Med. 26:303-314.*

*Scott, G.R. 1988. To morrow's animal plagues in perspective. p.28. In: Tierproduktion und Tiergesundheit in Entwicklungsländern im Blick auf das Jahr 2000. 25 Jahre Seminar für Tropenveterinärmedizin. J.E. Huhn (Ed.), Berlin.*

*Singh, K. and Schiere, J.B. 1993. Feeding of ruminants on fibrous crop residues. Aspects of treatment, feeding, nutrient evaluation, research and extension. Indian Council Agric. University, Wageningen, The Netherlands. pp. 486.*

*Sutmüller. P. 1961. A study of mineral nutrition in cattle under the conditions of an underdeveloped region. Koninklijk Instituut voor de Tropen, Amsterdam.*

*Udo, H.M.J. and Brouwer, B.O. 1993. A computerized method for systematically analy zing the livestock component of farming systems. Comp. Elect. Agric. 9: 335-356.*

*Udo, H.M.J.; Hermans, C. and Dawood, F. 1990. Comparison of two cattle production systems in Pabna district Bangladesh. Trop. Anim. Health and Prod., 22: 247-259.*

*Udo, H.M.J.; Meijer, J.; Dawood, F. and Dijkhuizen, A.A. 1992. The benefits of cattle in mixed farm systems in Pabna, Bangladesh. Asia-Australian J. Anim. Sci., 5: 495-503*

*Uilenberg, G.; Dobbelaere, D.A.E.; De Gee, A.L.W. and Koch, H.T. 1993. Progress in research on tick-borne diseases: Theileriosis and Heartwater. Vet. Quart. 15: 48-54.*

*Valk, Y.S. van der. 1987. Forms used by DDP in the extension services and some results so far. Ministry of Livestock Development, Kenya, May 1987.*

*Velzen, C.J. van. 1988. Adaptation of animals in foreign countries. In: Magazine for cat tle improvement. 2: 19-22. Veepro Holland. August 1988.*

*Vliet, A. van. 1995. Molecular characterisation and detection of Cowdria ruminaticum. Ph.D. Thesis, Utrecht. pp. 128.*

*Walshe, M.J. 1994. Dairy development, issues and options. p. 155. In: Dairy development and implementation. Sharing of experiences between Africa and Asia. E. Mann and B. Brooks (Eds.), FAO, Rome.*

*Walshe, M.J.; Grindle, A.J.; Nell, A.J. and Bachmann, M. 1991. "Dairy development in Sub-Saharan Africa: A study of issues and options". Technical paper number 135. Africa Technical Department Series, World Bank, Washington, D.C.*

*Wilson, R.T. and Clarke, S.E. 1976. Studies on the livestock of Southern Dafur, Sudan. II Production traits in cattle. Trop. Anim. Hlth. Prod. 8: 47-51.*

*Winrock International. 1992. Assessment of animal agriculture in sub-Saharan Africa. Winrock International Institute for Agricultural Development, Arkansas, USA. pp. 125.*

*Zerbini, E.; Gemeda, T.; Franceschini, R.; Sherington, J. and Wold, A.G. 1993. Reproductive performance of F1 crossbred dairy cows used for draught: Effect of work and diet supplementation. Anim. Prod. 57: 361-368.*

*Zerbini, E.; Gemeda, T.; Tegegne, A.; Gebre Wold A. and Franceschini, R. 1993. Effects of work and diet on progesterone secretion, short luteal phases and ovulations wit hout estrus in postpartum F1 crossbred dairy cows. Theriogenology, 40: 571-584.*

*Zwart, D. 1959. Goitre in goats on Dutch New Guinea. Tijdschr. Dierg. 84: 550-559.*

*Zwart, D. 1994. Problems for livestock smallholders in the tropics. p. 7. In: Application of biotechnology. 5th Symposium on Tropical Animal Health and Production, Utrecht.*

# EPILOGUE

In industrialized countries veterinary services in the food animal sector have evolved from individual treatment of diseased animals and from the control of major infectious diseases by eradication to collective prevention of diseases by vaccination and disease monitoring programs (Braun, et al., 1983). This resulted in a considerable improvement of animal health in many countries. In the 1970's these achievements were followed by herd fertility programs with regular scheduled farm visits (Noordhuizen, 1984). As soon as dairy farmers recognized the benefits of these herd fertility schemes, a strong request arose for similar programs in other operational farm management areas such as: health care, replacement rearing, nutrition, and milk production. This led to the development of integrated Herd Health and Production Management (HH & PM) programs implemented by veterinary practitioners (Noordhuizen, 1984). In a HH & PM program the technical and theoretical well known approaches used in individual animal health care, are broadened to incorporate the herd or farm as the unit of interest. The primary goal of these programs is to improve productivity and profit of the dairy enterprise by measuring, assessing and improving management performance.

In developing countries animal health services have been directed towards the implementation of disease surveillance and control programs that are intended for application on a national or regional scale. Departments of veterinary service of the Ministries of Agriculture in various countries in Africa and Central America have started herd health monitoring programs, commonly supported by international organizations for development cooperation. In many developing countries the phenomenon of local veterinary practitioners, managing a private veterinary practice, hardly exist. This is clearly demonstrated in many reports on livestock services for smallholders. In order to help livestock farmers in developing countries to move from a subsistence level of farming to a more production oriented system, the veterinary infrastructure has to be improved. The establishment of private veterinary practices with interest in animal husbandry is a prerequisite for achieving this goal. If this gets support from national governments and international organizations the implemention of HH & PM programs can become a valuable tool under those conditions.

Dairy farm management is very complex. It consists of: 1) planning on a short, medium, and long term basis, 2) execution of a number of operational management functions, such as: crop production, nutrition, health care, reproduction, milk production, herd replacement, fixed assets and labor, and cash flow, and 3) overall assessment or control. The eight operational management functions are all interrelated and driven by the management capabilities of the farmer (See Chapter 1).

Planning, execution and control are components of every industrial enterprise. However, the difference between a dairy farm and an industrial enterprise is that in the case of a dairy farm, the three management components are incorporated, in one person and in the case of an industrial enterprise divided among many individuals. The large-scale dairy farms with a more industrial enterprise organization are an exception. They are using many employees for different operational management functions.

HH & PM programs as described in this book consist of a complex of integrated veterinary, husbandry and economic activities, centered around regularly planned farm visits and on-farm data recording. They are based on a protocol approach of operational management functions and processes. In HH & PM programs pathophysiological and epidemiological knowledge of veterinary practitioners, and animal husbandry skills of farm advisors and agricultural economists have to be implemented into the management practices of the farmer. For that purpose a protocol was developed comprising four major components: 1) defining preset targets for individual herds, 2) description of materials and methods for execution and for reaching the preset targets, 3) decision making using information derived from data, farm and clinical inspections, and 4) follow-up in which actions, or recommendations of previous farm visits are evaluated. This protocol is used in all Chapters dealing with an operational management function.
Additionally, examples of problem solving are presented using a problem solving protocol (see Chapter 2, 5, 6 and 7).

In industrial enterprises inefficient management practices are diagnosed and corrected with the use of data. Modern dairy farms are industrial enterprises that should follow the same practice. The time is over that management decisions can be made on intuition. Data collection and processing form the skeleton of herd management and of HH & PM programs.
Herd records contain the information with which herd performance can be monitored, evaluated and analyzed and upon which a quantitative assessment of farm performance is based. One should keep in mind that records are only adequate when they permit the user to track performance and costs, to spot trends and problems, and to control resource utilization. Data on health, reproduction and production form the contemporary stethoscope in the hands of HH & PM practitioners. Data from external organizations such as DHIA and AI are providing production and reproductive data that have already been processed in performance figures can be instantly used to monitor and improve management practices.

Data sets from individual farms may serve as sentinel systems for disease or performance monitoring. Such data sets can also serve as the basis for research in several fields. Whether the use is for improved individual herd performance or for better understanding of general HH & PM aspects, the concern for data quality remains vital. Therefore, HH & PM practitioners must motivate dairy farmers to increase their efforts in data collection.
This is only possible when data are processed into performance indices and used as feedback information for farmers. The importance of record keeping has been stressed throughout the book.

From years back, veterinarians are ingrained in the germ theory of disease, largely because most disease etiology investigations have centered around Koch's postulates to prove causation. Therefore, most diagnostic efforts have been directed towards the pursuit of a germ. When a germ is found all pursuit of causative factors is terminated and all investigative efforts are shifted towards patient's relief of symptoms (Skidmore, 1996).

However, a clinical diagnosis should not be an end point but a starting point to search for underlying causal risk factors in management and in environmental conditions that are contributing to the disease and/or production deficiences. Therefore, treatment of a disturbance should always be accompanied by a change in managerial or environmental risk factors.

Farmer's are interested in improving overall management and generating profit and return from their dairy enterprise by utilizing various professional services provided by: nutritionists, agricultural economists, accountants, veterinarians, service and sales representatives and others. A tool that veterinarians can use to assist farmers in improving their management practices is by implementing HH & PM programs in their services that have an in-depth relationship with farm management. It may be very well possible that in the future the HH & PM protocol, described in this book, needs a shift towards a Hazard Analysis Critical Control Point (HACCP) assessment protocol (Noordhuizen and Welpelo, 1996).

In conclusion, the HH & PM practitioner should be involved in many aspects of farm management, and be concerned with improvement of farm productivity through better management. However one should realize that animal health is of primary importance to animal production. Consequently without an optimal health status of the herd it is impossible to improve animal productivity.

THE EDITORS

## REFERENCES

*Braun, R.K., J.P.T.M. Noordhuizen, G.A. Donovan, and A. Brand. A 1983. Goal oriented approach to herd health and production control. Proc. 15th Annual Convention of American Ass. of Bovine Practitioners. Nashville, Tennessee. pp.51-58.*

*Noordhuizen, J.P.T.M. 1984. Veterinary herd health and production control on dairy farms. Ph.D. Thesis, Veterinary Faculty, University of Utrecht, The Netherlands.*

*Noordhuizen, J.P.T.M. and J.H. Welpelo. 1996. Sustainable improvement of animal health care by systematic quality risk management. The Vet. Quart. 18 (4) 121-126.*

*Skidmore, A. L. 1996. Personal communication.*

# Curricula Vitae of Authors

**Geert Benedictus (1952)**

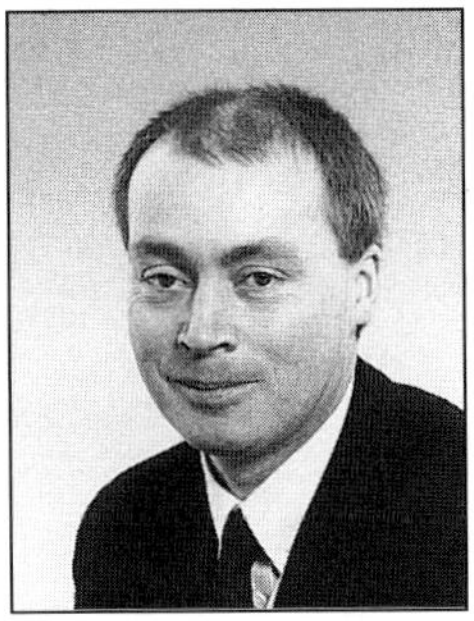

* Graduated from the Veterinary Faculty, of the University of Utrecht in 1976.
* Completed his PhD at the same University in 1985.
* Was director of a regional Animal Health Service Centre from 1991 to 1995.
* Currently division director of the National Animal health Service organization in the Netherlands for ruminants.

**Arie Brand (1931)**

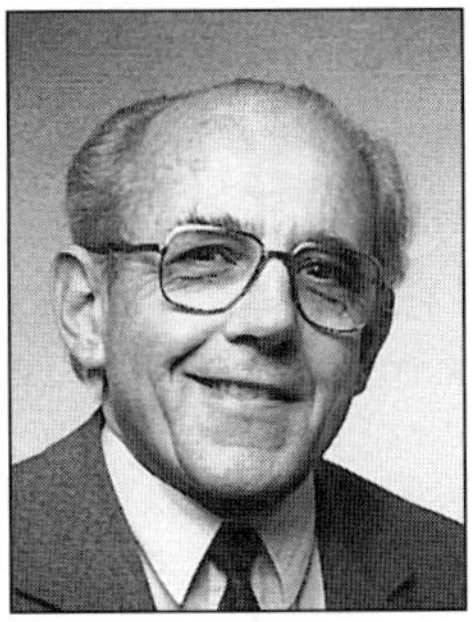

* Graduated from the Veterinary Faculty of the University of Utrecht in 1956.
* Worked as a food animal practitioner from 1956 to 1962. and as a researcher at the pharmaceutical company "Organon Ltd" from 1962 to 1966.
* Completed his PhD at the Department of Obstetrics, Gynecology and AI, Veterinary Faculty of Utrecht in 1970.
* Chair in Dairy Herd Health and Production Management, at the Veterinary Faculty of Utrecht in 1979.
* Currently visiting professor at the Faculty of Veterinary Science of the University of Zimbabwe.

**Alberto Brizzi (1955)**

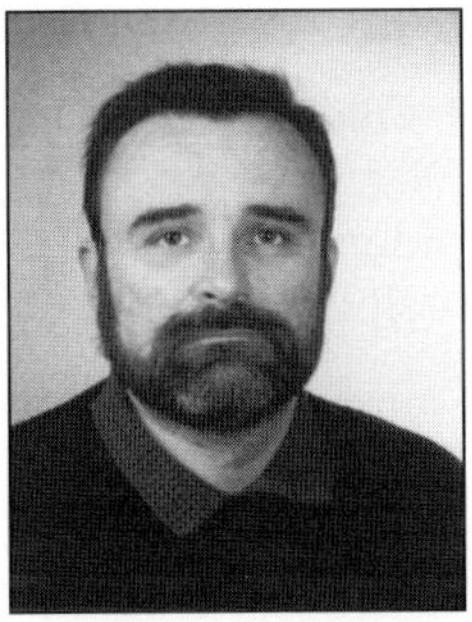

* Graduated in Veterinary Medicine at Bologna University, Italy, in 1980.
* From 1981 to 1984 active as bovine practitioner in Parma and Reggio Emilia, With special interests in dairy nutrition and Herd Health.
* Currently working as a private practitioner with specialization in claw diseases and Dairy Herd Health management.

**Aalt A. Dijkhuizen (1953)**

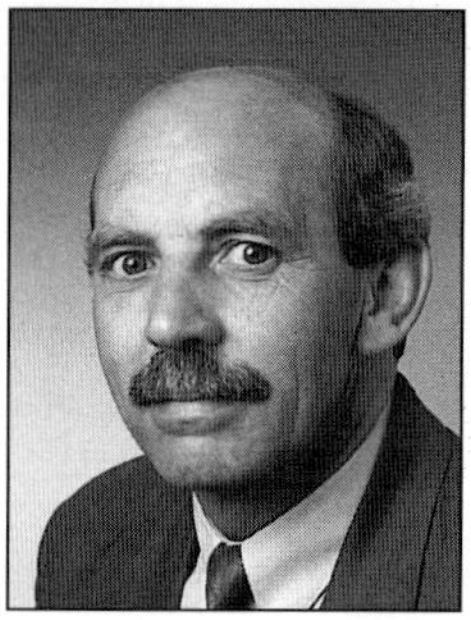

* Graduated in Agricultural Econonomics at Wageningen Agricultural University in 1977, with majors in Farm Management, Agricultural Policy and Animal Sciences.

* Completed his PhD at the Veterinary Faculty of the University of Utrecht in 1983.

* Is currently Professor in Animal Health Economics at Wageningen Agriculture University, Department of Farm Management.

**Carsten Enevoldsen (1953)**

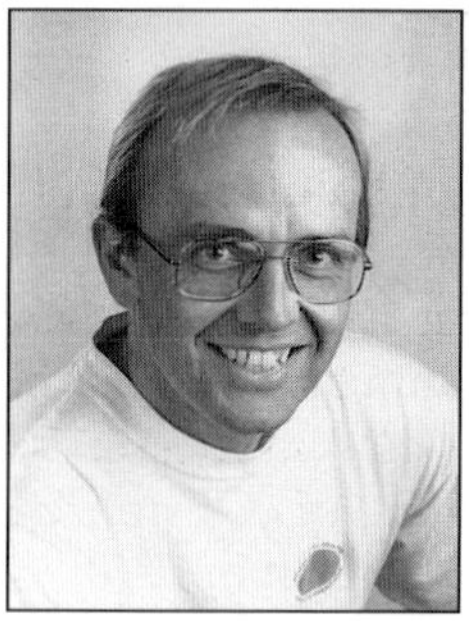

* Graduated as DVM at the Royal Veterinary & Agricultural University (RVAU) in Copenhagen, Denmark, in 1981. Was active in a mixed private practice from 1981 to 1985.

* Joined the Danish Institute of Animal Science (DIAS) in Foulum as Research Scientist from 1985 to 1988, and the Danish Research Academy as Scientist from 1988 to 1991. Spent 1 year as research fellow at Cornell University (USA) in the Department of Clinical Sciences.

* Completeded his PhD in epidemiology at RVAU, Copenhagen, Denmark, in 1993. Is currently Senior Research Scientist at DIAS in Foulum, Denmark.

**Hollis N. Erb (1948)**

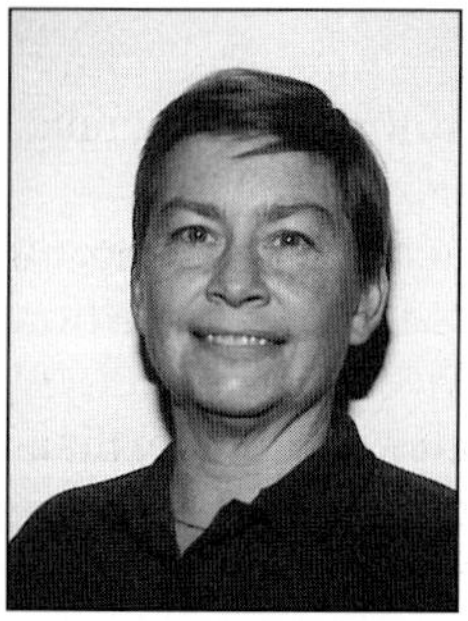

* Graduated at the University of California, Davis in 1974 with major in Veterinary Medicine.

* Completed PhD at the University of Guelph, Ontario, Canada, in 1979.

* Currently working as Professor of Epidemiology in the Department of Clinical Sciences at Cornell University.

**Klaas Frankena (1956)**

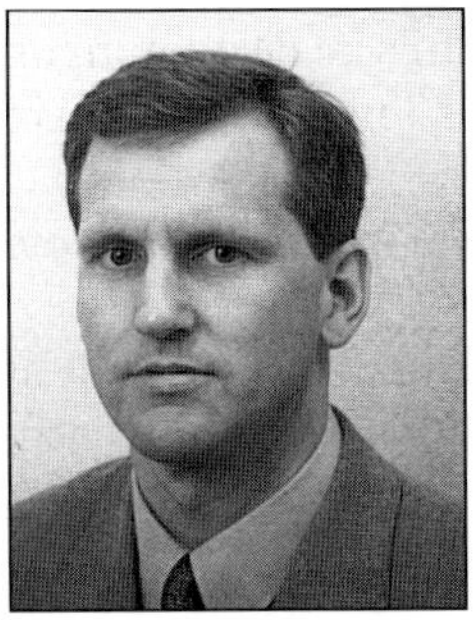

- Graduated from the Agricultural University of Wageningen with a major in Animal Sciences.
- Completed his PhD at the same University in 1987.
- From 1987 to 1995 assistant professor in Epidemiology in the Department of Animal Husbandry of The Agricultural University of Wageningen.
- Currently Associated Professor in Epidemiology in the same Department.

**David T. Galligan (1954)**

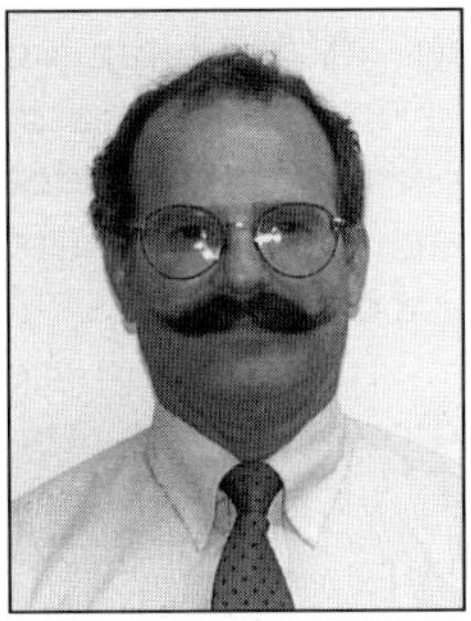

- Graduated in Veterinary Medicine at University of Pennsylvania in 1981.
- Completed his MBA at Wharton Graduate School, University of Pennsylvania, in 1985.
- Currently working as Associate Professor and Head of the section Animal Health Economics, at the School of Veterinary Medicine of the University of Pennsylvania.

**William Goodger (1941)**

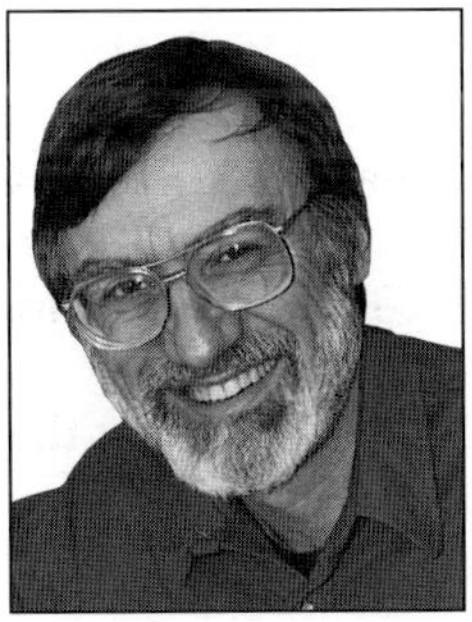

- Graduated from School of Veterinary Medicine of the Michigan State University in 1964.
- Completed a Professional Master's in Preventive Veterinary Medicine at the University of California, Davis, in 1977, and a MS in Agricultural Economics in 1980.
- Completed his PhD in epidemiology at the University of California, Davis, in 1981.
- Current position: Associated Professor of Epidemiology, University of Wisconsin, Madison, School of Veterinary Medicine.

**Chuck Guard (1948)**

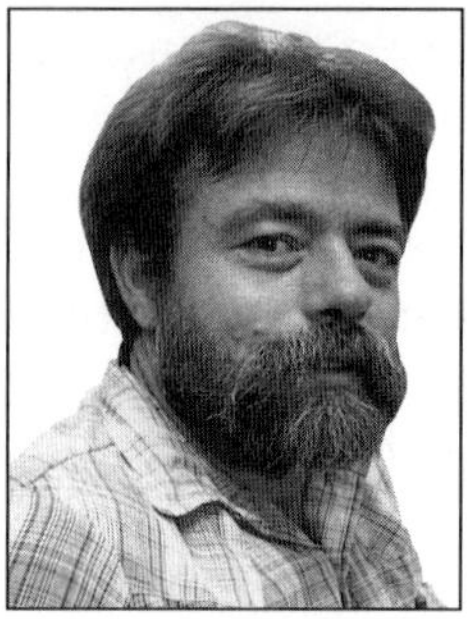

* Received a BS in engineering and a PhD in biology from Case Western reserve University in Cleveland Ohio in 1970 and 1975 respectively.
* Graduated as DVM at Cornell University, Ithaca, New York in 1980 and started his career in private practice.
* He joined the faculty of Veterinary Medicine at Cornell in 1982 as a member of the Ambulatory Clinic. He is currently associate professor of medicine, and director of the Ambulatory & Production Medicine Clinic.

**Ruud B.M. Huirne (1962)**

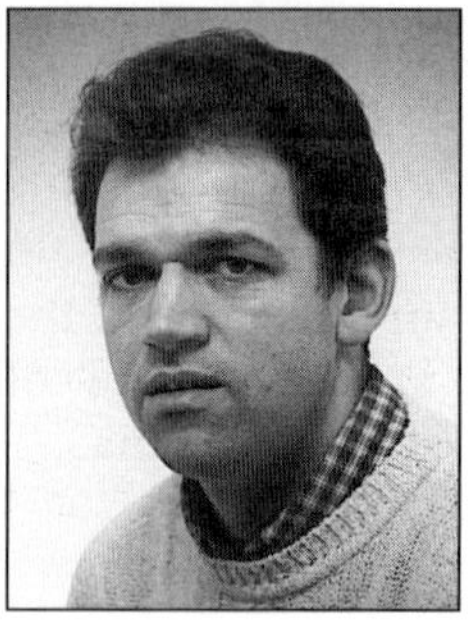

* Graduated in Agricultural Economics at Wageningen Agricultural University in 1986, with majors in Farm Management, animal Nutrition, and Operations Research.
* Completed his PhD at the Department of Farm Management at Wageningen Agricultural University in 1990.
* Currently working as Associate Professor at the Department of Farm Management of Wageningen Agricultural University.

**Michael F. Hutjens (1945)**

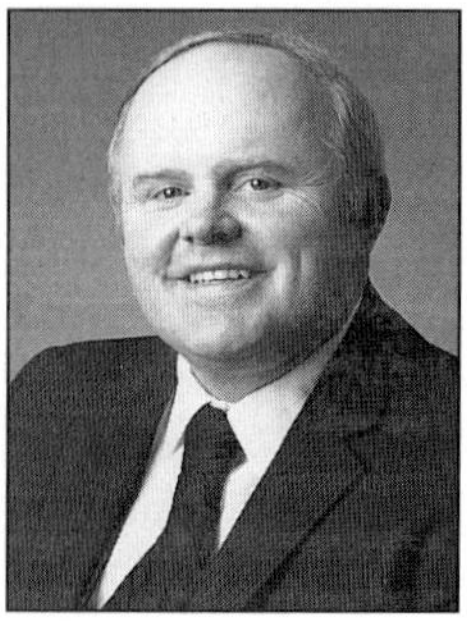

* Graduated with a B.S. (1967), M.S. (1969), and PhD. (1971) from the University of Wisconsin with majors in Dairy Science and Nutrition and a minor in Biochemistry.
* Employed at the University of Minesota from 1971 to 1979 in the department of Animal Science as an extension dairy specialist.
* Currently working as Professor of Animal Sciences at the University of Illinois as extension dairy specialist and teacher of dairy management.

**Alien Jalvingh (1965)**

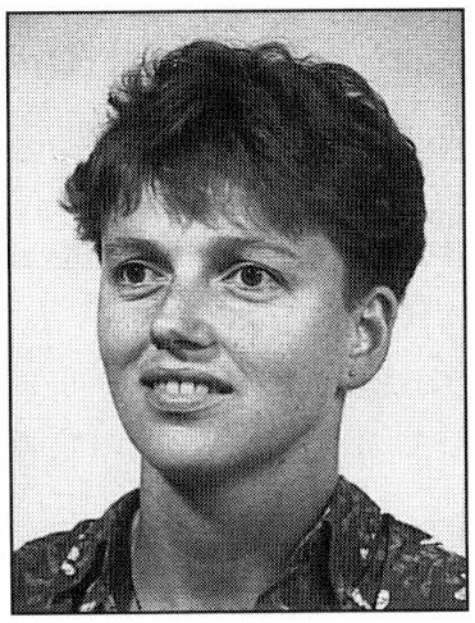

* Graduated in Animal Sciences at Wageningen Agricultural University in 1988, with majors in Animal Breeding and Farm Management.
* Completed her PhD at the Department of Farm Management and the Department of Animal Breeding of the same University in 1993.
* Currently working as a postdoc, made possible by a fellowship of the Royal Netherlands Academy of Arts and Sciences.

**Rijk de Jong (1941)**

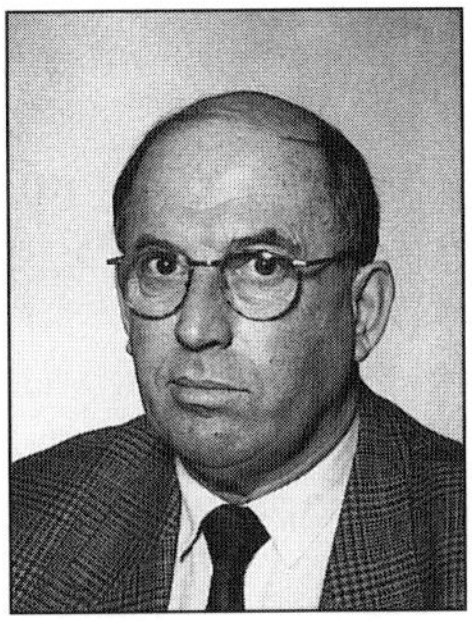

* Graduated from the Agricultural University of Wageningen, in 1969.
* Worked between 1969 and 1984 as a lecturer in Animal Science in Kenya, and carried out various evaluation and appraisal missions to Africa, South America, and Asia.
* From 1984 - 1996 he worked as a Scientific Project Officer at the Agricultural University of Wageningen.
* Completed his PhD in 1996, and is currently working as a livestock scientist in Kenya.

**Bram Kloosterman (1938)**

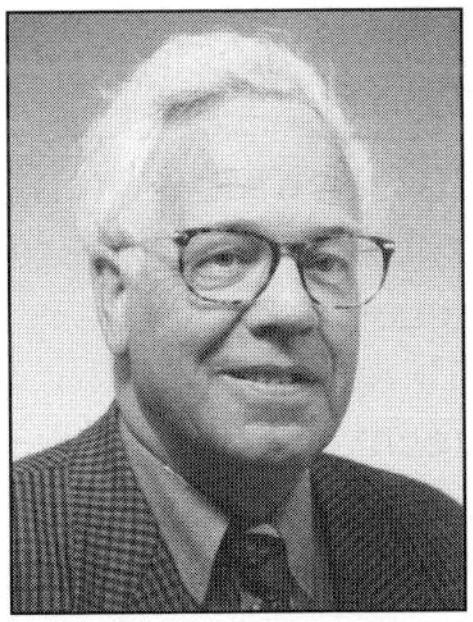

* Graduated in Animal Science from Wageningen Agricultural University with a major in Animal Nutrition.
* Completed his PhD. on gastrointestinal nematodes of cattle at the department of Health and Reproduction of the same university.
* Currently Associated Professor in health management of cattle in the same department.

**Wim D.J. Kremer (1957)**

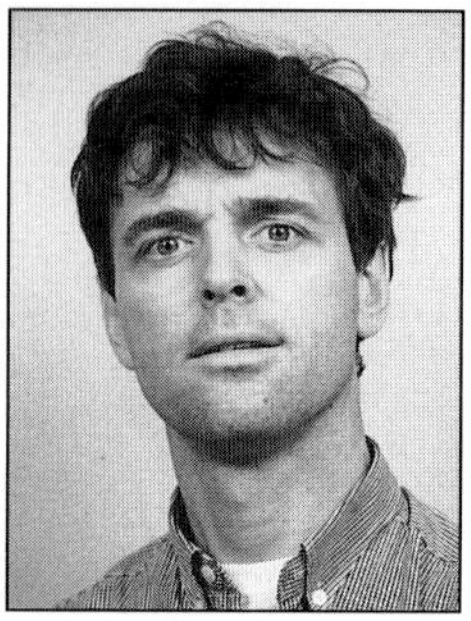

* Graduated as DVM from the Veterinary Faculty of the University of Utrecht, The Netherlands, in 1986.
* Completed his PhD at the University of Utrecht in 1993.
* Is currently head of the Ambulatory Clinic, Department of Herd Health & Reproduction of the Veterinary Faculty of the University of Utrecht, The Netherlands.

**Theo J.G.M. Lam (1960)**

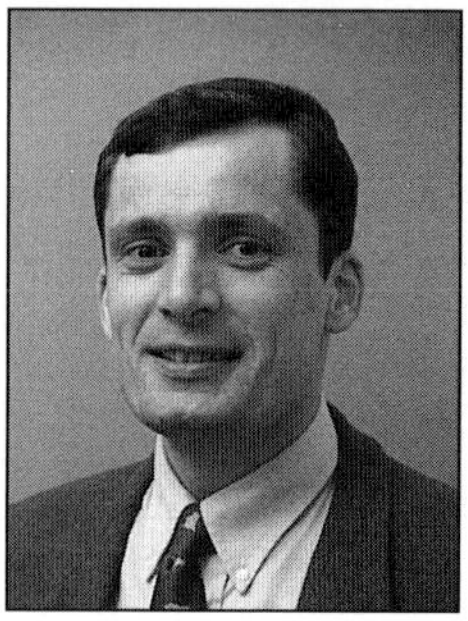

* Graduated as DVM from the Veterinary Faculty of the University of Utrecht, The Netherlands, in 1990.
* Was veterinarian in the ambulatory clinic of the Veterinary Faculty of Utrecht University from 1990 to 1992. Completed a MSc in veterinary epidemiology.
* Completed his PhD on bovine mastitis at the University of Utrecht in 1996.
* Is currently Assistent Professor in the department of Infectious Diseases & Immunology of the Veterinary Faculty of the University of Utrecht.

**Jos P.T.M. Noordhuizen (1947)**

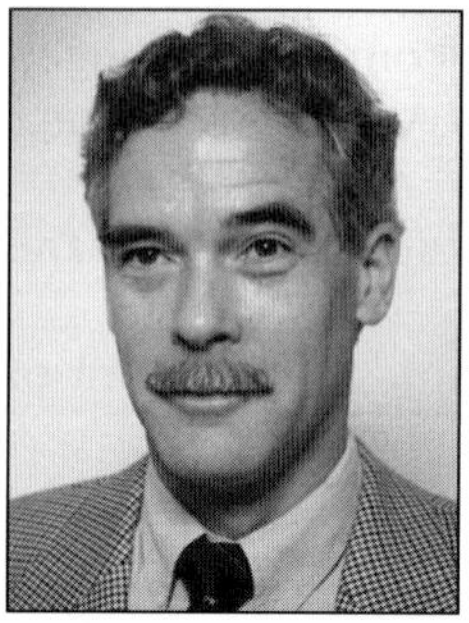

* Graduated from the Veterinary Faculty of the University of Utrecht in 1975.
* Was employed by the Veterinary Faculty of Utrecht in the Department of Obstetrics and Gynecology from 1978 to 1980 and worked in a mixed animal practice to 1981.
* Joined the Department of Herd Health and Ambulatory Clinic of the Veterinary Faculty of Utrecht in 1981 where he finished his PhD in 1984.
* Is since 1988 full Professor in Animal Husbandry with emphasis on Animal Health and Reproduction at the University of Wageningen, The Netherlands.

**Elsbeth N. Noordhuizen-Stassen (1953)**

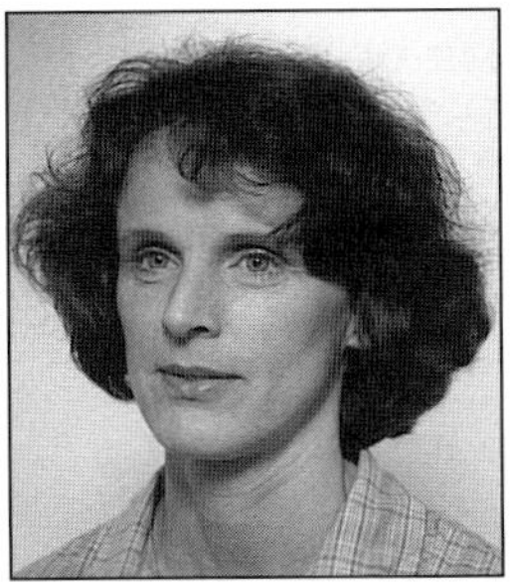

* Graduated from the veterinary Faculty of the University of Utrecht in 1978.
* Completed her PhD with distinction in 1984 at the University of Utrecht.
* Became Associated Professor at the Department of Herd Health and Reproduction with a major involvement in mastitis research in 1990.
* Was appointed Professor in Relationships between Man and Animal in 1996 at the Veterinary Faculty of Utrecht, The Netherlands.

**Christopher S.T. Nyabadza (1965)**

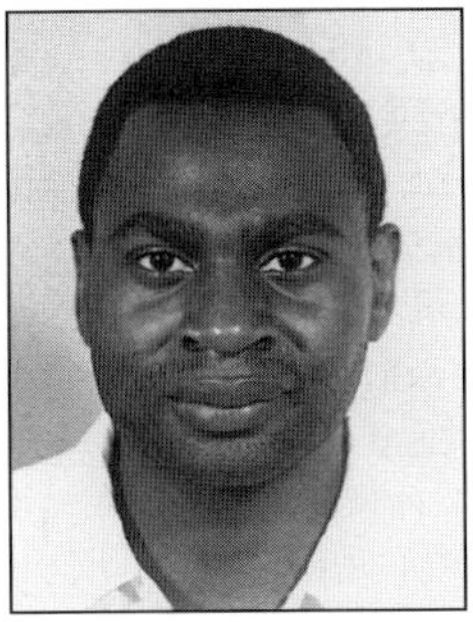

* Graduated from the University of veterinary Medicine in Brno, Czech Republic, in 1990.
* Completed a Master's in Veterinary Epidemiology at the Veterinary Faculty of the Utrecht University, The Netherlands, in 1996.
* Currently working as lecturer in the department of Clinical Veterinary Studies, Faculty of Veterinary Science, University of Zimbabwe, Harare, Zimbabwe.

**Thomas R. Overton (1969)**

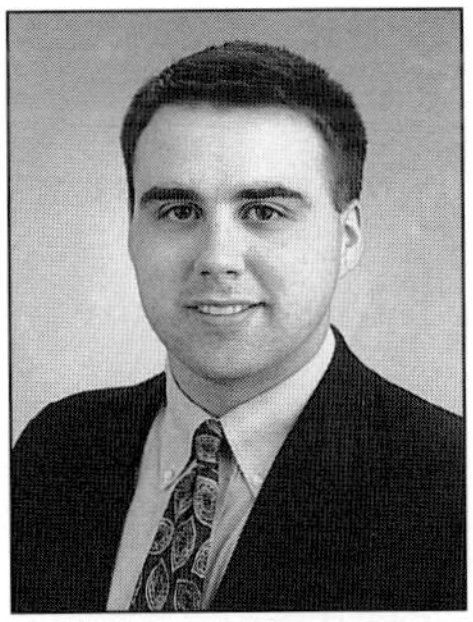

* Graduated with a B.S degree in Animal Sciences from Cornell University in 1990 with a major in dairy catle management.
* Master of Science from the University of Illinois in 1994.
* Currently research fellow at the University of Illinois.

**Kees A.M. Peeters (1959)**

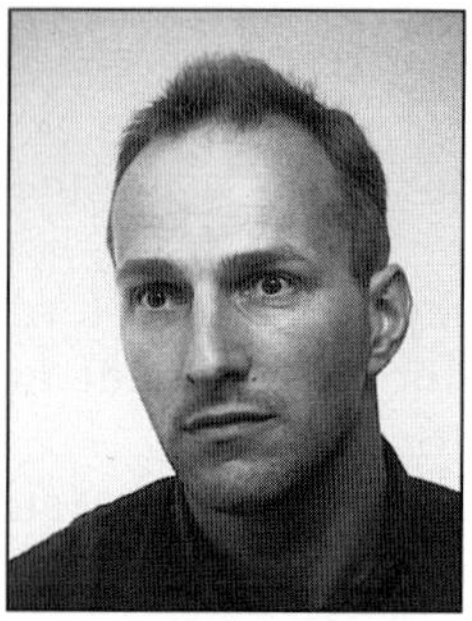

- * Graduated from Agricultural College in 1981.
- * Completed his veterinary study at the Veterinary Faculty of Utrecht in 1989.
- * Currently employed in a large animal practice with a main interest in dairy management.

**Wim H.M. van der Poel (1958)**

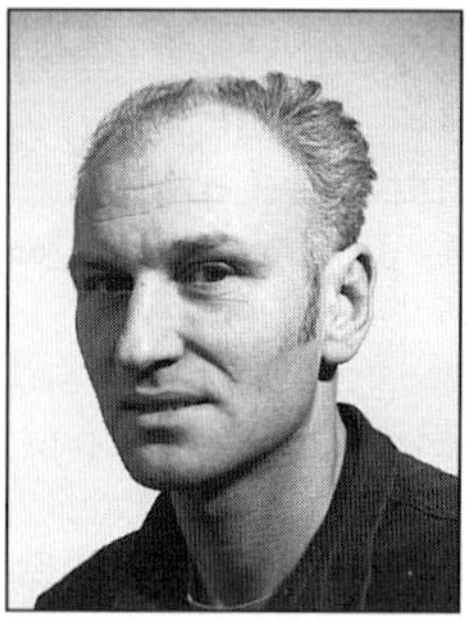

- * Graduated in Veterinary Medicine at the Faculty of Veterinary Medicine of the University of Utrecht in 1988.
- * Completed his PhD at the Department of Herd Health and Reproduction of the same University in 1995.
- * Currently working on research of viral zoonoses at the National Institute of Public Health and Environmental Protection in Bilthoven, The Netherlands.

**James D. Quigley III (1957)**

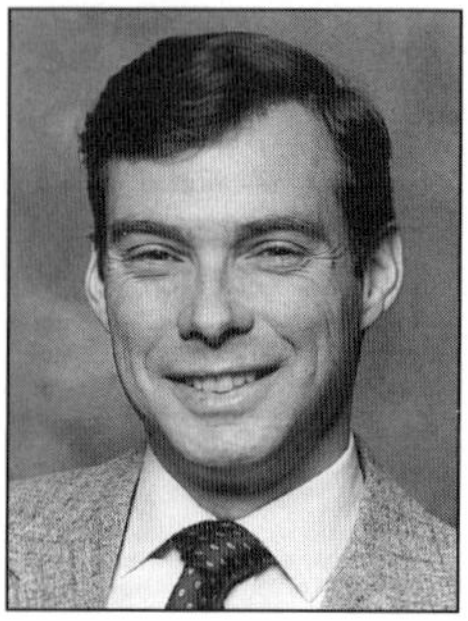

- * Graduated with a Bachelor of Science degree from the University of New Hampshire in 1979.
- * Completed a Master of Science degree with a major in Animal Sciences at the same University in 1983.
- * Obtained the PhD Degree at Virginia Tech University in 1985.
- * Was dairy research manager for a U.S. feed company from 1985 to 1988.
- * Was from 1988 Assistent Professor at the University of Tennessee, Knoxville, Department of Animal Sciences and since 1993 Associate Professor at the same University.

**Daniel T. Scholl (1961)**

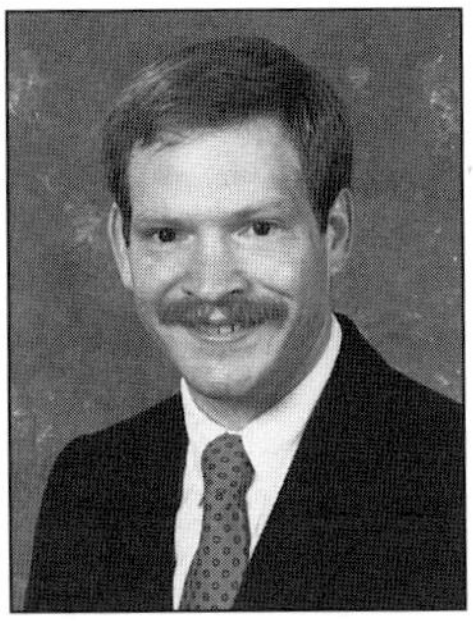

* Graduated with a Bachelor of Science Degree from the University of California at Davis, School of Veterinary Medicine, in 1985.
* Completed the Master of Preventive Veterinary Medicine Degree at Davis in 1988.
* Completed the PhD Degree in the Department of Herd Health and Reproduction, Faculty of Veterinary Medicine, University of Utrecht in 1992.
* Currently working as an Assistent Professor in the Department of epidemiology and Community Health, School of Veterinary Medicine, Louisiana State Univers.

**Ynte H. Schukken (1959)**

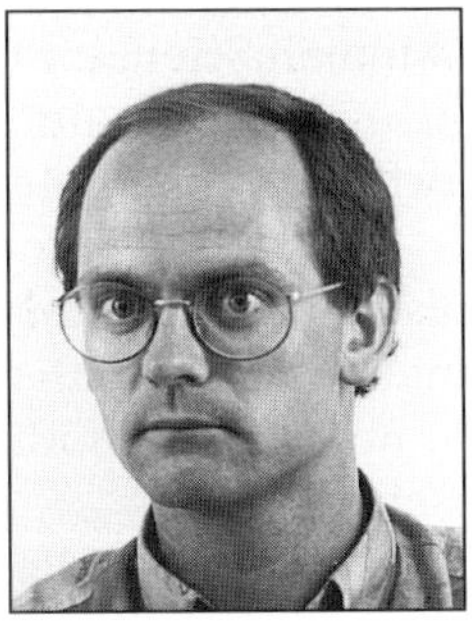

* Graduated as DVM at the Veterinary Faculty of the Utrecht University, The Netherlands, in 1985.
* Completed a MSc in Veterinary Epidemiology & Biostatistics at Cornell University, Ithaca New York, in 1987.
* Finished his PhD on dairy cattle mastitis epidemiology at the Veterinary Faculty of the Utrecht University in 1990.
* Currently Associate Professor in dairy herd health at the department of Herd Health & Reproduction of the Veterinary Faculty of Utrecht University.

**Andrew L. Skidmore (1957)**

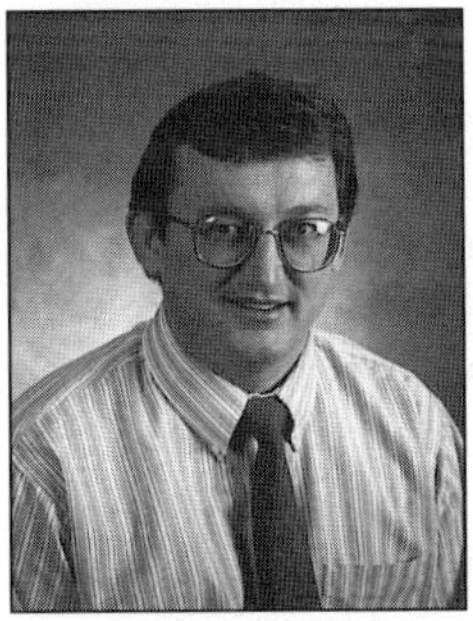

* Graduated from Kansas State University with a Bachelors of Science degree in 1982 and a Doctor of Veterinary Medicine degree in 1984.
* Graduated from Cornell University with PhD in 1990.
* Currently working as a farm business consultant at farm Credit of Western New York, ACA.

**Charles J. Sniffen (1937)**

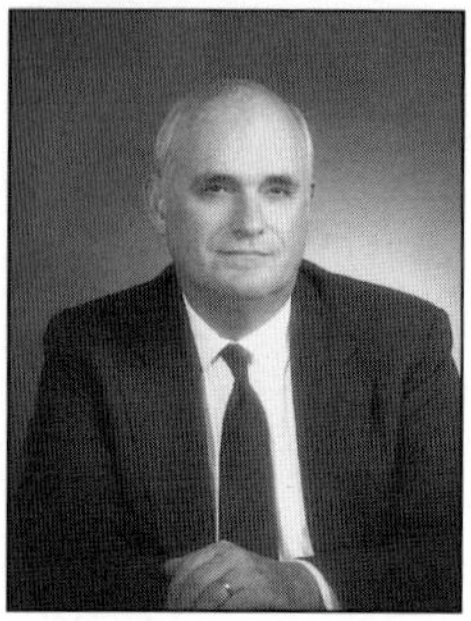

* Graduated from Ohio State University with a major in dairy science in 1960.
* Finished his Master of Science at the University of New Hampshire in 1967.
* Completed his PhD in ruminant nutrition at the University of Kentucky in 1970.
* Currently President of W.H. Miner Agricultural Research Institute, Chazy, New York.

**Mark A. Varner (1953)**

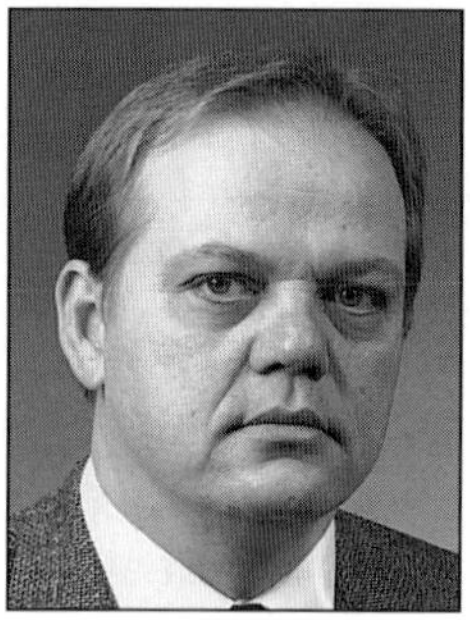

* Received his BSc in Animal Science at the University of Minnesota in 1975, and his MSc in Animal Science at Washington State University in 1977.
* Completed his PhD in physiology at North Carolina State University in 1981.
* Was employed as extension specialist and Assistent Professor at the Department of Animal Science of the University of Maryland from 1981 on, involved in both extension activities and research and teaching.
* He is employed as extension specialist and Associate Professor at the Department of Animal Science of the University of Maryland since 1993.

**Jacobus J. Verhoeff (1947)**

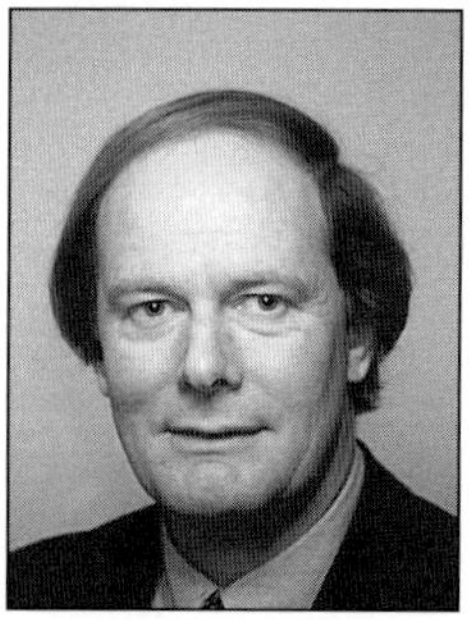

* Graduated from the Veterinary Faculty of the University of Utrecht in 1974.
* Completed his PhD study at the same university in 1983.
* From 1974 to 1990 he was employed at the Department of Herd Health and Ambulatory Clinic as an Associated Professor.
* Currently working as a coordinator of dairy extension activities and field research of the Animal Health Service Institute in the Netherlands.

**Dick Zwart (1930)**

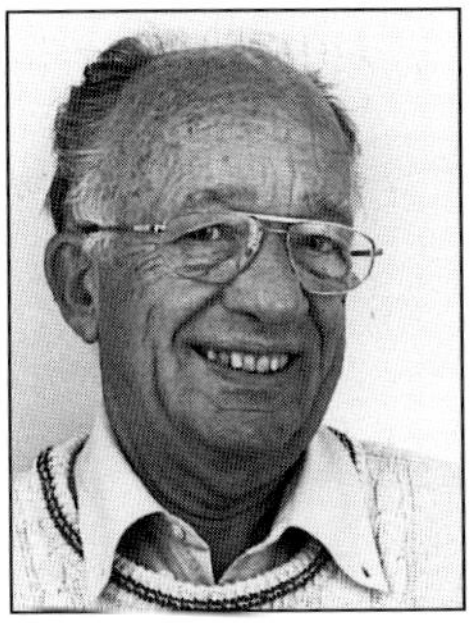

* Graduated from the Faculty of Veterinary Medicine, University of Utrecht in 1954.
* Completed a PhD study at the same University 1n 1962.
* Obtained a full professorhip in Tropical diseases and Protozoology at the University of Utrecht, Faculty of Veterinary Medicine in 1966.
* Was appointed as a full Professor in Tropical Animal Husbandry at the Agricultural University of Wageningen in 1986.

# INDEX